MW01178015

Hypercoagulable States

Fundamental Aspects, Acquired Disorders, and Congenital Thrombophilia

Edited by
M.J. Seghatchian
M.M. Samama
S.P. Hecker

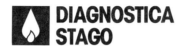

DIAGNOSTICA STAGO

CRC Press
Boca Raton   New York   London   Tokyo

Library of Congress Cataloging-in-Publication Data

Hypercoagulable states : fundamental aspects, acquired disorders, and
  congenital thrombophilia / edited by M.J. Seghatchian, M.M. Samama,
  Sydney Hecker.
      p.   cm.
  Includes bibliographical references and index.
  ISBN 0-8493-5804-3 (alk. paper)
  1. Blood coagulation disorders.   2. Thrombosis.   I. Seghatchian,
M.J.   II. Samama, Meyer M.   III. Hecker, Sydney.
  [DNLM: 1. Blood Coagulation Disorders--physiopathology.   2. Blood
Coagulation Disorders--complications.   3. Thrombosis--blood.
4. Thrombosis--physiopathology.   WH 322 H998 1996]
  RC647.C55H97 1996
  616.1'57—dc20
  DNLM/DLC
  for Library of Congress   95-26738
                                                                                                 CIP

© 1996 by CRC Press, Inc.

No claim to original U.S. Government works
International Standard Book Number 0-8493-5804-3
Library of Congress Card Number 95-26738
Printed in the United States of America 1 2 3 4 5 6 7 8 9 0
Printed on acid-free paper

FOREWORD

This concept of the pathogenesis of thrombosis is almost 200 years old and was first described by John HUNTER (1812) as follows:

> "Where there is a full power of life, the vessels are capable of keeping the blood in fluid state".

This idea was later stated in a more specific fashion in the Classical Triad of VIRCHOW (1856) describing the causes of thrombosis:

> "Abnormalities of the blood vessels. Alteration in the constituents of the blood. Aberration of blood flow."

These landmark statements were corroborated (1974) by SEVITT. He gave a clear description of the mechanisms by which venous thrombi are formed. WESSLER (1974) did the tests on the activation of blood coagulation with the classical experiment known as the WESSLER model, producing experimental venous thrombosis in animals.

Hemostasis is considered to be the body's first line of defence against thrombosis and bleeding. These are the two sides of the same "biological coin" of hemostasis. This defence mechanism is effectively achieved by suitable changes in the cell surface subsequent to activation, facilitating recruitment and rearrangement of appropriate components of plasma. Bioamplification and bioattenution of the clotting process then takes place on physiological surfaces in an organized manner. This involves at least 30 known proteins (receptors, enzymes, substrates, cofactors and inhibitors) that participate in ensuring that localised coagulation occurs on demand and that the subsequent fibrin is efficiently removed by fibrinolytic processes.

A mistake by "mother nature" however may occur. This is exemplified by : inherited deficiency or dysfunction of one of the three major natural defence systems (Heparins-Antithrombin; Protein C-Thrombomodulin-Protein S, Plasminogen-Plasminogen activator mechanisms). These can lead to a change in hemostatic balance, ranging from what is known as "normal basal physiological hypercoagulability" to uncontrolled thrombotic complications. In addition to this "Inherited Thrombophilia" which accounts for only about 15% of the documented episodes of thrombosis, there is a heterogeneous array of clinical disorders with increased risk of thromboembolism. These "Acquired Thrombophilias" often have an unknown pathophysiological basis and are due to multifactorial defects of the hemostatic defence system, predisposing to thrombosis in different sites or organs. Thus, the relationship between hypercoagulability and thrombosis is multifactorial.

The actual incidence of thomboembolic disease is thought to be about five times higher than the prevalence of malignant disease. Recognising the health care importance of thrombosis, workers in the biological sciences have made large efforts and contributions to understanding its pathogenesis and treatment. Close collaboration between the laboratory and the clinician is essential for a meaningful interpretation of abnormal values or significant medical history, which need to complement each other to minimize error in clinical interpretation.

Many new therapeutic modalities and an ever-increasing number of therapeutic agents have been added to our pharmacopoeia. The choice of an appropriate treatment strategy may be a dilemna for the clinician, even when the essential information is provided by basic scientists and clinical pharmacologists. A "designer product" is needed for some patients. The final decision must come from the clinician who has first hand knowledge of the patient's needs and is able to orchestrate the best plan on an individual basis.

In the past two decades considerable advances have been made in the development of highly sensitive and specific molecular markers for measuring activation processes in hemostasis in various pathophysiological conditions. The classical coagulation assays, used with ingenuity, still provide much useful information in various deficiency states associated with thrombophilia. The recently reported "APC-resistance thrombophilia" by DAHLBACK, assessed by APTT ratio is a good example of improvement of our detection capability of thrombotic tendency to approximately 20 to 60% of patients with a history of thrombosis. Nevertheless it is with molecular markers of the activation states of hemostasis that the task of distinguishing between altered basal physiological normal hemostasis from those seen subsequent to low grade thrombotic events and conditions which predispose to thrombotic complications is much facilitated.

A wealth of new information is also continuously being generated by large scale epidemiological studies. These clearly help to define normal ranges. This enables us to decide at what protein level the variation may give rise to the inherited/acquired coagulopathies and to what extent vascular/endothelial and/or other cellular components of blood play roles in modulating the clinical outcome of venous or arterial thrombosis. Some epidemiological studies have also proved useful in preventative decision making.

As always in a rapidly progressing field, information is widely scattered in the primary literature. In the case of hypercoagulability the concept, methodology, biochemistry, epidemiology and the development aspects of clinical diagnosis and management have produced an extremely wide range of publications difficult for the practising clinician or laboratory worker to access. Our decision to produce a book on hypercoagulability arose primarily from lack of a comprehensive text covering the needs and interests of many clinicians and scientists. Secondly, it came from our love of the subject we have taught to so many medical technologists, clinical scientists, medical students, residents and post doctoral fellows in hematology and blood transfusion medicine. In the planning stage of this book, we have decided on the idea of an integrated approach to cover both laboratory principles and clinical practices, making it as comprehensive as possible. We have attempted to bring together in one volume all the relevant available information which has some bearing in hypercoagulability, even though it may be incomplete. Molecular genetics was purposely avoided as excellent books on this topic have recently appeared.

As in all multi-author books, it is difficult to accommodate the anticipated needs of readers. However, the authors selected are a mixture of distinguished academics and clinicians, all experienced, with their own ideas about how to convey their messages. We were thrilled by their gracious acceptance of our invitation, for their contributions, and their kind acquiescence to our sometimes extensive editing. Because the editing was expected to be very time consuming we called upon S. Hecker to join us as Associate Editor. We are grateful for the forbearance of the authors who completed their chapters and then revised their work in timely fashion. Any success of this book will be due in no small measure to the efforts of our contributing authors, who have been close colleagues and friends of the editors for many years : a "gift" from friends to other present and future friends. The authors are all busy individuals of independent spirit. Thus, despite the recommendations for the style of the camera ready manuscript, large numbers of articles have been received in different format. We have attempted to harmonize the style as much as possible but for the sake of time saving we adopted in certain cases different style in references, figures and tables.

With the hope that readers may be from many different disciplines, we included an introductory chapter devoted to an overview covering the five major areas of interest : conceptual, analytical, physiological, epidemiological and clinical. This is followed by a set of chapters dealing with basic principles of the pathophysiology of the hemostatic components, followed by discussion of the important factors involved in the pathogenesis of thrombosis in relation to various clinical disorders or related disease states.

Emphasis throughout is placed on the clinical practices and characteristic laboratory features of patients with congenital disorders and individuals with high risk for thromboembolism. Due to the importance of special diagnostic procedures and therapeutic values of certain new blood products and drug therapies a set of chapters on this topic is also included. The overlap in some areas, though kept to a minimum, was unavoidable and may actually benefit some readers. It is our sincere hope that this book will fulfill the needs of basic scientists, clinicians, and even some experts by providing current information in this rapidly growing field.

We wish also to take the opportunity to express our appreciation to Dr. Ismaïl Elalamy, Dr. Marc Trossaërt and Nicole Galtier, Hôtel-Dieu/Paris, Joanne Foley and Juanita Powley (NBS)/London, and of course Marsha Baker of CRC Press/Florida, for their assistance in this venture from start to completion. We greatly appreciate the support and inspiration of all our contributors and their special efforts.

Dr. M. J. Seghatchian
NBS, Colindale, London

Dr. M. M. Samama
Hôtel-Dieu, University Hospital, Paris

CO-EDITOR

Dr. M.J. Seghatchian B.Sc., Ph.D. is Principal Clinical Scientist in charge of the Quality Assurance Laboratory at the North London Blood Transfusion Centre and Honorary Lecturer at Guy's Hospital Medical and Dental School. His basic training is in chemistry, specialising in radiation chemistry/polymerisation at CNRS, Orsay, obtaining in 1964 his doctorate in Physical Chemistry from the University of Paris, France. He also obtained in 1972 a Ph.D. in medical biochemistry from the University of London, England, following post-doctoral studies at Guy's Hospital on the application of radioisotopes in medicine and sptectroscopic techniques in drug enzyme interactions.

Since 1973, Dr. Seghatchian's interests focused on the regulatory control and standardisation aspects of the haemostatic components of blood, originating the integrated system of QA at NLBTC. As a visiting scientist, he worked for several years at the National Institute for Biological Standards and Control and the MRC Epidemiology and Medical Care Unit at Northwick Park Hospital, on the standardisation/automation of coagulation assays and methodological aspects of hypercoagulability. He has pioneered the chromogenic assay of Factors VIII/VII, and developed a new electrophoretic method for the characterisation of native and altered forms of Factor VIII/vWF, Protein C/Protein C inhibitor complexes and thrombogenic components of prothrombin complexes. In the capacity of visiting scientist, he collaborated with several leading scientists and clinicians in Sweden, France, Italy, U.S.A., Canada, and South America on the molecular abnormalities of haemostatic proteins, inhibitors of proteolytic enzymes, and heparin-induced thrombocytopenia. He has also acted as a WHO Expert Consultant on Coagulation for Mediterranean countries.

Dr. Seghatchian's current research interests include characterisation of the activity states of the haemostatic components implicated in haemapheresis procedures and hypercoagulability with particular reference to clinical and methodological aspects of platelet interaction with vitamin K dependent proteins, Factor VIII/vWF and vWF fragments. He has recently been active in the development of simple screening tests for platelet morphological/functional integrity using automated cell counters and assessing platelet activation/release reaction storage lesion by microplate and flowcytometry techniques.

Dr. Seghatchian is currently an editor of the journals *Transfusion Science, Thrombosis Research,* and *Clinical and Applied Thrombosis/Hemostasis.* He has co-edited a two-volume publication on Factor VIII/vWF (CRC Press, 1990) and Quality Assurance in Transfusion Medicine (CRC Press, 1992) and co-edited a book on vitamin K and vitamin K dependent protein (CRC Press, 1993) which deals with several methodological and epidemiological aspects of hypercoagulability. Dr. Seghatchian also acts as referee and an editorial advisory member for several scientific journals. He has published more than 200 scientific papers and abstracts, and delivered more than 40 guest lectures at national and international meetings. He is a founding member of both the British Society of Blood Transfusion and the British Society of Haemostasis and Thrombosis, and a member of several international societies. As the chairman, he has organised several symposiums on platelet activation and storage lesion and standardization aspects of hemostatic function testing in hypercoagulable states for BBTS Components Special Interest Group.

CO-EDITOR

Dr. Meyer-Michel Samama, M.D., is Professor of Haematology, Chief of the Laboratory of Haematology at the Hôtel-Dieu Hospital, and the Director of the Laboratory of Experimental Thrombosis of the Faculty of Medicine in Paris (University Paris VI).

Dr. Samama obtained his degree of Pharmacist-Biochemist in 1951 in Paris, received his medical training at the Broussais-Hôtel-Dieu University in Paris, and obtained his M.D. degree in 1968. In 1971 he became Associate Professor of Haematology and assumed his present position as the Director of the Laboratory of Haematology at the Hôtel-Dieu University Hospital in Paris. He became a full professor in 1981.

His main interest is in haematology with a specialty in hemostasis. His research work and interest in hemostasis and thrombosis started in 1955, and he has become an expert in the field of antithrombotic drugs.

His main contributions to this field concern congenital and acquired dysfibrinogenemia, congenital deficiencies of Proteins C and S, hypofibrinolysis and thrombosis, thrombolytic and antithrombotic drugs, and a recent interest in low molecular weight heparins.

Dr. Samama is past President of the French Group on Thrombosis and Hemostasis and the Chairman of the Council of the Fibrinolysis Study group; and he has served as President of the Mediterranean League against Thrombosis. He was also a member of the Council of the International Society of Thrombosis and Hemostasis. He has been active on the editorial boards of several medical journals, including *Hemostasis and Thrombosis Research*.

From 1969 to 1979 an average of 25 papers per year, including general reviews, were published by M.M. Samama and his group. During recent years this number has increased about two-fold.

He and his group have authored over 50 original published papers during the last three years in the field of thrombosis and hemostasis and he has co-authored several books and proceedings of scientific meetings.

He has received the Distinguished Career Award of the International Society of Thrombosis and Hemostasis (New York 1993).

ASSOCIATE EDITOR

Sydney Philip Hecker, M.D., M.S. (Med.) is the Medical Director of Health Plans, Palo Alto Medical Foundation in Palo Alto, California, U.S.A. He is Assistant Clinical Professor of Medicine Emeritus, Stanford University School of Medicine, Stanford, California.

Dr. Hecker obtained his M.D. degree from the University of Toronto, Canada, in 1952, and his Master of Science in Medicine degree from Georgetown University, Washington, D.C. in 1955. He has served visiting fellowships in angiology at the University of Zurich, Switzerland, and in the Coagulation Laboratory, Hôtel-Dieu, Paris.

Dr. Hecker practiced internal medicine with special interests in pulmonary diseases, angiology, and thrombosis from 1957 to 1990. He has been the Medical Director of Health Plans since 1986. Dr. Hecker was a Research Associate of the Palo Alto Medical Research Foundation between 1960-1980, a member of its Board of Directors from 1964-1986, and Chairman of the Research Committee from 1972-1979. Between 1960-1980, he published approximately 11 research papers and delivered approximately 20 invited lectures on thrombosis, vascular disease, and thrombolysis. He was Coordinator of the European Urokinase Study at the University Hospital, Basel, Switzerland, which published its results of a multicenter controlled trial of Urokinase in myocardial infarction in 1975. He was Director of the Non-Invasive Vascular Laboratory at the Palo Alto Medical Clinic between 1980-1990.

Dr. Hecker is a member of the Board of Directors of the Unified Medical Group Association, Chairman of its Pharmacy and Therapeutics Committee, Editor of its newsletter "Prescription Pad", and the UMGA Medication Formulary. He contributed to *"A Diagnostic Approach to Chest Disease"*, Lillington and Jamplis in 1965; and *"Healthcare Management Guidelines: Inpatient and Surgical Care"*, Milliman and Robertson, 1990.

Current research interests include participation in the asthma study of the Outcomes Measurement Project of the American Group Practice Association and as a member of the OMP Steering Committee.

CONTRIBUTORS

Nobuo Aoki
Professor
First Department of Medicine
Saitama Medical School
Moroyama-Machi, Iruma-Gunn
Saitama-Ken, Japan

T. Baglin
Addenbrooke's NHS Trust
Cambridge, UK

Kenneth A. Bauer
Professor
Molecular Medicine Unit
Beth Israel Hospital
Boston, Massachusetts

Edouard M. Bevers
Department of Biochemistry
Cardiovascular Research Institute
Maastritcht, The Netherlands

Henrik Birgens
Department of Medicine and Hematology
Herlev Hospital
Herlev, Denmark

John Bonnar
Professor, Head
Department of Obstetrics and Gynaecology
Trinity College
St. James Hospital
Dublin, Ireland

J. C. Bordet
Department of Haemostasis
Hôpital Edouard Herriot
Lyon, France

Henri Bounameaux
Head
Division of Angiology and Hemostasis
Department of Medicine
University Hospital of Geneva
Genève, Switzerland

Yves Cadroy
Department of Haemostasis
Hôpital Purpan
Toulouse, France

Jacques-Philippe Caen
IVS, Hôpital Lariboisière
Paris, France

David Chen
Atherosclerosis Program
Rehabilitation Insitute of Chicago
Chicago, Illinois, USA

Sergio Coccheri
Professor, Head
Department of Angiology and Blood
Coagulation
University Hospital S. Orsola
Bologna, Italy

Jean Philippe Collet
Laboratory of Cytometry
CNRS
Villejuif, France

Paul Comfurius
Department of Biochemistry
Cardiovascular Research Institute
Maastritcht, The Netherlands

Jacqueline Conard
Department of Biological Haematology
Hôtel-Dieu
Paris, France

Paul Brian Contino
Division of Molecular Medicine
The Mount Sinai Medical Center
New York, NY, USA

Björn Dahlbäck
Professor
Department of Clinical Chemistry
Malmö General Hospital
Malmö, Sweden

Marc Dechavanne
Professor
Department of Haemostasis
Hôpital Edouard Herriot
Lyon, France

M. P. M. de Maat
TNO Institute of Ageing and Vascular
Research
Gaubius Laboratory
Leiden, The Netherlands

R. Durst
Department of Haematology
Hadassah University Hospital
Jerusalem, Israël

Ismail Elalamy
Department of Biological Haematology
Hôtel-Dieu
Paris, France

Amiram Eldor
Professor - Director
Institute of Hematology
Tel Aviv, Israel

M. Peter Esnouf
Nuffield Department of Clinical Biochemistry
University of Oxford
Radcliffe Infirmary
Oxford, United Kingdom

S. Farid
Hines Veterans Affairs Hospital
Hines, Illinois, USA

Patrick J. Gaffney
Division of Haematology
NIBSC
Hertfordshire, United Kingdom

Robert Girot
Professor
Department of Biological Haematology
Hôpital Tenon
Paris, France

A. Goldfarb
Department of Haematology
Hadassah University Hospital
Jerusalem, Israël

Jenny Goudemand
Professor
Laboratory of Haematology
Hôpital C. Huriez
Lille, France

Stephen C. L. Gough
Division of Medicine
The General Infirmary
Leeds, United Kingdom

Jorgen Gram
Centralsygehuset I Esbjerb
Klinisk - Kemisk Afdeling
Esbjerg, Denmark

M. Greaves
Department of Haematology
The Central Sheffield
Royal Hallamshire Hospital
Sheffield, United Kingdom

David Green
Professor
Atherosclerosis Program
Rehabilitation Institute of Chicago
Chicago, Illinois, USA

M. C. Guillin
Department of Haematology
Hôpital Beaujon
Clichy, France

A. A. Halle
Loyola University Stritch School of Medicine
Maywood, Illinois, USA

A. Hamsten
Department of Clinical Chemistry
Karolinska Hospital
Stockholm, Sweden

Niels Ebbe Hansen
Department of Medicine and Haematology
Herlev Hospital
Herlev, Denmark

Frits Haverkate
TNO Institute of Ageing and Vascular
Research
Gaubius Laboratory
Leiden, The Netherlands

Gérard Helft
Department of Cardiology
Hôpital Necker
Paris, France

Marie-Hélène Horellou
Department of Biological Haematology
Hôtel-Dieu
Paris, France

Jorgen Jespersen
Centralsygehuset I Esbjerb
Klinisk - Kemisk Afdeling
Esbjerg, Denmark

S. Johnson
Loyola University Stritch School of Medicine
Maywood, Illinois, USA

Takatoshi Koyama
First Department of Medicine
Saitama Medical School
Moroyama-Machi, Iruma-Gunn
Saitama-Ken, Japan

Hau C. Kwaan
Professor
Hematology/Oncology Section
The Medical School

David A. Lane
Department of Haematology
Charing Cross and Westminster Medical
School, Hammersmith
London, United Kingdom

Thomas Lecompte
Professor
Laboratory of Haemostasis et Thrombosis
Centre Hospitalier Universitaire
Nancy, France

Cristina Legnani
Department of Angiology and Blood
Coagulation
University Hospital S. Orsola
Bologna, Italy

Gordon D. O. Lowe
Professor
Haemostasis, Thrombosis and Vascular
Medicine Unit
Royal Infirmary
Glasgow, United Kingdom

T. McKiernan
Loyola University Stritch School of Medicine
Maywood, Illinois, USA

J. Maclouf
INSERM
Hôpital Lariboisière
Paris, France

Harry L. Messmore Jr
Hines Veterans Affairs Hospital
Hines, Illinois, USA

George J. Miller
MRC Epidemiology and Medical Care Unit
The Medical College of St. Bartholomew's
Hospital
London, United Kingdom

Manouchehr Mirshahi
Laboratory Sainte-Marie
Hôtel-Dieu
Paris, France

Zohar Mishal
Laboratory of Cytometry
CNRS, Villejuif, France

Yale Nemerson
Professor
The Mount Sinaï Medical Center
New York, NY, USA

Robin J. Olds
Department of Pathology
University of Otago
Dunedin, New Zealand

Bjarne Østerud
Professor
Department of Biochemistry
University of Tromsø
Tromsø, Norway

Gualtiero Palareti
Department of Angiology and Blood
Coagulation
University Hospital S. Orsola
Bologna, Italy

Torben Plesner
Department of Hematology
Herlev Hospital
Herlev, Denmark

Colin R. M. Prentice
Professor
Division of Medicine
The General Infirmary
Leeds, United Kingdom

F. E. Preston
Professor
Department of Haematology
Royal Hallamshire Hospital
Sheffield, United Kingdom

E. A. Rachmilewitz
Department of Haematology
Hadassah University Hospital
Jerusalem, Israël

Robert D. Rosenberg
Professor
Molecular Medicine Unit
Beth Israel Hospital
Boston, Massachusetts

Meyer M. Samama
Professor
Department of Biological Haematology
Hôtel-Dieu
Paris, France

Pierre Yves Scarabin
INSERM U 258
Hôpital Broussais
Paris, France

Nicole Schlegel
Department of Biological Haematology
Hôpital Robert Debré
Paris, France

Jerard Seghatchian
North London Blood Transfusion Centre
Colindale
London, United Kingdom

Pierre Sié
Professor
Laboratory of Haematology
Université Paul-Sabatier
Toulouse, France

Edgar Smeets
Department of Biochemistry
Cardiovascular Research Institute
Maastritcht, The Netherlands

Claudine Soria
Diféma, Faculty of Medicine and Pharmacy
Rouen, France

Jeannette Soria
Laboratoire Sainte-Marie/Hôtel-Dieu
Paris, France

Swee Lay Thein
Institute of Molecular Medicine
John Radcliffe Hospital
Headington
Oxford, UK

Douglas A. Triplett
Professor and Assistant Dean
Department of Hematology
Ball Memorial Hospital
Muncie, Indiana, USA

M. C. Trzeciak
Department of Haemostasis
Hôpital Edouard Herriot
Lyon, France

Patrick Van Dreden
Diagnostica Stago
9, rue des Frères Chausson
92600 Asnières

Marc Vasse
Diféma, Faculty of Medicine and Pharmacy
Rouen, France

Elisabeth Verdy
Department of Biological Haematology
Hôpital Tenon
Paris, France

Marc Verstraete
Professor
Center for Molecular and Vascular Biology
Katholieke Universiteit Leuven
Leuven, Belgium

W. H. Wehrmacher
Department of Pathology and Medicine
Loyola University Stritch School of Medicine
Maywood, Illinois, USA

Björn Wiman
Professor
Department of Clinical Chemistry
Karolinska Hospital
Stockholm, Sweden

Robert F. A. Zwaal
Professor
Department of Biochemistry
Rijksuniversiteit Limburg
Maastricht, The Netherlands

HYPERCOAGULABLE STATES : FUNDAMENTAL ASPECTS ACQUIRED DISORDERS AND CONGENITAL THROMBOPHILIA

(Table of Contents)

C. **Therapeutic Aspects**

I

Introduction

HYPERCOAGULABLE STATES: AN OVERVIEW

M.J. Seghatchian* and M.M. Samama **

* NBS, Colindale, London ; ** Hôtel-Dieu, University Hospital, Paris

I. INTRODUCTION

This overview deals with conceptual, pathophysiological, analytical, epidemiological and clinical aspects of hypercoagulable states.

A. FUNDAMENTAL ASPECTS

The basic concept of hemostasis/thrombosis, "the opposite sides of the same biological coin", has been around for almost a century, since Morawitz presented, in 1905, an update on investigated theory of blood coagulation then available. Since then, a multitude of theories has been proposed by many scientists trying to understand how this physiological process works. Today, despite many advances in this evolving field of clinical and laboratory medicine, hypercoagulability still remains an attractive "unresolved" concept.

A range of triggering mechanisms such as trauma, septic shock, bacteremia and many other pathophysiological conditions initiate primary hemostasis and promote thrombus formation. In depth biochemical and functional analyses are required for proper assessment of the sequence of events. The basic principle of primary hemostasis is now well defined (see Figure 1a). Events such as endothelial cell, platelet and leucocyte activation, production of prostacyclin, nitric oxide (NO) and tissue plasminogen activator release as well as the newly understood regulatory anticoagulation system (protein C, protein S, thrombomodulin, C4b-binding protein); and the endothelial released tissue factor inhibitors, all play major roles in regulating the process of hemostasis/thrombosis (see Figure 1b and 1c). This list is not comprehensive in terms of triggering and/or bioamplification, bioattenuation, biomodulation/bioregulation. However, despite these refinements the modern coagulation scheme can be conceptually and experimentally defined as one pathway (Figure 2). Tissue factor is the major triggering factor and the activated platelet is the essential solid surface for bioamplification, bioattenuation processes in the intermediate stage. Thrombin orchestrates its own destruction (Figures 2,3).

B. CURRENT CONCEPT OF PRIMARY ANTICOAGULANT SYSTEM

Major advances have also been made in understanding the role of various inhibitors of coagulation enzymes. This is schematically shown in figure 2. The major activator of coagulation is currently believed to be tissue factor VIIa complexes (see Figure 2). The major inhibitors can be classified broadly as follows :

1. Primary inhibitors of proteolytic enzymes:

i - tissue factor pathway inhibitor (TFPI), acting on factor Xa factor VIIa/tissue factor ;

ii - antithrombin and heparin-like molecules enhancing the inhibitory potency of AT III on a whole range of coagulation proteases including factors Xa, IXa, XIa and VIIa ;

iii - C1-esterase inhibitor and α_2-macroglobulin acting on kallikrein and factor XIIa and thrombin;

iv - Thrombin and activated protein C (APC) with ability to inactivate factor Va and factor VIIIa, which can be blocked by α_1-antitrypsin, α_2-macroglobulin and specific inhibitors of APC (PCI).

2. Secondary inhibitors: The clinical significance of these inhibitors is still uncertain, though it is established that α_1-antitrypsin acts on factor XIa and trypsin; heparin cofactor II, probably of minor physiological importance, specifically inhibits thrombin; platelet factor XIa inhibitor and protein nexin 1 and 2/amyloid -protein precursor inhibit factors XIa, IXa and thrombin.

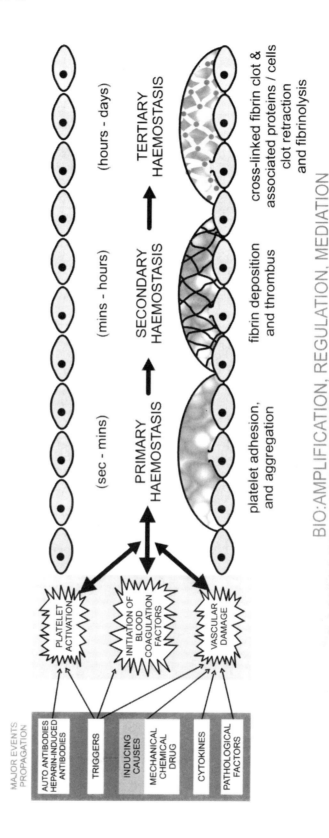

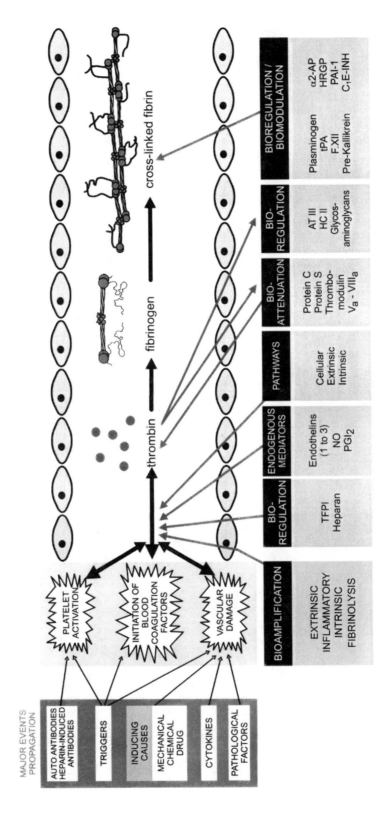

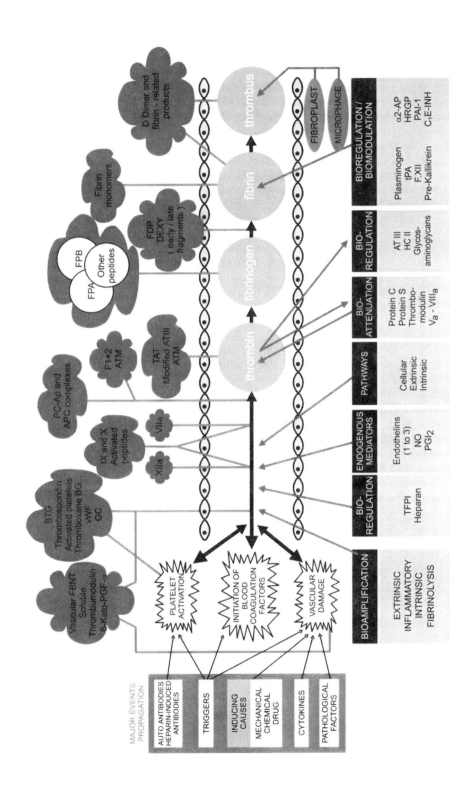

Figure 1(a, b, c) :
The hemostatic system is finely "tuned" to maintain the circulating blood in the fluid state and yet respond hemostatically in seconds to various vascular injuries to normal vessels. The participation of clotting proteins and platelets in hemostasis is better recognized than the involvement of leucocytes and other cells. Leucocytes/erythrocytes participate in clotting systems as cofactors by three general mechanisms. First, they express or secrete molecules that have procoagulant or anticoagulant properties. Second, they cause functional changes in vascular endothelial cells and each other inducing further bioregulatory effects. Third, they form aggregates and/or get trapped in fibrin obstructing the microcirculation under certain conditions. Activated platelets can localise leucocytes at sites of vascular injury and modulate their function.

The triggering mechanism, together with the role of platelet activation and vascular damage on hemostasis/thrombosis is shown in Figures 1a, b, c. In respect to platelet involvement, four distinct phases of platelet activation have been described, each of which is associated with one or more clinical bleeding disorders. These include:

i) **Platelet adhesion** which occurs in response to exposure either to natural thrombogenic surfaces e.g. subendothelium rich in collagen, fibronectin, von Willebrand factor or artificial surfaces such as vascular grafts. Direct measurement of platelet adhesion is not yet commonly used in the clinical laboratory though the ristocetin cofactor test is a good surrogate method reflecting abnormal interaction of vWF with platelet glycoprotein 1b. Several other markers of platelet activation exist as mentioned in Figure 1c.

ii) **Platelet aggregation** or self-association into a plug. This at low shear rate is mainly mediated by the interaction of fibrinogen with glycoprotein receptors (IIb, IIIa that are held together by micro molar concentrations of calcium). Excellent tests for platelet aggregation exist; since EDTA irreversibly dissociates IIb/IIIa complex, aggregation study is performed in citrated sample as it allows micro molar concentration of calcium to remain associated with the Gp IIb/IIIa complex, thereby maintaining its functional integrity.

iii) **Secretion** - In this process the content of two major granules, dense granules (adenosine diphosphate, adenosine triphosphate, serotonin and calcium) and α-granules (platelet factor 4, vWF, fibrinogen, βTG), are released into the immediate extracellular space at high concentration, contributing to the formation of plug.

iv) **Microvesiculation with the exposure of phosphatidylserine (PS) on platelet surface** - Platelets upon activation, microvesiculation or stimulation provide a specialised surface where coagulation and fibrinolytic proteins are biomodulated. This is a common feature of all activated cellular surfaces (e.g. endothelial cells and monocytes).

Endothelial cells also play major roles in clot formation and lysis processes:
i) They contain an ADPase which limits platelet activation.
ii) They produce two potent anti-platelet compounds; prostaglandin (PGI_2) and nitric oxide (NO) with ability to regulate hemostasis.
iii) They contain thrombomodulin which neutralises the thrombin procoagulant activity, as well as producing anticoagulant activity through the protein C pathway.
iv) They also contain large amounts of vWF multimers in the Weibel-Pelade bodies which upon release contribute to platelet clumping (e.g. in TTP and Sickle Cell Anaemia).
v) They release TPA as major regulatory protein and Plasminogen Activator Inhibitor (PAI-1).
vi) Finally, upon exposure to compounds such as thrombin, endotoxin, interleukin-1 or tumour necrosis factor not only promote protein C and fibrinolytic activation but also express tissue factor and play a major role in modulation of TFPI.

Thrombin generation and destruction are modulated by a series of bioamplification ; bioattenuation and bioregulation/biomodulation systems including some endogenous mediators and inflammatory substances (see Fig 1b). However, if on balance thrombin procoagulant activity overcomes the anticoagulant potential, fibrin formation will occur. Fibrin usually orchestrates its own destruction through a series of bioregulation/biomodulation mechanisms (Figure 1b). Large numbers of molecular markers of hemostasis/thrombosis are now available enabling us to assess with some degree of accuracy the state of hypercoagulability, facilitating possible intervention by appropriate drug therapy.

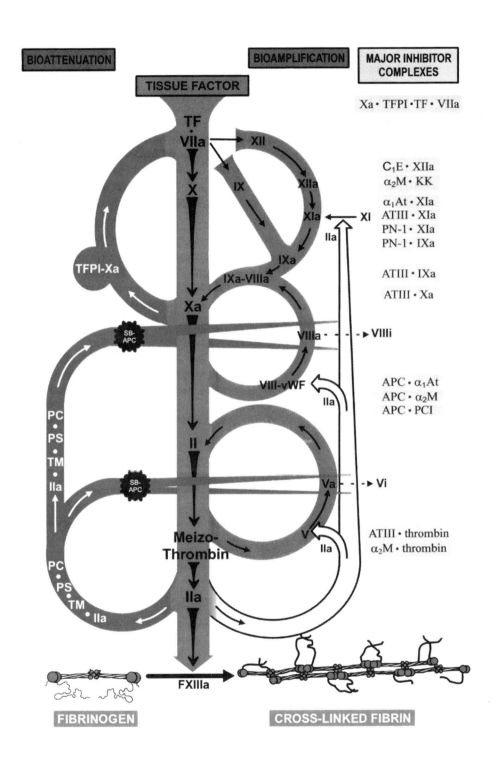

Figure 2 : A simple scheme describing coagulation from tissue factor release to fibrin formation, indicating major "Bioattenuation" loops (dark green) "Bioamplification" loops (light blue) and various plasma protease-inhibitor complexes (boxed yellow). In the current concept of coagulation, tissue factor (TF)-VIIa Complex (TF-VIIa) is the major activator of factor X, acting at three different levels:

i) Through ternary complex formation (TF-VIIa-Xa) leading to hypercoagulability and formation of low grade thrombin generation (shown as dark arrows). Free Xa has little biological significance as excess Xa is inhibited, in time, by tissue factor pathway inhibitor (TFPI), which is able to shut down the VIIa-tissue factor through formation of a quaternary complex (TF-VIIa-TFPI-Xa) : first loop of Bioattenuation process.

ii) Through factor IXa, so called "Josso Loop", where plasma factor VIII-vWF plays a major role in the Bioamplification process, enhancing by 1000 fold the rate of Xa generation. This reinforcement loop, which remains confined to platelet procoagulant surface, is not inhibited by TFPI.

iii) Through contact system, influencing the rate of factor IXa generation through factor XIa. This activation process is under the control of several proteolytic inhibitors (see below).

The two most important cofactors for Xa and IIa Bioamplication process are factor VIII and V respectively, which are activated by thrombin (IIa). Factor XI is also probably activated by thrombin as shown with large open arrows, contributing to the increased rate of the bioamplification process. Excess thrombin inactivates factors Va and VIIIa directly but also indirectly, through the formation of a quarternary complex (IIa-TM-PS-PC). This so called surface bound activated protein C (SB-APC), shown as scissors, down regulates thrombin generation by converting Va and VIIIa to Vi and VIIIi respectively (see also Figure 3). It should be noted that a partial cleavage of Prothrombin by Tenase complexes, on platelet procoagulant surfaces, leads to Meizo-Thrombin, which remains surface bound. Surface bound Meiza-Thrombin is capable of activating both factor V and protein C. It is only after a second cleavage of Prothrombin (II) thrombin (IIa) is released from the surface.

Large numbers of proteolytic inhibitors present in plasma, are able to modulate the course of coagulation at different stages. These include:

i) TF-VIIa-TFPI-Xa with specificity for factor Xa.

ii) C_1 Esterase Inhibitor; $\alpha_2 M$; $\alpha_1 At$, ATIII, which are able to keep contact phase enzymes under control.

iii) The newly identified protease inhibitor (protease Nexin 1-2, found primary in the brain), which can inhibit factors XIa and IXa. Protease Nexin is an essential intracerebral anticoagulant; where tissue factor can occur but there is virtually no TFPI or thrombomodulin to keep thrombin generation under control. (See Van Nostrand et al *Ann. New York Acad., Science*, 674, 243, 1992 for review.)

iv) Activated protein C is inhibited by several inhibitors ($\alpha_1 At$, $\alpha_2 M$, PCI) which block excessive anticoagulation. v. ATIII and $\alpha_2 M$ have the broadest specificity for various coagulation proteases (including IIa), accounting for 77% and 14% of the total inhibitory effect respectively.

C. LOOK BACK/LOOK FORWARD

From physiological and clinical points of view these variables of hemostasis are not independent entities, although from the laboratory standpoint they are often assessed in isolation. In this respect in induced hypercoagulability (whatever the origin) it is important to define thresholds of activation, which must reach a certain level to surpass the cellular and plasma inhibitory mechanisms, in time and place. It is pertinent to note that epidemiologically there is a major difference between males and females in regard to bleeding, hemorrhage and thrombosis. While "caveman" with the "hunting" lifestyle physiologically needed to be more protected from bleeding than thrombosis, the female because of the natural physiology of pregnancy and delivery had to be more protected from hemorrhage. It is also interesting to note that the risk factors for male and female for thrombosis are similar in post menopausal age groups

Another physiological evidence for natural protection is the difference that exists in terms of laboratory quantitation between thrombophilia and hemophilia. With less than 80% ATIII one is prone to thrombosis but with about 50% factor VIII one is not hemophilic. Moreover, although one usually focuses on visible initiation events (e.g. surgery, trauma, bacteremia), or some visible clinical endpoints (bleeding, embolism, thrombosis, necrosis) hemostatic abnormalities are often related to dysfunction of relatively invisible modulatory mechanisms. Pathophysiological abnormalities associated with hypercoagulability are the summation of cooperative interactions of many components of blood including endothelial abnormalities.

II. CONCEPTUAL ASPECTS

A. DEFINITION (CONCEPTS)

The term "hypercoagulable state" is a generic one that has emerged over a century to describe clinical conditions in which imbalance between procoagulant and anticoagulant forces leads to prothrombotic states. Today hypercoagulability means different things to clinicians and technologists. This controversy probably stems from the fact that hypercoagulability has no uniform clinical manifestation and usually is the summation of several triggering events. Moreover, there is lack of consensus on the appropriate laboratory diagnostic and monitoring tests of the specified therapeutic modality. This is of particular relevance to disseminated intravascular coagulation (DIC) which is considered as a continuum process, due to solid phase as opposed to liquid phase events. Patients with ATIII, protein C or protein S congenital deficiencies may have asymptomatic DIC. This may also occur during the early phase of oral anticoagulant treatment since protein C is decreased earlier than factors II, IX and X. Moreover while DIC was long considered a "ghost syndrome", because no real markers could relate its "confused" triggering mechanisms to "confused" laboratory/clinical findings, today a long list of triggering mechanisms and laboratory tests are available that reflect its initiation and propagation. These tests help determine the therapy.

Evidence is accumulating that not only activated platelets but also microvesiculation of red cells (once considered inert in coagulation) in various hemoglobinopathies can lead to thrombosis. Clot structure itself plays a major role in thrombophilia. This is very well illustrated in dysfibrinogeneamia. Thrombin and factor Xa binding to fibrin are today considered important in extension of thrombosis, requiring a 10 times higher dose of heparin, as opposed to the therapeutic dose of heparin for inhibition of fibrin associated factor Xa and thrombin.

A new definition of "thrombophilia" conceptually describes any congenital or acquired disorders with increased tendency to thrombosis. Nevertheless it is still unclear whether thrombophilia covers all attributes of prothrombotic states, except that all such conditions have a common property of predisposing to thrombotic events. There is still considerable confusion in the appropriate terminology. Currently three terms : thrombophilia, prothrombotic and prethrombotic are used as synonyms to describe hypercoagulability. It is important to note that the term "pre" thrombotic state is slightly different, and should be avoided as the term "pre" suggests an irreversible evolution toward clinical thrombosis. This is not true. There are many instances in which even a protracted thrombotic state never results in thrombosis. Today, it is feasible to differentiate between symptomatic and asymptomatic hypercoagulability.

B. CLASSIFICATION OF HYPERCOAGULABILITY

Thrombotic events can be subgrouped anatomically into venous, arterial or capillary (disseminated). In today's concept, the term hypercoagulability-induced thrombosis (classically applied to familial venous thrombosis) has broadened to cover all types of thrombosis, whether capillary, venous or arterial in nature. Many acquired clinical conditions involving abnormality in the vessel wall or the circulating blood are known today. Several other terminologies such as primary (congenital, familial, coagulative) and secondary (non-coagulative, acquired, physiological and drug or treatment-related) are still used in current literature as synonyms. Table I shows a broad subclassification of various conditions associated with hypercoagulability.

C. COAGULATIVE HYPERCOAGULABILITY (PRIMARY THROMBOPHILIA)

Primary thrombophilia is often caused by abnormality in one of the three major natural inhibitors (AT III, protein C and protein S) and/or in patients with resistance to activated protein C. Clinically this is usually characterised by an increased tendency to recurrent D.V.T. under age 40, in one or more family members. About 50% of patients with a history of thrombosis are asymptomatic, having an unknown triggering event(s). This places emphasis on the usefulness of accurate laboratory characterisation to help the clinicians in their decision making.

D . NON-COAGULATIVE AND COMBINED HYPERCOAGULABILITY

Several less defined coagulative hypercoagulabilities with less frequent thrombosis (e.g. heparin cofactor II) and non-coagulative thrombosis (e.g. homocystinuria) have been described. Acquired thrombophilias are more frequent and more difficult to diagnose as they are often reversible or transient. There is nevertheless a clear relationship between idiopathic thrombosis and cancer, economic class syndrome and advancing age, etc.

Combined congenital and acquired conditions such as pregnancy in patients with an inhibitor defect and/or subsequent to administration of anticoagulant therapy has also been reported. Oral contraceptives appear to enhance the thrombotic tendency in an individual with a coagulation inhibitor deficiency.

Table I : Some Conditions Associated with Suspected Hypercoagulable States

a/ **Primary thrombophilia** (deficiency/dysfunction)	b/ **Secondary/acquired disease/syndromes related):**	c/ **Physiological and treatment related hypercoagulability**
•Protein C/protein S •Antithrombin III •Plasminogen •Fibrinogen •Reduced plasminogen activator •Heparin cofactor II ? •APC Resistance (Factor V Leiden) •Increased Histidin rich glycoprotein ? •Mutation in Thrombomodulin	•Lupus Anticoagulant •Malignancy including : Trousseau syndrome ; non-bacterial thrombotic endocarditis ; thrombosis associated with DIC •Myeloproliferative disorders including Essential thrombocytemia •Haemoglobinopathies (S, C, D, ß-Thal) •Chronic Inflammatory Disease (Behcet; IBS) •Diabetes Mellitus •Homocystinuria Vascular Disease •Paroxysmal Nocturnal hemoglobinuria (PNH) •Thrombotic thrombocytopenic Purpura (TTP) •Hyper viscosity and hyperlipidemia •Congestive heart failure	•Pregnancy and the puerperum and pregnancy associated hypertension pre-eclampsia •Postperative state and immobilization •Obesity and advancing age •Administration of various chemotherapeutic agents (L-asparaginase, mitomycin ; adjuvant program for breast cancer •Estrogen administration (oral contraceptive use diethylstilbestrol for prostate cancer • Heparin/warfarin therapy • Blood products (PCC; PC; cytokines)

a/ A specific defect in one of the three anticoagulant system (heparin antithrombin III; protein C-thrombomodulin, protein S; plasminogen-plasminogen activator mechanism, defined as inherited thrombophilia. Available tests show that these entities cause only about 10% of documented episodes of thrombosis. This number increases to 30% of cases caused by a specific defect of the anticoagulant system if APC resistance is included.

b/ A heterogeneous array of clinical disorders exists in which there is increased risk of thromboembolism compared with the general population. These disorders are defined as acquired thrombophilia.

c/ The pathophysiologic basis of hypercoagulability in most of these conditions is not fully understood. Clearly, it is often multifactorial. The same comment is pertinent in secondary hypercoagulable states.

III. FIBRINOLYTIC ABNORMALITY AND THROMBOSIS

Hypofibrinolysis, including hypoplasminogenemia, dysplasminogenemia or PAI-1 increase..., hypofibrinogenemia or dysfibrinogenemia may lead to prothrombotic states.

Hypofibrinolysis, due to elevated levels of plasminogen activator inhibitor-1 (PAI-1) is often associated with thrombosis, though it is not expressed clinically in the absence of a thrombogenic stimulus. A decreased level of activators of the fibrinolytic system could also induce a predisposition to thrombosis. Similarly hypofibrinogenemia or dysplasminogenemia may be considered as a sign of hypercoagulability. It is worth noting that both t-PA and PAI-1 exhibit circardian variations. The former is at its lowest in morning, while the latter is at its peak and drops in the evening. Moreover platelets contain considerable amounts of PAI-1, therefore the sampling procedure must be carefully monitored to obtain reliable data for interpretation.

The assessment of the activation states based on functional activity versus concentration is a useful approach for the differential characterisation of various subtypes. Both familial hypoplasminogenemia with parallel decrease in immunological and functional properties (type I) and only functional alteration of the plasminogen molecule (type II) have been described. Recurrent DVT with or without pulmonary embolism may occur in both types. Only about 15% of patients with dysfibrinogenemia have an increased risk of thrombosis. In this condition the formed fibrin fails to be readily lysed by plasmin.

Genetic variability in the fibrinolytic system as well as environmental factors affecting synthesis or release of fibrinolytic agents, such as obesity, metabolic diseases or hypertriglyceridemia can influence the fibrinolytic system, affecting clinical outcome. For example, hereditary severe hypofibrinogenemia or afibrinogenemia may coexist with thrombosis. One possible explanation of this paradoxical observation is that thrombin is generated but not adsorbed on fibrin.

In sepsis the increased level of PAI-1 is related to endotoxin-induced synthesis release of PAI-1, whereas in nephritic disease there is an association between elevated PAI-1 and endothelial damage. This is supported with decrease in the ratio of VIII:c/vWF: Ag indicating the involvement of certain cells containing vWF:Ag (endothelials and platelets). The localised elevated PAI-1 levels also play essential roles in the initiation of thrombotic complications e.g. in preeclampsia, where increased levels of both PAI-1 and PAI-I mRNA are demonstrated.

IV. CELLULAR ABNORMALITY AND THROMBOPHILIA

There is a fundamental difference between the fluidity of blood in clotting tubes and that in the circulation. In the latter living cells, through a network of signals and interactions, mostly on cellular surfaces, respond to injury or frequent trauma that triggers the clotting process in a controlled way.

A. PLATELETS AND ENDOTHELIAL CELLS AS ESSENTIAL COMPONENTS OF BIOREGULATION

Our understanding of the bioregulation/biomodulation of hemostasis is still evolving. There is clear evidence for involvement of cellular pathways in the bioamplification, bioattenuation and bioregulatory/biomodulatory processes in thrombophilia. While activated platelets and shedded platelet microvesicles expressing sites for prothrombinase assembly enhance the rate of thrombin generation, nevertheless platelets also contain thrombomodulin which can convert the procoagulant activity of thrombin to an anticoagulant property. This occurs through the involvement of the protein C/protein S pathway which also requires phosphatidylserine (PS) on the membrane surface. As schematically shown in Figure 3, while free thrombin is a potent procoagulant enzyme for prothrombinase formation but thrombin bound thrombomodulin (surface bound thrombin) is a potent activator of protein C, a strong anticoagulant.

The importance of microvesiculation in hemostasis is seen in Scott Syndrome, a condition characterised by deficiency in procoagulant activity, and associated with decreased microvesiculation and bleeding. On the other hand, sickle cell anaemia is frequently associated with circulating erythrocyte-derived microvesicles and thrombotic episodes.

Endothelial cells also play a pivotal role in modulating hemostasis. They have a relatively strong anticoagulant luminal surface, but can rapidly acquire tissue factor procoagulant properties after immunological, chemical and/or physical injury. Exposure of vascular endothelial cells to the inflammatory cytokines, interleukin 1 (IL-1) and tumour necrosis factor (TNF), released by macrophages is known to up-regulate tissue factor synthesis as well as down-regulate thrombomodulin expression. Changes in the synthesis of heparin-like substances on endothelial surfaces is also considered responsible for imbalance between the procoagulant and anticoagulant mechanisms. Thus vessel wall abnormalities can induce a hypercoagulable state influencing indirectly protein C, antithrombin-thrombin and tissue factor - tissue factor inhibitor pathway (TFPI), No familial thrombotic deficiency for TFPI has been yet reported. Nevertheless endothelium is a major source of circulatory TFPI, which can be released (stored or novo synthesis) upon lipopolysaccharide or heparins (both unfractionated and LMW Heparins). Apart from the bioattenuation properties, endothelial cells have receptors for both single and double chains urokinase generating plasmin in strategically located areas to influence evolving fibrin formation.

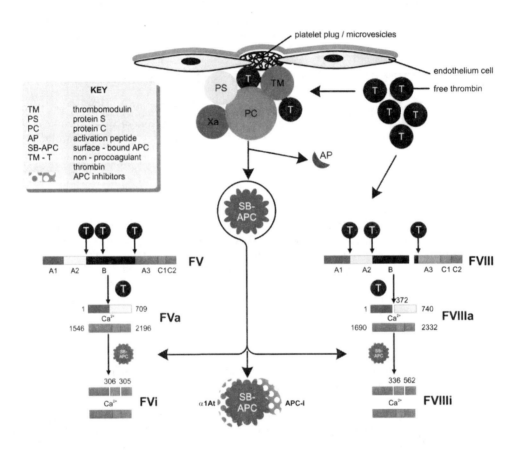

B. THE BIOREGULATORY ROLE OF LEUCOCYTES/ERYTHROCYTES

A large number of cell adhesion molecules are involved in the attachment of leucocytes and monocytes to endothelial cells. There is also a clear link between the inflammatory cytokines and atherosclerosis. Both endothelial cells and leucocytes contain ADPase which limits platelet activation and produces nitric oxide (NO) as a potent antiplatelet agent. Clearly the pathogenic mechanisms of hypercoagulable states predisposing to thrombotic complications are numerous, including several other aspects of functional alteration of the vessel wall, blood flow and hyperviscosity as well as classically impaired hemostatic function.

With the increase in clinical applications of artificial surfaces in biomaterials attention is focused on both their activation and thromboresistance properties. Thrombus formation on these surfaces is almost inevitable. Simultaneous therapy with anticoagulant, platelet aggregation inhibitors or plasminogen activators is essential. Nevertheless, while thrombus formation may be inhibited, continuous alterations in blood constituents cannot be avoided. This issue is reviewed in a separate chapter.

V. ANALYTICAL ASPECTS

The strategy for defining hypercoagulability, on the basis of laboratory findings, has also undergone conceptual changes. For a long time hypercoagulability in the laboratory was defined as an accelerated clotting time. Then it was realised that the sensitivity of coagulation assays was very low and that the abnormality in the fluid phase only reflects part of the story. The next moves were the assessment of coagulation in special clotting tubes to enhance sensitivity, the use of the thromboelastograph to assess activation states in whole blood, and the development of activation markers of hemostasis. Today, various experimental models are used in order to examine blood coagulation in a circulating flow system.

A. THE USEFULNESS OF THROMBOELASTOGRAPHY

Laboratory analysis of hemostatic abnormalities seeks not only to provide clues for coagulation disorders through abnormal clotting time but also to define other abnormalities such as defective fibrin formation; abnormal/altered fibrin polymerisation/dissolution and abnormal clot retraction. In these respects, the thromboelastograph has made important contributions. It allows coagulation in a special device using whole blood instead of plasma or platelet rich blood. It defines that thrombosis is an excess thrombin generation. Finally, the involvement of factor XIIIa, platelet and excess fibrinogen leads to short pulses after a lag phase, whereas the presence of tissue factor in the system not only shortens the lag phase of clotting but also gives a large pulse as an indicator of clot firmness. This is of particular relevance to the modern concept of fibrin structure recently presented by B. Blombäck.

B. ASSESSMENT OF THE ACTIVATION STATES

In many conditions, the abnormality in hemostasis is due to molecular dysfunctions. This is best evaluated by the assessment of the activation states, based on immunological assays. These enable measurement of the absolute concentration of coagulant proteins and the functional activity based on biochemical/biological assay. The ratio of functional activity to the concentration provides information on the activity state and differentiates between native (ratio of one), activated and inactivated forms with the ratio above and below unity respectively.

C. ACTIVATION MARKERS OF HEMOSTASIS

Advances in biochemistry of coagulation proteins made it possible to measure with high degree of accuracy and specificity molecular markers of coagulation and fibrinolysis (Figure 1c). Today methods of assessment of fibrinopeptide A and B and release of other activation peptides such as prothrombin fragment F1+2, activation peptides of FIX, FX and protein C; methods based on fibrinogen/fibrin fragments (e.g. D-dimer & E) ; direct assessment of proteolytic enzymes alone (VIIa, XIIa, XIa) or in complexes with proteolytic inhibitors such as Thrombin-Antithrombin (TAT), α_1-AT-proteases, α_2-M-proteases; activated protein C - protein C inhibitor complex and plasmin - antiplasmin (PAP) are providing new insights into pathophysiological states of hypercoagulability.

The main unanswered question is how to differentiate various stages of activation by these activation markers. For instance fibrinopeptide A increase means that excess thrombin, as compared to basal level, has been generated acting on fibrinogen. But could we consider a hypercoagulable mechanism restricted only to prothrombin activation leading to F1+2 without being associated with increased FPA or TAT complexes? It is important to note that thrombin has more than 25 substrates, all competing with each other on the basis of their characteristic biochemical properties and reaction rates. Another important factor which discriminates the usefulness of these markers is the half life *in vivo*. For example D-Dimer, which is now routinely measured, has a longer half life than F1+2 and FPA, which circulate only for a short period. The ratio between TAT and PAP complexes is a better indicator to define which of the two processes is in disequilibrium as compared to each other and/or other markers. New assays such as factor VIIa, factor XIIa and factor Xa in complexes with ATIII or XIIa - in complexes with $\alpha_2 M$, which measure the early or intermediate phases of activation of clotting are recently available but their usefulness requires further investigations. Finally, all these assays suffer from the quality of sample collection and poor, non-standardised venepuncture. Standardization remains an issue of paramount importance. Much also remains to be elucidated in regard to an appropriate anticoagulant cocktail for collection of blood samples for assessment of the activation markers of hemostasis.

D. ACTIVATION MARKERS OF PLATELET AND FIBRINOLYTIC SYSTEM

In parallel, major advances have been made in assessing activation states of platelets and in differentiation of various stages of activation; aggregation/adhesion and secretion/release reactions. These can be evaluated on the basis of exposure of activation markers of platelet membrane, microvesiculation and the platelet released products.

We have also witnessed major advances in the assessment of the components of fibrinolytic systems. Currently these new concepts and methods are applied to evaluation of the bioamplification and bioattenuation processes of hemostatic pathway but also help to determine the *in vivo* functional integrity of hemostasis. The clinical scientist and haematologist can meet the multiple challenges of improved sensitivity, specificity, precision and accuracy with the use of newer indexes of hypercoagulability. These allow accurate differentiation between native, mutant, activated and intermediate complexes and non-functional or partially active molecules observed by the classical diagnostic procedures.

A schematic representation of activation, regulation and/or thrombosis formation along with the various activation markers which are in use for the identification of the nature of hypercoagulability is shown in Figure 1c. Many new biochemical approaches and analyses to detect abnormalities in gene structure are used today in specialised centres : these methods can be successfully be applied to test the earlier classical hypothesis.

VI. EPIDEMIOLOGICAL/CLINICAL ASPECTS

Hypercoagulability leading to Deep Vein Thrombosis (DVT) or Arterial Thrombosis is a common disorder with a frequency of about 1:1000 individuals per year. Numerous acquired and inherited risk factors, such as surgery, prolonged immobilisation, malignancies, deficiencies of some important inhibitors of blood coagulation (protein C, protein S, ATIII) and poor anticoagulant response to activated protein C are associated with thrombosis. These are classified in Table I.

Despite increased understanding of most risk factors, the majority of episodes of DVT seem to occur spontaneously without any known predisposing condition. This suggests that there are additional mechanisms for the development of DVT yet to be discovered. The three key plasma subcomponents of coagulation pathway involved in hemostatic disorders are FVII; FVIII/vWF and fibrinogen. Deficiency of these proteins leads to increased tendency to bleed. On the other hand high levels of these proteins are epidemiologically associated with thrombosis.

In addition, elevated levels of factor VIII/vWF appear to be associated more with blood group A, B, and AB as compared to blood group O. Thus it is possible that a relationship also exists between blood group and thrombosis. These hypotheses have been recently tested epidemiologically by the Leiden group. Their results are summarised below :

A. ASSOCIATION OF FVIII/VWF AND BLOOD GROUP WITH DVT

In a sex and aged matched patient controlled study of 301 consecutive patients under 70 with a known episode of thrombosis, univariate analysis of blood group, vWF and factor VIII found a positive relationship between vWF levels, factor VIII levels and thrombotic risk. In multivariate analysis only factor VIII remained as a risk factor, and the dose-response relationship between factor VIII level and risk of thrombosis persisted (subjects with factor VIII levels over 150 IU/dl have a relative risk of 4.8 (95% Cl 2.3-10)). In contrast, the adjusted relative risk for blood group and for each vWF-stratum did not differ from unity. These results may fit in a similar mechanism as recently described for APC-resistance. In the latter, a mutated factor V is not efficiently inactivated by activated protein C, defined as « factor Va persistence ». If high levels of factor VIII lead to increased concentrations of activated factor VIII, a similar imbalance between procoagulant and anticoagulant factors would be the result as in APC-resistance. It remains to be elucidated which mechanism, genetic or environmental, leads to high factor VIII levels. These findings suggest an effect of blood group and vWF, both fully mediated through factor VIII. The 25% prevalence of factor VIII levels greater than 150 IU/dl among unselected consecutive thrombosis patients and the adjusted relative risk for thrombosis (of almost 5) leads the Leiden group to the conclusion that high factor VIII levels are common and present a clear increase in risk of thrombosis, similar to the risk conferred by deficiencies of the coagulation-inhibiting proteins and APC-resistance.

B. ASSOCIATION BETWEEN FVII, FIBRINOGEN AND DVT

High plasma levels of coagulation factor VII and fibrinogen are well known risk factors for arterial thrombosis. Additionally, Mspl and Haelll polymorphisms in the factor VII and fibrinogen genes have recently been reported to be associated with the increased concentration of both proteins in the plasma. However, no conclusion could be drawn with respect to an increase or decrease in thrombosis risk.

In a population-based case-controlled study of 199 patients with a confirmed episode of deep-vein thrombosis, the clinical importance of fibrinogen and FVII were investigated by the Leiden group.

For fibrinogen there was a positive level-related association between the plasma fibrinogen level and thrombotic risk. Subjects with a plasma fibrinogen greater than 5 g/L had an almost fourfold increased risk. The frequencies of the different Haelll genotypes were out of balance only for the thrombosis patients with a deficit of the H1H2 genotype. Possession of an H1H2 genotype was associated with a 40% reduction in thrombosis risk.

For factor VII, neither the plasma level nor the Mspl genotypes were related to deep-vein thrombosis, although possession of a M2 allele was clearly associated with significantly lower factor VII levels. The frequencies of the Mspl genotypes were the same for patients and control subjects and exhibited Hardy-Weinberg equilibrium. These findings support the concept that plasma fibrinogen, a determinant of arterial thrombosis is also a risk factor for venous thrombosis. Factor VII plasma concentration is unrelated to deep-vein thrombosis. These observations are supported by data from DNA analysis of polymorphisms.

C. ASSOCIATION BETWEEN SOME DEFICIENCY STATES AND DVT

Excluding thrombosis associated with malignancy, myeloproliferative diseases, hyperlipidemia and nephrotic syndrome, there are small numbers, about 10% of cases, in which an association between hypercoagulability and thrombotic episodes have been established. Their causes include: dysfibrinogenemia (1%), plasminogen deficiency (1-2%); antiphospholipids (2-3%), antithrombin deficiency (2-4%); protein C deficiency (5-8%); protein S deficiency (5-8%); fibrinolysis abnormalities (10-15%) and the largest recently reported thrombophilia (APC-resistance) which varies from 20% to 60% for some familial thrombophilias according to various authors. The mean high prevalence of APC-resistance in about 20% of cases, (due to factor V gene mutation) raises the question of whether it is worthwhile to screen for this abnormality. Screening might be done in patients with a personal or familial history of thrombotic events. Where the prevalence of thrombosis is relatively high, a large scale screening is probably of little clinical significance.

D. ASSOCIATION BETWEEN HYPERLIPIDEMIA AND THROMBOSIS

A number of epidemiological studies have been undertaken to determine the association between lipid in particular low density lipoprotein (LDL) with elevated risk of ischemic heart disease. Parallel investigations have been carried out to lower the level of oxidised LDL, the main artherogenic component of cholesterol, using new drugs and "optimal" use of vitamin E and C supplements as potent antioxidants. New trials are in progress to reduce IHD with low dose Warfarin with some promising results.

E. THROMBOGENICITY ASSOCIATED WITH BLOOD PRODUCTS

The use of blood products (e.g. prothrombin complex concentrate (PCC); FXI concentrate; platelet concentrates containing microvesicles) has been associated with thrombotic complications. PCC at high dose (>80 U/kg) can sometimes lead to thrombosis with fatal consequences. This is of particular relevance in patients with trauma or surgery and coexistent liver disease. The development of high purity factor IX concentrate has reduced the risk involved to some extent. However, *in vivo* the infusion of a single dose of either PCC or high purity FIX concentrates is associated with a considerable rise in FPA; F1+2 and TAT showing evidence of coagulation activation *in vivo*, but unaccompanied by clinical thrombosis. Infusion of FXI concentrate in some patients with vascular problems appears to be associated with thrombosis.

Increased levels of F1+2 and other activation markers of hemostasis have been noted in subjects with proven familial thrombosis due to ATIII, protein C and protein S deficiency. In the majority of cases the levels are very high in the presence of active thrombosis and fall subsequent to Warfarin therapy. While the use of these molecular markers facilitate improved diagnosis as compared to INR, we are still unable to define the role of activation markers in the diagnosis, prognosis or management of patients with thrombophilia with or without anticoagulant therapy.

V. CONCLUSION

Today the field of hypercoagulability has become a distinct discipline in its own right, though it is still in the stage of vigorous development. The introduction of new activation markers of hemostasis helped to establish the interrelationship of a large number of clinical/subclinical conditions associated with hypercoagulability. Improved and more standardised laboratory techniques, provide better diagnostic/prognostic approaches. The multifactorial triggering nature of some forms of hypercoagulability is recognized. We should remain ready to revise earlier beliefs as soon as possible. Thrombosis is a complex process involving interaction of many components such as platelets, red cells, leucocytes, macrophages, pro and anticoagulant/fibrinolytic proteins, protease inhibitors and endothelial cells, all acting in concert.

Cellular interactions play an important role in both physiological hemostasis and pathological thrombotic responses. All cellular components of blood including erythrocytes, through the expression of phosphatidylserine, contribute in the amplification of procoagulant and anticoagulant activities and regulate hemostasis in a variety of ways. The understanding of cofactor roles of various cellular components of blood will provide the basis for development of new approaches for intervention in thrombotic states. Of particular relevance is the critical role of leucocytes in inflammation processes, including the ability to migrate to the site of inflammation and release an impressive series of toxic agents such as proteases, reactive oxygen species, and cationic proteins, capable of killing invading pathogens. Evidence suggests that infection might be an important etiologic factor in the development of anti-neutrophil cytoplasm antibody (ANCA) which can cause endothelial cell damage but is an extremely useful diagnostic serological marker for a variety of well known primary vasculitic syndromes, including Wegener's granulomatosis and idiopathic necrotizing and crescentic glomerulonephritis, Churg-Strauss Syndrome, Henoch-Schönlein purpura and some nonvasculitic diseases such as rheumatoid arthritis, inflammatory bowel disease, and autoimmune hepatobiliary diseases. These observations provide the stimulus to study the relationship between inflammatory process induced hypercoagulability and also stimulated efforts to identify the pathogenic mechanisms that may lead to development of better therapeutic strategies. Clearly, further *in vivo* studies are needed to provide clinical support for the relevance of various cell-cell and cell-protein interaction and signalling in various pathophysiological conditions associated with hypercoagulability.

To sum up, the underlying mechanisms involved in triggering a thrombotic state and the appropriate mode of therapy remain a major scientific clinical challenge requiring a broad spectrum of assays for a better characterisation and assessment of the activation states of each component involved. For example disseminated intravascular coagulopathy is a spectrum of diseases in its own right covering a continuum of multifactorial events from localised thrombosis to recurring thrombosis and lysis with either asymptomatic low grade consumptive coagulopathy to symptomatic skin necrosis. There has been a resurgence of interest in the role of endothelium in modulating the essential active principles of thrombophilia. More development work is needed to ascertain the cause/effect relationship in hypercoagulability. The new generation markers of hemostatic balance provides tools for assessing biochemical imbalance between procoagulant and anticoagulant *in vivo*, prior to the appearance of thrombotic episode or DIC. Properly designed prospective studies will be required to explain why some individuals are more prone to clinically significant hypercoagulable state and how to intervene with appropriate therapy prior to an overt thrombosis. These issues are addressed in detail by our eminent contributors.

Further research on the complex interactive events occurring at the luminal surface of the vasculature and within the vessel wall is clearly needed. Meanwhile, alert clinicians confronted with the sheer diversity of conditions associated with thrombophilia must keep in mind a long list of differential diagnostic approaches.

We strongly believe that a state-of-the-art book on hypercoagulable states covering the concepts physiological, analytical, epidemiological and clinical aspects in one volume is timely and useful, as these topics usually appear in fragmentary fashion in specialised journals.

REFERENCES AND SUGGESTED READINGS

To avoid duplication and in an effort to save space in this introductory chapter, we have not cited references. Readers should consult each individual chapter for updated references.

ACKNOWLEDGEMENT

The authors wish to express their sincere thanks to Andy Miller for the graphic works.

Fundamental Aspects and Laboratory Approaches

A. Fundamental Aspects of Haemostasis/Thrombosis

TISSUE FACTOR, FLOW AND
THE INITIATION OF COAGULATION

Y. Nemerson and P.B. Contino
Mount Sinaï Medical School, New York

Tissue factor (TF) is a relatively small transmembrane protein that is present on the plasma membranes of many cell types, but is notably absent from endothelial cells, at least under ordinary circumstances. While its existence was first inferred over 150 years ago, its identity as a unique protein was not accepted until is was first purified to homogeneity[1]. The protein exists in three clear domains: a 219 residue extracellular structure that has significant structural homology with the class 2 cytokine receptor family, an extremely hydrophobic 23 residue transmembrane domain which is likely in a helical configuration, and a small cytoplasmic tail consisting of 21 residues which is of unknown significance. While TF has been frequently referred to as a "receptor", no such function has yet been ascribed to this molecule; i.e., TF is not associated with any signal transduction upon binding its ligand, factor VII and VIIa. Thus, while it is possible that TF is involved as a receptor, to date its only known function is as an essential enzyme activator that initiates coagulation *via* its interaction with factors VII and VIIa.

TF is a bifunctional cofactor in the sense that it supports two entirely different, but related reactions. Upon binding to TF, factor VII is labilized with respect to its activation by factor Xa[2] and by other complexes of TF and VIIa.[3,4] It appears that the latter reaction occurs on vesicle surfaces; however, whether TF in cell membranes has sufficient mobility to catalyze this reaction remains to be demonstrated. Put differently, it is possible that on cell surfaces TF:VII is converted to TF:VIIa by fluid-phase VIIa, although the rates of activation by VIIa appear to be much slower than those achieved by factor Xa. Whatever the cell-surface mechanism is, it is clear that factor VII when bound to tissue factor is rapidly converted to VIIa by virtue of cleavage of a single peptide bond. The physiological advantage of achieving initiation of coagulation on a membrane-bound enzymatic complex is that the site of initiation is localized to the site of vascular injury,

It has now become clear that blood coagulation is intimately involved in the thrombotic process. It is also widely believed that TF is the most potent physiological and pathophysiological initiator of coagulation. Accordingly, this molecule has received an enormous amount of attention and, in the fifteen years since it was first isolated[1] many hundreds of papers have been published regarding its biochemical, physiological and pathophysiological properties. Its biochemical function is that of an essential enzyme activator;[5,6] it is perhaps best viewed as the regulatory subunit of a holoenzyme that also contains a catalytic subunit, factor VIIa. Factor VII, the zymogen that gives rise to the enzymic species, factor VIIa, circulates in the plasma. Factor VIIa, uniquely amongst the enzymes involved in coagulation, has been detected in human plasma;[7-9] presumably it is present in the circulation and not an artifact of blood collection. Thus, the initiation of coagulation is accomplished by allowing the circulating blood to physically contact TF, which is located in normally inaccessible sites.

Because of its plasma-membrane location, TF also localizes the site of the initiation of coagulation. To date, with the possible exception of amniotic fluid embolism and extensive crush injuries, TF has not been identified in the circulation. Despite a large literature on cultured endothelial cell TF, there is little evidence that these cells express TF *in vivo*. A possible exception to this is the occasional endothelial cell that was immunohistochemically positive in placental sections[10], but only in the vicinity of inflammation. Because placenta may be specialized with respect to clotting its own vessels, it is likely inappropriate to generalize from this organ.

In general, then, it is reasonable to conclude that active TF remains on the cells in which it is synthesized, or, possibly in cellular detritus. Within the arterial wall, the adventitia is the major source of TF;[11] the smooth muscle cells have been shown to contain biochemically detectable TF,[12] whereas immunohistochemical stains have indicated little or no TF in the media[13,14]. Conversely, a flow study using everted vessels in a Baumgartner chamber revealed readily detectable TF activity[15] in the subendothelium. Regarding the localization of this molecule, different techniques have yielded different results.

Recently, the extracellular domain of TF has been crystallized and its structure has been solved. The molecule belongs to the cytokine superfamily of cell-surface receptors, but to date, no receptor function has been assigned to this molecule; i.e., no signal transduction has been detected upon binding of its ligand. The precise sites of interaction with factor VII, of course, cannot be deduced from the structure of TF; this must await solution of the crystal structure of TF:VIIa. This binary complex has been crystallized (Kichhoffer et al, submitted for publication); the crystals diffract to better than 3 Å, and the solution of its structure is close to completion. Only then will the contact sites between TF and factor VIIa be known explicitly and with high resolution.

A discrepancy between TF content and activity has been well-documented in the literature, but has received relatively little attention. Bach and Rifkin[16] suggested that the influx of Ca^{2+} upregulated cellular TF activity as brief exposure to an ionophore markedly increased cell-surface TF activity. Le et al.,[17] in a very convincing study, demonstrated that there were two classes of TF molecules on a cell surface: both bound VIIa, both showed TF:VIIa amidolytic activity, but only one activated factor X and only one was inhibited by Tissue Factor Pathway Inhibitor (TFPI). Thus, an immunohistochemical stain would have grossly overestimated the available TF as would a direct amidolytic assay for TF:VIIa. Other evidence for a disparity between procoagulant and immunoreactive TF has been published: Walsh and Geczy,[18] showed that treatment of human peripheral blood monocytes increased their activity ≈2-fold following stimulation with endotoxin and "low-dose" cyclohexamide, whereas the antigen level fell by approximately 70%, again indicating that immunologic assessment of cellular TF may be misleading.

The need for a better technique for the localization of vascular TF is also evident from other disparate results in the literature. One study utilizing *in situ* hybridization with TF mRNA along with immunohistochemistry found TF mostly in the adventitia, but some hybridization and staining was found in normal media (particularly the saphenous vein)[13]. The endothelium was negative by both techniques. Of particular interest was the detection of TF in atherosclerotic plaques, mostly in macrophages or in cells of unknown origin. More or less similar immunohistochemical results were obtained by Sueishi and colleagues[19] who studied human aortic atheroma: however, stainable TF was "ubiquitously present" in the intima, but again, not in the endothelium. In the placenta, TF was identified in the villous stroma, with the trophoblasts being negative[10]. Interestingly, a few endothelial cells near inflammatory sites stained positively. Taken together, these studies indicate that TF is present at low concentrations in the vascular media, but is mainly in the adventitia. As noted above, a flow study[15] indicated that TF activity was readily measurable in the normal arterial subendothelium. This result indicates that assays based on the procoagulant activity of TF may be considerably more sensitive than those based on immunohistochemical techniques. In this regard, Drake has claimed that cultured endothelial cells displayed positive immunoreactivity when they contained only 5% of their maximal TF activity[20]. These investigators, however, used a plasma clotting time assay, which is most likely neither precise nor sensitive. By measuring TF in a tubular flow reactor when the perfusate contained VIIa, X, Va and prothrombin, we can detect vanishingly small amounts of TF: surface densities in the range of 10^{-18} mols.cm^{-2} were readily detected as evidenced by thrombin generation (unpublished data). Because the surface density of TF that is required to initiate thrombosis *in vivo* is unknown, the pathophysiological meaning of any TF surface density is also unclear. It is for this reason that studies measuring surface tissue factor in a flow system must be performed.

Attempts to measure vascular TF by homogenizing or sonicating tissues are plagued with potential artifact. The reason for this lies in the effects of particle size and number on any biochemical reaction velocity: It is axiomatic that the rate of an enzymatic reaction cannot exceed the rate of collision between enzyme and substrate molecules. Thus, the upper limit of a reaction will be given by the collision frequency. Usually this rate is only a fraction of the collision frequency and this occurs because not every collision results in product formation; some collisions are abortive and result in a free enzyme and an unaltered substrate molecule. Ideally, this fraction may be expressed as a probability function and for an ensemble of molecules of similar size, the number of collisions is *independent* of the particle size; i.e., it is a property only of a particular enzyme substrate pair. The theory of collisions occurring with a target was developed by Smoluchowski[21] and results in the following expression:

$$C_f = 8\pi DRn \qquad (1)$$

where C_f is the collision frequency, R is the particle radius, D, the diffusion constant and n, the number of particles. This expression clearly states that the collision frequency is a direct function of the radius and the number of particles. Now, Stoke's law for a sphere moving in a liquid of viscosity η, gives the frictional coefficient ρ, as:

$$\rho = 3\pi\eta R \qquad (2)$$

Further, Einstein's expression for Brownian motion expresses diffusion, D, as:

$$D = \frac{kT}{\rho} \qquad (3)$$

where k is Boltzmann's constant and T, the absolute temperature in Kelvin. Combining equation 1,2 and 3 results in:

$$C_f = \frac{8kT}{3\eta}n \qquad (4)$$

This equation shows that C_f is, in fact, independent of the particle size. This occurs because of the inverse relationship between target size, R, and diffusion, D. Note that C_f, however, is still directly proportional to the number of particles, n. Equation 4, however, applies only when the particles are of equal size. Debye (1942, original reference unknown) shows, however, that the influence of differing particle size is small:

$$C_f = \frac{1}{4}(2 + \frac{R_1}{R_2} + \frac{R_2}{R_1})\frac{8kT}{3\eta}n \qquad (5)$$

where R_1 and R_2 are the radii of each species (note that eq. 5 reduces to eq. 4 when $R_1 = R_2$). It follows from equation 5 that relatively large changes in R have a small effect on collision frequency: if $R_1/R_2 = 3$, the frequency increases by a factor of only 4/3. If, however, the increase in size is accompanied by a similar decrease in n, e.g., a factor of 3, the resultant collisions will be reduced to only 0.44 of the original rate. The substance of this argument is that great care must be exercised in performing an apparently simple determination such as the total TF content of a given tissue. Because tissues are heterogeneous, it seems likely that comparing samples from different organs would be fraught with error because of differing particle sizes and numbers.

Arterial TF Following Balloon Injury: Recent studies have shown that the smooth muscle cells of the media of rat aorta possessed small, but potentially significant amounts of TF as determined by a specific bioassay[22]. The animals were subjected to a procedure that is similar to angioplasty of human coronary arteries. Interestingly, the measurable TF rose considerably shortly after balloon injury to this vessel. Furthermore, *in situ* hybridization for TF mRNA also showed a marked increase in the media following the injury. Importantly, frank thrombus was observed on the vessel wall following a second ballooning of the rat aorta, thus suggesting that if TF is involved, it must be present on or very near the surface of the injured vessel (unpublished results). Endothelial cells were not evaluated in this study as they are removed by the ballooning. It is somewhat difficult to assess the meaning of these experiments because, as noted above, the amount of TF required to initiate coagulation on vascular tissue is simply not known. The presence of thrombus on the luminal surface of the vessel, however, is presumptive evidence that the induced TF was accessible to the flowing blood.

Further, there are essential differences between classical, three-dimensional kinetics and the type of two-dimensional kinetics which occur on a vascular surface. When a viscous fluid flows through a rigid cylinder, the flow rate of the fluid near the surface is retarded by virtue of viscous interactions with the surface. This retardation is translated throughout the flowing fluid so that the flow profile assumes a parabolic shape. Thus, the flow velocity is greatest at the center of the tube and least near the wall. When the fluid contains a solute, the delivery of the solute to the wall is given by:

$$k = c_o (\gamma_w D^2 / L)^{1/3} \qquad (6)$$

$$\gamma_w = 4Q / (\pi r^3) \qquad (7)$$

where D is the diffusion coefficient of the protein (solute) in $cm^2 \cdot sec^{-1}$, and Q is the volumetric flow rate ($ml \cdot min^{-1}$). The coefficient, C_o, is equal to $3^{4/3}/\Gamma(1/3)$ (Γ is the mathematical "gamma function"). Thus, the transport rate for any species in solution can be readily estimated. The reason that the tube length is important is that only the molecules in close proximity to the wall are converted (by a wall-bound enzyme species) to product. This non-linearity (which is in contrast to 3-D catalysis) results in a zone of substrate depletion, the "substrate boundary layer," that increases in size with the tube length. The average thickness of this layer, δ, is given by Cussler[23] as:

$$\delta = \frac{2}{3}(4\pi r^2 \frac{DL}{Q})^{1/2} \qquad (8)$$

These treatments assume that the reactive surface is homogeneous and therefore might not apply to a sparse enzyme density on a surface. However, we[24] and others[25] have found this not to be true, that is the tubes with TF or prothrombinase behave as if they were homogeneously coated with enzyme.

Another property of surface catalysis that must be considered is that a 2-D surface is, in fact, saturable. For example, the binding capacity of a phosphatidylserine/phosphatidylcholine (30:70, w/w) membrane for Xa is about 12 $pmol \cdot cm^{-2}$.[26-29] With an equilibrium binding constant of $\approx$ 33 nM, the microcapillary surface is essentially saturated at 150 nM, the approximate plasma concentration of factor X. The fact that planes are saturable and finite means that if soluble substrates reach surface-bound enzymes only *via* surface diffusion, the reaction may not reach Vmax, which is predicated on infinite substrate concentration and hence, infinite collision frequency between substrate and enzyme.

The inherent saturability of a plane has a consequence pertinent to our experiments: that for a flux of factor X to the surface achieved at physiological flow conditions and factor X concentrations, maximal conversion to Xa occurs only when the surface is entirely saturated with TF. However, the surface density of TF required for half-maximal activation is very much less than half-saturation! This phenomenon was first elucidated by Berg and Purcell[30]. In essence, they showed that for low fluxes to the cell surface, surface coverage by a receptor (or an enzyme) of the order of 0.01% could capture half the molecules encountering the cell surface. Thus, increasing the surface coverage to homogeneity (100%), an increase of a factor of 10^4, would increase the capture by only a factor of two. The theoretical curve for capture *vs.* surface coverage is a rectangular hyperbola and therefore one can readily calculate the surface coverage that would yield one-half the rate obtained at total surface coverage, the $K_{1/2}$, mathematically analogous to the K_M of Michaelis-Menten kinetics. Therefore when the surface coverage is lower than the $K_{1/2}$ the rate of capture (or product formation in the case of a surface enzyme) will vary almost linearly with receptor or enzyme density. In contrast, when the surface density is much greater than the $K_{1/2}$, the reaction rates will be essentially independent of receptor or enzyme density. Thus, in order to evaluate changes in surface TF density, it is obviously necessary to know where on this curve the baseline density falls. This cannot be calculated and must be determined empirically.

The importance of the hyperbolic response to TF surface density is illustrated in Figure 1 (taken from a recent publication from our laboratory),[26] in which the rate of factor X activation is plotted *vs.* TF surface density. The data were derived from experiments utilizing a flow reactor developed by us[31]. Briefly, clean glass microcapillary tubes are filled with a suspension of phospholipid vesicles containing known amounts of TF. The vesicles spontaneously fuse on the inner surface of the capillary forming a continuous, stable bilayer with known amounts of TF. A solution of factors VIIa and X is then perfused through the capillary and the Xa content of the effluent is measured using a chromogenic assay. The illustrated experiments were done at tissue factor densities ranging from zero to 80 fmoles·cm^{-2}. It is obvious that a hyperbolic response is obtained; the $K_{1/2}$ was 1.7 and 3.3 fmoles·cm^{-2} at γ_w of 100 and 1600 sec^{-1}, respectively. These shear rates are typical of veins and small arteries and the factor X concentration is about physiological. As discussed above, the flux of factor X varies with γ_w; hence the $K_{1/2}$ at a constant substrate concentration also rises with γ_w.

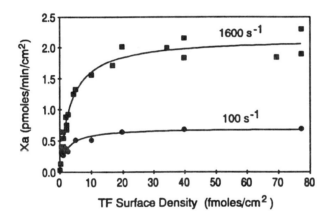

Figure 1. The rate of Xa production in the flow reactor as a function of TF surface density. The upper curve was derived at a wall shear rate of 1600 sec^{-1}, and the lower at 100 sec^{-1} (from reference 26).

The importance of this concept is that in the region of arterial narrowing, the γ_w increases, thus increasing the delivery of factor X (and all other proteins) to the surface. Thus, it is clearly possible that the exposed TF could be on the plateau (as in figure 1), but following narrowing of the vessel, the shift in substrate flux would shift the curve to the right. Accordingly, the TF could therefore become rate-limiting. Thus, changes in TF density could readily become significant on narrowed vessels, whereas it would be without kinetic effect on vessels of normal calibre. Put differently, changes in the surface density of TF are not interpretable without a complete analysis of the system including substrate flux to the surface and, hence, the γ_w. In addition, we propose to study thrombin generation by including factor V and prothrombin in the perfusate. The reason for doing this is that it is possible that only small amounts of Xa are required to reach the transport rate limited hydrolysis of prothrombin; i.e., thrombin generation. Indeed, we have preliminary evidence that the addition of TFPI to a flow reactor experiment in concentrations sufficient to reduce Xa production *almost completely* has essentially no effect on thrombin generation when the surface density is relatively high, in the range of that encountered on the surface of fibroblasts (unpublished data). This is also the rationale for investigating the role of anticoagulants that inhibit the coagulation process by different mechanisms, as indicated above.

The role of factors VIII and IX in factor X activation by vascular cells and tissue: It appears quite likely that coagulation, *in vivo*, is initiated by tissue factor, although this paradigm has not been exhaustively tested. While this formulation is consistent with the negligible bleeding associated with factor XII (Hageman factor) deficiency, it has been difficult to design experiments which yield results consistent with the clinical observation that patents lacking factors XI, VIII or IX have mild to very severe hemorrhagic disorders. Broze's laboratory[32] found that thrombin can activate factor XI, thereby providing a mechanism for the feed-back activation of this factor. These experiments were performed using purified coagulation factors; others, however, have challenged these results because no activation of factor XI was observed when plasma was added to the system[33]. Thus, the mechanism by which factor XI is activated remains obscure. Another problem associated with TF-dependent activation of coagulation concerns the role of factors VIII and IX. This is clearly important as there is no doubt that patents lacking either of these factors exhibit severely abnormal hemostasis. We have previously addressed this problem by assessing the rate of factor X activation utilizing the flow reactor contain TF. The perfusates always contained factor VIIa (10 nM), factor X (150 nM), factor IX (50 nM) and $CaCl_2$ (5 mM). The variable additions were factor VIII and TFPI. γ_w was varied from 100 sec^{-1} to 1600 sec^{-1}.

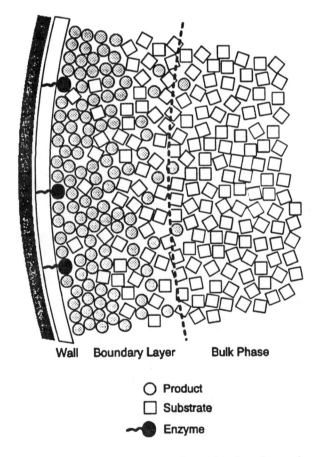

Figure 2. Schematic of the substrate and product gradients developed near the wall of a tubular flow reactor (from reference 26).

The results can be summarized as follows: 1) at the TF to phospholipid ratio used (1:100,000; mol/mol), the addition of factor VIII led to increased factor X activation in a shear-dependent manner; i.e., as γ_w increased, the effect of factor VIII increased. This is expected on hydrodynamic grounds as the delivery of factor VIII, a fairly large protein, would be marked enhanced by convection. 2) The addition of TFPI augmented the difference between "plus VIII" and "minus VIII" experiments. In effect, in the absence of factor VIII the direct TF:VIIa catalyzed activation of factor X was rapidly inhibited by TFPI, whereas Xa production in the presence of VIII and IX persisted longer[34]. This observation suggests that the VIIIa:IXa complexes persist on the lipid surface, thereby continuing the activation of factor X. These results were confirmed in a static system[35]. Mann's group published results which are consistent with this observation, but support a different interpretation: Xa cleaves one of the two activation bonds in factor IX, thereby making it better substrate for TF:VIIa[36]. These experiments were performed at very high factor IX concentrations, over 5 times the physiological concentration, thus casting some doubt on the significance of these findings.

We recently found in flow reactor experiments, that the level of Xa in the vicinity of the wall could be inferred to be of the order of 50-150 nM. Thus, using this artificial system, it is likely that factor IX would be attacked by Xa even at 50 nM, the approximate plasma concentration of factor IX. The reason that such high Xa levels are obtained follows from the dynamics of the flow reactor: as discussed above, there is a zone of substrate depletion near the wall and this "substrate boundary layer" can be estimated from classical hydrodynamic equations. Because this layer is caused by conversion of substrate to product at the wall, a symmetrical gradient (of opposite sign to the substrate gradient) of product is formed. Product generation estimated at the tube outlet averages the product concentration of the entire cross-section of the tube; in general the product gradient must be calculated, rather than determined. We, however, were able to measure the Xa concentration in the immediate vicinity of the wall by determining how much Xa was bound to this anionic lipid surface. Combining these data with the K_D of Xa and PS/PC (30/70) membranes, we arrived at the figure for Xa near the surface. A schematic of these discontinuities is shown in figure 2.

It should be emphasized that this concentration of Xa would exist even if it did not bind to the surface as its genesis resides in substrate conversion and is independent of product binding to the surface. Thus, one would expect this high level of Xa to exist at the surface of vascular tissue and cell monolayers. Its magnitude, of course, would depend on the rate of substrate conversion, which, in turn, would be a function of the TF surface density. This provides the rationale for testing vascular tissue for their TF activity which would provide data for the quantitative estimation of Xa in the vicinity of the cell surface. Until quantitative experiments such as these are reported, the levels of tissue factor expressed by various cells will not be interpretable.

REFERENCES

1. **Bach, R., Nemerson, Y. & Konigsberg, W.,** Purification and characterization of bovine tissue factor., *J.Biol.Chem.,* 256, 8324, 1981.
2. **Nemerson, Y. & Repke, D.,** Tissue Factor Accelerates the Activation of Coagulation Factor VII: The Role of a Bifunctional Coagulation Cofactor, *Thromb. Res.,* 40, 351, 1985.
3. **Rao, L.V. & Rapaport, S.I.,** Activation of factor VII bound to tissue factor: a key early step in the tissue factor pathway of blood coagulation, *Proc.Natl.Acad.Sci.U.S.A.,* 85, 6687, 1988.
4. **Neuenschwander, P.F., Fiore,M.M., and Morrissey, J.H.,** Factor VII Autoactivation Proceeds via Interaction of Distinct Protease-Cofactor and Zymogen-Cofactor Complexes, *Journal of Biological Chemistry,* 268, 21489, 1993.
5. **Nemerson, Y.,** Tissue factor and hemostasis, *Blood,* 71, 1, 1988.
6. **Nemerson, Y. & Gentry, R.,** An ordered addition, essential activation model of the tissue factor pathway of coagulation: evidence for a conformational cage, *Biochemistry,* 25, 4020, 1986.
7. **Seligsohn, U., Osterud, B., Brown, S.F., Griffin, J.H. & Rapaport, S.I.,** Activation of human factor VII in plasma and in purified systems: roles of activated factor IX, kallikrein, and activated factor XII, *J.Clin.Invest.,* 64, 1056, 1979.
8. **Fiore, M.M., Neuenschwander, P.F. & Morrissey, J.H.,** The biochemical basis for the apparent defect of soluble mutant tissue factor in enhancing the proteolytic activities of factor VIIa, *J Biol Chem,* 269, 143, 1994.
9. **Wildgoose, P., et al.,** Measurement of basal levels of factor VIIa in hemophilia A and B patients, *Blood,* 80, 25, 1992.
10. **Carson, S.D. & Ramsey, C.A.,** Tissue factor (coagulation factor III) is present in placental microvilli and cofractionates with microvilli membrane proteins, *Placenta.,* 6, 5, 1985.

11. **Maynard, J.R., Dreyer, B.E., Stemerman, M.B. & Pitlick, F.A.,** Tissue-factor coagulant activity of cultured human endothelial and smooth muscle cells and fibroblasts, *Blood,* 50, 387, 1977.

12. **Taubman, M.B., et al.,** Agonist-mediated tissue factor expression in cultured vascular smooth muscle cells. Role of Ca2+ mobilization and protein kinase C activation, *J Clin Invest,* 91, 547, 1993.

13. **Wilcox, J.N., Smith, K.M., Schwartz, S.M. & Gordon, D.,** Localization of tissue factor in the normal vessel wall and in the atherosclerotic plaque, *Proceedings of the National Academy of Sciences, U.S.A.,* 86, 2839, 1989.

14. **Drake, T.A., Morrissey, J.H. & Edgington, T.S.,** Selective cellular expression of tissue factor in human tissues. Implications for disorders of hemostasis and thrombosis, *American Journal of Pathology,* 134, 1087, 1989.

15. **Weiss, H.J., Turitto, V.T., Baumgartner, H.R., Nemerson, Y. & Hoffmann, T.,** Evidence for the presence of tissue factor activity on subendothelium, *Blood,* 73, 968, 1989.

16. **Bach, R. & Rifkin, D.B.,** Expression of tissue factor procoagulant activity: regulation by cytosolic calcium, *Proc Natl Acad Sci U S A,* 87, 6995, 1990.

17. **Le, D.T., Rapaport, S.I. & Rao, L.V.,** Relations between factor VIIa binding and expression of factor VIIa/tissue factor catalytic activity on cell surfaces, *J Biol Chem,* 267, 15447, 1992.

18. **Walsh, J.D. & Geczy, C.L.,** Discordant expression of tissue factor antigen and procoagulant activity on human monocytes activated with LPS and low dose cycloheximide, *Thromb. Haemostas.,* 66, 552, 1991.

19. **Sueishi, K., et al.,** Endothelial function in thrombosis and thrombolysis, *Jpn Circ J,* 56, 192, 1992.

20. **Drake, T.A., Cheng, J., Chang, A. & Taylor, F., Jr.,** Expression of tissue factor, thrombomodulin, and E-selectin in baboons with lethal Escherichia coli sepsis, *Am J Pathol,* 142, 1458, 1993.

21. **Smoluchowski, v.,** *Zeitshrift fur Pahysikalische Chemie,* 92, 129, 1917.

22. **Marmur, J.D., et al.,** Tissue factor is rapidly induced in arterial smooth muscle after balloon injury, *J Clin Invest,* 91, 2253, 1993.

23. **Cussler, E.** *Diffusion: Mass transfer in fluid systems* (Cambridge University Press, Cambridge, 1984).

24. **Gemmell, C.H., Broze, G.J., Jr., Turitto, V.T. & Nemerson, Y.,** Utilization of a continuous flow reactor to study the lipoprotein- associated coagulation inhibitor (LACI) that inhibits tissue factor, *Blood,* 76, 2266, 1990.

25. **Schoen, P., Lindhout, T., Willems, G. & Hemker, H.C.,** Continuous Flow and the Prothrombinase-Catalyzed Activation of Prothrombin, *Thromb.Haemost.,* 64, 542, 1990.

26. **Andree, H.A., Contino, P.B., Repke, D., Gentry, R. & Nemerson, Y.,** Transport rate limited catalysis on macroscopic surfaces: the activation of factor X in a continuous flow enzyme reactor, *Biochemistry,* 33, 4368, 1994.

27. **Nelsestuen, G. & Broderius, M.,** Interaction of Prothrombin and Blood-Clotting Factor X with Membranes of Varying Composition, *Biochemistry,* 16, 4172, 1977.

28. **Krishnaswamy, S., Jones, K. & Mann, C.,** Prothrombinase Complex Assembly, Kinetic Mechanism of Enzyme Assembly on Phospholipid Vesicles, *Journal of Biological Chemistry,* 263, 3823, 1988.

29. **Giesen, P.L.A., Willems, G.M., Hemker, H.C. & Hermens, W.T.,** Membrane-mediated assembly of the prothrombinase complex, *J.Biol.Chem.,* 266, 18720, 1991.

30. **Berg, H. & Purcell, E.,** Physics of chemoreception, *Biophysical Journal,* 20, 193, 1977.

31. **Contino, P., Repke, D. & Nemerson, Y.,** A continuous flow reactor system for the study of blood coagulation, *Thromb Haemost,* 66, 138, 1991.

32. **Gailani, D. & Broze, G.J., Jr.,** Factor XI activation in a revised model of blood coagulation, *Science,* 253, 909, 1991.

33. **Scott, C.F. & Colman, R.W.,** Fibrinogen blocks the autoactivation and thrombin-mediated activation of factor XI on dextran sulfate, *Proc Natl Acad Sci U S A,* 89, 11189, 1992.

34. **Repke, D., et al.,** Hemophilia as a defect of the tissue factor pathway of blood coagulation: effect of factors VIII and IX on factor X activation in a continuous-flow reactor, *Proc.Natl.Acad.Sci.U.S.A.,* 87, 7623, 1990.

35. **Komiyama, Y., Pedersen, A.H. & Kisiel, W.,** Proteolytic activation of human factors IX and X by recombinant human factor VIIa: Effects of calcium, phospholipids, and tissue factor, *Biochemistry,* 29, 9418, 1990.

36. **Lawson, J.H. & Mann, K.G.,** Cooperative activation of human factor IX by the human extrinsic pathway of blood coagulation, *J Biol Chem,* 266, 11317, 1991.

PLATELET PROCOAGULANT ACTIVITY AND MICROVESICLE FORMATION

R.F.A. Zwaal, P. Comfurius, E. Smeets, and E.M. Bevers
Cardiovascular Research Institute Maastricht, University of Limburg, Maastricht.

I. INTRODUCTION

In general terms, aberrations of normal hemostasis will lead either to thrombosis or to bleeding disorders. Whereas thrombosis, which may reflect or result from a hypercoagulable state, is usually accompanied by undue production of thrombin, bleeding disorders usually occur when thrombin formation is limited. Through its ability to activate blood platelets and to convert fibrinogen into insoluble fibrin, thrombin is widely appreciated as the key enzyme in hemostasis. Its rate and extent of formation upon vessel wall injury is controlled by the concerted action of different positive and negative feedback reactions,[1] in which blood platelets also play a critical role. The contribution of blood platelets to the hemostatic process is well recognized to occur in a variety of ways.[2] Interactions with subendothelial structures of damaged blood vessels (e.g. collagen) causes platelets to adhere to the vessel wall, which is followed by platelet aggregation to form a primary hemostatic plug. This process elicits platelet secretion of a variety of compounds that contribute to consolidation of the platelet aggregate. Perhaps one of the most important effects is the formation of catalytic platelet membrane surfaces on which coagulation factors assemble and interact, thereby increasing their local concentrations and favouring their mutual juxtapositions. While this leads to a dramatic increase in the rate of thrombin formation, it is also instrumental in negative feedback control as inactivation of coagulation factors can be catalyzed by the same membrane surface.

In recent years, it is increasingly recognized that formation of procoagulant membrane surfaces entails a rapid reorientation (flip-flop) of membrane phospholipids leading to exposure of anionic (procoagulant) phosphatidylserine at the cells' outer surface.[3-7] Moreover, this process seems to be tightly associated with shedding of microvesicles from the platelet plasma membrane.[4,8-11] Usually, the membrane surface of both microvesicles and remnant cells acquire the property of catalyzing phospholipid-dependent reactions in blood coagulation. In this chapter, we address the mechanisms involved in the formation of procoagulant membrane surfaces and shedding of microvesicles, and discuss its possible contribution to hypercoagulable states.

II. PHOSPHOLIPID-DEPENDENT REACTIONS IN BLOOD COAGULATION

Two sequential reactions of the coagulation cascade are strongly enhanced in the presence of lipid surfaces that contain anionic phospholipids.[1] The first reaction concerns the proteolytic conversion of the zymogen factor X into an active serine proteinase, factor Xa. This reaction is catalyzed by the tenase complex, which consists of an active proteolytic enzyme, factor IXa, that interacts with a non-enzymatic protein factor VIIIa on an anionic membrane lipid surface in the presence of Ca^{2+}. Once factor Xa is formed, it assembles together with another non-enzymatic protein, factor Va, and Ca^{2+} on the membrane to form the prothrombinase complex which efficiently converts prothrombin into thrombin. Kinetic studies have shown that negatively charged phospholipid membranes produce an effective decrease in the K_m of factor X and prothrombin, the substrates of these reactions, from far above to far below their respective plasma concentrations[12,13]. This enables both reactions to proceed at close to V_{max}, the level of which is primarily determined by the non-enzymatic protein cofactors VIIIa and Va, respectively [12-14]. The combined decrease in the K_m of these two consecutive reactions in the presence of anionic phospholipid surfaces can increase the rate of thrombin formation by several orders of magnitude.

0-8493-5804-3/96/$0.00+$.50

Although any negatively charged phospholipid may contribute to the formation of a catalytic surface, membranes containing phosphatidylserine exhibit the highest procoagulant activity.[15] Moreover, unlike other anionic phospholipids, phosphatidylserine is the only lipid that retains its procoagulant properties, irrespective of the ionic strength of the medium or the net charge of the lipid surface. Platelet membranes, like those of most other cells, contain two anionic phospholipid classes in appreciable quantities, i.e. phosphatidylserine and phosphatidylinositol. Of these two lipids, phosphatidylserine is considered to be solely responsible for the formation of procoagulant lipid surfaces in stimulated platelets, because of the weak procoagulant activity of phosphatidylinositol and its conversion in the phosphatidylinositol cycle upon cell activation. It should be mentioned that platelets are devoid of tissue thromboplastin, the phosphatidylserine-containing lipoprotein that stimulates factor VIIa to initiate the extrinsic coagulation pathway.

III. PLATELET PROCOAGULANT ACTIVITY

Unstimulated blood platelets are only slightly capable of promoting assembly and catalysis of the tenase- or prothrombinase complex. Activation of platelets is required to produce a differential increase of both procoagulant reactions[16-17] particularly due to the formation of factor Va and VIIIa binding sites,[6,18-21] the extent of which is dependent on the platelet activation procedure. Calcium-ionophore, a mixture of collagen and thrombin, and the complement membrane attack complex C5b-9, are the most potent stimulants of platelet procoagulant activity, increasing the cell's ability to produce some 20-fold enhancement of either factor Xa or thrombin formation, relative to unstimulated platelets.[6,16,17,22] Platelet activation by collagen alone produces a moderate rise in procoagulant activity (approx. 8-fold), which is approximately twice as high as that observed after platelet activation by thrombin. On the other hand, weak activators like ADP, epinephrine and platelet-activating factor do not appreciably enhance the procoagulant activity of platelets, irrespective of whether platelet aggregation and release occur. The presence of extracellular Ca^{2+} during platelet activation is required to evoke platelet procoagulant activity, which strongly suggests that a substantial increase in cytoplasmic Ca^{2+} is a prerequisite for the formation of a procoagulant surface. Also, mild stirring of the platelet suspension during stimulation enhances generation of procoagulant activity with collagen and/or thrombin, but not with ionophore or complement.

The time course of generation of platelet procoagulant activity does not parallel that of platelet release reactions and aggregation. For example, platelet secretion and aggregation induced by collagen and thrombin at 37°C is completed within 2 min, but full expression of procoagulant activity usually requires 5 min or more. It is well-established that formation of a procoagulant membrane surface can occur irrespective of platelet secretory events and aggregation, the more so as storage-pool deficient platelets and thrombasthenic platelets (which do not aggregate) are indistinguishable from normal platelets in their ability to become procoagulant.[23]

IV. EXPOSURE OF PHOSPHATIDYLSERINE
AT THE PLATELET OUTER SURFACE

During the last 20 years it has become evident that both halves of the lipid bilayer membrane of most, if not all, eukaryotic cells have distinctly different lipid compositions.[7,24,25] The outer leaflet of cell membranes is predominantly composed of cholinephospholipids, whereas the aminophospholipids (particularly phosphatidylserine) preferentially occupy the inner leaflet. While different mechanisms have been proposed to play a role in the generation and maintenance of membrane phospholipid asymmetry, it has become evident that an ATP- and sulfhydryl-dependent transporter (aminophospholipid translocase), that specifically shuttles aminophospholipids from the outer to the inner leaflet of cell membranes, plays an important part in this process[26,27] (Figure 1). Since aminophospholipid translocase is active in unstimulated platelets, the implicit absence of phosphatidylserine on the outer surface of these cells explains why they are hardly able to promote appreciable stimulation of phospholipid-dependent coagulation reactions. When platelets are lysed, their procoagulant effect is strongly increased to equal that of unilamellar liposomes prepared from their phospholipid extract. As expected, very similar results have been obtained with red cells, leukocytes and endothelial cells [28], that have comparable membrane phospholipid asymmetry.

Activation of blood platelets can lead to a progressive loss of the asymmetric distribution of membrane phospholipids, producing increased exposure of phosphatidylserine at the outer surface.[3,4] This process is presumably due to the induction of rapid transbilayer movements (flip-flop) of all major phospholipid classes, which leads to scrambling of the lipids over the bilayer membrane.[3,29] A rise in cytoplasmic Ca^{2+} also inhibits aminophospholipid translocase activity which prevents phosphatidylserine from being pumped back to the inner membrane leaflet, although mere inhibition of this lipid pump does not by itself result in a rapid loss of phospholipid asymmetry.[5,30] On the other hand, extrusion of cytoplasmic Ca^{2+} from activated platelets may reactivate phospholipid translocase, resulting in back-transport of surface-exposed phosphatidylserine to the inner membrane leaflet with progressive loss of platelet procoagulant activity.[5]

Whereas it has been suggested that lipid scrambling results from the formation of a membrane perturbing complex which is formed between Ca^{2+} and phosphatidylinositol-4,5-bis-phosphate (PIP-2)[31] recent evidence from our laboratory strongly suggests the involvement of a transmembrane protein (phospholipid scramblase), which is switched on after interaction with Ca^{2+} at the cytoplasmic side of the cell membrane[32] (Figure 1). The extent to which scrambling of membrane phospholipids with resulting surface exposure of phosphatidylserine occurs during platelet activation, closely parallels the cell's ability to stimulate tenase- or prothrombinase activity. It should be mentioned that Ca^{2+} influx in erythrocytes[5] and endothelial cells[33] can also lead to lipid scrambling and surface exposure of phosphatidylserine accompanied by expression of procoagulant activity, albeit at a slower rate than that observed with platelets.

V. PLATELET MICROVESICLE FORMATION

It has been known for several decades that platelet activation may be accompanied by formation of platelet-derived microparticles with clot-promoting activity.[34-36] The importance of this process for platelet procoagulant activity has long been underestimated, witnessed by the fact that these microparticles were often referred to as 'platelet dust'. Although it has been suggested earlier that they were derived from intracellular membranes and externalized upon secretion,[37] it has now become evident that these particles are formed at the cell surface by shedding from the plasma membrane. As a result, they contain the major membrane glycoproteins Ib, IIb and IIIa, as well as membrane cytoskeletal proteins filamin, talin and myosin heavy chain.[6,8,10] Electronmicroscopy has revealed these particles as unilamellar microvesicles with an average diameter of about 0.2 μM.[38] Their time-course of appearance is slower than that of platelet aggregation and secretion, but closely follows the time-course of generation of platelet procoagulant activity. Moreover, the extent of formation of microvesicles also depends on the platelet activation procedure in a similar fashion as the generation of platelet procoagulant activity, i.e. most pronounced following ionophore-, collagen + thrombin- or complement C5b-9 activation, moderate after collagen activation and low after activation by thrombin, ADP, or epinephrine. Usually, some 25-30% of the total platelet procoagulant activity and factor Va binding sites are associated with the microvesicle population, while the remainder resides with the remnant cells. Platelets activated by complement pore proteins C5b-9 form a notable exception in that most of the procoagulant activity and factor Va binding sites are associated with the microvesicles.[6]

Shedding of microvesicles appears to be closely linked to Ca-induced scrambling of membrane phospholipids. Since blebbing and shedding of microvesicles from the platelet surface entails eversion and fusion of apposing segments of plasma membrane, this process has been earlier suggested to lead to transient formation of nonbilayer lipid phases at the point where the plasma membrane fuses to form the budding vesicle[6] ; this would lead to a concomitant localized collapse in membrane phospholipid asymmetry and the appearance of phosphatidylserine in the cell's outer leaflet, including that of the microvesicle itself. Recently, however, it has been shown that microvesicle formation can be suppressed without affecting the transbilayer scrambling of the lipids.[39] Also, while the flip-flop process involves all major phospholipid classes, the rate of inward transbilayer migration of sphingomyelin was found to be appreciably slower than the transbilayer migration rate of the other (glycero)phospholipids.[29,39] This will produce a mass imbalance across the bilayer, increasing the surface pressure in the outer leaflet relative to the inner leaflet, a process which is known to result in

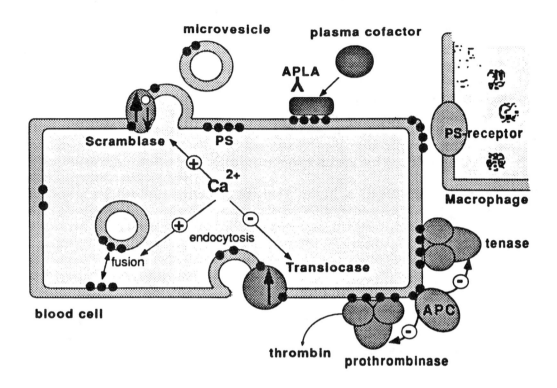

Figure 1. Cellular phenomena associated with phosphatidylserine topology in blood cell membranes. In unactivated cells, membrane phospholipid asymmetry is generated by an ATP-dependent lipid pump (translocase) that specifically shuttles aminophospholipids (e.g. phosphatidylserine) from the external to the internal leaflet of the lipid bilayer membrane. When phosphatidylserine is provided from an external source, translocase activity produces mass imbalance between the two leaflets of the lipid bilayer that may facilitate endocytosis. Influx of calcium can inhibit translocase and activates a non-ATP-dependent lipid transporter (scramblase) that produces rapid lipid flip-flop leading to loss of membrane phospholipid asymmetry, which results in surface exposure of phosphatidylserine (PS). Mass imbalance between the two membrane leaflets resulting from scramblase activity may facilitate formation of microvesicles that also expose phosphatidylserine. Moreover, calcium-influx produces fusion of storage granules with the plasma membrane followed by exocytosis. Surface exposed phosphatidylserine promotes assembly and catalysis of tenase and prothrombinase complexes leading to dramatic accalaration of thrombin formation, while this surface also exerts negative feedback by promoting C (APC) catalyzed inactivation of factors Va and VIIIa. In the antiphospholipid syndrome, certain plasma proteins (e.g. prothrombin, β_2-glycoprotein I) may interact with phosphatidylserine leading to exposure of cryptic epitopes toward which antiphospholipid-antibodies (APLA) are directed. Also, surface-exposed phosphatidylserine may trigger recognition by PS-receptors on macrophages leading to removal of the blood cells from the circulation.

outward bending of the plasma membrane. This may facilitate shedding of microvesicles to release the unequal surface pressure between the two membrane leaflets (Figure 1). Therefore, microvesicle formation is presumably the result and not the cause of transbilayer scrambling of membrane phospholipids. It should be noted that the ability to form microvesicles is certainly not unique to platelets. For example, ionophore-induced influx of Ca^{2+} into red blood cells[40] or complement C5b-9-induced Ca^{2+}-influx into endothelial cells[33] also leads to a partial loss of membrane phospholipid asymmetry and surface exposure of procoagulant phosphatidylserine, [5,33,41] accompanied by shedding of microvesicles from their respective plasma membranes.

VI. SCOTT SYNDROME

The above-described phenomena of Ca-induced scrambling of membrane phospholipids and shedding of plasma membrane-derived microvesicles is strongly decreased in platelets from a patient with a rare bleeding disorder. This disorder was first described by Weiss et al.[42] and is characterized by an isolated deficiency of platelet procoagulant activity, presently referred to as Scott syndrome. Although activation of these platelets produces normal release and aggregation, these platelets express a considerably lower number of binding sites for factors Va and VIIIa, relative to normal platelets.[43] Moreover, in response to various agonists, the patient's platelets were appreciably impaired in their ability to support both tenase- and prothrombinase activity, showed a decreased surface exposure of plasma membrane phosphatidylserine and were markedly deficient in their capacity to generate microvesicles. [6,44]

It is remarkable that this aberrant behaviour can also be demonstrated in the patient's red blood cells upon treatment with Ca-ionophore.[45] Unlike normal erythrocytes, no surface exposure of procoagulant phosphatidylserine and concurrent microvesicle formation occurs under these conditions. The fact that resealed ghosts from normal erythrocytes also scramble their lipids upon Ca-influx, whereas resealed ghosts from the patient's erythrocytes do not, lends further support to the notion that the bleeding disorder is due to a membrane defect. Although no obvious abnormality in membrane protein composition of the patient's platelets and erythrocytes is apparent by SDS-electrophoresis, this does not rule out that the aberrant membrane-related phenomena may reflect a mutation in an early stem cell that affects multiple hematologic lineages. In this context, it is of interest to mention that aminophospholipid translocase activity, as well as its inhibition by intracellular Ca^{2+}, is indistinguishable from that of normal cells.[45] Also, the PIP-2 levels in the patient's blood cells do not significantly deviate from that of normal cells, further refuting the proposal that this compound would be involved in lipid scrambling phenomena.

VII. PRO- AND ANTICOAGULANT ACTIVITY OF PLATELET-DERIVED MICROVESICLES

While membranes containing phosphatidylserine provide a catalytic surface for the tenase and prothrombinase complex, they are also capable of stimulating the proteolytic inactivation of factors Va and VIIIa by activated protein C in conjunction with protein S. Since protein C is activated by thrombin, after interaction with thrombomodulin on endothelial cells, activated protein C exerts efficient negative feedback by limiting thrombin formation at the site where platelet activation occurs.[46] The physiological importance of this process is illustrated in patients with partial protein C deficiency who suffer from recurrent thrombosis.

The capacity of activated platelets and platelet-derived microvesicles to support protein C-catalyzed inactivation of the factor Va has strong similarities to their ability to stimulate prothrombinase activity[47] (Figure 1). After platelet stimulation, about 25% of the protein C-catalyzed inactivation of factor Va appears to be associated with microvesicles shed from the cell surface, which is virtually identical to that observed for prothrombinase. Also, the ability of platelets to support protein C activity depends on the platelet activation procedure in a very similar fashion to their ability to support prothrombinase activity. These observations illustrate the efficiency of the negative feedback loop exerted by activated protein C, by restricting thrombin formation at the same membrane surface where it is formed.

VIII. SURFACE-EXPOSED PHOSPHATIDYLSERINE AS A SIGNAL FOR REMOVAL OF PROCOAGULANT MEMBRANES

There is increasing evidence to suggest that exposure of phosphatidylserine at the cell surface forms a signal in cell recognition processes. Introduction of phosphatidylserine in the outer leaflet of red blood cell membranes induces increased adherence of the cells to monocytes and macrophages, and leads *in vivo* to rapid clearance from the circulation by the liver and the spleen.[48] The clearance of senescent red cells from the circulation may at least in part also bear on this mechanism, as it has been shown that these cells gradually become less able to maintain membrane phospholipid asymmetry.[49] Surface exposure of phosphatidylserine may also be instrumental in the process of apoptosis, and the mechanism by which apoptotic cells are recognized by macrophages. It has been shown that apoptotic lymphocytes can be taken up by peritoneal macrophages after recognition by a receptor at the macrophage surface that specifically interacts with phosphatidylserine[50] (Figure 1). Similar mechanisms might be operative by the removal of activated platelets and microvesicles, thereby counteracting prolonged circulation of potentially thrombogenic surfaces.

IX. PLATELET-DERIVED MICROVESICLES AND ANTI-PHOSPHOLIPID SYNDROME?

Antiphospholipid antibodies comprise a rather heterogeneous group of circulating immunoglobulins, which are associated with an increased risk of arterial or venous thrombosis, thrombocytopenia and recurrent abortions.[51] The group of disorders characterized by the presence of these antibodies is referred to as 'anti-phospholipid syndrome'. Whereas it has been thought for a long time that these antibodies are directed toward phospholipids alone, recent evidence strongly suggests that these antibodies recognize neo-epitopes exposed by lipid-bound (plasma) proteins, e.g. β_2-glycoprotein I, prothrombin, protein C and protein S[52-55] (Figure 1). Thus, it appears that at least four different antiphospholipid antibodies exist that can be distinguished by their antigenic targets and anticoagulant activity *in vitro*. For example, while β_2-glycoprotein I exhibits a moderate inhibitory effect on prothrombinase activity in the presence of phosphatidylserine-containing lipid vesicles, inhibition is enhanced by a distinct subtype of so-called anticardiolipin antibodies that recognize a cryptic epitope which is exposed after interaction of this glycoprotein with the anionic phospholipid surface.[56] Interaction of the antibodies with lipid-bound plasma proteins occurs irrespective of whether phospholipid vesicles, activated platelets or platelet-derived microvesicles are used.

These observations may shed new light on the apparent controversy that thrombotic complications can be associated with circulation of antibodies in plasma that prolong clotting times *in vitro*. Endothelial cell damage and/or platelet activation and microvesicle formation *in vivo*, may provide the anionic phospholipid surface to which certain plasma proteins interact with exposure of neo-epitopes. Provided that these epitopes are exposed at a sufficiently high concentration during lengthy periods of time, the immune response could be addressed to these lipid-bound proteins to counteract excessive thrombin formation. This may represent a normal response of the immune system toward prolonged exposure of thrombogenic membrane surfaces, rather than reflecting a disorder of the immune system with formation of thrombogenic antibodies. The origin of this prolonged exposure may be due to persistent vascular damage and platelet activation, and/or to defects in the mechanisms by which phosphatidylserine-containing surfaces are removed from the circulation. Binding of antiphospholipid antibodies to thrombogenic surfaces will also mediate cell-cell interaction, promoting their removal from the circulation.

X. MICROVESICLES AND HYPERCOAGULABLE STATES

Prospective studies as to whether or not circulating microvesicles are reliable indicators of a hypercoagulable state are presently not available. However, there are reasons to surmise that circulating microvesicles may be associated with thrombotic episodes. It should be realized, however, that these vesicles do not initiate blood coagulation or thrombosis, but only accelerate thrombin formation once coagulation is started. This is for example illustrated by the observation that infusion of procoagulant phospholipid in rabbits is potentially thrombogenic, but only in combination with factor Xa in a dose that was not thrombogenic when given alone.[57] Also, the recent insight on the mode of action of antiphospholipid antibodies may be suggestive for a putative role of microvesicles in thrombotic disease, although experimental proof to support this notion is still lacking. Sickle cell aneamia is another example which is known to be frequently associated with circulating erythrocyte-derived micovesicles. Sickling of reversibly sickled cells by repeated cycles of de- and reoxygenation *in vitro*, has been shown to result in shedding of procoagulant microvesicles that have lost membrane phospholipid asymmetry and expose phosphatidylserine.[58] It is tempting to suggest that these microvesicles contribute to the thrombotic episodes that frequently accompany sickle cell crisis. Finally, platelet-derived microvesicles were recently shown to circulate *in vivo* in blood from patients with activated coagulation and fibrinolysis, whereas microvesicles were rarely found in healthy individuals, and if so in trace amounts.[59] While it remains to be established if and to what extent microvesicles contribute to thrombosis, these observations may indeed suggest that their circulation *in vivo* may reflect a hypercoagulable state.

REFERENCES

1. **Mann, K.G., Nesheim, M.E.. Church, W.R., Haley, P. and Krihnaswamy, S.,** Surface-dependent reactions of the vitamin K-dependent enzyme complexes. *Blood* , 1, 1990.
2. **Zucker, M.B. and Nachmias, V.T.** , Platelet activation. *Arteriosclerosis,* 5, 2, 1985.
3. **Bevers, E.M., Comfurius, P. and Zwaal, R.F.A.,** Changes in membrane phospholipid distribution during platelet activation. *Biochim. Biophys. Acta,* 736, 57, 1983
4. **Thiagarajan, P. and Tait, J.F.,** Collagen-induced exposure of anionic phospholipid in platelets and platelet-derived microparticles. *J. Biol. Chem.,* 266, 24302, 1991.
5. **Comfurius, P., Senden, J.M.G., Tilly, R.H.J., Schroit, A.J., Bevers, E.M. and Zwaal, R.F.A.,** Loss of membrane phospholipid asymmetry in platelets and red cells may be associated with calcium-induced shedding of plasma membrane and inhibition of amino-phospholipid translocase. *Biochim. Biophys. Acta,* 1026, 153, 1990.
6. **Sims, P.J., Wiedmer, T., Esmon, C.T., Weiss, H.J. and Shattil, S.J.,** Assembly of the platelet prothrombinase complex is linked to vesiculation of the platelet plasma membrane. Studies in Scott syndrome: an isolated defect in platelet procoagulant activity. *J. Biol. Chem,.,* 264, 17049, 1989
7. **Schroit, A.J. and Zwaal, R.F.A.,** Transbilayer movement of phospholipids in red cell and platelet membranes. *Biochim. Biophys. Acta,* 313, 1991.
8. **Sims, P.J., Faioni, E.M., Wiedmer, T. and Shattil, S.J.** , Complement proteins C5b-9 cause release of membrane vesicles from the platelet surface that are enriched in the membrane receptor for coagulation factor Va and express prothrombinase activity. *J. Biol. Chem.,* 263, 18205, 1988.
9. **Wiedmer, T., Shattil, S.J., Cunningham, M. and Sims, P.J.,** Role of calcium and calpain in complement-induced vesiculation of the platelet plasma membrane and in the exposure of the platelet factor Va receptor. *Biochemistry,* 29, 623, 1990.
10. **Fox, J.E.B., Austin, C.D., Reynolds, C.C. and Steffen, P.K.,** Evidence that agonist-induced activation of calpain causes the shedding of procoagulant-containing microvesicles from the membrane of aggregated platelets. *J. Biol. Chem.,* 266, 13289, 1991.
11. **Fox, J.E.B., Austin, C.D., Boyles, J.K. and Steffen, P.K.,** Role of the membrane skeleton in preventing the shedding of procoagulant-rich microvesicles from the platelet plasma membrane. *J. Cell Biol.,* 111, 483, 1990.
12. **Rosing, J., Tans, G., Govers-Riemslag, J.W.P., Zwaal, R.F.A. and Hemker, H.C.,** The role of phospholipids and factor Va in the prothrombinase complex. *J. Biol. Chem.,* 255, 274, 1980.
13. **Van Dieijen, G., Tans, G., Rosing, J. and Hemker, H.C.** , The role of phospholipid and factor VIIIa in the activation of bovine factor X. *J. Biol. Chem.,* 256, 3433, 1981.
14. **Nesheim, M.E., Taswell, J.B. and Mann, K.G.,** Isolation and characterization of single chain bovine factor V. *J. Biol. Chem.,* 254, 508, 1979.
15. **Rosing, J., Speijer, H. and Zwaal, R.F.A.,** Prothrombin activation on phospholipid membranes with positive electrostatic potential. *Biochemistry,* 27, 8, 1988.
16. **Comfurius, P., Bevers, E.M. and Zwaal, R.F.A.,** The involvement of cytoskeleton in the regulation of trans-bilayer movement of phospholipids in human blood platelets. *Biochim. Biophys. Acta,* 815, 143, 1985.
17. **Rosing, J., Rijn van , J.L.M.L., Bevers, E.M., Dieijen van, G., Comfurius, P. and Zwaal, R.F.A.** , Impaired factor X- and prothrombin activation associated with decreased phospholipid exposure in platelets from a patient with a bleeding disorder. *Blood,* 65, 1557, 1985.
18. **Tracy, P.B., Peterson, J.M., Nesheim, M.E., McDuffie, F.C. and Mann, K.G.,** Interaction of coagulation factor V and factor Va with platelets. *J. Biol. Chem.,* 254, 10345.
19. **Kane, W.H. and Majerus, P.W.,** The interaction of human coagulation factor Va with platelets. *J. Biol. Chem.,* 257, 3963, 1982.
20. **Ahmad, S.S., Rawala-Sheikh, R., Ashby, B. and Walsh, P.N.,** Platelet receptor-mediated factor X activation by factor IXa. High-affinity factor IXa receptors induced by factor VIII are deficient on platelets in Scott Syndrome. *J. Clin. Invest.,* 84, 824, 1989.
21. **Gilbert, G.E., Sims, P.J., Wiedmer, T., Furie, B., Furie, B.C. and Shattil, S.J.,** Platelet-derived microparticles express high affinity receptors for factor VIII. *J. Biol. Chem.,* 266, 17261, 1991.
22. **Fox, J.E.B., Reynolds, C.C. and Austin, C.D.,** The role of calpain in stimulus-response coupling: evidence that calpain mediates agonist-induced expression of procoagulant activity in platelets. *Blood,* 76, 2510, 1990.
23. **Bevers, E.M., Comfurius, P., Nieuwenhuis, H.K., Levy-Toledano, S., Enouf, J., Belluci, S., Caen, J.P. and Zwaal, R.F.A.,** Platelet prothrombin converting activity in hereditary disorders of platelet function. *Brit. J. Haematol.,* 63, 335, 1986.

24.   **Zwaal, R.F.A.,** Membrane and lipid involvement in blood coagulation. *Biochim. Biophys. Acta,* 515, 163-205, 1978.
25.   **Op den Kamp, J.A.F.** , Lipid asymmetry in membranes. *Ann. Rev. Biochem.,* 48, 47, 1979.
26.   **Seigneuret, M., and Devaux, P.F.,** ATP-dependent asymmetric distribution of spin-labeled phospholipids in the erythrocyte membrane: Relation to shape changes. *Proc. Natl. Acad. Sci. USA* 81, 3751, 1984.
27.   **Connor, J. and Schroit, A.J.,** Transbilayer movement of phosphatidylserine in erythrocytes: inhibition of transport and preferential labeling of a 31000-dalton protein by sulfhydryl reactive reagents. *Biochemistry,* 27, 848, 1988.
28.   **Zwaal, R.F.A. and Hemker, H.C.,** Blood cell membranes and haemostasis. *Haemostasis,* 11, 429, 1982.
29.   **Smeets, E.F., Comfurius, P., Bevers, E.M. and Zwaal, R.F.A.,** Calcium-induced transbilayer scrambling of fluorescent phospholipid analogs in platelets and erythrocytes. *Biochim. Biophys. Acta,* 1195, 281, 1994.
30.   **Bitbol, M., Fellmann, P. Zachowski, A. and Devaux, P.F.,** Ion regulation of phosphatidylserine and phosphatidylethanolamine outside-inside translocation in human erythrocytes. *Biochim. Biophys. Acta* 904, 268, 1987.
31.   **Sulpice, J-C., Zachowski, A., Devaux, P.F. and Giraud, F.,** Requirement for phosphatidylinositol 4,5-bisphosphate in the Ca2+-induced phospholipid redistribution in the human erythrocyte membrane. *J. Biol. Chem.,* 269, 6347, 1994.
32.   **Comfurius, P., Williamson, P.L., Smeets, E.F., Bevers, E.M. and Zwaal, R.F.A.** Manuscript in preparation.
33.   **Hamilton, K.K., Hattori, R., Esmon, C.T. and Sims, P.J.,** Complement proteins C5b-9 induce vesiculation of the endothelial plasma membrane and expose catalytic surface for assembly of the prothrombinase enzyme complex. *J. Biol. Chem.,* 265, 3809, 1990.
34.   **Wolf, P.,** The nature and significance of platelet products in human plasma. *Brit. J. Haematol.,* 13, 269, 1967.
35.   **Crawford, N.,** The presence of contractile proteins in platelet microparticles isolated from human and animal platelet-free plasma. *Br. J. Haematol.,* 21, 53, 1972.
36.   **Sandberg, H., Andersson, L.-O and Högland, S.,** Isolation and characterization of lipid-protein particles containing platelet factor 3 released from human platelets. *Biochem. J.,* 203, 303, 1982.
37.   **Sandberg, H., Bode, A.P., Dombrose, F.A., Hoechli, M. and Lentz, B.R.,** Expression of coagulant activity in human platelets: release of membranous vesicles providing platelet factor 1 and platelet factor 3. *Thromb. Res.,* 39, 63, 1985.
38.   **Zwaal, R.F.A., Comfurius, P., Bevers, E.M.,** Platelet procoagulant activity and microvesicle formation. Its putative role in hemostasis and thrombosis. *Biochim. Biophys. Acta,* 1180, 1, 1992.
39.   **Williamson, P., Kulick, A., Zachowski, A., Schlegel, R.A. and Devaux, P.F.,** Ca2+ induces transbilayer redistribution of all major phospholipids in human erythrocytes. *Biochemistry,* 31, 6355, 1982.
40.   **Allan, D. and Mitchell, R.H.,** Accumulation of 1,2 diacylglycerol in the plasma membrane may lead to echinocyte transformation of erythrocytes. *Nature,* 258, 348, 1975.
41.   **Chandra, R., Joshi, P.C., Bajpai, V.K. and Gupta, C.H.,** Membrane phospholipid organization in calcium-loaded human erythrocytes. *Biochim. Biophys. Acta,* 902, 253, 1987.
42.   **Weiss, H.J., Vivic, W.J., Lages, B.A., and Rogers, J.,** Isolated deficiency of platelet procoagulant activity. *Am. J. Med.,* 67, 206, 1979.
43.   **Weiss, H.J.,** Scott Syndrome: a disorder of platelet procoagulant activity. *Blood,* 3, 312, 1994.
44.   **Rosing, J., Bevers, E.M., Comfurius, P., Hemker, H.C., Dieijen van, G., Weiss, H.J. and Zwaal, R.F.A.,** Impaired factor X- and prothrombin activation associated with decreased phospholipid exposure in platelets from a patient with a bleeding disorder. *Blood,* 65, 1557, 1985.
45,   **Bevers, E.M., Wiedmer, T., Comfurius, P., Shattil, P., Weiss, S.J., Zwaal, R.F.A. and Sims, P.J.,** Defective Ca2+ induced microvesiculation and deficient expression of procoagulant activity in erythrocytes from a patient with a bleeding disorder: A study of the red blood cells of Scott syndrome. *Blood,* 79, 380, 1992.
46.   **Esmon, C.T.,** The protein-C anticoagulant pathway. *Arteriscleros. Thromb.* 12, 135, 1992.
47.   **Tans, G., Rosing, J., Thomassen, M.C.L.G.D., Heeb, M.J., Zwaal, R.F.A. and Griffin, J.H.,** Comparison of anticoagulant and procoagulant properties of stimulated platelets and platelet-derived microparticles. *Blood,* 77, 2641, 1991.
48.   **Schroit, A.J., Madsen, J.W. and Tanaka, Y.,** In vivo recognition and clearance of red blood cells containing phosphatidylserine in their plasma membranes. *J. Biol. Chem.,* 260, 5138, 1985.
49.   **Connor, J., Pak, C.C. and Schroit, A.J.,** Exposure of phosphatidylserine in the outer leaflet of human red blood cells. Relationship to cell density, cell age, and clearance by mononuclear cells. *J. Biol. Chem.,* 269, 2399, 1994.
50.   **Fadok, V.A., Voelker, D., Campbell, P.A., Cohen, J.J., Bratton, D.L. and Henson, P.M.,** Exposure of phosphatidylserine on the surface of apoptic lymphocytes triggers specific recognition and removal by macrophages. *J. Immunol.* 148, 2207, 1992.
51.   **McNeill, H.P. and Krilis, S.A.,** Antiphospholipid antibodies. *Aust, NZ, J,. Med.,* 21, 463, 1991.
52.   **Galli, M., Comfurius, P., Maassen, C., Hemker, H.C., De Baets, M.H., Breda-Van Vriesman, Barbui, T., Zwaal, R.F.A.,** Anticardiolipin antibodies (ACA) directed not to cardiolipin but to a plasma protein cofactor. *Lancet,* 335, 1544, 1990.
53.   **McNeill, H.P., Simpson, R.J., Chesterman, C.N. and Krilis, S.A.,** Anti-phospholipid antibodies are directed against a complex antigen that includes a lipid-binding inhibitor of coagulation: ß2-Glycoprotein I (apolipoprotein H). *Proc. Natl. Acad. Sci. USA* 87, 4120, 1990.
54.   **Bevers, E.M., Galli, M., Barbui, T., Comfurius, P. and Zwaal, R.F.A.,** Lupus anticoagulant IgG's (LA) are not directed to phospholipids only, but to a complex of lipid-bound human prothrombin. *Thromb. Haemostaa,* 66, 629, 1991.
55.   **Oosting, J., Derksen, R.H.W.M., Bobbink, I.W.G., Hackeng, T.M., Bouma, B.N. and de Groot, P.G.,** Antiphospholipid antibodies directed against a combination of phospholipids with prothrombin, protein C, or protein S: an explanation for their pathogenic mechanism. *Blood,* 81, 2618, 1993.
56.   **Galli, M., Comfurius, P., Barbui, T., Zwaal, R.F.A. and Bevers, E.M.,** Anticoagulant activity of ß2-glycoprotein-I is potentiated by a distinct subgroup of anticardiolipin antibodies. *Thromb. Haemostas.* 68, 297, 1992
57.   **Giles, A.L., Nesheim, M.E., Hoogendoorn, H., Tracy, P.B. and Mann, K.G.,** Stroma-free human platelet lysates potentiate the in vivo thrombogenicity of factor Xa by the provision of coagulant-active phospholipid. *Brit. J. Haematol.,* 51, 457, 1982.
58.   **Franck, P.F.H., Bevers, E.M., Lubin, B.H., Comfurius, P., Chiu, D.T., OpdenKamp, J.A.F., Zwaal, R.F.A., van Deenen, L.L.M. and Roelofsen, B.,** Uncoupling of the membrane skeleton from the lipid bilayer: The cause of accelerated phospholipid flip-flop leading to an enhanced procoagulant activity of sickled cells. *J. Clin. Invest.,* 75, 183, 1985.
59.   **Holme, P.A., Solum, N.O., Brosstad, F., Roger, M. and Abdelnoor, M.,** Demonstration of platelet-derived microvesicles in blood from patients with activated coagulation and fibrinolysis using a filtration technique and western blotting. *Thromb. Haemostas.,* 72, 666, 1994.

MONOCYTES AND HYPERCOAGULABLE STATES

B. Østerud

Institute of Medical Biology, University of Tromsø

I. INTRODUCTION

The mononuclear phagocytic cell line originates in the bone marrow, where the dividing cells, monoblasts and promonocytes, reside and monocytes are formed. The monocytes leave the bone marrow and are transported by the peripheral blood to the body´s organs and cavities, where they differentiate into macrophages. The total concentration of monocytes in blood amounts to 4% of the total leukocyte count. Apart from their phagocytic activity, monocytes and macrophages play a central role in the immune system by processing and presenting ingested antigenic material, synthesizing and secreting immunomodulatory factors (i.e. cytokines) and destroying target cells via a non-phagocytic mechanism.

In recent years it has become evident that monocytes and macrophages also participate in the molecular events leading to thrombin formation which is probably an integral part of their physiological and pathophysiological roles in wound repair, chronic inflammation, disseminated intravascular coagulation (DIC) in sepsis, postoperative thrombosis and atherosclerosis.

This report will not discuss the mechanism of initiation of blood coagulation and its regulation by tissue factor pathway inhibitor (TFPI) since comprehensive reviews are available[1-3] and also presented in this book. The intent is to provide insight into the multiple procoagulant activities monocytes/macrophages possess, and how these may account for the pathophysiological reactions in various diseases. Since tissue factor (TF) is apparently the most important procoagulant product of monocytes, the major part of this chapter concerns the induction and expression of this potent trigger of clot formation.

II. THE MECHANISM FOR EXPRESSION OF TF ACTIVITY IN MONOCYTES

A. TISSUE FACTOR

It is well established that a variety of monocyte stimulating agents induce production and expression of TF on the surface of monocytes. Some of the agents known are listed in Table I. Only a few of these are capable of inducing TF in monocytes in suspension (whole blood) in contrast to their reported effects on monocytes in cell cultures. Except for the lipopolysaccharides (LPS), C5a and the immune complexes, all of the other agents have probably only enhancing effect on the generation of tissue factor activity in monocytes in whole blood[4].

TF is a membrane glycoprotein of 295 amino acids, containing four N-linked glycosylation sites, and an organized extracellular domain, a 23 amino acids hydrophobic transmembrane region and a 21 amino acid cytoplasmatic tail. The extracellular domain functions as the receptor for factor VII/VIIa. The binding of factor VII/VIIa to the TF is apparently independent of the lipid composition in the membrane surrounding the TF antigen (for review see ref. 5). However, the potential of the cellular complex of TF/VIIa to catalyze the activation of factors IX and X is strongly limited to the association of the substrate with phosphatidylserine.[6, 7]

Table I : Agents that Induce or Enhance Monocyte Tissue Factor Activity

Lipopolysaccharides (LPS)   Lipoproteins
(oxidized-LDL)   C-reactive protein (CRP)
Immune-complexes   Lymphokines
C5a   Platelets
Tumor necrosis factor-α (TNF-α)   Granulocytes
Interferon-γ (IF-γ)   Allogenic cells
Interleukin-1β (IL-1β)   Phorbol ester (PMA)
Platelet factor 4 (PF4)   N-formyl-methionyl-
Lectins   phenylalanine (FMLP)
Platelet activating factor (PAF)
P-selectin

Monocyte levels of TF m-RNA are undetectable in freshly isolated monocytes of whole blood.[8] LPS upregulation of TF m-RNA is maximal within 1-2 hours and decreases to background values 6 hours after induction.[9] In cell cultures the TF m-RNA is induced at a slower rate[8]. LPS induction of the TF gene in monocytes requires transcriptional activation mediated by both activator protein-1 and nuclear factor kB.[10]

B. CELLULAR INTERACTIONS IN EXPRESSION OF TISSUE FACTOR ACTIVITY

Even before it was recognized that TF was produced in monocytes, it was found that platelets enhanced TF activity in leukocytes.[11] This was later confirmed in studies on isolated monocytes in cell cultures.[12] For almost 15 years we have used a simple whole blood system with heparin or hirudin as anticoagulants, to study the expression of TF under more physiological conditions. This technique revealed a fifty fold difference in expression of TF activity in monocytes in blood of different individuals.[13, 14] Since it was observed that those who generate very high TF activity (high responders) appeared to be members of families with a history of cardiovascular diseases (especially coronary heart disease), an intensive search for the explanation of this phenomenon has been performed as outlined below.

C. ROLE OF PLATELETS AND GRANULOCYTES IN LPS INDUCED TF ACTIVITY IN MONOCYTES

When partially platelet depleted white cells from high responders were cross combined with platelets (platelet rich plasma-PRP) from a low responder and then stimulated with LPS, this led to a marked drop (60-70%) in TF generation compared to the values obtained with autologous platelets.[15] The role of platelets in LPS induced TF activity was further established by stimulating white blood cells recombined with either platelet poor plasma (PPP) or PRP. Only about one third of TF activity was induced in the absence of platelets as compared to cells recombined with PRP.[15]

A mandatory role of granulocytes in provoking the platelet enhancement of TF activity induced by LPS was demonstrated using a plasma system with physiological concentrations of recombined mononuclear cells, granulocytes and platelets.[16] No difference was seen in the production of TNF by the monocytes which suggests that the granulocyte/platelet effect is not at the level of general monocyte activation.[16] Furthermore, the phorbol ester, PMA, and the central mediator of inflammatory reactions, tumor necrosis factor alpha (TNF-α) caused a several fold increase in LPS induced TF activity in a platelet and granulocyte dependent manner and was shown to be due to stimulation of both granulocytes and monocytes. The central role of platelets in LPS induced TF activity in monocytes was verified by the use of anti-CD15 antibody. Low concentrations of this antibody abolished the stimulatory effect of platelets and granulocytes. The inhibitory effect of the antibody was probably associated with CD-15´s role as a complementary ligand for P-selectin.[16] This has been confirmed by obtaining similar results with a specific antibody to P-selectin.[17]

D. ENHANCEMENT OF LPS INDUCED TF ACTIVITY BY PLATELET FACTOR 4 (PF4)

In a recent study it was shown that PF4, which is released from activated platelets, or the synthetic peptide hPF4 (58-70), amplified several fold LPS or LPS plus TNF-α induced TF activity in monocytes, whereas PF4 had no inducible effect by itself.[18] The PF4 effect was granulocyte dependent and a mononuclear anti-P-selectin antibody abolished almost all of the enhancing effect of hPF4 (58-70) on LPS induced TF activity in monocytes.[18,19] Thus, PF4 is an important platelet product that is indirectly involved in enhancing LPS induced TF activity in monocytes, probably through its interaction with granulocytes and increased release of platelet activating factor (PAF)[20] which propagates granulocyte activation. Activated granulocytes then interact with platelets in a P-selectin dependent reaction which then ultimately triggers a platelet product that interacts with monocytes and enhances LPS induced TF activity. This product might be P-selectin although there is strong evidence that P-selectin alone has no TF inducible effect on monocytes of whole blood.[18]

E. THE CATALYTIC ACTIVITY OF FACTOR VIIa/TF ON MONOCYTE CELL MEMBRANES

Although all TF is expressed on the surface of monocytes, its catalytic activity is only about 10% compared to the TF activity of lysed cells.[21] This difference in catalytic activity is probably not due to a special dependence on the TF apoprotein to be associated with certain phospholipids, i.e. ionic phospholipids. It rather reflects the necessity for the substrates, factors IX and X, to be bound to negatively charged phospholipids, primarily present in the inner layer of the cell surface membrane. Accordingly, cell lysis will convert inactive factor VII/TF complexes on the intact monocytes into complexes expressing catalytic activity.[22] Therefore, monocyte membrane damage under certain pathological conditions may result in a highly active form of TF in vivo.[23] However, this phenomenon cannot explain the enhancement of LPS induced TF activity in monocytes by platelets/granulocytes described above, since the cells were tested for TF activity after lysing the cells and adding optimal exogenous phospholipids.

III. MONOCYTE ASSOCIATED TF´S ROLE IN SEPTICEMIA

A. SHWARTZMAN REACTION

It has been suggested that the generalized Shwartzman reaction is provoked by the initial injection of LPS which causes formation of fibrin through clotting of blood by TF present on either monocytes or the damaged vessel wall. Presumably, the fibrin is immediately taken up by macrophages of the mononuclear phagocyte system or the endothelium system in the liver (RES). However, when the second injection of LPS is given, the RES no longer has the capacity to remove the fibrin aggregates produced, and as a result thrombin develops in the blood vessels. It has been more difficult to explain the observation that cortisone acetate, when substituted for the first of two LPS doses, also provokes the Shwartzman reaction in rabbits.[24] Glucocorticosteroids are known to have an inhibitory effect on monocyte/granulocyte stimulation of inflammatory reactions, among others.[25, 26]

Indeed, pretreating the rabbits with a dose of either LPS or glucocorticosteroids resulted in a several-fold increase in TF activity associated with the circulating monocytes after LPS was given the next day.[27, 28] The rise in monocyte TF activity correlated well with the degree of sickness of the animals. These results seemed to be consistent with studies of high doses of steroids in infectious disease and septic shock, in which steroids increased mortality, often from secondary infection.[29] Although TF is also well known to be induced in endothelial cells in vitro, no TF activity was found in the endothelium of animals in which the Shwartzman reaction was induced[30] or in saphenous veins transfused with LPS or thrombin.[31] However, extensive damage of the vessel wall caused by the release of oxygen radicals and lysosomal enzymes from activated granulocytes may also promote blood clotting through release and exposure of TF on cells of the damaged vessel wall. Today we do not know which system is most important for the generation of DIC, but the rapid exposure of TF on the surface of circulating monocytes suggests that these cells are crucial for the sudden occurrence of DIC in septic shock.

B. ROLE OF TISSUE FACTOR IN THE COAGULANT AND INFLAMMATORY RESPONSE TO E. COLI SEPSIS IN BABOONS AND CHIMPANZEES

Recent studies on primates support the concept that LPS induced TF and resultant activation of the coagulation system (DIC) is a significant pathophysiological contribution to the lethality of the syndrome. This was demonstrated by the efficacy of neutralizing monoclonal antibodies against TF to reverse lethality of Escherichia coli-induced septicemia in a primate model.[32] Expression of TF by the vascular endothelium was also not detected here as TF was mainly observed in the endothelium confined to the marginal zone of the spleen, where macrophages also expressing TF were present.[33] The importance of TF-dependent initiation of the coagulation pathway is further supported by the effect of the specific physiologic inhibitor of the TF pathway (TFPI) in animal models of septic shock.[34, 35] However, the observation that blocking thrombin generation by using an inactive factor Xa failed to reverse the lethality remains unexplainable, although the propagation of coagulation and consumption of fibrinogen was prevented.[36]

Another interesting aspect of the function of TF as a regulator of interleukin-6 (IL-6) production was demonstrated in experimental E. coli sepsis in baboons. Infusion of TFPI and subesequent attenuation of DIC response in animals given lethal doses of E.coli was associated with an attenuation of the IL-6 response.[37] It was therefore suggested that TF not only influences the coagulant response to E.coli, but may also amplify the inflammatory response. A further support for a link between IL-6 and coagulation activation was provided in experimental endotoxemia in chimpanzees.[38] In this study it was found that elimination of IL-6 attenuated coagulation activation in a low grade endotoxemia. Whether these obsevations are related to the regulation of TF expressed on the circulating monocytes in the blood of these animals remains to be clarified.

C. MENINGOCOCCAL SEPTICEMIA AND INFECTIONS IN EARLY INFANTS

Disseminated intravascular coagulation (DIC) is a common manifestation of fulminant meningococcal disease.[39] It is still unknown how the pathological reactions leading to DIC occur in these patients. Strong indications of a central role for hypercoagulable monocytes in this process were obtained when it was shown that the meningococcal infection was associated with greatly elevated levels of TF in the circulating monocytes.[40] Indeed, a close relationship was observed between the TF activity level in monocytes isolated from the patients blood on admission to hospital and the outcome of the disease. High levels, i.e. more than a 60-300 fold increase of monocyte TF activity, always prevailed in patients in whom the disease had a lethal outcome. It was also interesting that a new rise in TF of circulating monocytes 20-30 hours after admission coincided with extensive white cell aggregation and impaired blood circulation.[41]

The exact contribution of DIC to organ pathophysiology and outcome in patients with severe septicemia has yet to be defined. Most probable is dysfunction of various organs, particularly the kidneys, adrenals and muscles, along with peripheral gangrene of the extremities and skin hemorrhage from extensive coagulation system activation and inhibited fibrinolysis.

Flow cytometric studies revealed that when bacterial infection was present in young human infants, more than 60% of the monocytes examined showed fluorescence indicative of the presence of surface TF.[42] More than 60 % of the cells were found to be TF positive in certain instances where infection was highly probable but not proven. In addition, positive cells were found in three cases of isoimmune hemolytic disease of the newborn, whereas less than 25 % of monocytes derived from babies in the absence of discernible infection or isoimmune hemolytic disease expressed TF. From the same study it was not possible to make any general statement as to whether viral infections in the neonate induce TF expression in circulating monocytes.

IV. TF EXPRESSION IN MONOCYTES OF OTHER INFECTIOUS DISEASES

Several additional well-studied experimental models of human diseases add support for the concept that monocyte expressed TF might be responsible for one or more aspects of the pathophysiology of these disorders. Fibrin formation, linked to activation and infiltration of white blood cells, has been documented in association with experimental endocarditis, the hypereosinophilic syndrome, and familial Mediterranian fever (for review see ref. 43).

Circulating monocytes in rats, and in man, displayed increased TF activity during gram-negative peritonitis. The newly synthesized TF may induce microvascular thrombosis and precede thromboembolic complications. Peritoneal macrophages from rats and humans produce substantial amounts of TF during secondary bacterial peritonitis.[44] This TF is probably essential for the formation of fibrin deposits, which in turn is a prerequisite for the creation of intraabdominal adhesions. The documented mechanisms of fibrin deposition at the cellular level probably represent a fundamental host defence designed to delimit the offending infection. A simultaneous, significant decrease in TF content of standardized specimens from lung, aortic wall, liver, spleen, pancreas and jejunum was observed in rats with peritonitis.[45] This could reflect mobilization of macropages expressing TF in favour of the infectious focus, as samples from the colon of cecal-perforated animals showed a consistent increase compared to controls.

V. ENHANCED TF ACTIVITY IN CIRCULATING MONOCYTES AFTER TRAUMA AND SURGERY

Despite the conceivable relationship between thrombosis and monocyte production of TF activity, there have been few systematic studies of changes in patients´ monocyte TF activity levels as possible inducers of hypercoagulability. However, one study disclosed a strict correlation between enhanced monocyte TF activity and thromboembolic complications.[46] Seventeen splenectomized trauma patients and 6 surgical controls were assayed at 3 day post-injury intervals for levels of TF activity in circulating monocytes. Changes in monocyte TF were correlated to increases in the turnover of ^{125}I-fibrinogen. All trauma patients who exhibited significantly increased fibrinogen turnover experienced thromboembolic episodes and had monocytes whose TF activity was increased an average of 300% over surgical controls. It should be noted that the monocytes isolated from the blood of the patients had been subjected to cell cultures before testing for TF activity. It is therefore possible that the very high TF activity observed in these monocytes, may also stem from activation and induction of TF activity from allowing the cells to adhere to the plastic in flasks used to isolate monocytes.

Although it has been proposed that an increase of TF in monocytes after surgery is normal and that the increased TF in monocytes has no pathophysiological consequences[46], a significant rise in TF activity has been observed in circulating monocytes postoperatively. Thus, in 47 patients with and without cancer undergoing elective surgery, an average increase of 100% in TF activity of circulating monocytes was observed.[47] This paralleled an almost 4 fold increase in TF activity when the patients´ blood was subjected to LPS stimulation as compared to presurgery. Our experience is that high responders, those who generate very high TF activity in monocytes of LPS stimulated blood, are more susceptible to post-operative thrombotic complications than low responders.[48]

VI. HYPERCOAGULABILITY ASSOCIATED WITH MONOCYTES/MACROPHAGES IN CANCER PATIENTS

A large body of evidence suggests that the hemostatic system is frequently activated in cancer patients. The exact mechanism of enhanced activation of the coagulation system still remains unresolved. However, independent of whether TF is located in the tumor cells or tumor associated macrophages, TF is probably the major trigger of coagulation (for review see Chapter 8 in this book). A strong correlation between circulating fibrinogen peptide A (FPA) levels and unstimulated mononuclear TF activity was found in patients with lung carcinoma.[50] Another study showed increased procoagulant activity in monocytes (both unstimulated and endotoxin induced) in ovarian (stages III and IV) but not in uterine (stages I and II) carcinoma.[51] These results suggest that in advanced malignancy, activation of host monocytes to produce TF may also occur at sites far removed from the primary tumor. However, convincing evidence is lacking that tumor induced cytokines can stimulate peripheral monocytes to generate procoagulant activity and trigger thrombosis.

Combined procoagulant and proteolytic activity in promyelocytes has been suggested as the cause of observed bleeding in patients with acute promeylocytic leukemia.[52] The production of procoagulant activity of these cells was established by Northern blot analysis which revealed that a substantial proportion of the patient´s blast cells constitutively expressed TF transcripts.[53] In contrast, myeloid precursor cells derived from normal bone marrow lacked TF mRNA, consistent with their absence of procoagulant activity.

VII. THE HYPERCOAGULABILITY OF MACROPHAGES IN ATHEROSCLEROTIC PLAQUES

Monocytes are essential in the development of atherosclerotic lesions. These cells, when differentiated to macrophages in the vessel wall, function as the phagocytizing cells of oxidized-LDL. The resultant generation of foam cells is an early event in the atherogenic process (for review see ref. 54). These cells also express TF[55], and the fatal outcome of plaque rupture is most likely triggered by exposed TF which causes an instant thrombus formation. The importance of TF in this regard has been demonstrated through prevention of arterial reocclusion after thrombolysis with recombined TFPI.[56]

As indicated earlier in this chapter, the high responder phenomenon appears to be associated with a high risk of coronary heart disease. Although there is no hard data on the role of activation of the blood coagulation system and subsequent thrombin formation in atherogenesis, platelets are important.[54] Theoretically, monocyte associated TF, even at low levels, may turn out to play an important role in the platelet mediated reactions known to be associated with the development of atherosclerosis. It is the author´s personal opinion that this mechanism is an important pathological reaction that may account for the many individuals who experience myocardial infarction despite normal blood lipids.

There have been several reports that various lipoproteins may induce TF activity in adherent monocytes. This is probably not the whole truth since LDL preparations with virtually no LPS contamination failed to induce TF activity.[57] These preparations also failed to enhance LPS induced TF activity in the monocytes of the cultures. Interestingly, oxidized LDL significantly enhanced LPS-induced TF activity in adherent monocytes, but even oxidized LDL failed to induce TF activity in the absence of LPS. Oxidized LDL is found in atherosclerotic lesions and is known to promote atherogenesis. Therefore, monocytes exposed to oxidized LDL in the intimal lesion of the vessel wall may express increased levels of TF that can contribute to a hypercoagulability state and to the thrombotic events associated with atherosclerosis.

VIII. OTHER HYPERCOAGULABILITY PROPERTIES OF MONOCYTES

Although TF is the most potent trigger of blood coagulation activation and obviously the most important procoagulant activity of circulating monocytes, there is a growing concept that peripheral blood monocytes may provide the appropriate membrane surface for the assembly and function of virtually all the coagulation complexes involved in thrombin production (for review see ref. 58). Thus, strong evidence documents that amplification of the tissue factor response is accomplished by the assembly and function of the prothrombinase complex, a complex of the cofactor Va and the enzyme factor Xa that, bound to the monocyte´s surface in the presence of calcium ions, effectively cleaves prothrombin to thrombin.[59] Factor Va may be provided through the activation of the plasma procofactor factor V by a protease associated with the monocyte membrane.[60] The prothrombinase complex may be found on resting monocytes, but LPS stimulation significantly enhances prothrombin activation.[61] Faciliation of more factor Xa in addition to TF/VIIa activation of factor X directly, may take place through the functional interactions of factors VIIIa and IXa with the monocyte surface.[62]

Monocytes are among the most efficient cells in the vasculature to initiate and amplify coagulation through a regulated function of different membrane receptors. Apparently, many of the various reactions earlier thought to be entirely associated with activated blood platelets may take place on the surface of the monocytes.

It has been suggested that monocytes can also directly activate factor X to Xa after binding of this zymogen to an organized membrane receptor.[63] The factor X receptor on monocytes was identified as CD11b/CD18, which is the same receptor that also binds fibrinogen[64], although fibrinogen and factor X appear to bind to spatially separate sites on CD11b/CD18 (for review see ref. 65). The process of factor X activation, which was induced by incubating ADP with freshly isolated monocytes, was not affected by neutralizing, anti-TF MoAbs.[63] Such an alternative activation mechanism of the coagulation system might have been important in the early phase of triggering blood clotting in order to generate factor Xa for obligatory activation of factor VII to VIIa. However, extensive studies have not confirmed this activation mechanism of factor X.[66]

Monocytes/macrophages also produce coagulation factors. Peritoneal macrophages from mice were shown to synthesize factors VII, X, prothrombin and V.[67, 68] Factor V has also been detected in human monocytes[69] and factor VII m-RNA has been assigned to human macrophages.[70] Today, hardly any knowledge exists about the physiological role of the plasma coagulation factors generated in these cells.

REFERENCES

1. **Rapaport, S.I., and Rao, L.V.M.,** Initiation and regulation of tissue factor-dependent blood coagulation, *Arterioscler, Thromb.*, 12, 1111, 1992.
2. **Sandset, P.M., and Abildgaard, U.,** Extrinsic pathway inhibitor -the key to feedback control of blood coagulation initiated by tissue thromboplastin, *Haemostasis*, 21, 219, 1991.
3. **Rapaport, S.I.,** The extrinsic pathway inhibitor: A regulator of tissue factor-dependent blood coagulation, *Thromb. Haemost.*, 66, 6, 1991.
4. **Østerud, B.,** unpublished data, 1992.
5. **Edgington, T.S., Mackman, N., Brand, K., and Ruf, W.,** The structural biology of expression and function of tissue factor, *Thromb. Haemost.*, 66, 67, 1991.
6. **Krishnaswamy, S., Field, K.A., Edgington, T.S., Morrissey, J.H., and Mann, K.G.,** Role of the membrane surface in the initiation of human coagulation factor X, *J. Biol. Chem.* ,267, 26110, 1992.

7.   **Krishnaswamy, S.,** The interaction of human factor VIIa with tissue factor, *J. Biol. Chem.,* 267, 23696, 1992.
8.   **Gregory, S.A., Morrissey, J.H., and Edgington, T.S.,** Regulation of tissue factor gene expression in the monocyte procoagulant response to endotoxin, *Mol. Cell. Biol.,* 9, 2752,1989.
9.   **Halvorsen, H., Anderssen, T., and Østerud, B.,** unpublished data, 1994.
10.   **Mackman, N., Brand, K., and Edgington, T.S.,** Lipopolysaccharide-mediated trascriptional activation of the human tissue factor gene in THP-1 monocytic cells requires both activator protein 1 and nuclear factor kB sites, *J. Exp. Med.,* 174, 1517, 1991.
11.   **Niemetz, J., and Marcus, A.J.,** The stimulatory effect of platelets and platelet membranes on the procoagulant effect of leukocytes, *J. Clin. Invest.,* 54, 1437, 1974.
12.   **Lorenzet, R., Niemetz, J, Marcus, A.J., and Brockman, M.J.,** Enhancement of mononuclear procoagulant activity by platelet 12-hydroxy-eicosatetraenoic acid, *J. Clin. Invest.,* 78, 418, 1986.
13.   **Østerud, B., and Eskeland, T.,** The mandatory role of complement in the endotoxin-induced synthesis of tissue thromboplastin in blood monocytes, *FEBS Lett.,* 149, 75, 1982.
14.   **Østerud, B.,** The high responder phenomenon: Enhancement of LPS induced tissue factor activity in monocytes by platelets and granulocytes, *Platelets,* In press 1994.
15.   **Østerud, B., Olsen, J.O., and Wilsgård, L.,** The role of arachidonic acid release and lipoxygenase pathway in lipopolysaccharide-induced thromboplastin activity in monocytes, *Blood Coagulation and Fibrinolysis,* 3, 309, 1992.
16.   **Halvorsen, H., Olsen, J.O., and Østerud, B.,** Granulocytes enhance LPS-induced tissue factor activity in monocytes via an interaction with platelets, *J. Leuk. Biol.,* 54, 275, 1993.
17.   **Halvorsen, H., Østerud, B.,** unpublished data, 1993.
18.   **Sissener, C., Lia, K., Rekdal, Ø., Halvorsen, H. and Østerud, B.,** Platelet factor 4 (PF4) and the synthetic peptide hPF4 (58-70) enhance LPS-induced tissue factor activity in monocytes, *Thromb. Haemost.,* 69, 734 (abstract), 1993.
19.   **Sissener, C.,** The carboxyterminal tridecapeptide of platelet factor 4: Synthesis and effects on human monocytes and granulocytes, *Thesis,* University of Tromsø, pp 1-107, 1994.
20.   **Østerud, B.,** Platelet activating factor enhancement of lipopolysaccharide-induced tissue factor activity in monocytes: requirement of platelets and granulocytes, *J. Leuk. Biol.,* 51, 462, 1992.
21.   **Østerud, B.,** unpublished data, 1984.
22.   **Le, D., Rapaport, S.I., and Rao, L.V.M.,** Relations between factor VIIa binding and expression of factor VIIa/tissue factor catalytic activity on cell surfaces, *J. Biol. Chem.,* 262, 15447, 1992.
23.   **Walsh, J.O., and Geczy, C.L.,** Discordant expression of tissue factor antigen and procoagulant activity on human monocytes activated with LPS and low dose cycloheximide, *Thromb. Haemost.,* 66, 552, 1991.
24.   **Thomas, L., and Good, R.A.,** Bilateral cortical necrosis of kidneys in cortisone-treated rabbits following injection of bacterial toxins, *Proc. Soc. Exp. Biol. Med.,* 76, 604, 1951.
25.   **Motsay, G.J., Alho, A., and Jaeger, T., Dietzman, R.H., and Lillehei, R.C.,** Effects of corticosteroids on the circulation in shock: experimental and clinical results, *Fed. Proc.,* 29, 1861, 1970.
26.   **Hammerschmidt, D.E., White, J.G., Craddoch, P.R., and Jacob., H.S.,** Corticosteroids inhibit complement-induced granulocyte aggregation: A possible mechanism for their efficacy in shock states, *J. Clin. Invest.,* 63, 789, 1979.
27.   **Østerud, B., Olsen, J.O., and Tindall, A.,** The generalized Shwartzman reaction: Effects of steroids and endotoxin on thromboplastin synthesis by monocytes, in *Mononuclear Phagocytes. Charcteristics Physiology and Function,* van Furth, R., Ed., Martinus Nijhoff, Boston, 1985, 705.
28.   **Østerud, B., Tindall, A., and Olsen, J.O.,** Effect of steroids during Escherichia coli endotoxemia in rabbits, *Haemostasis* ,19, 292, 1989.
29.   **Bone, R.C., Fisher, C.J.Jr., Clemmer, T.P., Slotman, G.J., Craig, A.M., Balk, R.A., and the Methylprednisolone Severe Sepsis Study Group,** A Controlled Clinical Trial of High-Dose Methylprednisolone in the Treatment of Severe Sepsis and Septic Shock, *New Eng. J. Med.,* 317, 653, 1987.
30.   **Østerud, B., Tindall., Brox, J.H., and Olsen, J.O.,** Thromboplastin content in the vessel wall of different arteries and organs of rabbits, *Thromb. Res.,* 42, 323, 1986.
31.   **Solberg, S., Østerud, B., Larsen, T., and Sørlie, D.,** Lack of ability to synthesize tissue factor by endothelial cell in intact human saphenous veins, *Blood Coagulation and Fibrinolysis,* 1, 595, 1990.
32.   **Taylor, F.B.Jr., Chang, A., Ruf, W., Morrissey, J.H., Hinshaw, L., Catlett, R., Blick, K., and Edgington, T.S.,** Lethal E. coli septic shock is prevented by blocking tissue factor with monoclonal antibody, *Sirc. Shock,* 33, 127, 1991.
33.   **Drake, T.A., Cheng, J., Chang, A., and Taylor, F.B.Jr.,** Expression of tissue factor, hrombomodulin, and E-selectin in baboons with lethal E. coli sepsis, *Am. J. Pathol.,* 142, 1458, 1993.
34.   **Sandset, P.M., Warn-Cramer, B.J., Rao, L.V.M., Maki, S., and Rapaport, S.I.,** Immunodepletion of extrinsic pathway inhibitor (EPI) sensitizes rabbits to endotoxin-induced intravascular coagulation and the generalized Shwartzman reaction, *Blood,* 78, 1496, 1991.
35.   **Creasey, A.A., Chang, A.C.K., Feigen, L., Wun, T.C., Taylor, F.B.Jr., and Hinshaw, L.B.,** Tissue factor pathway inhibitor (TFPI) reduces mortality from E. coli septic shock, *J. Clin. Invest.,* 91, 2850, 1993.
36.   **Taylor, F.B.Jr., Chang, A.C.K., Peer, G.T., Mather, T., Blick, K., Catlett, R., Lockhart, M.S., and Esmon, C.T.,** DEGR-factor Xa block disseminated intravascular coagulation initiated by Escherichia coli without preventing shock or organ damage. *Blood,* 78, 364, 1991.
37.   **Taylor, F.B.Jr.,** Role of tissue factor in the coagulant and inflammatory response to LD_{100} E. coli sepsis and in the early diagnosis of DIC in the baboon, in DIC. *Pathogenesis, diagnosis and therapy of disseminated intravascular fibrin formation,* Muller-Berghaus, G., Madlener, K., Blomback, M., and ten Cate, J.W., Experta Medica, 1993, 19.

38. **van der Poll, T., Levi, M., Hack, C.E., ten Cate, H., van Deventer, S.J.H., Eerenberg, A.J.M., de Groot, E.R., Jansen, J., Gallati, H., Buller, H.R., ten Cate, J.W., and Aarden, L.A.**, Elimination of interleukin 6 attenuates coagulation activation in experimental endotoxemia in chimpanzees, *J. Exp. Med.*, 179, 1253, 1994.

39. **McGehee, W.G., Rapaport, S.I., and Hjort, P.F.**, Intravascular coagulation in fulminant meningococcocemia, *Ann. Intern. Med.*, 67, 250, 1967.

40. **Østerud, B., and Flægstad, T.**, Increased thromboplastin activity in monocytes of patients with meningococcal infection: Related to un unfavourable prognosis, *Thromb. Haemost.*, 49, 5, 1983.

41. **Østerud, B.**, Leukocytes, adhesive proteins and disseminated intravascular coagulation: treatment of DIC with plasma/ leukapheresis?, in *DIC. Pathogenesis, diagnosis and therapy of disseminated intravascular fibrin formation*, Muller-Berghaus, G., Madlener, K., Blomback, M., and ten Cate, J.W., Eds,. Experta Medica, 1993, 33.

42. **Rivers, R.P.A., Cattermole, H.E.J., and Wright, I.**, The expression of surface tissue factor apoprotein by blood monocytes in the course of infections in early infancy, *Pediatr. Res.* , 31, 567, 1992.

43. **Edwards, R.L., and Rickles, F.R.**, The role of leukocytes in the activation of blood coagulation, *Sem. Haematol.*, 29, 202, 1992.

44. **Almdahl, S.M., Brox, J.H., and Østerud, B.**, Mononuclear phagocyte thromboplastin and endotoxin in patients with secondary bacterial peritonitis, Scand. J. Gastroenterol. 22, 914, 1987.

45. **Almdahl, S.M., and Østerud, B.**, Experimental gramnegative septicaemia: Thromboplastin generation in mononuclear phagocytes from different anatomical sites, *Thromb. Res.*, 47, 37, 1987.

46. **Miller, C.L., Graziano, C.G., Lim, R..C., and Chin, M.**, Generation of tissue factor by patient monocytes: Correlation to thromboembolic complications, *Thromb. Haemost.*, 46, 489, 1981.

47. **Østerud, B., and Due, J.H.**, Blood coagulation in patients with benign and malignant tumors before and after surgery. Special reference to thromboplastin generation in monocytes, *Scand. J. Haematol.*, 32, 258, 1984.

48. **Østerud, B.**, unpublished data, 1992.

49. **Rao, L.V.M.**, Tissue factor as a tumor procoagulant, Cancer and *Metastasis Rev.*, 11, 249, 1992.

50. **Edwards, R.L., Rickles, F.R., and Cronlund, M.**, Abnormalities of blood coagulation in patients with cancer. Mononuclear cell tissue generation, *J. Lab. Clin. Med.*, 98, 912, 1981.

51. **Semeraro, N., Montemorro, P., Conese, M., Giordano, D., Stella, M., Restaino, A., Cagnazzo, G., and Colucci, M.**, Procoagulant activity of mononuclear phagocytes from different anatomical sites in patients with gynecological malignancies, *Int. J. Cancer*, 45, 251, 1990.

52. **Wijermans, P.W., Rebel, V.I., Ossenkoppele, G.J., Huijggens, P.C., and Langenhuijsen, M.M.**, Combined procoagulant activity and proteolytic activity of acute promyelocytic leukemic cells; Reversal of bleeding disorder by cell differentiation, *Blood*, 73, 800, 1989.

53. **Bauer, K.A., Conway, E.M., Bach, R., Koningsberg, W.H., Griffin, J.D., and Demetri, G.**, Tissue factor gene expression in acute myeloblastic leukemia, *Thromb. Res.*, 56, 425, 1989.

54. **Ross, R.**, Atherosclerosis: A defense mechansim gone awry, Am. J. Pathol., 143, 987, 1993.

55. **Wilcox, J.N., Smith, K.M., Schwartz, S.M., and Gordon, D.**, Localization of tissue factor in the normal vessel wall and in the atherosclerotic plaque, *Proc. Natl. Acad. Sci. USA*, 86, 2839, 1989.

56. **Haskel, E.J., Torr, S.R., Day, K.C., Palmier, M.O., Wun, T-C., Sobel, B.E., and Abendschein, D.R.**, Prevention of arterial reocclusion after thrombolysis with recombinant lipoprotein-associated coagulation inhibitor, *Circulation*, 84, 821, 1991.

57. **Brand, K., Bank, C.L., Mackman, N., Terkeltaub, R.A., Fan, S.-T. and Curtiss, L.K.**, Oxidized LDL enhances lipopolysaccharide-induced tissue factor expression in human adherent monocytes, *Arterioscler. Thromb.*, 14, 790, 1994.

58. **Tracy, P.B., Robinson, R.A., Worfolk, L.A., and Allen, D.H.**, Procoagulant activities expressed by peripheral blood mononuclear cells, *Meth. Enzymol.*, 222, 281, 1993.

59. **Tracy, P.B., Eide, L.L., and Mann, K.G.**, Human prothrombinase complex assembly and function on isolated peripheral blood cell populations, *J. Biol. Chem.*, 260, 2119, 1985.

60. **Allen, D.H., and Tracy, P.B.**, Blood, 78, Suppl. 1 (Abstract 240), 1991.

61. **Robinson, R.A., Worfolk, L.A., and Tracy, P.B.**, Endotoxin enhances the expression of monocyte prothrombinase activity, *Blood*, 79, 406, 1992.

62. **McGee, M.P., and Li, L.C.**, Functional difference between intrinsic and extrinsic coagulation pathways. Kinetics of factor X activation on human monocytes and alveloar macrophages, *J. Biol. Chem.*, 266, 8079, 1991.

63. **Altieri, D.C., Morrissey, J.H., and Edgington, T.S** Adhesive receptor Mac-1 coordinates the activation of factor X on stimulated cells of monocytic and myeloid differentiation: An alternative initiation of the coagulation protease cascade, *Proc. Natl. Acad. Sci. USA*, 85, 7462, 1988.

64 **Altieri, D.C., and Edgington, T.S.**, The saturable high affinity association of coagulation factor X to ADP stimulated human monocytes defines a novel function of the Mac-1 receptor, *J. Biol. Chem.*, 263, 7007, 1988.

65. **Altieri, D.C.**, Coagulation assembly on leukocytes in transmembrane signaling and cell adhesion, *Blood*, 81, 569, 1993.

66. **Østerud, B.**, unpublished data, 1989.

67. **Østerud, B., Lindahl, U., and Seljelid, R.**, Macrophages produce blood coagulation factors, *FEBS Lett.*, 120, 41, 1980.

68. **Østerud, B., Bøgwald, J., Líndahl, U., and Seljelid, R.**, Production of blood coagulation factor V and tissue thromboplastin by macrophages in vitro, *FEBS Lett.*, 127, 154, 1981.

69. Synthesis of coagulation factor V by cultured aortic endpthelium, *Blood*, 63, 1467, 1984.

70. **McGee, M.P., and Wallin, R., Devlin, R**, Identification of mRNA coding for factor VII protein in human alveolar macrophages. Coagulant expression may be limited due to postribosomal processing, *Thromb. Haemost.*, 61, 170, 1989.

THE PROTEIN C ANTICOAGULANT PATHWAY AND HEPARIN-ANTITHROMBIN MECHANISM

K.A. Bauer* and R. D. Rosenberg**
* Veterans Affairs Medical Center, West Roxbury, Massachusetts
** Massachusetts Institute of Technology, Cambridge

The blood coagulation mechanism consists of a series of linked proteolytic reactions in which zymogens are converted to trypsin-like enzymes. The end result of these transformations is the generation of thrombin, which is able to act upon fibrinogen and platelets to produce the hemostatic plug. For coagulation system enzymes to be generated at any significant rate, a zymogen, a cofactor, and a converting enzyme must form a multimolecular complex on a natural surface. These transformations are suppressed if the converting enzyme is inhibited, the protein cofactor is destroyed, or the surface receptors essential for the assembly of the macromolecular complex are sequestered. Several natural anticoagulant mechanisms are able to exert damping effects upon each step of the coagulation cascade via the mechanisms outlined above. Two of these systems are the heparin-antithrombin and protein C anticoagulant mechanisms (see Figure 1), which regulate the serine proteases and activated cofactors, respectively.

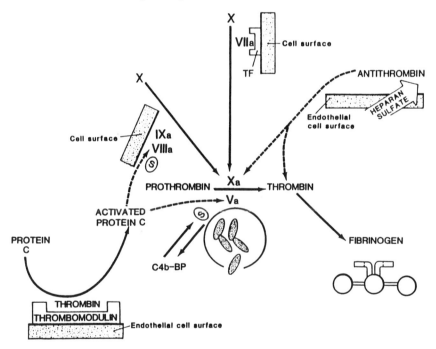

Figure 1. A schematic of the protein C anticoagulant pathway and heparin-antithrombin mechanism. Factor X can be activated by the extrinsic (factor VIIa-tissue factor {TF}) or the intrinsic (factor IXa-VIIIa-activated cell surface complex) pathways. Factor Xa binds to the factor Va on activated platelets and mediates the conversion of prothrombin to thrombin under physiologic conditions. Thrombin is then able to act upon fibrinogen to form a fibrin clot; the initial step in this conversion results in the liberation of fibrinopeptide A (FPA). Thrombin and factor Xa are inactivated by antithrombin bound to heparan sulfate molecules associated with the vascular endothelium resulting in the formation of factor Xa-antithrombin and thrombin-antithrombin complexes. Protein C is activated by thrombin bound to the endothelial cell receptor thrombomodulin. Once activated, protein C functions as a potent anticoagulant by inactivating factors VIIIa and Va. Protein S enhances the binding of activated protein C to phospholipid-containing membranes and is able to accelerate the inactivation of factors VIIIa and Va by this enzyme. The complement component, C4b-binding protein (C4b-BP), complexes with protein S resulting in a reduction of protein S functional activity.

I. PROTEIN C ANTICOAGULANT PATHWAY

In 1960, Mammen et al.[1] showed that a blood coagulation inhibitor, termed "autoprothrombin IIa," is generated when thrombin is added to prothrombin. In 1976, Stenflo[2] isolated a new vitamin K-dependent protein which he termed protein C. Subsequently, Seegers et al.[3] provided immunologic evidence that the component described as autoprothrombin IIa and that designated as protein C were the same protein.

A. THE STRUCTURE OF PROTEIN C AND PROTEIN S

Human protein C is a vitamin K-dependent plasma glycoprotein of Mr 62,000. The entire amino acid sequence of the mature 461 amino acid human glycoprotein has been deduced from the cloning of its cDNA.[4,5] Protein C consists of a heavy chain of Mr 41,000 and a light chain of Mr 21,000, which are joined by a single disulfide bridge (Figure 2). It is synthesized by liver cells [6] and circulates in human plasma at a concentration of about 4 µg/mL.[7,8] A single chain form of the zymogen has been identified that constitutes approximately 20 percent of the total protein C in the human circulation.[9,10] This suggests that the zymogen is initially synthesized as a single polypeptide chain and subsequently cleaved to generate a two chain structure. There are two forms of the protein C molecule, termed a and b, which result from differing amounts of N-linked carbohydrate.[11] All forms can be activated to species that possess anticoagulant activity.

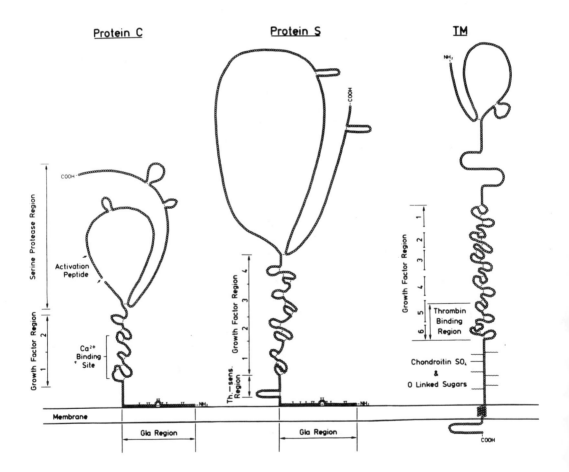

Figure 2. Schematic representation of the structures of protein C, protein S, and thrombomodulin. The Gla residues are indicated by small Y-shaped symbols. Reprinted from reference 95 with permission of the American Society of Biochemistry and Molecular Biology, Inc.

The human gene that codes for protein C is 12 kb in size and contains 9 exons.[4,12] It is located on chromosome 2.[13,14] The promotor region exhibits a TATA box 27 base pairs upstream from exon 1. Transcription of the gene is initiated at a consensus transcription start site approximately 70 base pairs upstream from the ATG translation initiation codon with the resultant mRNA containing 99 bases that code for a basic signal peptide, 27 bases that code for a linking propeptide, 1,257 bases that code for the light and heavy chains of the circulating zymogen as well as a connecting dipeptide, Lys-Arg, 296 bases of 3' non-coding sequence, and 38 bases with a polyadenylation segment. Comparison of the structures of the genes that encode vitamin K-dependent coagulation zymogens shows that only protein C and factor IX have highly similar exon size and sequence. However, there is little similarity in the size and structure of the introns for these two genes.

Both protein C and activated protein C possess γ-carboxyglutamic acid (Gla) residues in the amino-terminal region of the light chain (Figure 2). These residues are required for calcium-dependent binding of the proteins to cell membranes.[15] After the Gla domain, there follows a stack of hydrophobic residues and two epidermal growth factor (EGF) repeats, and the protease domain. The presence of β-hydroxyaspartic acid, which results from another post-translational modification in the EGF domain of the light chain, also appears to be required for calcium-dependent conformational changes in the molecule.[16,17]

In order to perform its anticoagulant function, human protein C is converted to a component with serine protease activity, activated protein C, by thrombin bound to vascular thrombomodulin in the presence of calcium ions (see below). The scission of a single Arg_{12}-Leu_{13} bond at the amino-terminal end of the heavy chain of the zymogen releases an activation peptide of approximately Mr 1,400.[18] The activation process is dependent on a calcium-binding site in the EGF region of protein C, rather than on the vitamin K-dependent Gla domain.[19,20] Occupancy of a single calcium-binding site produces a conformational change in the molecule that allows it to be readily activated by the thrombin-thrombomodulin complex, but makes it resistant to activation by thrombin alone.[21-24] The active site serine residue on activated protein C is located on the heavy chain.[25] Similar to other trypsin-like proteases, activated protein C has a specificity for Arg-containing residues on some synthetic substrates, factor VIIIa, and factor Va.

Human protein S is a vitamin K-dependent glycoprotein of Mr 70,000[26,27] that is synthesized by hepatocytes, vascular endothelial cells, and megakaryocytes.[6,28-30] Activated protein C complexes with protein S[31-33] on platelet[34,35] or endothelial cell membranes[36], and then the complex catalyzes the inactivation of factor VIIIa and factor Va. In human plasma, protein S is normally present at a concentration of 20-25 μg/mL.[37,38] Approximately 60 percent of the protein S is reversibly bound to a regulatory component of the classical complement pathway, C4b-binding protein, and 40 percent is free.[37,39-41] Only the free form of protein S functions as a cofactor for activated protein C.[41,42]

C4b-binding protein (Mr 570,000) is present in normal plasma at a concentration of approximately 150 μg/mL. It is a multimeric protein with a spider-like appearance on electron microscopy[43], consisting of seven identical α-chains and one β chain linked by disulfide bonds.[44-46] C4b-binding protein forms a non-covalent 1:1 stoichiometric complex with protein S.[39]

The binding site for protein S on C4b-binding protein is located on the β chain, while those for C4b are on the α-chains.[40,43] The K_D for the protein S-C4b-binding protein interaction changes from approximately 10^{-7} mol/L in the absence of calcium[40] to 5×10^{-10} mol/L in the presence of calcium.[47] Other, unidentified plasma proteins may also be involved in regulating the protein S-C4b-binding protein interaction and the level of free protein S.[47] Protein S in complex with C4b-binding protein retains the ability to interact with activated protein C, thereby competitively inhibiting the anticoagulant activity of free protein S.[48]

The structure of protein S has been deduced from the cloning of its cDNA.[49-51] The cDNA encodes 108 bases of 5' non-coding sequence, a 24 amino acid signal peptide, a 17 amino acid propeptide, a mature single chain protein S molecule of 635 amino acids, and 1,132 bases of 3' non-coding sequence. In contrast to the other vitamin K-dependent coagulation proteins, protein S is not a zymogen. The amino terminal region is homologous to other vitamin K-dependent plasma proteins and contains 11 Gla residues (Figure 2). Following the Gla domain, there is a thrombin-sensitive region within a disulfide loop, containing two protease-sensitive bonds,[37,52] followed by four EGF repeats. Thrombin-cleaved protein S requires higher calcium ion concentrations to bind to negatively charged phospholipid membranes[53,54], and is unable to mediate the anticoagulant activity of activated protein C.[55] This suggests that the thrombin-sensitive region of protein S is important for maintaining the proper conformation of the Gla domain. A β-hydroxyaspartic acid residue is located in the first EGF domain[56], and one β-hydroxyasparagine residue is present in each of the other EGF repeats.[57] In contrast to the EGF-like domains of protein C, these regions of protein S bind calcium with much higher affinity and this is important for maintaining the stability and conformation of the molecule.[58,59] The carboxy terminal end of protein S lacks sequences found in serine proteases and is somewhat homologous with sex hormone-binding proteins.[60,61] A region within this domain (residues 605-614) appears to be involved in the molecule's interaction with C4b-binding protein[62,63]; a surface-exposed sequence of protein S (residues 420-434) also appears to be important for this interaction.[64]

The human genome contains the expressed protein S gene, (α), and a pseudogene (β). Both are located on chromosome 3.[14,65,66] The protein S α gene spans over 80 kb and contains 15 exons and 14 introns.[67-69] The sequence of the β gene is homologous with exons II through VIII and the 3' untranslated region of the α gene.[67-69]

B. MECHANISM OF ACTIVATED PROTEIN C GENERATION

Thrombin is the only physiologically relevant serine protease that converts significant amounts of protein C to activated protein C.[70] However, the rate of activated protein C generation is extremely slow when blood is allowed to clot under in vitro conditions.[71,72] This finding brought into question whether physiologically relevant levels of activated protein C could be produced within the human body. It seemed possible that a cofactor might exist on the surface of endothelial cells which could accelerate the thrombin-dependent activation of protein C. When protein C and thrombin were perfused together through the coronary microcirculation, significant amounts of activated protein C were generated during a single pass.[73] Perfusion of either protein C or thrombin alone failed to generate any activated protein C. These data were most consistent with a model in which thrombin binds to a high affinity receptor on the endothelium and the enzyme receptor complex is then able to rapidly convert protein C to activated protein C. In fact, cultured endothelial cells, but not other cell types, possess a high affinity site for thrombin which enhances the conversion of protein C to activated protein C by about 30-fold as compared with free thrombin.[73,74] The endothelial cell binding site was purified and named thrombomodulin.[75] Thrombomodulin (Mr 100,000) forms a 1:1 complex with thrombin, which is then able to rapidly convert protein C to activated protein C. The interaction of thrombin with thrombomodulin appears to induce a reversible conformational change in the enzyme that permits it to activate protein C rapidly in the presence of divalent ions. Moreover, the thrombin-thrombomodulin complex exhibits a somewhat diminished ability to clot fibrinogen, activate factor V, or trigger platelet activation.[76,77] Thus, thrombomodulin has the ability to accelerate the rate of thrombin-dependent protein C conversion as well as to partially inhibit the procoagulant activities of the enzyme.

Cloning the cDNA for thrombomodulin[78,79] showed that it resembled other coated pit receptors such as the LDL receptor. Figure 2 depicts the overall structure of thrombomodulin with its five separate domains. It exhibits a short C-terminal intracytoplasmic tail, a membrane spanning region, a serine-threonine-rich area to which chondroitin sulfate chains are linked, six EGF β type repeats, and an N-terminal lectin like domain.

The interaction between thrombomodulin and thrombin occurs mainly via the fifth EGF β (third loop) and sixth EGF β (second and third loop) regions of the receptor and the negative exosite of the enzyme (residues Thr_{147}-Ser_{158} of the B chain).[80-86] The site of interaction on the enzyme overlaps with, but is not identical to that used to complex with the fibrinogen substrate.[87] The formation of the thrombin-thrombomodulin complex leads to a conformational change in the active site of the enzyme as well as at some distance from this region.[88] The interaction between thrombomodulin and protein C takes place mainly between the fourth EGF β region (especially residues 333-350) and the Gla-containing as well as the two EGF regions of protein C.[84,86,89] It appears that glutamic acid residue 349 in the fourth EGF domain of the receptor is particularly critical for the calcium-dependent interaction with the Gla regions of protein C.[90] The serine-threonine-rich region of thrombomodulin is also of some importance to the above interactions. This region of the endothelial cell receptor is endowed with a covalently linked chondroitin sulfate chain with a highly sulfated terminal monosaccharide sequence.[82,86,91-94] The presence of the glycosaminoglycan chain augments the binding affinity of thrombin to thrombomodulin by about 2-5 fold, increases the K_M of activated protein C generation by about 30 percent and lowers the calcium ion optima for the above interactions by about threefold.[82,86,91-94] The serine-threonine-rich region also serves as a spacer segment positioning the binding sites on thrombomodulin away from the membrane surface and thereby optimizing the function of the receptor.[82] Thus, thrombin binds tightly to endothelial cell thrombomodulin, altering the specificity of the complexed enzyme such that it is then able to rapidly cleave protein C, which has assembled at a neighboring site on the receptor.

C. MECHANISM OF ACTION OF THE PROTEIN C ANTICOAGULANT PATHWAY

There are approximately 100,000 thrombomodulin molecules per vascular endothelial cell.[95] In the microvasculature, the surface area of endothelium in contact with blood is considerably greater than in large vessels.[96] Hence it is likely that protein C activation occurs primarily in the microvasculature. Thrombin bound to thrombomodulin complexes more rapidly with antithrombin than does free thrombin.[97,98] After thrombin interacts with antithrombin, the complex dissociates from thrombomodulin, thus allowing the receptor to bind additional thrombin. There is also evidence that thrombin bound to thrombomodulin is internalized by cells,[99] but the importance of this effect is controversial.[100]

Once evolved, activated protein C is able to inactivate two cofactors of the coagulation cascade, factor Va and factor VIIIa, by limited proteolysis.[101-103] The procofactors, factor V and factor VIII, are relatively resistant to proteolysis by activated protein C.

Activated protein C suppresses prothrombin activation by factor Xa on the platelet surface by cleaving peptide bonds of membrane bound-factor Va,[101,104] which acts as platelet surface receptor for factor Xa. Of note, when factor Xa binds to factor Va, it protects factor Va from the proteolytic action of activated protein C.[105] Activated protein C can also destroy the biologic activity of factor VIIIa[102,103,106-108] on cell membranes, thereby modulating factor Xa generation mediated by factor IXa.

Protein S is involved in activated protein C-dependent destruction of factor Va and factor VIIIa. In purified systems, protein S enhances the binding of activated protein C to cell membranes but the cleavage of factor Va and factor VIIIa by the enzyme is accelerated less than four-fold.[31-33,109-112] Protein S in the free form is required for activated protein C to exert its anticoagulant activity in plasma.[41,113] Activated protein C and protein S form a 1:1 stoichiometric complex in the presence of calcium ions and a phospholipid surface.

The relatively small increase in the rate of inactivation of factor VIIIa and factor Va by activated protein C in the presence of protein S has led investigators to search for other cofactors in the protein C anticoagulant pathway. Recently patients with hereditary resistance to the anticoagulant action of activated protein C in a clotting assay were identified,[114] raising the possibility of the existence of an additional cofactor for this enzyme besides protein S. While the molecular basis of this disorder is frequently a factor V mutation ($Arg_{506}Gln$) that renders the activated form of the molecule resistant to inactivation by activated protein C,[115] factor V can act as a cofactor for the enzyme in inactivating factor VIIIa.[116] Other potential mechanisms by which protein S could limit thrombin generation independent of activated protein C have been investigated. In experiments in purified systems, protein S is able to bind to factor Va and this results in the inhibition of prothrombinase activity.[117]

Activated protein C is cleared from the circulation with a half-life of approximately 15 minutes.[118] It is neutralized by several protease inhibitors in human plasma, a Mr 57,000 protease inhibitor designated protein C inhibitor,[119] α_1-antitrypsin,[120-122] α_2-macroglobulin,[123] α_2-antiplasmin,[124] and plasminogen activator inhibitor-1.[125] These inhibitors neutralize activated protein C at a relatively slow rate, though the activity of the protein C inhibitor is enhanced by high concentrations of heparin.[126] Several of these activated protein C-inhibitor complexes have been identified in plasmas of patients or animals with heightened intravascular coagulation.[127-131] Studies of human protein C inhibitor, human α_1-antitrypsin, and the corresponding activated protein C-inhibitor complexes in rabbits demonstrate half-lives of 23 hours, 62 hours, and 20 and 72 minutes, respectively.[132] Pharmacokinetic studies of the clearance of human activated protein C in guinea pigs show two distinct mechanisms.[133] These are the formation of activated protein C-protease inhibitor complexes and subsequent elimination by hepatic receptors, and the direct catabolism of the enzyme by the liver by a nonsaturable pathway.

D. PATHOPHYSIOLOGICAL STUDIES OF THE PROTEIN C ANTICOAGULANT PATHWAY

Evidence obtained from animal studies and clinical observations indicates that the protein C-thrombomodulin mechanism functions in vivo to suppress thrombotic phenomena. Infusion of a small amount of thrombin into dogs induces protein C activation before there are any observable changes in the levels of factor V, fibrinogen, or platelets.[118] Activated human protein C can prevent the accretion of radiolabeled fibrinogen onto preformed jugular venous thrombi in dogs.[134] This enzyme can also inhibit platelet-dependent thrombus formation on prosthetic vascular grafts under arterial flow conditions in primates.[135] A monoclonal antibody directed against protein C is able to induce thromboembolism in mice.[136]

The administration of large amounts of activated human protein C into baboons just before the infusion of 100 percent lethal doses (LD_{100} doses) of Escherichia coli allows animals to survive and prevents the development of disseminated intravascular coagulation and organ damage.[137] Prior blockade of endogenous protein C activation with a monoclonal antibody to protein C converts a sublethal dose of infused Escherichia coli organisms (10 percent of the LD_{100} level) into a lethal dose. Furthermore, baboons receiving C4b-binding protein and a sublethal dose of bacteria develop disseminated intravascular coagulation and organ damage that can be prevented by protein S supplementation.[138]

In the baboon sepsis model, the administration of a competitive inhibitor of factor Xa binding to factor Va (i.e., active site blocked-factor Xa) blocked the development of disseminated intravascular coagulation similar to activated protein C.[139] However, unlike activated protein C, the animals still developed organ damage and ultimately died, which suggests that this anticoagulant may limit inflammation in vivo.

Based on experiments in dogs and pigs, occlusion of the left anterior descending coronary artery for short periods results in the generation of relatively high amounts of activated protein C in the ischemic region without deleterious effects on cardiac function.[140] Administration of a monoclonal antibody that inhibits protein C activation to animals undergoing an identical experimental protocol causes impaired recovery of left ventricular function. These studies indicate a potential role for activated protein C in preventing ischemic injury.

II. THE HEPARIN-ANTITHROMBIN MECHANISM

At the beginning of the 20th century, thrombin was observed to lose activity gradually when added to defibrinated plasma or serum.[141,142] On the basis of these data it was postulated that a specific inactivator of this proteolytic enzyme, antithrombin, was present within the blood. In 1916 McLean[143] isolated heparin from the liver and discovered the potent anticoagulant properties of this substance. Its inhibitory effect on purified procoagulants was clarified by Brinkhous and colleagues,[144] who showed that heparin was effective as an anticoagulant only in the presence of a plasma component that they termed "heparin cofactor." During the 1950's, kinetic studies conducted by Waugh and collaborators[145] and Monkhous and colleagues[146] suggested that plasma antithrombin activity and plasma heparin cofactor activity are intimately related. In 1968 Abildgaard[147] was able to isolate small amounts of an α_2-globulin from human plasma that functioned in both capacities. Subsequently, Rosenberg and Damus[148] purified large quantities of this human inhibitor and showed that plasma antithrombin activity and plasma heparin cofactor activity reside in the same molecule.

A. ANTITHROMBIN STRUCTURE AND MECHANISM OF ACTION

Human antithrombin is a plasma glycoprotein of Mr 58,000 and its concentration in normal human plasma is about 140 µg/ml.[149] It is a single polypeptide chain composed of 432 amino acids.[150] The location of functionally important domains such as the enzyme binding region (reactive site), the potential heparin binding sites, the conformation-sensitive tryptophan, and the S-S crosslinks (see below) are shown in Figure 3.

The human gene that codes for antithrombin is 15 kilobases in size and contains 7 exons.[151-155] It is located on chromosome 1.[156,157] The promotor region does not possess a TATA box at -25 or a CAAT box at -70 to -80.[158] However, the 5' flanking region contains an 8 base pair segment that exhibits high homology to the J_κ-C_κ enhancer of murine and human IgG κ chain genes.[159] This control element appears to be critical for the efficient synthesis of antithrombin and IgG κ light chains within tissue-specific environments. Transcription of the antithrombin gene is initiated at a unique site 72 base pairs upstream from the ATG translation initiation codon,[155,160] and the resultant mRNA contains 96 bases that code for the signal peptide, 1296 bases that code for the amino acid sequence of the native protein, and about 175 bases of 3' non-translated region including a polyadenylation segment.[161] Alternate splicing of the primary transcripts may take place at two sites within the first intron. This process leads to either a native antithrombin molecule with its signal peptide or to a truncated product consisting of the N-terminal 14 amino acids of the signal peptide as well as the five C-terminal amino acids encoded by a portion of the first intron. This latter polypeptide appears to remain within the cell, but its function remains enigmatic.

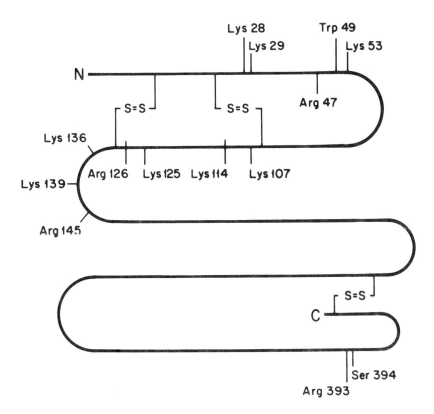

Figure 3. Critical sites within antithrombin. Arg_{393}-Ser_{394} is the reactive site of antithrombin. Trp_{49} is the conformation-sensitive aromatic residue. The various lysine and arginine residues are potential sites for the binding of the different domains of heparin to the protease inhibitor.

Antithrombin neutralizes thrombin by forming a 1:1 stoichiometric complex between the two components via an interaction between a reactive site arginine in antithrombin and an active center serine in thrombin.[148] The above process involves generation of a stable tetrahedral intermediate between enzyme and inhibitor that resists the bond cleavage that normally occurs with substrate. Complex formation occurs at a relatively slow rate in the absence of heparin. However, when the polysaccharide is present, it binds to lysyl residues on antithrombin and dramatically accelerates the rate of complex formation.[148,162] This heparin-induced acceleratory phenomenon is due to an allosteric alteration in the protease inhibitor, which renders it more readily available for interaction with thrombin or other coagulation enzymes.[163] The thrombin-antithrombin complex is cleared by receptors in the liver,[164] and has a half-life in the circulation of less than 15 min.[165]

The reactive site of antithrombin is positioned near the C-terminal end of the protein at Arg_{393} (P1 site)-Ser_{394} (P1' site).[166] The three dimensional structures of reactive bond-cleaved α_1-antitrypsin and antithrombin show that both P1-P16 regions (N-terminal to the cleaved reactive site) represent central β-strands of six membered β sheets within the central cores of the proteins.[167-171] Based upon modeling studies, the native structure of the two protease inhibitors could be reconstructed by extracting the P1-P16 region from the beta strand complex and reattaching it to the P1' residue. This indicated that partial insertion of the same region into the central core of both proteins might be involved in stabilizing a reactive bond conformation, which "traps" proteases in a tetrahedral intermediate rather than permitting bond cleavage as occurs with substrates. This model was confirmed by adding various P1-P14 peptides to several plasma protease inhibitors, which blocked insertion of the different reactive site loops, allowed the above bonds to be cleaved by added proteases, and prevented these macromolecules from functioning as enzyme inhibitors. Thus, the available evidence indicates that the serine active centers of coagulation enzymes bind to the reactive site residues of antithrombin, the interaction induces a partial insertion of the amino terminal region of the reactive site into the core of the inhibitor which arrests cleavage of the reactive site bond, and the hemostatic enzymes are thereby "trapped" in a stable complex with protease inhibitor.

The two major heparin binding domains of antithrombin have been defined by various approaches. The first region (residues 28-53) was pinpointed by characterizing naturally occurring variants of antithrombin and chemically modified protease inhibitors with regard to heparin interactions, and proteolytic cleavage patterns in the presence and absence of polysaccharide.[172-179] Residues Lys_{28}, Lys_{29}, and Lys_{53} lie within this region, and could serve as positive binding sites for heparin. The second region (residues 107-156) was identified by characterizing selectively reduced or chemically modified antithrombin as well as evaluating the effects of antibodies against specific domains of the protease inhibitor.[180-182] Residues Lys_{107}, Lys_{114}, Lys_{125}, Lys_{136}, Lys_{139}, Arg_{129} and Arg_{145} are present within this region and could be involved in binding polysaccharide. The presence of a small pool of plasma antithrombin, which is not glycosylated at Asn_{135} and has increased heparin affinity, is further evidence for the close proximity of this residue to the heparin-binding domain.[183,184] Computer-generated modelling of antithrombin based upon the crystal structure of α_1-antitrypsin suggest that certain of the critical positively charged residues of region I and region II described above align to form a long stretch of positive residues which could bind sulfate groups of heparin or heparan sulfate.[167]

Many hemostatic enzymes of the coagulation cascade, factors IXa, Xa, XIa, and XIIa, are inactivated by antithrombin in a manner similar to that outlined for thrombin.[185-187] Heparin is able to dramatically accelerate each of these protease-protease inhibitor interactions. The magnitude of the polysaccharide-dependent acceleration of factor XIa-antithrombin interactions has been the subject of considerable controversy.[188] Saturation of antithrombin with heparin accelerates the above interaction to a very considerable extent. The addition of high molecular weight kininogen, which binds to factor XIa, further augments the rate of factor XIa neutralization by the heparin-antithrombin complex.[189,190]

Thus, the heparin-antithrombin mechanism is the major pathway of neutralization for most of the activated factors of the coagulation cascade in plasma except for factor XIIa, in which C1 inhibitor may play an important role. Careful studies of the interaction between purified factor VIIa or activated protein C and the heparin-antithrombin complex reveal only slow inactivation of these enzymes.[191,192] However, the binding of factor VIIa to tissue factor in the presence of calcium results in a greater than 30-fold increase in the rate of enzyme inhibition by antithrombin.[193,194] Other steps of the coagulation cascade that do not involve serine proteases are only minimally affected by heparin.

The overall mechanism by which heparin accelerates hemostatic enzyme-antithrombin complex formation has been investigated by determining the binding parameters and kinetic constants of the various heparin-antithrombin-hemostatic enzyme interactions. The relative importance of the binding of heparin to protease inhibitor, to enzyme, or to both, with respect to the polysaccharide-dependent acceleration of the various hemostatic enzyme-antithrombin interactions has been controversial. One group[195,196] showed that heparin-dependent enhancement in the rates of neutralization of thrombin, factor IXa, or factor Xa by antithrombin requires binding of the polysaccharide to the protease inhibitor, but not necessarily to the enzyme. Other investigators concluded that the approximation mechanism whereby heparin brings the enzyme close to antithrombin by binding to both proteins simultaneously, is of greater relative importance than the direct binding of polysaccharide to protease inhibitor.[197,198] This discrepancy may be due to differences in the molecular weights of the heparin used in these studies since heparin fractions of higher molecular weight accelerate certain of the hemostatic enzyme-protease inhibitor interactions to a greater degree than do lower molecular weight fractions due to multiple binding sites for antithrombin as well as more potent approximation phenomena.[199-201] Thus, the somewhat different conclusions about reaction mechanisms may reflect the use of different heparin preparations.

Trace amounts of heparin catalyze the interaction of large quantities of hemostatic enzyme and antithrombin.[196] This is because the neutralization of hemostatic enzyme by the heparin-antithrombin complex results in the release of the polysaccharide from the protease inhibitor, allowing it to bind to other antithrombin molecules. Furthermore, the binding of heparin to the hemostatic enzyme-antithrombin complex is 100 to 1,000-fold weaker than the interaction of mucopolysaccharide with free protease inhibitor, favoring the binding to antithrombin molecules that can inhibit enzymes. Thus, heparin is able to function as a catalyst and thereby initiate multiple rounds of protease-protease inhibitor complex formation.

B. STRUCTURE AND BIOSYNTHESIS OF HEPARIN AND HEPARAN SULFATE

Heparin is a highly sulfated glycosaminoglycan, which is present in mast cells, and is therefore widely distributed throughout a variety of organs including the liver, heart, lungs, kidneys, and intestine.[200] The biosynthesis of the polysaccharide is initiated by attachment of a carbohydrate-protein linkage region to the serine residues of the polypeptide serglycin, which contains extended sequences of alternating residues of serine and glycine.[201] After formation of the carbohydrate-protein connecting sequence, the polymer chain of the polysaccharide is assembled by the alternate attachment of N-acetylglucosamine and glucuronic acid. This simple copolymer is then modified by a concerted process which leads to different modifications in various segments of the polysaccharide chain. These include: partial N-deacetylation of glucosamine residues which permits exposed amino groups to accept sulfate ions in a transfer reaction with 3' phosphoadenylsulfate; variable epimerization of glucuronic acid residues to iduronic acid moieties; partial ester-sulfation of iduronic acid residues and, to a lesser extent, glucuronic acid residues at the C-2 position; and variable ester-sulfation of glucosamine moieties at the C-3 and the C-6 positions.[202-205] The final heparin proteoglycan product contains variable numbers of polysaccharide chains of Mr 30,000-100,000.[206,207]

Mammalian cells also synthesize a second type of heparin-like proteoglycan, a heparan sulfate proteoglycan, which consists of a core protein of specific structure with covalently attached glycosaminoglycans of 50-150 disaccharide units. The glycosaminoglycan side chains exhibit a structural diversity similar to heparin, which arises from differing arrangements of disaccharide units composed of alternating N-sulfate or N-acetylglucosamine residues, with or without, 6-0 or 3-0 ester groups, and glucuronic acid or iduronic acid residues with or without, 2-0-ester sulfate groups. One distinction between heparin and heparan sulfate proteoglycans is based upon the structure of the core protein. The heparin core protein is small and relatively simple in structure, with extended runs of Ser-Gly attachments sites, whereas heparan sulfate core proteins are large and more diverse in structure, with isolated Ser-Gly attachment sites and membrane spanning regions or glycolipid anchors. Other distinctions between heparin and heparan sulfate proteoglycans are the location of the glycoconjugate within the cell (heparin proteoglycan is found within mast cell granules, whereas heparan sulfate proteoglycans are located on cell surfaces or in the surrounding matrix), and the relative amounts of N-acetylglucosamine and glucuronic acid present in the carbohydrate chains (heparin is more extensively modified, with larger amounts of N-sulfate glucosamine residues, with and without 3-0- and 6-0-ester sulfate groups, and iduronic acid residues, with and without 2-0-ester sulfate groups, whereas heparan sulfate is less extensively modified with more N-acetylglucosamine residues and glucuronic acid residues).

Heparin and heparan sulfate potentiate the action of antithrombin by binding to the protease inhibitor. Only a small fraction of commercial heparin is able to bind to antithrombin, but is responsible for virtually all of the anticoagulant activity of the complex carbohydrate.[208] Oligosaccharides of eight or more monosaccharide units accelerate factor Xa-antithrombin interactions, but do not catalyze neutralization of other hemostatic enzymes.[209] Oligosaccharides of approximately 16 or more residues accelerate thrombin-antithrombin as well as factor IXa-antithrombin interactions. Kinetic examination of these species[209] suggests that oligosaccharides of approximately 16 residues display the capacity to neutralize thrombin rapidly by activating antithrombin, whereas larger oligosaccharides contain an additional structural element required for approximating free enzyme with protease inhibitor.

The domain of heparin that accelerates factor Xa-antithrombin interactions contains an octacsaccharide with a unique tetrasaccharide sequence. It is composed of a nonsulfated iduronic acid residue on the nonreducing end, followed by an N-acetyl glucosamine 6-0-sulfate group, a glucuronic acid moiety, and an N-sulfated/O-sulfated glucosamine residue on the reducing end.[210-215] Less is known about the structure and nature of the critical groups in larger heparin oligosaccharides that enhance interactions of thrombin with antithrombin.

Until recently, mast cells were thought to be the sole site of synthesis of anticoagulantly active heparin.[216] These cellular elements are located beneath the endothelium and have intracellular granules that contain heparin. Mast cells have not convincingly been shown to discharge heparin into the circulation under in vivo conditions. Endothelial cells synthesize heparan sulfate proteoglycans that contain the critical structures required to bind antithrombin and activate the protease inhibitor.[217-219] Heparan sulfate species with anticoagulant activity have been isolated from calf cerebral microvessels and aortae and these proteoglycans contain the critical monosaccharide sequences required for enhancing the activity of antithrombin toward thrombin and factor Xa.[220,221] Proteoglycans of this type have also been isolated from mast cell free-retinal microvessels and shown to function in a manner similar to comercial heparin. Cultured endothelial cells are known to synthesize heparan sulfate moieties that contain the critical oligosaccharides required for anticoagulant activity.[222,223]

Heparan sulfate proteoglycans (HSPG) have been isolated and their cDNAs cloned from rat microvascular endothelial cells.[224,225] The anticoagulantly active heparan sulfate proteoglycans (HSPG^{act}) that bind to antithrombin constitute approximately 5 percent of total heparan sulfate proteoglycans. The anticoagulantly inactive heparan sulfate proteoglycans (HSPG^{inact}), which do not interact with protease inhibitor, represent about 95 percent of total heparan sulfate proteoglycans. The core proteins of HSPG^{act} and HSPG^{inact} contain the same two major components with Mr of 50,000 and 30,000, respectively, and possess virtually identical primary structures. The HSPG^{act} is a previously unidentified species, termed ryudocan, whereas the HSPG^{inact} represents the rat homolog of syndecan. The latter species is a known proteoglycan which was originally thought to be limited in its distribution to epithelial cells.[225] The two cDNAs encode integral membrane proteins of 202 amino acids (ryudocan) and 313 amino acids (syndecan), respectively, that have extraordinarily homologous transmembrane and intracellular domains, but very distinct extracellular regions. These two core proteins and perhaps other members of this multigene family appear to constitute the major integral membrane proteins that bear anticoagulantly active heparan sulfate chains synthesized by endothelial cells.

The anatomic location of endothelial cell-associated heparan sulfates has been visualized by light and electron microscopy or rat aorta.[226] Only small quantities of antithrombin perfused through the aorta interact with the luminal side of the endothelium (about 1 percent), and most of this binds beneath the endothelial cells. This suggests a model in which endothelial cells produce HSPG^{act} that are initially positioned within cell membranes, proteoglycans are then liberated by plasmalemmal proteases, and free HSPG^{act} then accumulate predominantly in the basement membrane.

C. PHYSIOLOGIC ROLE OF THE HEPARIN-ANTITHROMBIN MECHANISM

The physiologic relevance of the endogenous heparin-antithrombin mechanism was demonstrated using isolated rat hind-limb preparations.[227] Perfusion of thrombin and antithrombin through the vascular tree accelerated thrombin-antithrombin complex formation 10- to 20-fold when compared with the calculated reaction rate of the two components in solution.[228] The antithrombin-accelerating activity in the hindlimb vasculature was proved to be heparan sulfate proteoglycan as perfusion of the hindlimb vasculature with heparinase prior to the hemostatic components reduced the amount of enzyme-inhibitor complex generated within the animal to uncatalyzed levels. Heparan sulfate components could not be detected in the buffer, which indicates that the anticoagulantly active molecules are tightly associated with the endothelium. Similar perfusion experiments have also been performed with normal mice and litter mates who are genetically deficient in mast cells.[229] Both strains of mice exhibited an identical 20-fold acceleration of thrombin-antithrombin interactions, which were eliminated by the prior infusion of Flavobacterium heparinase. These latter findings strongly suggest that endothelial cell heparan sulfate proteoglycans are wholly responsible for the acceleration of antithrombin action and that mast cell heparin plays little, if any, role in this phenomenon.

Thus, it appears probable that a small fraction of plasma antithrombin is normally bound to HSPG[act] associated with endothelial cells of the blood vessel wall. On the one hand, the small amounts of luminal HSPG[act] could be critically placed to bind antithrombin, accelerate the action of the protease inhibitor, and thereby regulate hemostatic mechanism activity at the blood-vessel wall interface. The much larger quantities of abluminal HSPG[act] could serve as a potential reservoir which could be brought into play with extensive damage to the overlying endothelium. On the other hand, HSPG[act] which accumulate on the abluminal surface of the endothelial cells could also act to modulate the ambient function of the coagulation cascade. Plasma antithrombin should have relatively free access to this locale as suggested by numerous studies which document the extraordinary permeability of the endothelial cell layer.[230] Indeed, the presence of ^{125}I-antithrombin bound to subendothelium after ex vivo perfusion testifies to the ready accessibility of this region to protease inhibitor. Thus, antithrombin would be critically placed to neutralize hemostatic enzymes and thereby protect natural surfaces against thrombus formation. Furthermore, the catalytic nature of anticoagulantly active heparan sulfate species would ensure the continual regeneration of the nonthrombogenic properties of the blood vessel wall. Potential defects in the above mechanism in humans might lead to arterial or venous thrombosis.

REFERENCES

1. **Mammen, E. F., Thomas, W. R., Seegers, W. H.**, Activation of purified prothrombin to autoprothrombin I or autoprothrombin II (platelet cofactor II) or autoprothrombin IIa, *Thromb Diath Haemaorrh*, 5,218, 1960.
2. **Stenflo, J.**, A new vitamin K-dependent protein, *J Biol Chem*, 251,255, 1976.
3. **Seegers, W. H., Novoa, E., Henry, R. L., Hassouna, H. I.**, Relationship of "new" vitamin K-dependent protein C and "old" autoprothrombin IIA, *Thromb Res*, 8,543, 1976.
4. **Foster, D., Davie, E.**, Characterization of cDNA coding for human protein C, *Proc Natl Acad Sci USA*, 81,4766, 1984.
5. **Beckmann, R., Schmidt, R., Santerre, R., Plutzky, J., Crabtree, G., Long, G.**, The structure and evolution of a 461 amino acid human protein C precursor and its messenger RNA, based upon the DNA sequence of cloned human liver cDNAs, *Nucl Acids Res*, 13,5233, 1985.
6. **Fair, D., Marlar, R., Levin, E.**, Human endothelial cells synthesize protein S, *Blood*, 67,1168, 1986.
7. **Griffin, J. H., Mosher, D. F., Zimmerman, T. S., Kleiss, A. J.**, Protein C, an antithrombotic protein, is reduced in hospitalized patients with intravascular coagulation, *Blood*, 60,261, 1982.
8. **Miletich, J. P., Sherman, L., Broze, G. J., Jr.**, Absence of thrombosis in subjects with heterozygous protein C deficiency, *N Eng J Med*, 317,991, 1987.
9. **Miletich, J. P., Leykam, J. F., Broze, G. J.**, Detection of single chain protein C in human plasma, *Blood*, 62,306a, 1983.
10. **Heeb, M. J., Schwarz, H. P., White, T., Lammle, B., Berrettini, M., Griffin, J. H.**, Immunoblotting studies of the molecular forms of protein C in plasma, *Thromb Res*, 52,33, 1988.
11. **Miletich, J. P., Broze, G. J., Jr.**, Beta protein C is not glycosylated at asparagine 329. The rate of translation may influence the frequency of usage at asparagine-X-cysteine sites, *J Biol Chem*, 265,11397, 1990.
12. **Plutzky, J., Hoskins, J. H., Long, G. L., Crabtree, G. R.**, Evolution and organization of the human protein C gene, *Proc Natl Acad Sci USA*, 83,546, 1986.
13. **Rocchi, M., Roncuzzi, L., Santamaria, R., Archidiacono, N., Dente, L., Romeo, G.**, Mapping through somatic cell hybrids and cDNA probes of protein C to chromosome 2, factor X to chromosome 13 and alpha$_2$-acid glycoprotein to chromosome 9, *Human Genetics*, 74,30, 1986.
14. **Long, G. L., Marshall, A., Gardner, J. C., Naylor, S. L.**, Genes for vitamin K-dependent plasma protein C and protein S are located on chromosomes 2 and 3 respectively, *Somat Cell and Molec Genet*, 14,93, 1988.
15. **Fernlund, P., Stenflo, J.**, Amino acid sequence of the light chain of bovine protein C, *J Biol Chem*, 257,12170, 1982.
16. **Drakenberg, T., Fernlund, P., Roepstorff, P., Stenflo, J.**, β-hydroxyasparatic acid in vitamin K-dependent protein C, *Proc Natl Acad Sci USA*, 80,1802, 1983.
17. **Ohlin, A.-K., Linse, S., Stenflo, J.**, Calcium binding to the epidermal growth factor homology region of bovine protein C, *J Biol Chem*, 263,7411, 1988.
18. **Kisiel, W.**, Human plasma protein C. Isolation, characterization, and mechanism of activation by α-thrombin, *J Clin Invest*, 64,761, 1979.
19. **Johnson, A. E., Esmon, N. L., Laue, T. M., Esmon, C. T.**, Structural changes required for activation of protein C are induced by Ca^{2+} binding to a high affinity site thatn does not contain gamma-carboxyglutamic acid, *J Biol Chem*, 258,5554, 1983.
20. **Ohlin, A.-K., Landes, G., Bourdon, P., Oppenheimer, C., Wydro, R., Stenflo, J.**, β-hydroxyaspartic acid in the first epidermal growth factor-like domain: its role in Ca^{2+} binding and biological activity, *J Biol Chem*, 263,19240, 1988.

21. **Amphlett, G. W., Kisiel, W., Castellino, F. J.**, Interaction of calcium with bovine plasma protein C, *Biochemistry*, 20,2156, 1981.
22. **Esmon, N. L., DeBault, L. E., Esmon, C. T.**, Proteolytic formation and properties of gamma-carboxyglutamic acid-domainless protein C, *J Biol Chem*, 258,5548, 1983.
23. **Sugo, T., Dahlback, B., Holmgren, A., Stenflo, J.**, Calcium binding of bovine protein S. Effect of thrombin cleavage and removal of the γ-carboxyglutamic acid-containing region, *J Biol Chem*, 261,5116, 1986.
24. **Stearns, D. J., Kurosawa, S., Sims, P. J., Esmon, N. L., Esmon, C. T.**, The interaction of a Ca^{2+}-dependent monoclonal antibody with the protein C activation peptide region. Evidence for obligatory Ca^{2+} binding to both antigen and antibody, *J Biol Chem*, 263,826, 1988.
25. **Stenflo, J., Fernlund, P.**, Amino acid sequence of the heavy chain of bovine protein C, *J Biol Chem*, 257,12180, 1982.
26. **DiScipio, R. G., Hermodson, M. A., Yates, S. G., Davie, E. W.**, A comparison of human prothrombin, factor IX (Christmas factor), factor X (Stuart factor), and protein S, *Biochemistry*, 16,698, 1977.
27. **DiScipio, R. G., Davie, E. W.**, Characterization of protein S, a γ-carboxyglutamic acid containing protein from bovine and human plasma, *Biochemistry*, 18,899, 1979.
28. **Fair, D., Marlar, R.**, Biosynthesis and secretion of factor VII, protein C, protein S, and the protein C inhibitor from a human hepatoma cell line, *Blood*, 67,64, 1986.
29. **Stern, D., Brett, J., Harris, K., Nawroth, P.**, Participation of endothelial cells in the protein C-protein S anticoagulant pathway: the synthesis and release of protein S, *J Cell Bio*, 102,1971, 1986.
30. **Ogura, M., Tanabe, N., Nishioka, J., Suzuki, K., Saito, H.**, Biosynthesis and secretion of functional protein S by a human megakaryoblastic cell line (MEG-01), *Blood*, 70,301, 1987.
31. **Walker, F. J.**, The regulation of activated protein C by a new protein: a possible function for bovine protein S, *J Biol Chem*, 255,5521, 1980.
32. **Walker, F. J.**, Regulation of bovine activated protein C by protein S: the role of the cofactor protein in species specificity, *Thromb Res*, 22,321, 1981.
33. **Walker, F. J.**, Regulation of protein C by protein S: the role of phospholipid in factor Va inactivation, *J Biol Chem*, 256,11128, 1981.
34. **Suzuki, K., Nishioka, J., Matsuda, J., Murayama, M., Hashimoto, S.**, Protein S is essential for the activated protein C-catalyzed inactivation of platelet-associated factor Va, *J Bio chem*, 96,455, 1984.
35. **Harris, K. W., Esmon, C. T.**, Protein S is required for bovine platelets to support activated protein C binding and activity, *J Biol Chem*, 260,2007, 1985.
36. **Stern, D., Nawroth, P., Harris, K., Esmon, C.**, Cultured bovine aortic endothelial cells promote activated protein C-protein S-mediated inactivation of factor Va, *J Biol Chem*, 261,713, 1986.
37. **Dahlback, B.**, Purification of human vitamin K-dependent protein S and its limited proteolysis by thrombin, *Biochem J*, 209,837, 1983.
38. **Fair, D., Revak, D. J.**, Quantitation of human protein S in the plasma of normal and warfarin-treated individuals by radioimmunoassay, *Thromb Res*, 36,527, 1984.
39. **Dahlback, B., Stenflo, J.**, High molecular weight complex in human plasma between vitamin K-dependent protein S and complement component C4b-binding protein, *Proc Natl Acad Sci USA*, 78,2512, 1981.
40. **Dahlback, B.**, Purification of human C4b-binding protein and formation of its complex with vitamin K-dependent protein S, *Biochem J*, 209,847, 1983.
41. **Comp, P. C., Nixon, R. R., Cooper, M. R., Esmon, C. T.**, Familial protein S deficiency is associated with recurrent thrombosis, *J Clin Invest*, 74,2082, 1984.
42. **Dahlback, B.**, Inhibition of protein Ca cofactor function of human and bovine proteins by C4b-binding protein, *J Biol Chem*, 261,12022, 1986.
43. **Dahlback, B., Smith, C. A., Muller-Eberhard, H. J.**, Visualization of human C4b-binding protein and its complexes with vitamin K-dependent protein S and complement protein C4b, *Proc Natl Acad Sci USA*, 80, 1983.
44. **Hillarp, A., Dahlback, B.**, Novel subunit in C4b-binding protein required for protein S binding, *J Biol Chem*, 263,12759, 1988.
45. **Hillarp, A., Dahlback, B.**, Cloning of cDNA coding for the β-chain of human complement component C4b-binding protein: sequence homology with the a chain, *Proc Natl Acad Sci USA*, 87,1183, 1989.
46. **Dahlback, B.**, Protein S and C4b-binding protein: components involved in the regulation of the protein C anticoagulant system, *Thromb Haemostas*, 66,49, 1992.
47. **Dahlback, B., Frohm, B., Nelsestuen, G.**, High affinity interaction between C4b-binding protein and vitamin K-dependent protein S in the presence of calcium. Suggestion of a third component in blood regulating the interaction, *J Biol Chem*, 265,16082, 1990.
48. **Nishioka, J., Suzuki, K.**, Inhibition of cofactor activity of protein S by a complex of protein S and C4b-binding protein, *J Biol Chem*, 265,9072, 1990.
49. **Lundwall, A., Dackowski, W., Cohen, E., et al.**, Isolation and sequence of the cDNA for human protein S, a regulator of blood coagulation, *Proc Natl Acad Sci USA*, 83,6716, 1986.
50. **Hoskins, J., Norman, D. K., Beckman, R. J., Long, G. L.**, Cloning and characterization of human liver cDNA encoding a protein S precursor, *Proc Natl Acad Sci USA*, 84,349, 1987.
51. **Ploos van Amstel, H. K., van der Zanden, A. L., Reitsma, P. H., Bertina, R. M.**, Human protein S cDNA encodes Phe-16 and Tyr 222 in consensus sequences for the post-translational processing, *FEBS Lett*, 222,186, 1987.
52. **Dahlback, B., Lundwall, A., Stenflo, J.**, Localization of thrombin cleavage sites in the amino-terminal region of bovine protein S, *J Biol Chem*, 261,5111, 1986.
53. **Walker, F. J.**, Regulation of vitamin K-dependent protein S. Inactivation with thrombin, *J Biol Chem*, 259,10335, 1984.
54. **Schwalbe, R. A., Ryan, J., Stern, D. M., Kisiel, W., Dahlback, B., Nelsestuen, G. L.**, Protein structural requirements and properties of membrane binding by γ-carboxyglutamic acid-containing plasma proteins and peptides, *J Biol Chem*, 264,20288, 1989.
55. **Suzuki, K., Nishioka, J., Hashimoto, S.**, Regulation of activated protein C by thrombin-modified protein S, *J Biochem*, 94,699, 1983.
56. **Fernlund, P., Stenflo, J.**, β-hydroxyaspartic acid in vitamin K-dependent proteins, *J Biol Chem*, 258,12509, 1983.
57. **Stenflo, J., Lundwall, A., Dahlback, B.**, β-hydroxyasparagine in domains homologous to the epidermal growth factor precursor in vitamin K-dependent proteins, *Proc Natl Acad Sci USA*, 84,368, 1987.
58. **Dahlback, B., Hildebrand, B., Linse, S.**, Novel type of very high affinity calcium-binding sites in b-hydroxy asparagine-containing epidermal growth factor-like domains in vitamin K-dependent protein S, *J Biol Chem*, 265,18481, 1990.

59. **Dahlback, B., Hildebrand, B., Malm, J.**, Characterization of functionally important domains in vitamin-K dependent protein S using monoclonal antibodies, *J Biol Chem*, 265,8127, 1990.
60. **Gershagen, S., Lundvall, A., Fernlund, P.**, A cDNA coding for human sex hormone binding globulin. Homology to vitamin K-dependent protein S, *FEBS Lett*, 243,293, 1987.
61. **Baker, M. E., French, F. S., Joseph, D. R.**, Vitamin K-dependent protein S is similar to rat androgen-binding protein, *Biochem J*, 243,293, 1987.
62. **Walker, F. J.**, Characterization of a synthetic peptide that inhibits the interaction between protein S and C4b-binding protein, *J Biol Chem*, 264,17645, 1989.
63. **Weinstein, R. E., Walker, F. J.**, Enhancement of rabbit protein S anticoagulant cofactor activity in vivo by modulation of the protein S C4b-binding protein interaction, *J Clin Invest*, 86,1928, 1990.
64. **Fernandez, J. A., Heeb, M. J., Griffin, J. H.**, Identification of residues 413-433 of plasma protein S as essential for binding to C4b-binding protein, *J Biol Chem*, 268,16788, 1993.
65. **Ploos van Amstel, H. K., van der Zanden, A. L., Bakker, E., Reitsma, P. H., Bertina, R. M.**, Two genes homologous with protein S cDNA are located on chromosome 3, *Thromb Haemostas*, 58,982, 1987.
66. **Watkins, P., Eddy, R., Fukushima, Y., et al.**, The gene for protein S maps near the centromere of human chromosome 3, *Blood*, 71,238, 1988.
67. **Ploos van Amstel, H. K., Reitsma, P. H., van der Logt, C. P. E., Bertina, R. M.**, Intron-exon organization of the active protein S gene PS alpha and its pseudogene PSb: duplication and silencing during primate evolution, *Biochemistry*, 29,7853, 1990.
68. **Edenbrandt, C. M., Lundwall, A., Wydro, R., Stenflo, J.**, Molecular analysis of the gene for vitamin K-dependent protein S and its pseudogene. Cloning and partial gene organization, *Biochemistry*, 29,7861, 1990.
69. **Schmidel, D. K., Tataro, A. V., Phelps, L. G., Tomczak, J. A., Long, G. L.**, Organization of the human protein S genes, *Biochemistry*, 29,7845, 1990.
70. **Kisiel, W., Davie, E. W.**, Protein C, *Methods Enzymol*, 80,320, 1981.
71. **Kisiel, W., Ericsson, L. H., Davie, E. W.**, Proteolytic activation of protein C from bovine plasma, *Biochemistry*, 15,4893, 1976.
72. **Salem, H., Broze, G., Miletich, J., Majerus, P.**, Human coagulation factor Va is a cofactor for the activation of protein C, *Proc Natl Acad Sci USA*, 80,1584, 1983.
73. **Esmon, C. T., Owen, W. G.**, Identification of an endothelial cell cofactor for thrombin-catalyzed activation of protein C, *Proc Natl Acad Sci USA*, 78,2249, 1981.
74. **Owen, W., Esmon, C.**, Functional properties of an endothelial cell cofactor for thrombin-catalyzed activation of protein C, *J Biol Chem*, 256,5532, 1981.
75. **Esmon, N. L., Owen, W. G., Esmon, C. T.**, Isolation of a membrane bound cofactor for thrombin-catalyzed activation of protein C, *J Biol Chem*, 257,859, 1982.
76. **Esmon, C. T., Esmon, N. L., Harris, K. W.**, Complex formation between thrombin and thrombomodulin inhibits both thrombin-catalyzed fibrin formation and factor V activation, *J Biol Chem*, 257,7944, 1982.
77. **Esmon, N. L., Carroll, R. C., Esmon, C. T.**, Thrombomodulin blocks the ability of thrombin to activate platelets, *J Biol Chem*, 258,12238, 1983.
78. **Jackman, R. W., Beeler, D. L., VanDeWater, L., Rosenberg, R. D.**, Characterization of a thrombomodulin cDNA reveals structural similarity to the low density lipoprotein recpetor, *Proc Natl Acad Sci USA*, 83,8834, 1986.
79. **Jackman, R., Beeler, D., Fritze, L., Soff, G., Rosenberg, R.**, Human thrombomodulin gene is intron depleted: nucleic acid sequences of the cDNA and gene predict protein structure and suggest sites of regulatory control, *Proc Natl Acad Sci USA*, 84,6425, 1987.
80. **Olsen, P. H., Esmon, N. L., Esmon, C. T., Laue, T. M.**, Ca^{2+} dependence of the interactions between protein C, thrombin, and the elastase fragment of thrombomodulin. Analysis by ultracentrifugation, *Biochemistry*, 31,746, 1992.
81. **Ye, J., Liu, L. W., Esmon, C. T., Johnson, A. E.**, The fifth and sixth growth factor-like domains of thrombomodulin bind to the anion-binding exosite of thrombin and alter its specificity, *J Biol Chem*, 267,11023, 1992.
82. **Tsiang, M., Lentz, S. R., Sadler, E.**, Functional domains of membrane-bound human thrombomodulin, EGF-like domains four to six and the serine/threonine-rich domain are required for cofactor activity, *J Biol Chem*, 267,6164, 1992.
83. **Suzuki, K., Nishioka, J.**, A thrombin-based peptide corresponding to the sequence of the thrombomodulin-binding site blocks the procoagulant activities of thrombin, *J Biol Chem*, 266,18498, 1991.
84. **Hayashi, T., Zushi, M., Yamamoto, S., Suzuki, K.**, Further localization of binding sites for thrombin and protein C in human thrombomodulin, *J Biol Chem*, 265,20156, 1990.
85. **Suzuki, K., Nishioka, J., Hayashi, T.**, Localization of thrombomodulin-binding site within human thrombin, *J Biol Chem*, 265,13263, 1990.
86. **Parkinson, J. F., Nagashima, M., Kuhn, I., Leonard, J., Morser, J.**, Structure-function studies of the epidermal growth factor domains of human thrombomodulin, *Biophys Res Commun*, 185,567, 1992.
87. **Wu, Q. Y., Sheehan, J. P., Tsiang, M., Lentz, S. R., Birktoft, J. J., Sadler, J. E.**, Single amino acid substitutions dissociate fibrinogen-clotting and thrombomodulin-binding activities of human thrombin, *Proc Natl Acad Sci USA*, 88,6775, 1991.
88. **Ye, J., Esmon, N. L., Esmon, C. T., Johnson, A. E.**, The active site of thrombin is altered upon binding to thrombomodulin. Two distinct structural changes are detected by fluorescence, but only one correlates with protein C activation, *J Biol Chem*, 266,23016, 1991.
89. **Hogg, P. J., Ohlin, A. K., Stenflo, J.**, Identification of structural domains in protein C involved in its interaction with thrombin-thrombomodulin on the surface of endothelial cells, *J Biol Chem*, 267,703, 1992.
90. **Zushi, M., Gomi, K., Honda, G., et al.**, Aspartic acid 349 in the fourth epidermal growth factor-like structure of human thrombomodulin play a role in its Ca^{2+}-mediated binding to protein C, *J Biol Chem*, 266,19886, 1991.
91. **Parkinson, J. F., Grinnell, B. W., Moore, R. E., Hoskins, J., Vlahos, C. J., Bang, N. U.**, Stable expression of a secretable deletion mutant of recombinant human thrombomodulin in mammalian cells, *J Biol Chem*, 265,12602, 1990.
92. **Bourin, M. C.**, Thrombomodulin: a new proteoglycan, *Ann Biol Clin*, 49,199, 1991.
93. **Nawa, K., Sakano, K., Fujiwara, H., et al.**, Presence and function of chondroitin-4-sulfate on recombinant human soluble thrombomodulin, *Biochem Biophys Res Commun*, 171,729, 1990.
94. **Parkinson, J. F., Garcia, J. G., Bang, N. U.**, Decreased thrombin affinity of cell-surface thrombomodulin following treatment of cultured endothelial cells with beta-D-xyloside, *Biochem Biophys Res Commun*, 169,177, 1990.
95. **Esmon, C. T.**, The roles of protein C and thrombomodulin in the regulation of blood coagulation, *J Biol Chem*, 264,4743, 1989.

96. **Busch, C., Cancilla, P., DeBault, L., Goldsmith, J., Owen, W.,** Use of endothelium cultured on microcarriers as a model for the microcirculation, *Lab Invest*, 47,498, 1982.
97. **Hofsteenge, J., Taguchi, H., Stone, S. R.,** Effect of thrombomodulin on the kinetics of the interaction of thrombin with substrates and inhibitors, *Biochem J*, 237,243, 1986.
98. **Jakubowski, H. V., Kline, M. D., Owen, W. G.,** The effect of bovine thrombomodulin on the specificity of bovine thrombin, *J Biol Chem*, 261,3876, 1986.
99. **Maruyama, I., Majerus, P. W.,** Protein C inhibits endocytosis of thrombin-thrombomodulin complexes in A549 lung cancer cells and human umbilical vein endothelial cells, *Blood*, 69,1481, 1987.
100. **Beretz, A., Freyssinet, J. M., Gauchy, J., et al,** Stability of the thrombin-thrombomodulin complex on the surface of endothelial cells and from human saphenous vein or from the cell line EA.hy 926, *Biochem J*, 259, 35, 1989.
101. **Walker, F. J., Sexton, P. W., Esmon, C. T.,** The inhibition of blood coagulation by activated protein C through the selective inactivation of activated factor C, *Biochim Biophys Acta*, 571,333, 1979.
102. **Vehar, G., Davie, E.,** Preparation and properties of bovine factor VIII (antihemophilic factor), *Biochemistry*, 19,401, 1980.
103. **Marlar, R. A., Kleiss, A. J., Griffin, J. H.,** Mechanism of action of human activated protein C, a thrombin-dependent anticoagulant enzyme, *Blood*, 59,1067, 1982.
104. **Dahlback, B., Stenflo, J.,** Inhibitory effect of activated protein C on activation of prothrombin by platelet-bound factor Xa, *Eur J Biochem*, 107,331, 1980.
105. **Nesheim, M. E., Canfield, W. M., Kisiel, W., Mann, K. G.,** Studies of the capacity of factor Xa to protect factor Va from inactivation by activated protein C, *J Biol Chem*, 257,1443, 1982.
106. **Kisiel, W., Canfield, W. M., Ericsson, L. H., Davie, E. W.,** Anticoagulant properties of bovine plasma protein C following activation by thrombin, *Biochemistry*, 16,5824, 1977.
107. **Fulcher, C., Gardiner, J., Griffin, J., Zimmerman, T.,** Proteolytic inactivation of human factor VIII procoagulant protein by activated protein C and its analogy with factor V, *Blood*, 63,486, 1984.
108. **Eaton, D., Rodriquez, H., Vehar, G.,** Proteolytic processing of human facotr VIII. Correlation of specific cleavages by thrombin, factor Xa, and activated protein C with activation and inactivation of factor VIII coagulant activity, *Biochemistry*, 25,505, 1986.
109. **Gardiner, J. E., McGann, M. A., Berridge, C. W., Fulcher, C. A., Zimmerman, T. S., Griffin, J. H.,** Protein S as a cofactor for activated protein C in plasma and in the inactivation of purified factor VIII:C, *Circulation*, 70,II-205 (Abstr), 1984.
110. **Walker, F. J., Chavin, S. I., Fay, P. J.,** Inactivation of factor VIII by activated protein C and protein S, *Arch Biochem Biophys*, 252,322, 1987.
111. **Solymoss, S., Tucker, M. M., Tracy, P. B.,** Kinetics of inactivation of membrane bound Va by activated protein C, *J Biol Chem*, 263,14884, 1988.
112. **Bakker, H. M., Tans, G., Janssen-Claessen, T., et al.,** The effect of phospholipids, calcium ions and protein S on rate constants of human factor Va inactivation by activated human protein C, *Eur J Biochem*, 208,171, 1992.
113. **Bertina, R. M., van Wijngaarden, A., Reinalda-Poot, J., Roort, S. R., Bom, V. J. J.,** Determination of plasma protein S-the plasma factor of activated protein C, *Thromb Haemostas*, 53,268, 1985.
114. **Dahlback, B., Carlsson, M., Svensson, P. J.,** Familial thrombophilia due to a previously unrecognized mechanism characterized by poor anticoagulant response to activated protein C: prediction of a cofactor to activated protein C, *Proc Natl Acad Sci USA*, 90,1004, 1993.
115. **Bertina, R. M., Koeleman, B. P. C., Koster, T., et al.,** Mutation in blood coagulation factor V associated with resistance to activated protein C, *Nature*, 369,64, 1994.
116. **Shen, L., Dahlback, B.,** Factor V and protein S as synergistic cofactors to activated protein C in degradation of factor VIIIa, *J Biol Chem*, 269,18735, 1994.
117. **Heeb, M. J., Mesters, R. M., Tans, G., Rosing, J., Griffin, J. H.,** Binding of protein S to factor Va associated with inhibition of prothrombinase that is independent of activated protein C, *J Biol Chem*, 268,2872, 1993.
118. **Comp, P. C., Jacocks, R. M., Ferrell, G. L., Esmon, C. T.,** Activation of protein C in vivo, *J Clin Invest*, 70,127, 1982.
119. **Suzuki, K., Deyashiki, Y., Nichioka, J., et al.,** Characterization of a cDNA for human protein C inhibitor. A new member of the plasma serine protease inhibitor superfamily, *J Biol Chem*, 262,611, 1987.
120. **Heeb, M. J., Griffin, J. H.,** Physiologic inhibition of human activated protein C by α_1-antitrypsin, *J Biol Chem*, 263,11613, 1988.
121. **Heeb, M. J., Espana, F., Griffin, J. H.,** Inhibition and complexation of activated protein C by two major inhibitors in plasma, *Blood*, 73,446, 1989.
122. **Heeb, M. J., Mosher, D., Griffin, J. H.,** Activation and complexation of protein C and cleavage and decrease of protein S in plasma of patients with disseminated intravascular coagulation, *Blood*, 73,455, 1989.
123. **Hoogendoorn, H., Toh, C. H., Nesheim, M. E., Giles, A. R.,** α_2-macroglobulin binds and inhibits activated protein C, *Blood*, 78,2283, 1991.
124. **Heeb, M. J., Gruber, A., Griffin, J. H.,** Identification of α_2-macroglobulin (α_2M) and α_2-antiplasmin (α_2AP) as Ca^{++}-dependent inhibitors of activated protein C (APC), *Thromb Haemostas*, 65,781 (abstract), 1991.
125. **Sakata, Y., Curriden, S., Lawrence, D., Griffin, J. H., Loskutoff, D. J.,** Activated protein C stimulates the fibrinolytic activity of cultured endothelial cells and decreases antiactivator activity, *Proc Natl Acad Sci USA*, 82,1121, 1985.
126. **Suzuki, K., Nishioka, J., Hashimoto, S.,** Protein C inhibitor. Purification from human plasma and characterization, *J Biol Chem*, 258,163, 1983.
127. **Espana, F., Griffin, J. H.,** Determination of functional and antigenic protein C inhibitor and its complexes with activated protein C in plasma by ELISA's, *Thromb Res*, 55,671, 1989.
128. **Espana, F., Vicente, V., Tabernero, D., Scharrer, I., Griffin, J. H.,** Determination of plasma protein C inhibitor and of two activated protein C-inhibitor complexes in normals and in patients with intravascular coagulation and thrombotic disease, *Thromb Res*, 59,593, 1990.
129. **Espana, F., Gruber, A., Heeb, M. J., Hanson, S. R., Harker, L. A., Griffin, J. H.,** In vivo and in vitro complexes of activated protein C with two inhibitors in baboons, *Blood*, 77,1754, 1991.
130. **Hoogendoorn, H., Nesheim, M. E., Giles, A. R.,** A qualitative and quantitative analysis of the activation and inactivation of protein C in vivo in a primate model, *Blood*, 75,2164, 1990.

131. **Toh, C. H., Hoogendoorn, H., Scully, M. F., Giles, A. R.**, Quantification of activated protein C (APC) in complex with α_2-macroglobulin (α_2-M) by ELISA in patients with disseminated intravascular coagulation (DIC), *Blood (Suppl. 1)*, 78,74a, 1991.

132. **Laurell, M., Stenflo, J., Carlson, T. H.**, Turnover of *I-protein C inhibitor and *I-α_1-antitrypsin and their complexes with activated protein C, *Blood*, 76,2290, 1990.

133. **Berger, H., Jr., Kirstein, C. G., Orthner, C. L.**, Pharmacokinetics of activated protein C in guinea pigs, *Blood*, 77,2174, 1991.

134. **Emerick, S. C., Bang, N. U., Yan, S. B., et al.**, Antithrombotic properties of activated human protein C, *Blood (suppl 1)*, 66,349a (abstract), 1985.

135. **Gruber, A., Griffin, J. H., Harker, L. A., Hanson, S. R.**, Inhibition of platelet dependent thrombus formation by human activated protein C in a primate model, *Blood*, 73,639, 1989.

136. **Kurosawa-Ohsawa, K., Kimura, M., Kume-Iwaki, A., Tanaka, T., Tanaka, S.**, Antiprotein C monoclonal antibody induces thrombus in mice, *Blood*, 75,2156, 1990.

137. **Taylor, F. B., Jr., Chang, A., Esmon, C. T., D'Angelo, A., Vigano-D'Angelo, S., Blick, K. E.**, Protein C prevents the coagulopathic and lethal effects of Escherichia coli infusion in the baboon, *J Clin Invest*, 79,918, 1987.

138. **Taylor, F., Chang, A., Ferrell, G., et al.**, C4b-Binding protein exacerbates the host response to Escherichia Coli, *Blood*, 78,357, 1991.

139. **Taylor, F. B., Jr., Chang, A. C. K., Peer, G. T., et al.**, DEGR-factor Xa blocks disseminated intravascular coagulation initiated by Escherichia Coli without preventing shock or organ damage, *Blood*, 78,364, 1991.

140. **Snow, T. R., Deal, M. T., Dickey, D. T., Esmon, C. T.**, Protein C activation following coronary artery occlusion in the in situ porcine heart, *Circulation*, 84,293, 1991.

141. **Contejean, C.**, Recherches sur les injections intraveineuses de peptone et leur influence sur la coagulabilite' du sang chez le chien, *Archives de Physiologic Normale et Pathologique*, 7,45, 1895.

142. **Morowitz, P.** *The Chemistry of Blood Coagulation*, Springfield, IL: Charles C. Thomas, 1968

143. **McLean, J.**, The thromboplastic action of cephalin, *Am J Physiol*, 41,250, 1916.

144. **Brinkhous, K. M., Smith, H. P., Warner, E. D., Seegers, W. H.**, The inhibition of blood clotting: an unidentified substance which acts in conjunction with heparin to prevent the conversion of prothrombin to thrombin, *Am J Physiol*, 125,683, 1939.

145. **Waugh, D. F., Fitzgerald, M. A.**, Quantitative aspects of antithrombin and heparin in plasma, *Am J Physiol*, 184,627, 1956.

146. **Monkhouse, F. C., France, E. S., Seegers, W. H.**, Studies on the antithrombin and heparin cofactor activities of a fraction absorbed from plasma by aluminum hydroxide, *Circ Res*, 3,397, 1955.

147. **Abildgaard, U.**, Highly purified antithrombin III with heparin cofactor activity prepared by disc gel electrophoresis, *Scand J Clin Lab Invest*, 21,89, 1968.

148. **Rosenberg, R. D., Damus, P. S.**, The purification and mechanism of action of human antithrombin-heparin cofactor, *J Biol Chem*, 248,6490, 1973.

149. **Murano, G., Williams, L., Miller-Andersson, M., Aronson, D., King, C.**, Some properties of antithrombin III and its concentration in human plasma, *Thromb Res*, 18,259, 1980.

150. **Petersen, E. E., Dudek-Wojciechowska, G., Sottrup-Jensen, L., Magnusson, S.**, The primary structure of antithrombin III (heparin cofactor). Partial homology between alpha$_1$-antitrypsin and antithrombin III, in *The Physiological Inhibitors of Coagulation and Fibrinolysis*, Collen D, Wiman B, Verstraete M, eds, Biomedical Press, Elsevier/North Holland, 1979.

151. **Bock, S. C., Wion, K. L., Vehar, G. A., Lawn, R. M.**, Cloning and expression of the cDNA for human antithrombin III, *Nucl Acids Res*, 10,8113, 1982.

152. **Prochownik, E. V., Markham, A. F., Orkin, S. H.**, Isolation of a cDNA clone for human antithrombin III, *J Biol Chem*, 258,8389, 1983.

153. **Chandra, T., Stackhouse, R., Kidd, V. J., Woo, S. L. C.**, Isolation and sequence characterization of a cDNA clone of human antithrombin III, *Proc Natl Acad Sci USA*, 80,1845, 1983.

154. **Prochownik, E. V., Bock, S. C., Orkin, S. H.**, Intron structure of the human antithrombin III gene differs from that of other members of the serine protease inhibitor superfamily, *J Biol Chem*, 260,9608, 1985.

155. **Bock, S. C., Marrinan, J. A., Radziejewska, E.**, Antithrombin III Utah: proline-407 to leucine mutation in a highly conserved region near the inhibitor reactive site, *Biochemistry*, 27,6171, 1988.

156. **Winter, J. H., Bennett, B., Watt, J. L., et al.**, Confirmation of linkage between antithrombin III and Duffy blood group and assignment of AT3 to 1q22-q25, *Ann Hum Genet*, 46,29, 1982.

157. **Kao, F. T., Morse, H. G., Law, M. L., Lidsky, A. , Chandra, T., Woo, S. L. C.**, Genetic mapping of the structural gene for antithrombin III to human chromosome 1, *Human Genetics*, 67,34, 1984.

158. **Bock, S. C., Levitan, D. J.**, Characterization of an unusual DNA length polymorphism 5' to the human antithrombin III gene, *Nucleic Acids Res*, 11,8569, 1983.

159. **Prochownik, E. V.**, Relationship between an enhancer element in the human antithrombin III gene and an immunoglobulin light-chain gene enhancer, *Nature*, 316,845, 1985.

160. **Prochownik, E. V., Orkin, S. H.**, In vivo transcription of a human antithrombin III 'minigene', *J Biol Chem*, 259,15386, 1984.

161. **Prochownik, E. V., Smith, M. J., Markham, A.**, Two regions downstream of AATAAA in the human antithrombin III gene are important for cleavage dependent-polyadenylation, *J Biol Chem*, 262,9004, 1987.

162. **Gettins, P. G., Fan, B., Crews, B. C., Turko, I. V., Olson, S. T., Streusand, V. J.**, Transmission of conformational change from the heparin binding site to the reactive centre of antithrombin, *Biochemistry*, 32,8385, 1993.

163. **Jordan, R. E., Beeler, D., Rosenberg, R. D.**, Fractionation of low molecular weight heparin species and their interaction with antithrombin, *J Biol Chem*, 254,2902, 1979.

164. **Perlmutter, D. H., Glover, G. I., Rivetna, M., Schasteen, C. S., Fallon, R. J.**, Identification of a serpin-enzyme complex receptor on human hepatoma cells and human monocytes, *Proc Natl Acad Sci USA*, 87,3753, 1990.

165. **Pizzo, S. V.**, Serpin receptor-1: a hepatic receptor that mediates the clearance of antithrombin III-proteinase complexes, *Am J Med*, 87 (Suppl 3B),10s-14s, 1989.

166. **Bjork, I., Jackson, C. M., Jornvall, H., Lavine, K. K., Nordling, K., Salsgiver, W. J.**, The active site of antithrombin, *J Biol Chem*, 257,2406, 1982.

167. **Huber, R., Carrell, R. W.**, Implications of the three-dimensional structure of α_1-antitrypsin for structure and function of serpins, *Biochemistry*, 28,8951, 1989.

168. **Mourey, L., Samama, J. P., Delarue, M., et al.**, Antithrombin III: structural and functional aspects, *Biochimie*, 72,599, 1990.
169. **Engh, R. A., Wright, H. T., Huber, R.**, Modeling of the intact form of the α_1-proteinase inhibitor, *Protein Engineering*, 3,469, 1990.
170. **Schulze, A. J., Baumann, U., Knof, S., Jaeger, E., Huber, R., Laurell, C.-B.**, Structural transition of α_1-antitrypsin by a peptide sequentially similar to β-strand s4A, *Eur J Biochem*, 194,51, 1990.
171. **Bjork, I., Ylinenjarvi, L., Olson, S. T., Bock, P. E.**, Conversion of antithrombin from an inhibitor of thrombin to a substrate with reduced heparin affinity and enhanced conformational stability by binding of a tetradecapeptide corresponding to the P1 to P14 region of the putative reactive-bond loop of the inhibitor, *J Biol Chem*, 267,1976, 1992.
172. **Bjork, I., Olson, S. T., Shore, J. D.**, Molecular mechanisms of the accelerating effect of heparin on the reactions between antithrombin and clotting proteinases, in *Heparin. Chemical and Biological Properties. Clinical Applications*, Lane DA, Lindahl U, eds, Edward Arnold, London, 1989.
173. **Olson, S. T., Bjork, I.**, Regulation of thrombin by antithrombin and heparin cofactor II, in *Thrombin: Structure and Function*, Berliner LJ, eds, Plenum, New York City, 1991.
174. **Bjork, I., Nordling, K.**, Evidence of a chemical modification for the involvement of one or more tryptophanyl residues of bovine antithrombin in the binding of high affinity heparin, *Eur J Biochem*, 102,497, 1979.
175. **Blackburn, M. N., Sibley, C. C.**, The heparin binding site of antithrombin III, *J Biol Chem*, 255,824, 1980.
176. **Villanueva, G. B., Perret, V., Danishefsky, I.**, Tryptophan residue at the heparin binding site in antithrombin III, *Arch Biochem Biophys*, 203,453, 1980.
177. **Karp, G. I., Marcum, J. A., Rosenberg, R. D.**, The role of tryptophan residues in heparin-antithrombin interactions, *Arch Biochem Biophys*, 233,712, 1984.
178. **Liu, C.-S., Chang, J.-Y.**, The heparin binding site of human antithrombin III. Selective chemical modification at Lys114, Lys125, and Lys287 impairs its heparin cofactor activity, *J Biol Chem*, 262,17356, 1987.
179. **Liu, C.-S., Chang, J.-Y.**, Probing the heparin-binding domain of human antithrombin III with V8 protease, *Eur J Biochem*, 167,247, 1987.
180. **Sun, X.-J., Chang, J.-Y.**, Heparin binding domain of human antithrombin III inferred from the sequential reduction of its three disulfide linkages, *J Biol Chem*, 264,11288, 1989.
181. **Chang, J.-Y.**, Binding of heparin to human antithrombin III activates selective chemical modification at Lysine 236, *J Biol Chem*, 264,3111, 1989.
182. **Smith, J. W., Dey, N., Knauer, D. J.**, Heparin binding domain of antithrombin III: characterization using a synthetic peptide directed polyclonal antibody, *Biochemistry*, 29,8950, 1990.
183. **Peterson, C. B., Blackburn, M. N.**, Isolation and characterization of an antithrombin III variant with reduced carbohydrate content and enhanced heparin binding, *J Biol Chem*, 260,610, 1985.
184. **Brennan, S. O., George, P. M., Jordan, R. E.**, Physiological variant of antithrombin lacks carbohydrate side chain at Asn 135, *FEBS Lett*, 219,431, 1987.
185. **Rosenberg, J. S., McKenna, P., Rosenberg, R. D.**, Inhibition of human factor IXa by human antithrombin-heparin cofactor, *J Biol Chem*, 250,8883, 1975.
186. **Kurachi, F., Fujikawa, K., Schmier, G., Davie, E. W.**, Inhibition of bovine factor IXa and factor Xa by antithrombin III, *Biochemistry*, 15,373, 1976.
187. **Stead, N., Kaplan, A. P., Rosenberg, R. D.**, Inhibition of activated factor XII by antithrombin-heparin cofactor, *J Biol Chem*, 251,6481, 1976.
188. **Beeler, D. L., Marcum, J. A., Schiffman, S., Rosenberg, R. D.**, Interaction of factor XIa and antithrombin in the presence and absence of heparin, *Blood*, 67,1488, 1986.
189. **Scott, C. F., Schapira, M., Colman, R. W.**, Effect of heparin on the inactivation rate of human factor XIa by antithrombin-III, *Blood*, 60,940, 1982.
190. **Olson, S. T., Shore, J. D.**, High molecular weight-kininogen and heparin acceleration of factor XIa inactivation by plasma proteinase inhibitors, *Thromb Haemostas*, 62,381 (abstract), 1989.
191. **Godal, H. C., Rygh, M., Laake, K.**, Progressive inactivation of purified factor VII by heparin and antithrombin III, *Thromb Res*, 5,773, 1974.
192. **Broze, G. J., Jr., Majerus, P. W.**, Purification and properties of human coagulation factor VII, *J Biol Chem*, 225,1242, 1980.
193. **Lawson, J. H., Butenas, S., Ribarik, N., Mann, K. G.**, Complex-dependent inhibition of factor VIIa by antithrombin III and heparin, *J Biol Chem*, 268,767, 1993.
194. **Rao, L. V. M., Rapaport, S. I., Hoang, A. D.**, Binding of factor VIIa to tissue ¨factor permits rapid antithrombin III/heparin inhibition of factor VIIa, *Blood*, 81,2600, 1993.
195. **Jordan, R. E., Oosta, G. M., Gardner, W. T., Rosenberg, R. D.**, The binding of low-molecular-weight heparin to hemostatic enzymes, *J Biol Chem*, 255,10073, 1980.
196. **Jordan, R. E., Oosta, G. M., Gardner, W. T., Rosenberg, R. D.**, The kinetics of hemostatic enzyme-antithrombin interactions in the presence of low-molecular-weight heparin, *J Biol Chem*, 255,10081, 1980.
197. **Olson, S. T., Shore, J. D.**, Transient kinetics of heparin-catalyzed protease inactivation by antithrombin III. The reaction step limiting heparin turnover in thrombin neutralization, *J Biol Chem*, 261,13151, 1986.
198. **Shore, J. D., Olson, S. T., Craig, P. A., Choay, J., Bjork, I.**, Kinetics of heparin action, *Ann NY Acad Sci*, 556,75, 1989.
199. **Jordan, R. E., Favreau, L. V., Braswell, E. H., Rosenberg, . R. D.**, Heparin with two binding sites for antithrombin or platelet factor, *J Biol Chem*, 277,400, 1982.
200. **Engelberg, H.**, *Heparin: Metabolism, Physiology and Clinical Application*, Charles C. Thomas, Springfield, Illinois, 1963.
201. **Ruoslahti, E.**, Structure and biology of proteoglycans, *Annu Rev Cell Biol*, 4,229, 1988.
202. **Silbert, J. E.**, Biosynthesis of heparin. 3. Formation of a sulfated glycosaminoglycan with a microsomal preparation from mast cell tumors, *J Biol Chem*, 242,5146, 1967.
203. **Lindahl, U., Hook, M., Backstrom, G., et al.**, Structure and biosynthesis of heparin-like polysaccharides, *Fed Proc*, 36,19, 1977.
204. **Backstrom, G., Hook, M., Lindahl, U., et al.**, Biosynthesis of heparin. Assay and properties of the microsomal uronosyl C-5 epimerase, *J Biol Chem*, 254,2975, 1979.
205. **Roden, L., Horowitz, M. I.**, Structure and biosynthesis of connective tissue proteoglycans, in *The Glycoconjugates*, Horowitz MI, Pigman W, eds, Academic Press, New York, 1977.

206. **Yurt, R. W., Leid, R. W., Jr., Austen, K. F.,** Native heparin from rat peritoneal mast cell, *J Biol Chem*, 252,518, 1978.

207. **Robinson, H. C., Horner, A. A., Hook, M., Ogren, S., Lindahl, U.,** A proteoglycan form of heparin and its degradation to single chain molecules, *J Biol Chem*, 253,6687, 1978.

208. **Lam, L. H., Silbert, J. E., Rosenberg, R. D.,** The separation of active and inactive forms of heparin, *Biochem Biophys Res Commun*, 69,570, 1976.

209. **Oosta, G. M., Gardner, W. T., Beeler, D. L., Rosenberg, R. D.,** Multiple functional domains of the heparin molecule, *Proc Natl Acad Sci USA*, 78,829, 1981.

210. **Rosenberg, R. D., Armand, G., Lam, L.,** Structure-function relationship of heparin species, *Proc Natl Acad Sci USA*, 75,3065, 1978.

211. **Rosenberg, R. D., Lam, L.,** Correlation between structure and function of heparin, *Proc Natl Acad Sci USA*, 76,1218, 1979.

212. **Leder, I. G.,** A novel 3-0 sulfatase from human urine acting on methyl-2-deoxy-2-sulfamino-alpha-D-glucopyranoside-3-sulfate, *Biochem Biophys Res Commun*, 94,1183, 1980.

213. **Lindahl, U., Backstrom, G., Hook, M., Thunberg, L., Fransson, L. A., Linker, A.,** Structure of the antithrombin-binding site of heparin, *Proc Natl Acad Sci USA*, 76,3198, 1979.

214. **Choay, J., Petitou, M., Lormeau, J. C., Sinay, P., Casu, B., Gatti, G.,** Structure-activity relationship in heparin: a synthetic pentasaccharide with high affinity for antithrombin III and eliciting high antifactor Xa activity, *Biochem Biophys Res Commun*, 116,492, 1983.

215. **Atha, D. H., Stephens, A. W., Rimon, A., Rosenberg, R. D.,** Sequence variation in heparin octasaccharides with high affinity for antithrombin III, *Biochemistry*, 23,5801, 1984.

216. **Dvorak, H. F., Orenstein, N. S., Galli, S. J., Dvorak, A. M.,** Cutaneous basophils and hypersensitivity, in *The Mast Cell: Its Role in Heal th and Disease*, Pepys J, Edwards AM, eds, Pitman Medical Publishers, Kent, England, 1979.

217. **Damus, P. S., Hicks, M., Rosenberg, R. D.,** Anticoagulant action of heparin, *Nature*, 246,355, 1973.

218. **Teien, A. N., Abildgaard, U., Hook, M., Lindahl, U.,** The anticoagulant effect of heparan sulfate and dermatan sulfate, *Thromb Res*, 11,107, 1977.

219. **Thomas, D. P., Merton, R. E., Barrowcliffe, T. W., Mulloy, B., Johnson, E. A.,** Anti-factor Xa activity of heparan sulfate, *Thromb Res*, 14,501, 1979.

220. **Marcum, J. A., Fritze, L. M. S., Galli, S. J., Karp, G., Rosenberg, R. D.,** Microvascular heparinlike species with anticoagulant activity, *Am J Phys*, 245,H725, 1983.

221. **Marcum, J. A., Rosenberg, R. D.,** Anticoagulantly active heparin-like molecules from vascular tissue, *Biochemistry*, 23,1730, 1984.

222. **Marcum, J. A., Rosenberg, R. D.,** Heparinlike molecules with anticoagulant activity are synthesized by cultured endothelial cells, *Biochem Biophys Res Commun*, 126,365, 1985.

223. **Marcum, J. A., Atha, D. H., Fritze, L. M. S., Nawroth, P., Stern, D., Rosenberg, R. D.,** Cloned bovine aortic endothelial cells synthesize anticoagulantly active heparan sulfate protoeglycan, *J Biol Chem*, 261,7507, 1986.

224. **Kojima, T., Leone, C. W., Marchildon, G. A., Marcum, J. A., Rosenberg, R. D.,** Isolation and characterization of heparan sulfate proteoglycans produced by cloned rat microvascular endothelial cells, *J Biol Chem*, 267,4859, 1992.

225. **Kojima, T., Shworak, N. W., Rosenberg, R. D.,** Molecular cloning and expression of two distinct cDNA-encoding heparan sulfate proteoglycan core proteins from a rat endothelial cell line, *J Biol Chem*, 267,4870, 1992.

226. **de Agostini, A. I., Watkins, S. C., Slayter, H. S., Youssoufian, H., Rosenberg, R. D.,** Localization of anticoagulantly active heparan sulfate proteoglycans in vascular endothelium: antithrombin binding on cultured endothelial cells and perfused rat aorta, *J Cell Biol*, 111,1293, 1990.

227. **Marcum, J. A., McKenney, J. B., Rosenberg, R. D.,** The acceleration of thrombin-antithrombin complex formation in rat hindquarters via heparinlike molecules bound to the endothelium, *J Clin Invest*, 74,341, 1984.

228. **Lau, H. K., Rosenberg, R. D.,** The isolation and characterization of a specific antibody population directed against the thrombin-antithrombin complex, *J Biol Chem*, 255,5885, 1980.

229. **Marcum, J. A., McKenney, J. B., Galli, S. J., Jackman, R. W., Rosenberg, R. D.,** Anticoagulantly active heparin-like molecules from mast cell-deficient mice, *Am J Physiol*, 19,H879, 1986.

230. **Simonescu, N.,** Cellular aspects of transcapillary exchange, *Physiol Rev*, 63,1536, 1983.

STUDY OF THE PROTHROMBOTIC STATE USING PERFUSION SYSTEMS

Y. Cadroy
Laboratoire Hématologie et Génétique, Hôpital Purpan, Toulouse

Normal hemostasis is a well-balanced system of procoagulant and anticoagulant activities. Hypercoagulability is a state of imbalance where procoagulant activities exceed the anticoagulant capacity of the hemostatic system. Laboratory markers indicative of platelet activation *(e.g., β-*thromboglobulin) or thrombin generation *(e.g.,* prothrombin fragment 1+2, thrombin-antithrombin III complexes, fibrinopeptide A) have been helpful in defining this state.

The prothrombotic state is a condition in which thrombosis occurs in circumstances which, normally, would not induce its formation. A prothrombotic state cannot be merely defined by the elevation of biological markers of hypercoagulability: each marker is the reflection of a specific imbalance in a precise area of the hemostatic system, and an elevation in one marker does not necessarily imply that this specific imbalance will be sufficient to promote the development of a thrombosis. A prothrombotic state could be better defined using thrombosis models, provided they are able to determine whether a particular clinical condition favors the development of thrombosis.

The great majority of thrombosis models have been developed in animals. These models are helpful not only for testing various therapeutic strategies for preventing the development of thrombosis, but also for investigating prothrombotic states. However, the clinical relevance of the results obtained with these animal models is always questionable since, besides obvious species differences, the prothrombotic state is created experimentally and does not totally reflect the complexity of the clinical situation in man.

Perfusion chambers have been developed to study thrombogenesis under well-controlled conditions, regarding notably the blood flow rate and the nature of the thrombogenic surface. In these models, vessel segments, cells of the vessel wall or their extracellular matrix, or purified proteins of the vessel wall coated on plastic surfaces, are exposed to non-anticoagulated or anticoagulated blood in various flow conditions to mimic arterial- and venous-type thrombus formation. These perfusion chambers have been used to investigate the influence of prothrombotic states in promoting thrombus formation in animals, but also directly in humans. This chapter describes the main perfusion systems and reviews the findings obtained using these models in the exploration of various prothrombotic situations.

I. PERFUSION CHAMBERS

A. DESCRIPTION OF PERFUSION CHAMBERS

A perfusion chamber is designed to study the interaction of blood with a thrombogenic surface in well-controlled blood flow conditions. Different types of perfusion chambers have been developed. Three will be discussed here. The first two chambers have been used in both animals (rabbit and dog) and humans whereas the third has been used exclusively in the baboon. Their main characteristics are summarized in Table I.

1. Annular Perfusion Chamber

The annular perfusion chamber, developed by Baumgartner et al,[1] is composed of a central rod in an outer cylinder. The thrombogenic surface is an everted vessel segment positioned on the central rod to be exposed to the flowing blood. The vessel segments are rabbit aortas or human umbilical arteries which are de-endothelialized by the balloon catheter technique or by exposure to air. The wall shear rates depend on the flow rate (from 10 to 50 mL/min) and on the distance between the vessel and the inner wall of the outer cylinder of the chamber: they range from 50 to 3,300 s^{-1}.

2. Parallel-Plate Perfusion Chamber

The parallel-plate perfusion chamber, developed by Sakariassen et al,[2,3] is composed of two plates and a coverslip holder made of polymethyl methacrylate (Figure 1). Blood circulates in a rectangular slit and interacts with a coverslip positioned on the coverslip holder. The coverslip may be coated with various materials such as cultured endothelium or the corresponding extracellular matrix or purified proteins (e.g., human type III collagen). The dimensions of the flow slit and the flow rate (5, 10 or 20 mL/min) determine the wall shear rate, which may range from 50 to 5200 ss^{-1}.

Table I : Characteristics of the Main Perfusion chambers

Perfusion Chamber	Thrombogenic Surface	Shear Rate (s^{-1})	Blood	Species	Quantification of Thrombus Formation
ANNULAR	Subendothelium of Rabit Aorta Human Umbilical Artery	50-3300	Anticoagulated & Non-anticoagulated	Rabbit & Human	Morphometry & Immunological Determination of Fibrin Isotopes (Radiolabeled platelets) Measurement of Pressure Difference
PARALLEL-PLATE	Cultured Endothelium ECM of Endothelium ECM of Fibroblasts Human Collagen	50-5200	Anticoagulated & Non-anticoagulated	Dog, Rabbit & Human	Morphometry Immunological Determination
CYLINDRICAL	Subendothelium of Baboon Aorta Rat Collagen Synthetic Vascular Graft (Dacron)	100-800	Non-anticoagulated	Baboon	Isotopes (radiolabeled Platelets and Fibrinogen) : Dynamic assessment of Thrombus Formation with Scintillation Camera.

3. Circular Perfusion Chamber

The circular perfusion chamber was developed by Hanson for the study of the interaction of blood with endarterectomized baboon aortas,[4] rat type I collagen,[5] or synthetic vascular graft material such as Dacron.[6] The shear rates range approximately from 100 to 800 s^{-1}.

Another circular perfusion chamber consisting of a cannular segment coated with collagen followed by two regions of larger diameter exhibiting flow recirculation have been developed to study the formation of arterial- and venous-type thrombi simultaneously.[5] The collagen was chosen as an appropriate substrate to simulate vascular injury, whereas the larger diameter regions were designed to produce disturbed flow and stasis, characteristic of venous thrombosis.

B. PERFUSION

These chambers are used *in vitro* with anticoagulated blood or *ex vivo* with non-anticoagulated blood. Whole blood is usually anticoagulated with citrate or with a low molecular weight heparin. The latter anticoagulant has the advantage of preventing any thrombin formation during the handling of the blood while preserving the possibility of a local formation of thrombin at the thrombogenic surface; thus, the role of coagulation in thrombogenesis may be studied.[7] The anticoagulated whole blood is recirculated by a roller pump over the thrombogenic surface usually for 10 min at 37°C. Studies using anticoagulated blood have been performed only with the annular and the parallel-plate perfusion chambers.[8]

When the perfusions are performed with nonanticoagulated blood, the annular and the parallel-plate perfusion chambers are placed between the carotid artery and jugular vein in rabbit,[1] or in dog,[9]

respectively, and the blood is drawn by a roller pump set distally to the chamber. In humans, non-anticoagulated blood is taken from an antecubital vein by an infusion set and drawn directly by a roller pump placed distally to the chamber. The cylindrical chamber is inserted into a chronic exteriorized arterio-venous shunt placed between the femoral artery and vein of baboons; the blood flow rate is controlled with a clamp or by a roller-pump placed distally to the chamber to produce a flow rate of 100-200 mL/min or 20 mL/min, respectively.[5,6] The perfusion lasts 5 or 10 min with the first two perfusion chambers and is much longer (40 min to a few hours) with the cylindrical perfusion chamber used in the baboon.

Notice that blood is not recirculated but discarded once it has flowed over the thrombogenic surface in the ex *vivo* perfusions performed in humans, whereas in those performed in animals, blood is recirculated and thus subject to normal dilution, filtration and inactivation in the host animal.

C. QUANTIFICATION OF THROMBUS FORMATION

Different approaches have been used to quantify thrombus formation. Concerning the models using the annular and the parallel-plate perfusion chambers, thrombus formation is usually measured by quantitative morphometry analysis performed on semi-thin sections of Epon embedded materials cut perpendicularly to the direction of the blood flow.[8] The position of the cut along the axis of the blood flow is critical since the deposition of fibrin and platelets is axially dependent. This axial-dependence is determined by the nature of the prothrombogenic surface: on procoagulant rabbit aorta, platelet and fibrin deposition decrease axially, whereas on nonprocoagulant collagen, platelet deposition decreases axially and fibrin deposition tends to increase axially.[10] Standard morphometry quantifies the percentage of platelet adhesion and of platelet aggregates defined as thrombi when the aggregates are more than 5 μm high. Computer-assisted morphometry is necessary to quantify the volume and the height of the thrombus.[11] Fibrin deposition can also be measured by morphometry analysis, but it is difficult to accurately determine the thickness of the fibrin meshes. An interesting alternative for quantifying the total amount of fibrin deposited is the immunological determination of fibrin-degradation products of plasmin-digested thrombi.[8,12] With these models, thrombus formation is always measured as an end-point.

In baboons, thrombus formation is quantified in a dynamic fashion and in real time with a scintillation camera using ^{111}In-radiolabeled autologous platelets and ^{125}I-radiolabeled homologous fibrinogen.[5,6] Thus, this method detects possible embolizations of thrombi. Red blood cell incorporation in thrombus may also be determined by measuring the total thrombus hemoglobin.[13]

D. THROMBUS FORMATION

Depending on the blood flow rate and the nature of the thrombogenic surface, both arterial- and venous-type thrombus formation can be investigated with these experimental models. Acute arterial-type thrombosis can be mimicked when vessel subendothelium, purified collagen, or synthetic vascular graft are perfused at high shear rates: thrombi are primarily composed of platelets. Venous-type thrombi form when vessel subendothelium or stimulated endothelium expressing tissue factor is perfused under low shear flow.[10,12,14,15] Also, a fibrin- and red-cell-rich thrombus forms in the expanded flow regions of the cylindrical chamber inserted in the arterio-venous shunt in baboons.[5,13]

E. PERFUSION AND ACTIVATION OF THE HEMOSTATIC SYSTEM

When the chambers are inserted *ex vivo* into shunts and perfused with native, non-anticoagulated blood, it is important to determine whether the procedure of perfusion itself does not activate the hemostatic system. This is particularly important when one wants to study the influence of hypercoagulable or prothrombotic states on thrombogenesis.

Biological markers indicative of thrombin formation and platelet activation have been measured in blood drawn from antecubital veins of healthy volunteers, at the blood flow inlet of the parallel-plate perfusion chamber, just after the venipuncture, and at the end of a 5 or 10 min perfusion period (Table II). Except for the plasma levels of prothrombin fragment 1+2, the other markers (β-thromboglobulin, thrombin-antithrombin III complexes and fibrinopeptide A) increased significantly during the perfusion; they remained within the normal range at 5 min, but were beyond the normal range at 10 min. Thus, we can consider that thrombin formation and platelet activation are negligible at the flow inlet of the perfusion chamber for perfusions ≤5 min.

The chronic femoral arterio-venous shunt does not activate platelets since plasma levels of platelet factor 4, β–thromboglobulin were not increased by the shunt placement.[16] The plasma levels of fibrinopeptide A were also very low.[5]

Table II : Plasma Levels of β-thromboglobulin, Prothrombin Fragment1+2,
Thrombin-Antithrombin III Complexes and Fibrinopeptide A
at the Flow Inlet of the Chambers Following 0, 5 and 10 min Perfusions

	Time (min)			
	0	**5**	**10**	**Normal limit[a]**
βTG (Ul/mL)	20.4 ± 2.4	25.7 ± 3.1*	54.7 ± 11.1*	< 42
F1+2 (nmol/L)	1.09 ± 0.21	0.99 ± 0.22	0.73 ± 0.15	< 1.11
T-AT (µg/L)	2.4 ± 0.1	3.0 ± 0.2*	4.5 ± 1.1*	< 4.1
FPA (µg/L)	1.2 ± 0.3	2.2 ± 0.4*	3.8 ± 0.6*	< 3

Mean + 1 SEM (n=4-11)
* $P \leq 0.05$ compared with corresponding values at zero min.
[a]Normal Limit as given by manufacturers of kits (in part from ref.15. With permission).

II. PERFUSION CHAMBERS AND PROTHROMBOTIC STATE

Different types of hypercoagulable or prothrombotic states have been studied using perfusion chambers, either in animals or directly in humans, and either with anticoagulated or native non-anticoagulated blood. The main characteristics of the different studies are presented in Tables III and IV.

A . ERYTHROCYTOSIS

The role of elevated red blood cell concentration in promoting the development of thrombosis has long been suspected. Thromboembolic disorders occur in patients with polycythemia vera,[17] but in these patients, high hematocrit is usually associated with other abnormalities, including thrombocytosis, which may potentiate the effect of high hematocrit in promoting thrombosis. No experimental study has examined the prothrombotic state of patients with primary polycythemia.

In patients with secondary polycythemia, the thrombotic risk appears much lower.[17] Clinical studies suggest that there is a positive relationship between elevated hematocrit and thrombotic risk, but somewhat contradictory results have been found.[18-24]

The role of normal red blood cells in platelet adhesion and thrombus formation was first assessed using the annular and parallel-plate perfusion chambers, short perfusion time (5 min), high shear rate and human anticoagulated blood.[25,26] Platelet deposition and thrombus formation on the subendothelium of rabbit aorta increased with increasing hematocrit, suggesting that high hematocrit may favor arterial thrombosis. These results have been mainly attributed to changes in the rheologic properties of the blood: when the hematocrit increases, the red blood cell motion enhances the transport of platelets toward the vessel wall.

Table III : Investigations of Prothrombotic States Using Perfusion System :
Characteristics of the Different Studies.

Prothrombotic State	Perfusion Chamber	Species	Thrombogenic Surface	Shear Rate (S⁻¹)	Perfusion Time (min)	Blood
Erythrocytosis						
Turitto & Weiss[25]	Annular	Human	Rabbit Sub	50,200,2600	5 & 10	Anticoagulated (citrate)
Cadroy & Hanson[13]	Cylindrical	Baboon	Rat Collagen I Expanded Flow Regions	100 & 800	30 & 40	Non-anticoagulated
Thrombocytosis Cadroy et al [5]	Cylindrical	Baboon	Rat Collagen I	100	40	Non-anticoagulated
Hyperlipoproteinemia						
Badimon et al [34]	Annular	Rabbit	Rabbit Sub	2600	5 & 20	Anticoagulated (citrate)
Tandon et al [35]	Annular	Human	Rabbit Sub	800	30	Anticoagulated (citrate)
Cadroy et al [36]	Parallel-Plate	Human	Human Collagen III	2600	3	Non-anticoagulated
Diabetes Mellitus Nievelstein et al [41]	Parallel-Plate	Human	ECM End & Fibroblast ECM of End-PMA	300 & 1300	1-20	Anticoagulated (citrate)

Abbreviations : Sub = Subendothelium ; End = Endothelium ; ECM = Extracellular Matrix ; Umb Art = Umbilical Artery ; LMWH = Low Molecular Weight Heparin.

The effect of high hematocrit on arterial-type and venous type thrombus formation has also been studied in baboons, using the cylindrical perfusion chamber comprising a collagen coated segment and two expanded flow regions, a long perfusion period (40 min), and native non-anticoagulated blood.[13] Baboons were bled or transfused to obtain three groups with low (20 to 25%), normal (35 to 40%) and high (50 to 55%) hematocrit. The results showed that the volume of venous-type thrombus increased threefold between the normal and high hematocrit groups, indicating that erythrocytosis favors the development of venous thrombosis. However, the role of red blood cells in promoting arterial-type thrombosis was not as clear in this study as in those reported above. A positive relationship was found between hematocrit and thrombus formation on collagen at high shear rate after 5 min of blood exposure but not at later time points. Furthermore, at lower shear rate (100 s⁻¹), platelet thrombus volume was negatively correlated with hematocrit. These results, although possibly related to the slightly smaller size of the baboon red blood cells as compared to human ones,[26] could account for the discordant conclusions given by clinical studies on the role of erythrocytes in thrombus formation.

B. THROMBOCYTOSIS

The prothrombotic state of patients with primary thrombocytosis, who are prone to develop cerebral and digital ischaemia, has not been investigated using experimental thrombosis models. The role of secondary thrombocytosis in promoting thrombosis is more questionable.[27] However, in patients undergoing coronary angioplasty, a positive correlation between platelet count and the risk of developing coronary thrombosis has been demonstrated.[28]

Using the annular perfusion chamber and native human blood, Baumgartner et al found a positive relationship between blood platelet count and thrombus formation on rabbit subendothelium.[29] In addition, platelet thrombus volume on collagen-coated segments increased with increasing platelet count in the baboon.[5]

C. HYPERLIPOPROTEINEMIA

Hyperlipoproteinemia is a major risk factor for atherosclerosis and thrombosis. It is associated with enhancement of platelet activity: in platelet aggregation tests, platelets appear more sensitive to aggregating agents.[30] Contradictory results have been found regarding a possible increase in plasma β-thromboglobulin.[31,32] Plasma factor VII was enhanced, but plasma levels of fibrinopeptide A did not differ between normal subjects and patients with hypercholesterolemia (type IIa), hypertriglyceridemia (type IV) or mixed hyperlipoproteinemia (type IIb).[33]

Three studies have examined whether hyperlipidemia promotes thrombosis in experimental thrombosis models using perfusion chambers. The first study was performed in rabbits fed a cholesterol-rich diet resulting in a high cholesterol plasma level (15 g/L) : as compared to normal rabbits (plasma cholesterol = 0.66 g/L), there was a threefold increase in thrombus formation on the subendothelium of rabbit aorta exposed to blood flowing in the annular perfusion chamber at high wall shear rate (2600 s^{-1}).[34] However, this extremely high plasma cholesterol level is not classically reached in humans; plasma concentrations of 3-4 g/L are more commonly found. Two other studies were directly performed using blood from patients presenting different types of hyperlipoproteinemia. The first was done with the annular perfusion chamber, rabbit subendothelium, and anticoagulated blood,[35] and the second using the parallel-plate perfusion chamber, type III human collagen fibrils and native non-anticoagulated blood.[36] These two studies, which gave concordant results, showed that patients with type IIa and IIb hyperlipoproteinemia had increased platelet adhesion at high wall shear rates. However, thrombus volumes were comparable to normal healthy volunteers. Thus, the effect of hyperlipoproteinemia on thrombus formation appears dependent on the plasma cholesterol level and is detectable at very high lipid plasma levels.

Interestingly, we found that in one patient with type V dyslipidemia, a rare lipid disorder characterized by a high level of chylomicrons, platelet adhesion and thrombus volume were dramatically reduced to 21.1% and 0.8 $\mu m^3/\mu m^2$ as against 53.2±8.5% and 10.9±3.1 $\mu m^3/\mu m^2$ in healthy controls. This finding may be due to a direct effect of chylomicrons on platelet function.[30] It is also possible that chylomicrons, which are voluminous particles, may impede the interaction of platelets with the vessel wall. The rate of thrombotic events does not appear to be increased in this type of dyslipidemia.[37]

D. DIABETES MELLITUS

Platelets of patients with diabetes mellitus were shown to have an increased ability to form thromboxane A$_2$ and therefore to be hypersensitive to aggregating agents.[38] Plasma levels of fibrinogen, factor VII, and von Willebrand factor were increased. Thrombin generation was promoted with increased plasma concentration of fibrinopeptide A, independent of the type of diabetes or the presence of vascular complications.[39] The concentration of type I plasminogen activator inhibitor was also elevated, giving a state of hypofibrinolysis.[40]

The prothrombotic state of patients with insulin dependent diabetes mellitus has been evaluated in flow situations using the parallel-plate perfusion system.[41] Anticoagulated blood was recirculated over non-procoagulant (extracellular matrix of cultured human endothelial cells and human fibroblasts) and procoagulant (extracellular matrix of stimulated cultured human endothelial cells producing tissue factor) surfaces at wall shear rates of 300 and 1,300 s^{-1}. The thrombogenesis of patients with insulin-dependent type I diabetes mellitus with or without vascular disease, and age- and sex-matched controls was comparable.

E. NEPHROTIC SYNDROME

The nephrotic syndrome is frequently associated with thromboembolic complications. The hypercoagulable state is mostly characterized by a hypersensitivity of platelets to aggregating agents,[42] decreased plasma levels of antithrombin III[43] and a hyperfibrinogenemia.[44] Thrombin generation and fibrinopeptide A levels are also elevated.[44,45]

Anticoagulated blood of patients with nephrotic syndrome was perfused over various thrombogenic surfaces positioned in the annular or the parallel-plate perfusion chambers.[45] On proaggregant surfaces (i.e., de-endothelialized human umbilical artery segments and collagen-coated coverslips), platelet adhesion was normal but platelet thrombus formation was enhanced, though modestly, at both 300 and 1,300 s^{-1}. On a procoagulant surface (i. e., endothelial extracellular matrix expressing tissue factor), the fibrin formation and deposition were strongly increased at 1,300 s^{-1}. This finding was correlated with the plasma level of fibrinogen. In addition, an increased deposit of fibrin could be reproduced when plasma fibrinogen levels in normal blood were artificially increased. Thus, hyperfibrinogenemia was shown to be a major risk factor for thrombosis in this system; it may represent the main factor responsible for the prothrombotic state of patients with a nephrotic syndrome.

Table IV : Investigations of Prothrombotic States Using Perfusion Systems :
Characteristics of the Different Studies

Prothombotic State	Perfusion Chamber	Species	Thrombogenic Surface	Shear Rate (S⁻¹)	Perfusion Time (min)	Blood
Nephrotic Syndrom						
Zwaginga et al [45]	Annular Parralel-Plate	Human	Human Umb Art Sub Equine Coll ECM of End-PMA	300 & 1300 300 1300	5	Anticoagulated (Citrate) Anticoagulated (LMWH)
Antiphospholipid Antibodies						
Escolar et al [47]	Annular	Human	Rabbit Sub	800	10	Anticoagulated (Citrate)
Oosting et al [48]	Parralel-Plate	Human	ECM of End-TNF+APL	1300	5	Anticoagulated (LMWH)
Oestrogen Contraceptives						
Inauen et al [50]	Annular	Human	Rabbit Sub	650	5	Non-Anticoagulated
Inauen et al [51]	Annular	Human	Rabbit Sub	650	5	Non-Anticoagulated
Smoking						
Pilitto et al [52]	Annular	Human	Rabbit End	800	10	Anticoagulated (Citrate)
Roald et al [53]	Parrallel-Plate	Human	Human Collagen III	650 & 2600	5	Non-Anticoagulated
Desmopressin						
Sakariassen et al [55]	Annular	Human	Human Umb Art Sub	2500	3	Anticoagulated (Citrate)

Abbreviations : Sub = Subendothelium ; End = Endothelium ; ECM = Extracellular Matrix ; Umb Art = Umbilical Artery ; LMWH = Low Molecular Weight Heparin ; APL = Antiphospholipid Antibodies

F . ANTIPHOSPHOLIPID ANTIBODIES

The relationship between the presence of antibodies directed against negatively charged phospholipids and thrombosis in patients with systemic lupus erythematosus (SLE) is well established. These patients have a hypercoagulable state with increased thrombin generation: the plasma concentration of prothrombin fragments 1+2 and fibrinopeptide A is elevated independent of prior histories of thromboembolic diseases.[46]

A first study examined the effect of plasma from SLE patients with antiphospholipid antibodies in promoting thrombus formation in the annular perfusion chamber model at a wall shear rate of 800 s⁻¹: platelet deposition and platelet thrombus formation were significantly enhanced 1.5- and 2.5fold as compared to normal plasma or SLE plasma without antiphospholipid antibodies. This effect was reproduced with purified immunoglobulins.[47]

Another study examined whether the incubation of antiphospholipid antibodies from SLE patients with cultured endothelial cells enhanced the thrombogenicity of the corresponding extracellular matrix.[48] Antiphospholipid antibodies by themselves had negligible action but they markedly potentiated the action of tumor necrosis factor in making the matrix thrombogenic: this thrombogenicity was related to the greater expression of tissue factor by the endothelium in presence of antiphospholipid antibodies.

G . OESTROGEN CONTRACEPTIVES

Oestrogen contraceptives increase the risk of thromboembolic disease. Women who take oestrogen contraceptives have a hypercoagulable state, characterized notably by increased plasma levels of coagulation factors (notably fibrinogen, factors II, Vll, Vlll, IX and X), decreased antithrombin III and protein S and increased thrombin generation[49].

Native, non-anticoagulated blood of women taking oral contraceptives was perfused for 5 min at a wall shear rate of 650 s⁻¹ over the subendothelium of rabbit aorta positioned in the annular chamber model.[50] Thrombus volume and fibrin deposition were respectively two- and four-fold increased in women taking long-term treatment (more than 1 year) of relatively high doses of oestrogen (50 µg/day ethinyl estradiol) as compared to women not taking any medication. There was no correlation between abnormal values of blood coagulation (fibrinogen, antithrombin III, fibrinopeptide A) and fibrin deposition or thrombus volume, suggesting that these biological parameters were not indicative for this increased thrombogenesis. In a further study, the same authors showed that with lower doses (20 μg/day ethinyl oestradiol) or shorter treatment, the thrombogenesis was less markedly affected.[51]

H. SMOKING

Epidemiological studies have clearly shown the link between occlusive arterial disease and heavy cigarette smoking. The prothrombotic state induced by smoking has been investigated in two studies. In the first study, anticoagulated blood collected prior to and after smoking was recirculated over rabbit aorta placed in annular perfusion chambers.[52] Acute smoking caused platelet deposition and activation on the endothelium, whereas there was no platelet deposition before smoking.

Roald *et al* examined the effect of smoking on collagen induced thrombogenesis in flowing human non-anticoagulated blood.[53] The average thrombus volume in blood from smokers was nearly two-fold that observed in blood from non-smokers when the perfusion was made at 2,600 s^{-1}; there were no differences at a lower shear rate (650 s^{-1}).

I. DESMOPRESSIN

Clinical findings have questioned whether the administration of 1-deamino(8-d-arginine)vasopressin (DDAVP) or desmopressin would promote a prothrombotic state since, in rare cases, its administration has been followed by myocardial infarction.[54]

The prothrombotic effect of the administration of desmopressin in normal volunteers has been studied by Sakariassen *et al* using the annular perfusion chamber, segments of human umbilical arteries as thrombogenic surface, anticoagulated blood and a wall shear rate of 2,500 s^{-1}.[55] Platelet adhesion and platelet thrombus aggregates were increased 1.5 and 2 times, respectively, 90 min after the administration of desmopressin. Interestingly, the enhanced platelet adherence, but not the increase in platelet thrombus aggregates, was related to the quantitative increase in von Willebrand factor antigen.

Another study has shown that desmopressin increases the thrombogenicity of the extracellular matrix of cultured human endothelial cells: platelet deposition on the matrix perfused for 5 min at 800 s^{-1} was significantly higher when the endothelial cells synthesizing the matrix were pretreated with desmopressin for 3 hours.[56]

III. CONCLUSION

The results presented in this chapter show that models of experimental thrombosis using perfusion chambers may be helpful in assessing the prothrombotic state encountered in various clinical situations. Other prothrombotic states can be explored with these models. For example, it will be interesting to see if these models can be used to determine whether patients with deficiencies in antithrombin III, protein C or protein S have a prothrombotic state. However, it is not sure whether these tests, like those measuring biological markers of the hypercoagulable state, will be able to assess the prothrombotic state of individual patients.

In the future, easier methods of quantifying thrombus formation should be developed. A method that measures the pressure difference between the chamber entrance and exit has been described: the pressure difference decreases with time when thrombotic masses progressively occlude the lumen of the chamber.[57] This global method does not discriminate between the deposition of platelets, fibrin, leucocytes, and red cells, but may however be very valuable for a wider clinical use of the model.

Finally, most of the studies have been performed in laminar flow conditions. This rheologic condition may not quite reflect the type of flow present at sites of thrombosis. Thus, "stenotic" chambers are currently being developed to study thrombus formation in conditions mimicking vascular stenosis. Results produced with these new chambers may possibly be more relevant to *in vivo* thrombogenesis.

REFERENCES

1. **Baumgartner, H.R. and Muggli, R.,** Adhesion and aggregation: morphological demonstration and quantitation in vivo and in vitro, in *Platelets in biology and pathology,* Gordon J.L., Ed., North Holland, Amsterdam, 1976, 23.
2. **Sakariassen, K.S., Aarts, P.A.M.M., de Groot, P.G., Houdjik, W.P.M. and Sixma J.J.,** A perfusion chamber developed to investigate platelet interaction inflowing blood with human vessel wall cells, their extracellular matrix, and purified components, *J. Lab. Clin. Med.,* 102, 522,1983.
3. **Sakariassen, K.S., Joss R., Muggli R., Kuhn H., Tschopp T.B., Sage H. and Baumgartner H.R.,** Collagen type III induced ex vivo thrombogenesis in humans: role of platelets and leucocytes in deposition of fibrin, *Arteriosclerosis, 19,* 276, 1990.
4. **Kelly, A.B., Marzec, U.M., Krupski, W., Bass, A., Cadroy, Y., Hanson, S.R. and Harker, L.A.,** Hirudin interruption of heparin-resistant arterial thrombus formation in baboons, *Blood,* 77, 1006, 1991.
5. **Cadroy, Y., Horbett, T.A. and Hanson, S.R.,** Discrimination between platelet-mediated and coagulation mediated mechanisms in a model of complex thrombus formation in vivo, *J. Lab. Clin. Med.,* 113, 436, 1989.
6. **Hanson, S.R., Kotze, H.F., Savage, B. and Harker, L.A.,** Platelet interactions with Dacron vascular grafts: a model of acute thrombosis in baboons, *Arteriosclerosis,* 5, 595, 1985.
7. **Zwaginga, J.J., Sixma, J.J. and de Groot, P.G.,** Activation of endothelial cells induces platelet thrombus formation on their matrix. Studies of new in vitro thrombosis model with low molecular weight heparin as anticoagulant, *Arteriosclerosis,* 10, 49, 1990.
8. **Sakariassen, K.S., Muggli, R. and Baumgartner, H.R.,** Measurements of platelet interaction with components of the vessel wall in flowing blood, *Methods Enzymol,* 169, 37, 1989.
9. **Roux, S.P., Sakariassen, K.S., Turitto, V.T. and Baumgartner H.R.,** Effect of aspirin and epinephrine on experimentally induced thrombogenesis in dogs : a parallelism between in vivo and ex vivo thrombosis models, *Arterioscler. Thromb.,* 11,1182, 1991.
10. **Sakariassen, K.S., Weiss, H.J. and Baumgartner, H.R.,** Upstream thrombus growth impairs downstream thrombogenesis in non-anticoagulated blood: effect of procoagulant artery subendothelium and non-procoagulant collagen, *Thromb. Haemostas.,* 65, 596,1991.
11. **Sakarlassen, K.S., Kuhn, H., Muggll, R. and Baumgartner, H.R.,** Growth and stability of thrombi in flowing citrated blood : assessment of platelet-surface interactions with computer-assisted morphometry. *Thromb. Haemostas.,* 60, 392, 1988.
12. **Diquélou, A., Dupouy, D., Gaspln, D., Constans, J., Sié, P., Boneu, B., Sakariassen, K.S., Cadroy, Y.,** Role of endothelial tissue factor in human thrombogenesis: a comparative study between the apical surface of stimulated endothelium and their extracellular matrix, submitted to publication.
13. **Cadroy, Y. and Hanson, S.R.,** Effects of red blood cell concentration on hemostasis and thrombus formation in a primate model, *Blood,* 75, 2185, 1990.
14. **Clozel, M., Kuhn, H. and Baumgartner, H.R.,** Procoagulant activity of endotoxin-treated human endothelial cells exposed to native human flowing blood, *Blood,* 73, 729, 1989.
15. **Diquélou, A., Lemozy, S., Dupouy, D., Boneu, B., Sakarlassen, K.S. and Cadroy, Y.,** Effect of blood flow on thrombin generation is dependent on the nature of the thrombogenic surface, *Blood,* 84, 7, 2205, 1994.
16. **Savage, B., McFadden, P., Hanson, S.R. and Harker, L.A.,** The relation of platelet dlelnsity to platelet age: survival of low-and high-density 1 Indium-labeled platelets in baboons, *Blood,* 68, 386, 1986.
17. **Berk, P.D., Goldberg, J.D., Donovan, P.B., Frlchtman, S.M., Berlin, S.l. and Wasserman, L.R.,** Therapeutic recommendation in polycythemia vera based on PVSG protocols, *Semin. Haematol.,* 23, 132, 1986.
18. **Burch, G.E. and DePasquale, N.P.,** The hematocrit in patients with myocardial infarction, *J.A.M.A.,* 180, 63, 1962.
19. **Conley, C.L., Russell, R.P., Thomas, C.B and Tumulty, P.A.,** Hematocrit value in coronary artery disease, *Arch Intern Med,* 113,170, 1964.
20. **Hershberg, P.l., Wells, R.E. and McGandy, R.B.,** Hematocrit and prognosis in patients with acute myocardial infarction, *J.A.M.A.,* 219, 855, 1972.
21. **Lowe, G.D.O., Machado, S.G., Krol, W.F., Barton, B.A. and Forbes, C.D.,** White blood cell count and hematocrit as predictors of coronary recurrence after myocardial infarction, *Thromb. Haemostas.,* 54, 700,1985.
22. **Schlant, R.C., Forman, S., Stamler, J. and Canner, P.L.,** The natural history of coronary heart disease. Prognostic factors after recovery from MI in 2789 men, *Circulation,* 66, 401, 1982.
23. **Harrison, M.J.G., Kendall, B.E., Pollack, S. and Marshall, J.,** Effect of hematocrit on carotid stenosis and cerebral infarction, *Lancet,* 2, 114, 1981.
24. **Lowe, G.D.E., Forbes, D.S., Jaap, A.J.,** Relation of atrial fibrillation and high hematocrit to mortality in acute stroke, *Lancet,* 1, 784, 1983.
25. **Turitto, V.T. and Weiss H.J.,** Red blood cells: their dual role in thrombus formation, *Science,* 207, 541, 1980.
26. **Aarts, P.A.M.M., Bolhuis, P.A., Sakariassen, K.S., Heethaar, R.M. and Sixma, J.J.,** Redblood cell size is important for adherence of blood platelets to artery subendothelium, *Blood,* 62, 214, 1983.
27. **Hirsh, J. and Dacie, J.V.,** Persistent post-splenectomy thrombocytosis and thromboembolism: a consequence of continuing anemia, *Br. J. Haematol.,* 7, 44, 1966.
28. **Barnathan, E.S., Schwartz, J.S., Taylor, L., Laskey, W.K., Kleavaland, J.P., Kussmaul, W.G. and Hirshfeld Jr, J.W.,** Aspirin and dipyridamole in the prevention of acute coronary thrombosis complicating coronary angioplasty, *Circulation,* 76, 125, 1987.
29. **Baumgartner, H.R., Turitto, V. and Weiss, H.J.,** Effect of shear rate on platelet interaction with subendothelium in citrated and native blood. 11. Relationships among platelet adhesion, thrombus dimensions, and fibrin formation, *J. Lab. Clin. Med.,* 95, 208, 1980.
30. **Brook, J.G. and Aviram, M.,** Platelet lipoprotein interactions. *Semin. Thromb. Hemost.,* 14, 258, 1988.
31. **Zahavi, J., Betteridge, J.D., Jones, N.A.G., Galton, D.J. and Kakkar, V.V.,** Enhanced in vivo platelet release reaction and malondialdehyde formation in patients with hyperlipidemia, *Am. J. Med.,* 70, 59, 1981.
32. **Pumphrey, C.W. and Dawes, J.,** Plasma ß-thromboglobulin as a measure of platelet activity. Effect of risk factors and findings in ischemic heart disease and after acute myocardial infarction, *Am. J. Cardiol, .* 50, 1258, 1982.
33. **Nossel, H.L., Smith, F.R., Seplowitz, A.H., Dell, R.B., Sciacca, R.R., Merskey, C. and Goodman, D.S.,** Normal levels of fibrinopeptide A in patients with primary hyperlipidemia, *Circ. Res.,* 45, 347, 1979.
34. **Badimon, J.J., Badlmon, L., Turitto, V.T. and Fuster, V.,** Platelet deposition at high shear rates is enhanced by high plasma cholesterol levels. In vivo study in the rabbit model, *Arterioscler. Thromb. 11,* 395, 1991.

35. **Tandon, N., Hoeg, J.M., Rodbard, D. and Jamleson, G.A.,** Perfusion studies on the formation of mural thrombi with cholesterol-modified and hypercholesterolemic platelets, J. *Lab. Clin. Med.,* 105, 157, 1985.

36. **Cadroy, Y., Lemozy, S., Diquélou, A., Ferrières, J., Douste-Blazy, P., Boneu, B. and Sakarlassen, K.S.,** Human type 11 hyperlipoproteinemia enhances platelet collagen adhesion in flowing non-anticoagulated blood, *Arterioscler. Thromb.,* 13, 1650, 1993.

37. **Fruchart, J.C. and Sheperd, J.,** Lipoproteins in disease: Classification of the hyperlipoproteinemias, in *Human plasma lipoproteins,* de Gruyter, W., New York, 1989, 3.

38. **Mustard, J.F. and Packham, M.A.,** Platelets and diabetes mellitus (editorial), *N. Engl. J. Med.,* 311, 665,1984.

39. **Ford, 1., Singh, T.P., Kitchen, S., Makris, M., Ward, J.D. and Preston, F.E.,** Activation of coagulation in diabetes mellitus in relation to the presence of vascular complications, *Diabetic Med.,* 8, 322, 1990.

40. **Juhan-Vague, 1. Alessi, M.C.,** Plasminogen activator inhibitor 1 and atherothrombosis, *Thromb. Haemostas.,* 70, 138, 1993.

41. **Nievelstein, P.F.A.M., Sixma, J.J., Ottenhof-Rovers, M., Wynne, H.J., de Groot P.G. and Banga, J.D.,** Platelet adhesion and aggregate formation in type I diabetes under flow condition, *Diabetes,* 40,1410, 1991.

42. **Machleidt, C., Mettang, T., Starz, E., Weber, J., Risler, T. and Kuhlmann, U.,** Multifactorial genesis of enhanced platelet aggregability in patients with nephrotic syndrome, *J. Clin. Int.,* 36, 1119, 1989.

43. **Kaufmann, R.H., Veltkamp, J.J., van Tilburg, N.H., van Es, L.A.,** Acquired antithrombin III deficiency and thrombosis in the nephrotic syndrome, *Am. J. Med.,* 65,607, 1978.

44. **Sagripanti, A., Cupisti, A., Ferdhegini, M., Pinori, E. and Barsotti, G.,** Molecular markers of hemostasis activation in nephrotic syndrome, *Nephron,* 51, 25, 1989.

45. **Zwaginga, J.J., Koomans, H.A., Sixma, J.J. and Rabelink, T.J.,** Thrombus formation and platelet-vessel wall interaction in the nephrotic syndrome under flow conditions, *J. Clin. Invest.,* 93, 204, 1994.

46. **Ginsberg, J.S., Demers, C., Brlll-Edwards, P., Johnston, M., Bona, R., Burrows, R.F., Weltz, J. and Denburg, J.A.,** Increased thrombin generation and activity in patients with systemic lupus erythematosus and anticardiolipin antibodies : evidence for a prothrombotic state, *Blood,* 81, 2958,1993.

47. **Escolar, G., Font, J., Reverter, J.C., Lopez-Soto, A., Garrldo, M., Cervera, R., Ingelmo, M., Castillo, R. and Ordlnas, A.,** Plasma from systemic lupus erythematosus patients with antiphospholipid antibodies promotes platelet aggregation. Studies in a perfusion system, *Arterioscler. Thromb.,* 12, 196, 1992.

48. **Oostlng, JD, Derksen, R.H.W.M., BlokziJl, L., Sixma, J.J., de Groot, P.**G., Antiphospholipid antibody positive sera enhance endothelial cell procoagulant activity. Studies in a thrombosis model, *Thromb. Haemostas.,* 68, 278, 1992.

49. **Wessler, S., Gltel, S.N.,** Thrombotic complications of oral contraceptives, in *Hemostasis and Thrombosis. Basic principles and clinical practice,* 2nd ed., Colman, R.W., Hirsh, J., Marder, V.J. and Salzman, E.W., Eds., J.B. Lippincott Company, Philadelphia, 1987, 1158.

50. **Inauen, W., Baumgartner, H.R., Haeberll, A. and Straub, P.W.,** Excessive deposition of fibrin, platelets and platelet thrombi on vascular subendothelium during contraceptive drug treatment, *Thromb. Haemostas.* 57, 306, 1987.

51. **Inauen, W., Stocker, G., Haeberll, A. and Straub, P.W.,** Effects of low and high dose oral contraceptives on blood coagulation and thrombogenesis induced by vascular subendothelium exposed to flowing human blood, *Contraception,* 43, 435, 1991.

52. **Pittilo, R.M., Clarke, J.M.F., Harrls, D., Mackle, I.J., Rowles, P.M., Machln, S.J. and Woolf, N.,** Cigarette smoking and platelet adhesion, *Br. J. Haematol.,* 58, 627, 1984.

53. **Roald, H.E., Orvlm, U., Bakken, I.J., Barstad, R.M., Klerulf, P. and Sakariassen, K.S.,** Modulation of thrombotic responses in moderated stenosed arteries by cigarette smoking and aspirin ingestion. *Arterioscler. Thromb.,* 14, 617, 1994.

54. **Mannuccl, P.M. and Lusher, J.M.,** Desmopressin and thrombosis, *Lancet,* 2, 675, 1989.

55. **Sakarlassen, K.S., Cattaneo, M., van der Berg, A., Ruggerl, Z.M. and Sixma, J.J.,** DDAVP enhances platelet adherence and platelet aggregate growth on human artery subendothelium, *Blood,* 64, 229, 1984.

56. **Galvez, A., Diaz-Ricart, M., Gomez G., Escolar, G., Castlllo, R. and Ordinas, A.,** DDAVP increases the thrombogenicity of the extracellular matrix of cultured human endothelial cells, *Thromb. Haemostas.,* 69, 1049 (abstr 1803), 1993.

57. **Baumgartner, H.R. and Sakariassen, K.S.,** Factors controlling thrombus formation on arterial lesions, *Ann. NY. Acad. Sci.,* 454,162, 1985.

Fundamental Aspects and Laboratory Approaches

B. Diagnostic Strategies and Laboratory Approaches

LABORATORY DIAGNOSIS OF HEREDITARY THROMBOPHILIA

F.E. Preston and M. Greaves
Haematology, Royal Hallamshire Hospital, Sheffield

Clinical risk factors for venous thromboembolism have been recognised for many years. Although it has long been suspected that other basic physiological abnormalities may be additional risk factors for thrombosis, the identification of these has until recently been somewhat elusive. Within recent years the emergence of familial thrombophilia and also the antiphospholipid syndromes as important causes of thrombosis has focused attention on the vital physiological role of coagulation inhibitors, and as a direct consequence of this our understanding of fundamental pathophysiological mechanisms which predispose to venous thromboembolism have been considerably advanced. Nowadays, an increasing number of laboratory investigations are required for the investigation of individuals with thrombophilia, (a predisposition to venous thromboembolism). These include tests of haemostasis and, in selected individuals, of molecular genetic analysis. This chapter is devoted to the investigation and diagnosis of individuals with familial thrombophilia.

I. FAMILIAL THROMBOPHILIA

Normally, the haemostatic mechanism consists of finely balanced interactions between cellular and fluid components of the vascular system and represented, somewhat artificially, by the coagulation and fibrinolytic systems. Familial thrombophilia could theoretically be caused by any genetically determined defect which produces increased fibrin formation through accelerated thrombin production or impaired fibrin dissolution. The former could be a consequence of either enhanced procoagulant or reduced inhibitor activity. The same effect could also occur through impaired fibrinolysis, either through increased fibrinolytic inhibition or reduced profibrinolytic activity. Other possible causes of inherited thrombophilia are genetically determined abnormalities of fibrinogen which result in abnormal fibrin formation.

The demonstration of an isolated abnormality of coagulation in an individual with thrombosis is not, by itself, sufficient evidence of an association between the two. In order to establish a causal relationship between any abnormality of coagulation or fibrinolysis and familial thrombophilia, it is necessary for a number of criteria to be satisfied. It is clearly important to demonstrate, through family studies, that the observed laboratory abnormality is an inherited defect and that within the pedigree the abnormality cosegregates with thrombosis. Since index cases are highly selected it is also important to demonstrate that the significant relationship between laboratory abnormality and thrombosis persists even after the proband has been excluded from the analysis. If the above criteria are applied to possible candidate risk factors for familial thrombophilia, a true relationship between the laboratory abnormality and increased thrombotic risk has been established for only a very small number. These are deficiencies of protein C, protein S, antithrombin and, the recently described activated protein C (APC) resistance.

Inherited deficiency of plasminogen is of some interest since a relationship between this disorder and thrombosis remains unproven despite a number of reports of venous thromboembolism in individuals with both familial hypo- (type I) and dysplasminogenaemia (type II) [1,2,3,4]. However, in virtually all of the pedigrees in which the association was reported, the thrombotic manifestations were confined to the propositus and this led to doubts as to whether familial hypoplasminogenaemia was a risk factor for thrombosis[4].

Further evidence to support this view was obtained by Shigekiyo[5] in 1992, who reported that in two large unrelated pedigrees with familial type I plasminogen deficiency a history of thrombosis was obtained in only 3 of 21 affected individuals. There was no significant difference in the incidence of thrombosis between those who did and those who did not have the disorder.

Similar reservations may be expressed about a possible relationship between familial dysplasminogenaemia (type II plasminogen deficiency) and venous thromboembolism. In the large pedigree described by Aoki and co-workers[2], and which included a female with an extremely low plasminogen level and who was therefore probably homozygous for the disorder, a history of thrombosis was obtained only in the proband. The severely affected female is now in her twenties and remains thrombosis-free[6]. To date there is little convincing evidence to support the view that in isolation either familial hypo- or dysplasminogenaemia are risk factors for venous thromboembolism.

Although a relationship between defective fibrinolysis and venous thrombosis might be anticipated there are, to date, no convincing data to support this view. One family has been described in which thrombosis appeared to cosegregate with impaired fibrinolytic activity of the vessel wall[7], but there has been no confirmation of this defect using more recently developed assays of tissue plasminogen activator (tPA) and plasminogen activator inhibitor. Although Mannucci and Tripodi[8] have described families in which thrombosis was considered to relate to impaired release of tissue plasminogen activator following venous occlusion or the administration of deamino-D-arginine vasopressin (DDAVP) clear evidence of a causal relationship between genetically determined abnormalities of synthesis or release of tPA or plasminogen activator inhibitor are still awaited. Similarly, there is no convincing evidence that familial abnormalities of histidine-rich glycoprotein are associated with an increased thrombotic risk[9].

Heparin cofactor II, a thrombin inhibitor, is another potential candidate which has failed to meet the necessary criteria for acceptance as a risk factor for thrombosis. Although both arterial and venous thrombosis has been reported in pedigrees with familial heparin cofactor II deficiency[10,11], more detailed studies have failed to demonstrate a convincing relationship between the disorder and thromboembolism. Bertina and his coworkers[12], for example, demonstrated that familial heparin cofactor II deficiency is equally prevalent amongst healthy subjects and those with a history of thrombosis. On the available evidence inherited heparin cofactor II deficiency cannot be considered a risk factor for venous thromboembolism.

Abnormalities of the recently described lipoprotein-associated coagulation inhibitor (LACI) which inhibits the factor VIIa tissue factor complex could be reasonably assumed to be associated with thrombosis but to date, there has been no evidence to support this view. In an attempt to identify an association between thrombosis and genetically determined abnormalities of LACI, Reitsma[13] performed sequence analysis of the exons from the LACI gene from samples obtained from 30 individuals with familial thrombophilia. However, no mutations were detected.

There have been a number of reports of thrombosis associated with dysfibrinogenaemia and Gladson[3], in their study of patients with venous thromboembolism, reported that the defect was responsible for 1% of unexplained thrombosis in young adults. In many instances the situation is somewhat analogous to that associated with plasminogen deficiency in that thrombosis is confined to the proband. However, in some pedigrees there does appear to be a genuine association between thrombophilia and the coagulation defect. The pedigrees of fibrinogen Vlissingen[14] and fibrinogen Frankfurt IV, which share the same mutation, are of particular interest since the defect is associated with both venous and arterial thrombosis. Any relationship between familial dysfibrinogenaemia and thrombophilia might thus depend on the underlying genetic defect.

A marked thrombotic tendency is present in individuals with the rare autosomal recessive disorder homocystinuria, and by the age of 30 almost half of affected individuals will have experienced a thrombotic event[15]. Both venous and arterial thrombosis may occur and it is now believed that homocysteinaemia is an independent risk factor for arterial vascular disease. The mechanism(s) by which homocysteine induces thrombosis is not entirely clear but one possible mechanism could be inhibition of protein C activation by homocysteine at endothelial cell surfaces[16]. It is of interest to speculate whether a thrombotic risk is associated with the heterozygous state for cystathione beta synthase deficiency, the enzyme deficiency mainly responsible for homocystinuria.

Although a number of groups have suggested that an association exists between genetically determined factor XII deficiency and thrombosis[17,18], there are to date insufficient published data to support this view.

II. PROTEIN C DEFICIENCY

Protein C is a vitamin K-dependent glycoprotein which is synthesised by the liver. By degrading the activated clotting factors V and VIII it functions as one of the major inhibitors of the coagulation system. The inhibitor was first isolated from plasma by Stenflo in 1976[19]. It was designated protein C on account of it being the third protein to be eluted from the ion exchange chromatogram. During 1976 also, Seegers and coworkers[20] demonstrated that the activated form of the inhibitor was identical to the anticoagulant autoprothrombin IIA that they themselves had described 16 years previously. The anticoagulant properties of protein C are achieved through activation on endothelial cell surfaces by a thrombin-thrombomodulin complex[21]. In addition to inactivating factors Va and VIIIa, activated protein C (APC) also destroys platelet prothrombinase activity by degrading platelet-bound factor Va at the receptor for factor Xa. The inhibitory effects of APC are achieved through the cofactor activity of another vitamin K-dependent inhibitor, protein S.

The diagnosis of familial thrombophilia requires the demonstration, by laboratory testing, of an unequivocal presence of an accepted risk factor for thrombophilia, a positive family history and exclusion of an acquired defect. Although it might reasonably be anticipated that a detailed clinical history will predict a diagnosis of familial thrombophilia, this was not borne out in a study conducted by Heijboer et al in 1990[22] of 277 consecutive, unselected patients with deep vein thrombosis. Although a positive family history was obtained in 67 of the 277 subjects, a specific abnormality was confirmed in only 11 of these. In this study, although an inherited defect was demonstrated in approximately one quarter of the subjects studied this was only predicted by a clinical history in 4%. One possible explanation for these findings is that we are currently unable to diagnose all genetically determined factors which predispose to thrombosis. It should be appreciated that the study by Heijboers et al (1990)[22] antedated the discovery of activated protein C and its subsequent recognition as the commonest cause of familial thrombophilia.

On the basis of phenotypic analysis, employing functional and immunological assays, familial protein C deficiency can be classified into two types. These comprise the commoner type 1 defects which are characterised by parallel reductions of functional and immunoreactive protein C and the type II variants in which protein C levels by functional assays are substantially lower than those obtained with immunoreactive assays, the latter often being within the normal range.

The correct identification of heterozygotes for any familial disorder of haemostasis is clearly of great clinical importance and necessitates the evaluation of an individual's result against an accurately derived reference range. For this reason, laboratories involved in this diagnostic area are strongly recommended to establish their own normal ranges.

In healthy individuals, protein C levels range from 0.65 U/ml to 1.45U/ml. However, this oversimplifies the true situation since protein C concentrations are greatly influenced by a number of factors, particularly age, sex and oral contraceptive usage[23,24]. The variation with age is most marked in young adult males in whom protein C levels show a significant increase between the age bands 15-19 years and 45-49 years[23]. Protein C levels are lower in premenopausal women than in men but the use of oral contraceptives is associated with an increase of 0.05-0.08 U/ml of protein C activity[23]. These physiological variations have important diagnostic implications and if ignored may result in the misclassification of individuals under investigation. It is for this reason that Tait and his colleagues (1993)[23] recommended the use of age and sex restricted reference ranges when interpreting protein C results. Although we agree with these sentiments, the establishment of restricted normal ranges by individual laboratories is probably an unachievable goal, since the majority of UK laboratories do not establish their own, even approximately derived, normal values.

Most heterozygotes have protein C levels of approximately 50% of normal but another diagnostic dilemma relates to the overlap of protein C activity which occurs between heterozygotes with relatively high protein C levels and normal individuals with protein C concentrations at the lower end of the normal range. Consequently, the latter group may be misdiagnosed as having protein C deficiency while true heterozygotes may be considered normal. In a study from The Netherlands, Allaart and her colleagues (1993)[25] reported considerable overlap between the protein C activities of 60 genetically confirmed heterozygotes and 83 normal individuals not on anticoagulant therapy. When normal frequency distribution curves were fitted for both groups the degree of overlap was such that 15% of heterozygotes would have escaped identification and 5% of normal individuals would have been misclassified as having protein C deficiency. From the above observations it is clear that most diagnostic laboratories will be unable to identify, with certainty, heterozygotes for protein C deficiency, since this requires the additional sophistication of DNA analysis. For this reason Allaart and co-workers[25], and also Pabinger et al (1992)[26] explored the possibility of optimising the discrimination between heterozygotes and normal individuals through additional assays and a combination of these. Although the former group reported that discrimination was improved using the combined measurement of factor II antigen with either protein C antigen or activity a degree of overlap was still apparent. It is doubtful whether such a procedure will be adopted by nonspecialist laboratories.

III. PROTEIN C AND ORAL ANTICOAGULATION

The laboratory diagnosis of familial protein C deficiency in warfarinised individuals is a particularly difficult problem since protein C, a vitamin K-dependent protein, is also affected by this drug. Thus, plasma levels of protein C are reduced in an identical manner to those of the other vitamin K dependent clotting factors II, VII, IX and X. Since protein C has a short half life of approximately 6 hours its plasma concentration falls rapidly following the introduction of coumarin therapy. This almost certainly has some bearing on the development of coumarin-induced skin necrosis which has been reported in a few patients with protein C deficiency[27,28]. It is likely that the initial rapid fall in protein C causes a temporary dissociation between protein C levels and those of the other vitamin K-dependent clotting factors The ensuing hypercoagulable state results in thrombosis within the subcutaneous microvasculature.

In stably anticoagulated patients the degree of reduction of protein C, and other vitamin K-dependent proteins, is proportional to the degree of intensity of anticoagulation and discrepant values are obtained between functional and immunoreactive assays. The discrepant results relate to the presence of decarboxylated forms of the vitamin K-dependent proteins which have markedly impaired functional activity but have normal or near normal immunoreactivity. Consequently, in orally anticoagulated patients, functional protein C activities are lower than the corresponding protein C antigen levels.

One approach to the diagnosis of protein C deficiency in orally anticoagulated patients is to examine the relationship between protein C levels and those of other vitamin K-dependent clotting factors. In order to assess this it is necessary to establish normal ranges for each of these proteins, including protein C, in patients without familial thrombophilia but who are stably anticoagulated. Subjects with protein C deficiency could therefore be expected to have protein C levels which are disproportionally low, relative to the vitamin K-dependent clotting factors.

In a study designed to examine the validity of this concept, Allaart and her colleagues measured functional and immunoreactive forms of the vitamin K-dependent proteins, including protein C, in anticoagulated patients with DNA proven protein C deficiency and compared the results with those obtained from anticoagulated protein S deficient control subjects. Using the same approach as they had adopted for non-anticoagulated heterozygotes for protein C deficiency they studied the degree of overlap in the results of different laboratory tests in the two groups. They observed that if the analysis is confined to protein C assays alone then protein C activity levels show a higher degree of overlap than protein C antigen levels. As with non-anticoagulated protein C deficient heterozygotes discrimination between the groups is increased if an additional assay is included in the analysis. Allaart et al discovered that the best discrimination between heterozygotes and normal individuals occurred with the combination of protein C antigen by ELISA and factor VII activity. This combination also produced the smallest percentage (10%) of heterozygotes above the lower limit of the normal (anticoagulated) range. Although this approach undoubtedly produces a useful degree of discrimination between heterozygotes and normal individuals, it should be appreciated that a certain diagnosis of protein C deficiency by this method is not possible. For those laboratories wishing to engage in this diagnostic area the best approach is to establish their own individual control values in anticoagulated patients, using those assays and methods with which they are particularly familiar.

IV. PROTEIN S DEFICIENCY

The vitamin K-dependent protein S is a non-enzymatic co-factor of activated protein C[29]. It is synthesised by the liver and also by endothelial cells[30]. In addition, it is also found in platelet alpha granules[31].

In plasma, protein S circulates in two forms. Approximately 65% of the total protein S is complexed with C4b-binding protein (C4bBP) and as such is unavailable as a co-factor for activated protein C. The remaining 35%, designated free protein S, remains uncomplexed and is the active moiety of the total circulating protein[32,33,34]. The bio-availability of protein S is closely linked to the concentration of C4bBP and through its interaction with protein S it acts as an important regulatory protein in the APC-PS inhibitory pathway. Thus, high affinity binding between protein S and C4bBP results in low levels of free protein S when the acute phase reactant C4bBP is increased or when total protein S is reduced. Conversely, low concentrations of C4bBP result in increased levels of free protein S[35,36]. On the basis of phenotypic data, familial protein S deficiency can be subdivided into three main types. Type 1 defects are characterised by a reduction in total protein S. Since this is mainly bound to C4bBP free protein S is also greatly reduced. In type II defects impaired protein S function relates to an abnormal molecular structure[37]. Although it can be anticipated that such abnormalities exist the picture has recently become confused by the observation that functional protein S assays are markedly affected by activated protein C (APC) resistance and that previously reported pedigrees with apparent type II protein S deficiency have been rediagnosed as having familial APC resistance[38,39]. Type III protein S deficiency is the least common inherited disorder and occurs as a consequence of altered binding characteristics between protein S and C4bBP. Low levels of free protein S occur as a consequence of the equilibrium between free and complexed protein S being shifted toward the bound form[40].

A precise diagnosis of familial protein S deficiency is somewhat hampered by the necessity to employ immunoreactive assays for both free and total protein S. Although functional protein S assays are available the recent demonstration that they are markedly affected by APC resistance indicates the necessity for some reappraisal of this methodology.

Although DNA analysis may be used to identify some heterozygotes with protein S deficiency, this approach is usually less rewarding than when applied to the detection of familial protein C or antithrombin deficiency. There are two highly homologous genes for protein S, both being located on chromosome 3[41]. The active gene, PS alpha, possesses 15 exons whereas the pseudogene, PS beta, comprises a number of missense, nonsense and splice site mutations which render gene expression impossible[41].

The prevalence of protein S deficiency within the general population is still uncertain since to date the published studies have focused solely on subjects and pedigrees with a history of thrombosis. For subjects presenting with venous thromboembolism the prevalence of protein S deficiency is within the range 4.8-8%,[42,43,3]. From individuals identified in this manner, Gladson et al (1988)[3] calculated the prevalence of protein S deficiency to be approximately 1 in 29 000 but for the reasons described earlier in respect of protein C deficiency, this is likely to be an underestimate.

In normal subjects the plasma concentrations of total protein S antigen are within the range 0.67-1.25 U/ml and free protein S antigen 0.23-0.49 U/ml with slightly higher values occurring in men[34]. In establishing a diagnosis of familial protein S deficiency it is essential to exclude acquired deficiencies of the coagulation inhibitor and also to take into consideration important physiological changes which might give rise to diagnostic confusion. In this regard the most important are the changes which occur during pregnancy when protein S concentrations fall progressively with lowest values occurring between 18 and 28 weeks [45,44]. Protein S levels are also reduced, but to a lesser extent, in women taking oral contraceptives[46]. Markedly reduced protein S levels are observed in those receiving oestrogens for growth retardation[47]. Reduced levels of protein S are commonly observed in individuals with disseminated intravascular coagulation[34,48], renal disease[49] and in association with lupus anticoagulants and/or other antiphospholipid antibodies[50]. Individuals with liver disease also have reduced protein S levels but interestingly, the degree of reduction of both free and total protein S is less than that of the other vitamin K-dependent proteins[34,48]. As with protein C, the diagnosis of familial protein S deficiency in orally anticoagulated individuals is extremely difficult since protein S levels are reduced in parallel with the other vitamin K-dependent proteins. In order to establish a diagnosis it is necessary to adopt an approach similar to that described previously in respect of protein C. As with protein C deficiency, in orally anticoagulated individuals a diagnosis of familial protein S deficiency cannot be established with certainty without recourse to genetic analysis. Protein S levels may be reduced in subjects with sickle cell disease and in male cigarettte smokers[51].

V. FAMILIAL ANTITHROMBIN DEFICIENCY

Antithrombin, a glycoprotein with a molecular weight of approximately 50 000 and synthesised by the liver, is the most important physiological inhibitor of the serine proteases. Its name is somewhat misleading since it inhibits not only thrombin but also the activated clotting factors IXa, Xa, XIa and XIIa. The inhibitory activity of antithrombin occurs through the formation of a 1:1 stoichiometric complex involving arginine of antithrombin and serine at the active site of the target serine protease. The rate of complex formation between antithrombin and serine protease is markedly accelerated by both heparin and heparan sulphate proteoglycans, the latter being located at endothelial cell surfaces. The observations that heparin and heparan sulphate proteoglycans exert similar effects and through similar mechanisms on antithrombin/serine protease complex formation[52] led Rosenberg (1989)[53] to postulate that the inhibition of serine proteases by antithrombin occurs at endothelial cell surfaces following an initial binding of a fraction of plasma antithrombin to heparan sulphate proteoglycans at the endothelial cell surface.

The clinical importance of antithrombin deficiency was first recognised in 1965 by Egeberg[54] who reported, in a Norwegian family, the association between familial antithrombin deficiency and venous thromboembolism. Although this relationship has been confirmed by numerous groups in pedigrees from many different parts of the world[55,56,57], the prevalence of familial antithrombin deficiency within the general population remains unclear with estimates varying widely from 1:2000 to 1:40000[58,56,3,57]. More recently Tait et al, 1991[59], reporting on asymptomatic Scottish blood donors, suggested that the prevalence of antithrombin deficiency in this group was 1:350. As with prevalence studies of familial protein C deficiency these widely differing estimates largely relate to differences in study design and selection bias. Most groups do, however, agree that familial antithrombin deficiency accounts for approximately 2-5% of patients under the age of 45 years presenting with venous thromboembolism.

Following a study of almost 10 000 healthy blood donors, Tait et al in 1993[60], concluded that the distribution of antithrombin within the general population is approximately gaussian with a mean value of 105.6 i.u./dl. Lower values were observed in premenopausal women than in men of the same age, but in later life the position is reversed with higher values being observed in postmenopausal women than either premenopausal women or in men of corresponding age. Oral contraceptive usage is associated with a small reduction in antithrombin in younger women but not in those over 30 years of age[60]. The minor effects exerted by age and sex were considered by the authors to be insufficient to warrant the establishment of separate reference ranges but great care should be exercised in the interpretation of borderline normal or abnormal results. As with other familial disorders, the accurate identification of heterozygotes may necessitate detailed family screening with or without gene analysis. Based on the results of functional and immunoreactive assays, familial antithrombin deficiency is generally classified into two main groups. Type 1 deficiency, is characterised by parallel reductions of both functional and immunological assays which reflects impaired synthesis of a structurally normal protein. This type is by far the commonest cause of antithrombin deficiency, accounting for 80-90% of reported cases[61]. Type II antithrombin deficiency, which accounts for the remainder, reflects the production of a structurally abnormal protein and is usually recognised by discrepant phenotypic results, characterised by reduced functional antithrombin activity associated with a normal or near normal antithrombin antigen level.

Within the last decade, our understanding of the molecular basis of antithrombin deficiency has been greatly facilitated by advances made in the molecular biology and functional characterisation of this important coagulation inhibitor[62,63,64]. Of particular importance was the recognition that the antithrombin molecule possesses two important functional domains, viz. a heparin-binding domain and a thrombin-binding domain. Type II defects could therefore occur as a consequence of point mutations which affected the heparin and/or the thrombin binding properties of the inhibitor molecule.

Many antithrombin variants have been described since the disorder was first reported by Sas et al in 1974[65]. To simplify the growing complexity of type II antithrombin deficiency states, a number of groups have proposed classification systems[66,67,68], but since these systems differ between themselves, the problem is still not completely resolved. We consider that the system proposed by Lane et al (1992)[68] is the most acceptable and is summarised as follows:

   a) subtype IIa: functional abnormalities affecting both reactive (thrombin-binding) site and heparin-binding site.
   b) subtype IIb: functional abnormalities limited to the reactive site.
   c) subtype IIc: functional abnormalities limited to the heparin-binding site.

Two laboratory methods are commonly employed for the diagnosis of antithrombin deficiency. These are assays for heparin cofactor activity and progressive antithrombin activity. The progressive antithrombin activity is a measure of the proteinase activity of antithrombin in the absence of heparin. Heparin cofactor activity determines the rate of inactivation of factor Xa or thrombin by antithrombin in the presence of heparin. Employment of the two assays allows a distinction to be made between the different type II subtypes. Since the heparin cofactor assay reflects both of the functional domains of the antithrombin molecule, reduced heparin cofactor activity is a diagnostic feature of all antithrombin variants, irrespective of which of the two functional domains is affected. The progressive antithrombin assay is more specific in that impaired activity by this assay is indicative of an abnormality at the thrombin binding site. Progressive antithrombin activity is thus normal in variants with reduced heparin binding[68]. Crossed immunoelectrophoresis, performed in the presence of heparin, is of value in distinguishing abnormalities affecting the heparin binding site from reactive site defects[69].

It is important to appreciate that the distinction between variants resulting from abnormalities of the heparin binding and those involving reactive sites is of some clinical relevance since substantial differences exist in respect of their relative thrombotic risk[66,69]. The risk of venous thromboembolism in individuals with defects affecting the reactive site of the molecule is approximately 50-60%, which is similar to that asociated with a type 1 defect. Examples of such type IIb defects are Antithrombin: Sheffield, Glasgow, Northwick Park and Hamilton[69,61]. By contrast, the thrombotic risk associated with variants resulting from defects of the heparin binding site is substantially lower at 6%.

VI. ACTIVATED PROTEIN C (APC) RESISTANCE

APC resistance, a disorder which interferes with anticoagulant properties of activated protein C, was first described by Dahlbäck and colleagues in 1993[70]. This same group also demonstrated the familial nature of the disorder and also suggested that it was the commonest cause of inherited thrombophilia. These observations were confirmed by Koster et al (1993)[71], who reported a seven-fold increase in the risk of deep vein thrombosis in affected individuals. Moreover, the abnormality was also detected in 5% of healthy age and sex-matched control subjects. More recently, Bertina and his colleagues (1994)[72] have provided unequivocal evidence that APC resistance is strongly associated with heterozygous (or homozygous) inheritance of a single nucleotide transition (G1691A) in the factor V gene, resulting in the amino acid substitution of Arg[506] Gln at the factor V heavy chain APC cleavage site, Arg[506]-Gly 507. Confirmation of the genetic basis for APC resistance has also been provided by Voorberg et al (1994)[73], Zöller and Dahlbäck (1994)[74], and Beauchamp et al (1994)[75]. The loss of the APC cleavage site in factor V effectively reduces the anticoagulant properties of activated PC and shifts the haemostatic balance in favour of thrombin generation. Bertina et al (1994)[72] also reported that the allelic frequency of this FV mutation in the Dutch population is 2%, and that as a genetically determined risk factor for venous thromboembolism, it is at least 10 times more common that familial deficiences of PC, PS and AT. Using a different molecular genetic approach, the Sheffield group has independently characterised the molecular genetic basis of APC resistance and has demonstrated the factor V gene, G1691A mutation in 5/144 unrelated, healthy individuals[75]. In all cases the presence of the mutation was associated with APC resistance. Beauchamp et al 1994[75], have also confirmed the observation that protein S function is dependent upon APC and that APC resistance is associated with impaired functional protein S activity[38.]

The diagnosis of APC resistance is based on the prolongation in the activated partial thromboplastin time (APTT), following the addition of activated protein C. The results are expressed as a ratio of the clotting times obtained in the presence and absence of APC (APC Ratio). APC resistance is characterised by a low APC ratio. Particularly low values are seen in association with homozygosity for the genetic defect. Currently, it is not possible to test for the defect if the APTT in the absence of APC is prolonged. The test therefore cannot be performed in patients receiving intravenous heparin or anticoagulants.

REFERENCES

1.   **Lottenberg, R., Dolly, F.R., Kitchen, C.S.** Recurring thromboembolic disease and pulmonary hypertension associated with severe hypoplasminogenaemia. *Am.J.Hematol.,* 19: 181-193, 1985.
2.   **Aoki, N., Moroi, M., Sakata, Y., et al.** Abnormal plasminogen. A hereditary molecular abnormality found in a patient with recurrent thrombosis. *J.Clin.Invest.,* 61: 1186-1195, 1978.
3.   **Gladson, C.L., Scharrer, I., Hach, V., et al.** The frequency of type heterozygous protein S and protein C deficiency in 141 unrelated young patients with venous thrombosis. *Thromb.Haemost.,* 59: 18-22, 1988.
4.   **Dolan, G., Greaves, M., Cooper, P., et al.** Thrombovascular disease and familial plasminogen deficiency: a report of three kindreds. *Brit.J.Haematol.,* 70: 417-421, 1988.
5.   **Shigekiyo, T., Uno, Y., Tomonari, A., et al.** Type I congenital plasminogen deficiency is not a risk factor for thrombosis. *Thromb.Haemost.,* 67: 189-192, 1992.
6.   **Aoki, N.,** Personal communication, 1992.
7.   **Johansson, L., Hedner, U., Nilsson, I.M.** A family with thromboembolic disease associated with deficient fibrinolytic activity in vessel wall. *Acta.Med.Scand.,* 203: 477-480, 1978.
8.   **Mannucci, P.M., Tripodi, A.,** Inherited factors in thrombosis. *Blood Rev.,* 2: 27-35, 1988.
9.   **Engesser, L., Kluft, C., Briet, E., et al.** Familial elevation of plasma histidine-rich glycoprotein in a family with thrombophilia. *Br.J.Haematol.,* 67: 355-358, 1987.
10. **Tran, T.H., Narbet, G.A., Duckert, F.** Association of heparin cofactor II deficiency with thrombosis. *Lancet,* 2: 413-414, 1985.
11. **Sie, T., Tichou, J., Dupouy, D., et al.** Constitutional heparin cofactor II deficiency associated with recurrent thrombosis. *Lancet,* 2: 414-416, 1985.
12. **Bertina, R.M., van der Linden, I.K., Engesser, L., et al.** Hereditary heparin cofactor II deficiency and the risk of development of thrombosis. Thromb.Haemost., 57: 196-200, 1987.
13. **Reitsma, P.H.,** Personal communication, 1992.
14. **Koopman, J., Haverkate, F., Briet E., et al.** A congenitally abnormal fibrinogen (Vlissingen) with a 7-base deletion

in the gamma-chain gene, causing defective calcium binding and impaired fibrin polymerization. *J.Bio.Chem.,* 266: 13456-13461, 1991.

15. **Mudd, S.H., Skovby, F., Levy, H.L., et al.** The natural history of homocystinuria due to cystathionine beta-synthase deficiency, *Am.J.Hum.Genet.,* 37: 1-31, 1985.
16. **Rodgers, G.M., Conn, M.T.,** Homocysteine, an atherogenic stimulus, reduces protein C activation by arterial and venous endothelial cells. *Blood,* 75: 895-901, 1990.
17. **Mannhalter, C., Fischer, M., Hopmeier, P., et al.** Factor XII activity and antigen concentrations in patients suffering from recurrent thrombosis. *Fibrinolysis,* 1: 259-263, 1987.
18. **Lammle, B., Wuillemin, W.A., Huber, I., et al.** Thromboembolism and bleeding tendency in congenital factor XII deficiency - a study on 74 subjects from 14 Swiss families. *Thromb.Haemos.,* 65: 117-121, 1991.
19. **Stenflo, J.,** A new vitamin K dependent protein-purification from bovine plasma and preliminary characterisation, *J.Biol.Chem.,*251: 353-355, 1976.
20. **Seegers, W.H., Novoa, E., Henry, R.L., et al.** Relationship of 'new' vitamin K dependent protein C and 'old' autoprothrombin II-A. *Thromb.Res.,* 8: 543-552, 1978.
21. **Esmon, C.T., Owen, W.G.** Identification of an endothelial cell cofactor for thrombin-catalyzed activation of protein C. *Proc.Natl.Acad.Sci.USA.,* 78: 2249-2252, 1981.
22. **Heijboer, H., Brandjes, D.P.M., Buller, H.R., et al.** Deficiencies of coagulation-inhibiting and fibrinolytic proteins in outpatients with deep-vein thrombosis. *N.Engl.J.Med.,* 323: 1512-1516, 1990.
23. **Tait, R.C., Walker, I.D., Islam, S.I.A.M., et al.** Protein C activity in healthy volunteers, influence of age, sex, smoking and oral contraceptives. *Thromb.Haemost.,* 70(2): 281-285, 1993.
24. **Dolan, G., Neal, K., Cooper, P., Brown, P., Preston, F.E.** Protein C, antithrombin III and plasminogen: Effect of age, sex and blood group. *Brit.J.of Haematol.,* 86: 798-803, 1994.
25. **Allaart, R.C.F., Poort, S.R., Rosendaal, F.R., et al.** Increased risk for venous thrombosis in carriers of hereditary protein C deficiency defect. *Lancet,* 341: 134-138, 1993.
26. **Pabinger, I., Allaart, C.F., Hermans, J., et al.** Hereditary protein C deficiency: Laboratory values in transmitters and guidelines for the diagnostic procedure. *Thromb.Haemost.,* 68: 470-474, 1992.
27. **Broekmans, A.W., van der Linden, I.K., Veltkamp, J.J., et al.** Prevalence of isolated protein C deficiency in patients with venous thrombotic disease and in the population. *Thromb.Haemost.,* 50: 350 (Abstract), 1983.
28. **Samama, M., Horellou, M.H., Soria, J., et al.** Successful progressive anticoagulation in a severe protein C deficiency and previous skin necrosis at the initiation of oral anticoagulant treatment. *Thromb.Haem.,* 51: (Letter), 132-133, 1984.
29. **Walker, F.J.,** Regulation of activated protein C by protein S. The role of phospholipid in factor Va inactivation. *J.Biol.Chem.,* 256: 11128-11131, 1981.
30. **Fair, D.S., Marlar, R.A., Levine, E.G.** Human endotheliel cells synthesize protein S. *Blood,* 67: 1168-1171, 1986.
31. **Schwartz, H.P., Heeb, M.J., Wencel-Drake, J.S., Griffin, J.H.** Identification and quantitation of protein S in human platelets. *Blood,* 66: 1452, 1985.
32. **Dahlbäck, B.** Purification of human C4b-binding protein and formation of its complex with vitamin K-dependent protein S. *Biochem.J.,* 209: 847-856, 1983.
33. **Dahlbäck, B.** Inhibition of protein C cofactor function of human and bovine protein S by C4b-binding protein. *J.Bio.Chem.,* 261: 12022-12027, 1986.
34. **Bertina, R.M., van Wijngaarden, A., Reinalda Poot, J.** Determination of plasma protein S - the protein cofactor of activated protein C. *Thromb.Haemost.,* 53: 268-272, 1985.
35. **Griffin, J.H., Fernandez, J.A., Gruber, A.** Critical reevaluation of free protein S (PS) and C4b-binding protein (C4BP) levels and implications for thrombotic risk. *Thromb.Haemost.* 65: 711 (Abstract), 1991.
36. **Comp, P.C., Forristall, J., West, C.D., et al.** Free protein S levels are elevated in familial C4b-binding protein deficiency. *Blood,* 76: 2527-2529, 1990.
37. **Mannucci, P.M., Valsecchi, C., Krachmalnicoff, A., et al.** Familial dysfunction of protein S. *Thromb.Haemost.,* 62: 763-766, 1989.
38. **Faioni, E.M., et al.** Resistance to activated protein C in nine thrombophilic families: Interference in a protein S functional assay. *Thromb.Haemost.,* 70: 1067-1071, 1993.
39. **Cooper, P.C., Hampton, K.K., Makris, M., et al.** Further evidence that activated protein C resistance can be misdiagnosed as inherited functional protein S deficiency. *Brit.J.of Haematol.,* 88: 201-203, 1994.
40. **Comp, P.C., Doray, D., Patton, D., et al.** An abnormal plasma distribution of protein S occurs in function protein S deficiency. *Blood,* 67: 504-508, 1986.
41. **Ploos van Amstel, H.K., Reitsma, P.H., van der Logt, C.P. et al.** Intron-exon organization of the active human protein S gene PS alpha and its pseudogene PS beta: duplication and silencing during primate evolution. *Biochemistry.,* 29: 7853-7861, 1990.
42. **Pabinger, I., Karnik, R., Lechner, K., et al.** Coumarin induced acral skin necrosis associated with hereditary protein C deficiency. *Blut,* 52: 365-370, 1986.
43. **Broekmans, A.W., Bertina, R.M., Reinalda-Poot, J., et al.** Protein S deficiency and venous thromboembolism. A study in three Dutch families. *Thromb.Haemost.,* 53: 273-277, 1985.
44. **Malm, J., Laurell, M., Dahlbäck, B.** Changes in the plasma levels of vitamin K-dependent proteins C and S and of C4b-binding proteins during pregnancy and oral contraception. *Br.J.Haematol.,* 68: 437-443, 1988.
45. **Comp, P.C., Thurnau, G.R., Welsh, J., et al.** Functional and immunological protein S levels are decreased during pregnancy. *Blood,* 68: 881-885, 1986.
46. **Boerger, L.M., Morris, P.C., Thurnau, G.R., et al.** Oral contraceptives and gender affect protein S status. *Blood,* 69: 692-694, 1987.
47. **Huisveld, I.A., Greven, E.C.G., Bouma, B.N.** Protein C and protein S levels in tall girls treated with ethinyloestradiol. *Thromb.Haemost.,* 58: 406 (Abstract), 1987.
48. **D'Angelo, A., Vigano-D'Angelo, S., Esmon, C.T., et al.** Acquired deficiences of protein S. *J.Clin.Invest.,* 81: 1445-1454, 1988.
49. **Comp, P.C., Vigano-D'Angelo, A., Thurnau, G.R., et al.** Acquired protein S deficiency occurs in pregnancy, the nephrotic syndrome and systemic lupus erythematosus. *Blood,* 66: 348a (Abstract), 1985.
50. **Malia, R.G., Hill, M., Cooper, P., Greaves, M., Preston, F.E.** Measurement of Protein S in patients with the lupus anticoagulant. *Thromb.Haemost.,* 65: 1831, 1991.
51. **Scott, B.D., Esmon, C.T., Comp, P.C.** The natural anticoagulant protein S is decreased in male smokers. *Am.Heart J.,* 122: 76-80, 1991.

52.   **Marcum, J.A., McKenny, J.B., Rosenberg, R.D.** Acceleration of thrombin-anithrombin complex formation in rat hind quarters via heparin-like molecules bound to the endotheliem. *J.Clin.Invest.,* 74: 341-350, 1984.

53.   **Rosenberg, R.D.** Biochemistry of heparin antithrombin interactions, and the physiologic role of the natural anticoagulant mechanism. *Am.J.Med.,* 97 (Suppl. 3b): 2-9, 1989.

54.   **Egeberg, O.** Inherited antithrombin deficiency causing thrombophilia. *Thromb.Diath.Haemorrh.,* 13: 516-530, 1965.

55.   **Thaler, E., Lechner, K.,** Antithrombin III deficiency and thromboembolism. *Clin.Haematol.,* 10: 369-390, 1981.

56.   **Rosenberg, R.D.** Actions and interactions of antithrombin and heparin. *N.Eng.J.Med.,* 292: 146-151, 1975.

57.   **Vykidal, R., Korninger, C., Kyrir, P.A., et al.** The prevalence of antithrombin III deficiency in patients with a history of venous thromboembolism. *Thromb.Haemost.,* 54: 744-745, 1985.

58.   **Abildgaard, U.** Antithrombin and related inhibitors of coagulation. *In Poller L (Ed) Recent Advances in blood coagulation.* Churchill Livingstone, Edinburgh, 3: 151-173, 1981.

59.   **Tait, R.C., Walker, I.D., Perry, D.J., et al.** Prevalence of antithrombin III deficiency subtypes in 4000 healthy blood donors. *Thromb.Haemost.,* 65: 534 (Abstract), 1991.

60.   **Tait, R.C., Walker, I.D., Islam, S.I.A.M., McCall, F. et al.** Influence of demographic factors on antithrombin III activity in a healthy population. *Brit.J.of.Haematol.,* 84: 476-480, 1993.

61.   **Prochownik, E.V.** Molecular genetics of inherited antithrombin III deficiencies. *Am.J.Med.,* 87 (Suppl. 3B): 15-18, 1989.

62.   **Bock, S.C.,Wion, K.L., Vehar, G.A., et al.** Cloning and expression of the cDNA for human antithrombin III. *Nucleic Acids Res.,* 10: 8113-8125, 1982.

63.   **Prochownik, E.V., Markham, A.F., Orkin, S.H.** Isolation of the cDNA clone for the human antithrombin III. *J.Bio.Chem.,* 128: 8389-8394, 1983.

64.   **Chandra, T., Stackhouse, R., Chidd, V.J., et al.** Isolation and sequence characterisation of a DNA clone of human antithrombin III. *Proc.Natl.Acad.Sci.USA.,* 58: 1094, 1983.

65.   **Sas, Y., Blasko, G., Banhegyi, D, et al.** Abnormal antithrombin III (antithrombin III 'Budapest') as a cause of a familial thrombophilia. *Thromb.Diath.Haemorr.,* 32: 105-115, 1974.

66.   **Finazzi, G., Caccia, R., Barbui, T.** Different prevalence of thromboembolism in the subtypes of congenital antithrombin III deficiency: review of 404 cases. *Thromb.Haemost.,* 58: 1094, 1987.

67.   **Hultin, M.B., McKay, J., Abildgaard, U.** Antithrombin Oslo: type 1b classification of the first reported antithrombin-deficient family with a review of hereditary antithrombin variants. *Thromb.Haemost.,* 59: 468-473, 1988.

68.   **Lane, D.A., Olds, R.R., Thein, S-L.** Antithrombin III and its deficiency states. *Blood Coagulat.Fibrinol.,* 3: 315-342, 1992.

69.   **Lane, D.A., Caso, R.** Antithrombin III: structure, genomic organisation, function and inherited deficiency. *In Tuddenham E.G.D. (Ed) Clinical Haematology, vol 4(2). The molecular biology of coagulation,* Baillière-Tindall, London. 961-998, 1989.

70.   **Dahlbäck, B., et al.** Familial thrombophilia due to a previously unrecognised mechanism characterised by poor anticoagulant response to activated protein C. Prediction of a cofactor to activated protein C. *Proc.Natl.Acad.Sci.USA.,* 90: 1004-1008, 1993.

71.   **Koster, T., et al.** Venous thrombosis due to poor anticoagulant response to activated protein C: Leiden Thrombophilia Study. *Lancet,* 342: 1503-1506, 1993.

72.   **Bertina, R.M., et al.** Mutation in blood coagulation factor V associated with resistance to activated protein C. *Nature,* 369: 64-67, 1994.

73.   **Voorberg, J., et al.** Association of idiopathic venous thromboembolism with single point-mutation at Arg[506] of factor V. *Lancet,* 343: 1535-1536, 1994.

74.   **Zöller, B., Dahlbäck, B.,** Linkage between inherited resistance to activated protein C and factor V gene mutation in venous thrombosis. *Lancet,* 343: 1536-1538, 1994.

75.   **Beauchamp, N.J., et al.** High prevalence of a mutation in the factor V gene within the UK population: relationship to activated protein C resistance and familial thrombosis. *Brit.J.Haem.,* 1994.

DIAGNOSIS OF ACTIVATION STATES
OF CIRCULATING PLATELETS

M.C. Trzeciak, J.C. Bordet and M. Dechavanne
Hôpital Edouard Herriot, Lyon.

At the site of tissue injury, platelets undergo a variety of morphological and biochemical modifications. These changes include :

1) A change in shape with the formation of pseudopodia.

2) The secretion of stored granules, namely dense granules, α-granules and lysosomes.

3) The expression of new epitopes and binding sites for coagulation proteins on the cell surface.

In vitro, this activation process can be triggered by numerous agonists such as thrombin, collagen, epinephrine, ADP and platelet-activating factor.

Several assays have been proposed for the detection of in vivo platelet activation. They consist of the evaluation of morphological platelet changes, alteration of platelet function, biochemical platelet modifications and the release of platelet products into the plasma or urine [Table I]. This brief review will summarize the results obtained by clinical investigation with the most reliable markers of platelet activation.

I. MEASUREMENT OF PLASMA CONCENTRATIONS
OF SECRETED PLATELET PROTEINS

Following platelet activation a number of granule-bound proteins are secreted. Plasma levels of two specific platelet proteins, platelet factor 4 (PF4) and ß-thromboglobulin (ß-TG) may provide an index of platelet release in vivo.

PF4 is secreted from platelets as a tetramer of molecular weight 31,120 daltons and then bound to a proteoglycan carrier. The PF4-proteoglycan carrier complex binds to endothelial cells and activated platelets. Unfractionated heparin, but not low molecular weight heparin, induces the release of endothelium bound PF4. Unbound PF4-proteoglycan complex circulates in blood with a half-life of 3-4 minutes.

ß-TG designates 3 proteins immunologically indistinguishable, each of molecular weight 36,000 daltons, but with different isoelectric points. They all circulate as a tetramer with a half-life of 100 minutes. They are filtered in the glomeruli, taken up and cleared within proximal tubular cells.

A. ASSAYS

Technical problems related to sample collection and processing limit the clinical use of the measurement of these two markers. Blood must be drawn with only slight or no stasis. The first ml is discarded. A plastic tube containing 2.7 ml of blood is mixed with 0.3 ml of an aqueous anticoagulant mixture (78 mM EDTA, 10 mM theophyllin, 0.33 µg/ml, prostaglandin E_1, pH 7.4, mOsm 290 or 57 mM EDTA, 0.83 mM chloro-adenosin, 260 mM procaïne, pH 6.0, mOsm 740).[37,38] The aqueous anticoagulant mixture is stored at -70°C and then thawed just before blood sampling. The tube containing blood is inverted one time and cooled immediately in an icewater bath for 30 min then centrifuged at 900 g for 30 min at 4°C. The middle layer containing platelet poor plasma is carefully harvested with a disposable pipette[39] and aliquots are frozen at -20°C until assay. PF4 and ß-thromboglobulin are measured by radioimmunoassay or enzyme-linked immunoassay.[40-42]

8493-5804-3/96/$0.00+$.50
© 1996 by CRC Press

Table I : Different assays proposed to detect platelet activation

		Ref.
Count and morphological changes of platelets		
Density distribution		1
Circulating platelet aggregates		2
Platelet survival time		3,4,5
Platelet function		
platelet adhesiveness		6
spontaneous platelet aggregation in whole blood		7
in platelet rich plasma		8
shear platelet aggregation		9
in vitro agonist-induced platelet aggregation		10,11
Biochemical assays		
ß-thromboglobulin	in plasma, platelet,	12
	in urine	13,14
platelet factor 4	in plasma, platelet	12
thrombospondin in plasma		15,16
P-selectin in plasma		17
glycocalicin in plasma		18
ATP - ADP content in platelets		19
serotonin content in platelets		20,21
thromboxane A_2 metabolites in plasma, urine		22
Changes in the platelet membrane glycoproteins		
changes in GP IIb-IIIa - active conformation of GP IIb-IIIa		23
- ligand binding to GP IIb-IIIa		24
- receptor-induced conformational change in the ligand		25,26
- ligand-induced conformational change in GP IIb-IIIa		27
changes in GP Ib		28
exposure of granule protein :		
α granule membrane protein : P-selectin		29
lysosomal membrane protein		30,31
dense granule membrane protein		32
secreted platelet protein (TSP)		3,34
Expression of binding sites for coagulation proteins		35
Microparticles		25,36

B. NORMAL VALUES

In healthy individuals, the plasma concentration of PF4 is 3.3 ± 1.7 ng/ml, whereas the ß-TG level is 23.4 ± 6.6 ng/ml (mean ± 1 standard deviation.[16] The mean value in males is not significantly different from that in female.[37] After an in vitro release reaction, ß-TG and PF4 appear simultaneously in the plasma.[43]

However in vivo, the two proteins are cleared from the plasma at different rates. This explains that the normal ratio of ß-TG/PF4 is greater than 2.3[41] and in the case of platelet activation during blood sampling or processing the ratio tends to be equal to 1. Older healthy individuals have increased levels of plasma ß-TG and PF4 compared to younger healthy subjects, indicating an in vivo platelet activation.[44] Physical exercise increases the plasma levels of these two markers, but cigarette smoking has no effect.

C. RESULTS IN PATHOLOGICAL STATES

In patients with impaired renal function without thrombosis the level of ß-TG is elevated and PF4 normal.[45] During treatment with unfractionated heparin only plasma PF4 concentrations are increased.[43]

Both markers of the platelet release reaction are elevated in several pathological states. For the diagnosis of acute deep vein thrombosis, the sensitivity (35 %) and specificity (80 %) of the plasma ß-TG assay are low[13]. In acute myocardial infarction and unstable angina the relationship between an individual's ß-TG or PF4 levels and the severity, extent of vascular disease or recurrence of myocardial infarction is not clear.[46-48] In patients with stable angina, ß-TG and PF4 levels are elevated only in patients with prior infarction. ß-TG correlates positively with the extent of left ventricular regional dysfunction and conversely with the ejection fraction, suggesting platelet activation at the site of the injured cardiac wall.[49] Aspirin is associated with a reduction of ß-TG and PF4 levels.[47] During cardiopulmonary bypass in patients who underwent open heart surgery there is a similar release of both platelet specific proteins that tends to increase until the end of extracorporeal circulation.[46]

Patients with diabetes mellitus, presenting an increased risk of developing coronary artery disease, also have an increased mean of ß-TG and PF4 plasma levels.[50] There is no correlation between the plasma levels of these markers and the stages of either retinopathy, macroangiopathy or nephropathy.[51,52] The levels of both platelet specific proteins in diabetic patients without evidence of vascular disease are comparable to the levels found in patients with vascular disease. This suggests that platelet stimulation might precede the development of vascular disease. An adequate blood glucose control is accompanied by a reduction of ß-TG levels, although the values remain higher than those measured in a control group.[53]

Patients with active malignant diseases or myeloproliferative disorders have elevated ß-TG plasma levels and to a lower extent elevated PF4 levels.[54] The same parameters are normal in patients with secondary thrombocytosis.[55] Patients with essential thrombocythaemia show a marked increase in plasma ß-TG concentration while the plasma PF4 concentration is normal or slighty increased.[56] In sickle cell anemia, the ß-TG level is frequently elevated but the ß-TG/PF4 ratio is significantly lower in patient groups compared to controls. This increase can be due to an artefactual in vitro release.[57]

In thrombocytopenic patients, ß-TG is increased in the case of intravascular platelet consumption, normal in autoimmune thrombocytopenia and not measurable in amegakaryocytic thrombocytopenia.[58] With the exception of thrombocytopenic patients with acute leukemia, severe infections such as septicemia or pneumonia are associated with elevated levels of ß-TG.[59]

To summarize, measurements of ß-TG and PF4 must be considered as an interesting tool to investigate the pathogenic role of platelets in vascular diseases. However, the plasma levels of these two proteins do not have any predictive value for the recurrence of thrombosis. Moreover, one has to be very careful during blood sample collection and processing to prevent in vitro ß-TG and PF4 release. These limitations have prevented their routine clinical use.

II. MEASUREMENTS OF THROMBOXANE METABOLITES

During their adhesion to the subendothelium, mostly to deep vessel wall collagen (types I & III) or during intra-vascular aggregation mainly induced by thrombin generation, stimulated platelets produce prostaglandin endoperoxides and thromboxane A_2 (TxA_2). These metabolites participate with ADP in the chain reaction of platelet activation. They are synthesized from free arachidonic acid, mainly by activated phopholipase A_2, which occurs during the secretion of granule content (irreversible phase of platelet aggregation) and to a small degree by a phospholipase C/diglyceride-monoglyceride lipase pathway.

The formation of the endoperoxides followed by that of TxA_2 are dependent upon cyclooxygenase (or prostaglandin H synthase), which is an enzyme that can be completely inhibited by nonsteroidal anti-inflammatory drugs (NSAIDS) such as indomethacin or aspirin. The common use of aspirin, the most widely consumed drug in the world, considerably limits the diagnosis of platelet activation by methods of thromboxane metabolite measurements. Salicylate level determinations are often recommended aid in the interpretation of metabolite measurements. Aspirin inhibits secondary ADP induced aggregation and platelet responses to collagen, but fails to inhibit thrombin induced aggregation like that which occurs during certain arterial thrombi formation. It also has beneficial effects on unstable angina and other heart failures[60]. It can be said that thomboxane is one marker of the irreversible state of platelet aggregation, but not of the primary phase of platelet activation. Therefore, thromboxane measurements alone are not sufficient evidence to provide a diagnosis of platelet activation in patients having taken NSAIDS.

A . THROMBOXANE METABOLITES

Thromboxane A_2 is a short half-lived molecule in biological fluid (32 sec at 37°C in plasma) which rapidly breaks down within seconds into the stable thromboxane B_2 (TxB_2). TxB_2 determinations in plasma have been used to evaluate endogenous TxA_2 generation, but it is well recognized that artificial formation of thromboxane can occur during blood sampling.[61,62] The measurement of TxB_2 in urine might have been a noninvasive method, but urinary TxB_2 levels are thought to represent to a large extent kidney synthesis[22]. This representation is very controversial.[63] In vivo, TxB_2 is rapidly metabolized through two major pathways. The first is by ß-oxidation mainly in the liver resulting in 2,3-dinor-TxB_2. The second is by dehydrogenation into 11-dehydro-TxB_2 (11-d$HTxB_2$ is also named 11-keto-TxB_2)[64] which most probably occurs in the liver, lungs, kidneys and to a smaller extent (may be non-enzymatically) in the blood, during and after its collection.[62,65] A combination of these two enzymatic pathways leads to the formation of 11-dehydro-2,3-dinor-TxB_2 (or 11-keto-2,3-dinor-TxB_2) [Figure 1].

Furthermore, 11-d$HTxB_2$ has a longer plasma half-life than TxB_2, 17 min and 3 min respectively.[66] Measurement of 11-d$HTxB_2$ and 2,3-dinor-TxB_2 found in urine, provide an index of the total body production and an index of platelet activation. For example, an elevation of these urinary metabolites precedes and is contemporary with myocardial infarction. The level of 11-d$HTxB_2$ then returns to normal values within 24 hrs.[67]

Infusion studies of [$^3H_8$]-TxB_2 have shown 2,3-dinor-TxB_2 to be the major urinary metabolite,[64] but it is not the main physiological metabolite. Found in the greatest amount in urine, 11-d$HTxB_2$ has a longer plasma half-life and is excreted more rapidly than 2,3-dinor-TxB_2.[68-72] In a pathological state such as myocardial infarction the urinary 11-d$HTxB_2$ level varies more rapidly and to a greater degree than 2,3-dinor-TxB_2.[67] Thus, today 11-d$HTxB_2$ determinations from plasma or urine seem to be the best index of in vivo generation of platelet TxA_2.

B . ASSAYS

Quantitation of plasma TxB_2 metabolites (TxB_2-M) can be done from venous blood collected in the presence of indomethacin and EDTA at a final concentration of 50 µM and 7 mM, respectively. Plasma is obtained from 5 ml of blood which is immediately centrifuged at 4°C and then kept frozen at -70°C until analysis. Urine aliquots of 20 ml, obtained after one micturition (overnight specimen for example) are also immediately kept frozen until analysis. For a daily determination we recommend the addition of an antioxidant to the flask before fractionation (butylhydroxytoluene 50 µM).

During the past two decades several prostanoid assays have been developed in many laboratories using gas chromatography associated first with flame ionization detection (GC-FID) and more recently with mass-spectrometry (GC-MS). They also use either low or high pressure liquid chromatography, thin layer chromatography or affinity chromatography, which are all purification steps associated with radio- or enzymo-immunoassays (RIA or EIA). Stable-isotope dilution assays using gas chromatography-mass spectrometry in the negative chemical ionization mode (GC-NICI-MS and GC-NICI-MS/MS) are still the referenced method used.

Normally prostanoids are analysed as pentafluorobenzyl-ester-methyloxime-trimethylsilyl ether derivatives after many steps of extraction and purification.[73] Such a method is costly due to expensive equipment and the length of time needed to prepare the samples. Other analytical methods such as capillary isotachopheresis[74] and supercritical fluid chromatography[75] are now under investigation.

Extractions and clean-up procedures must be done in order to eliminate other lipids in the measurement of TxB_2 metabolites (TxB_2-M) or other prostanoids in biological fluids. In the case of plasma samples, to ensure there is displacement of the prostanoid fraction that can be associated with albumin, a precautionary measures are used to enhance the specificity of the assay and avoid artefactual reactivity EIA methods. Purification steps also avoid antibody cross-reactivities. There are commercially available

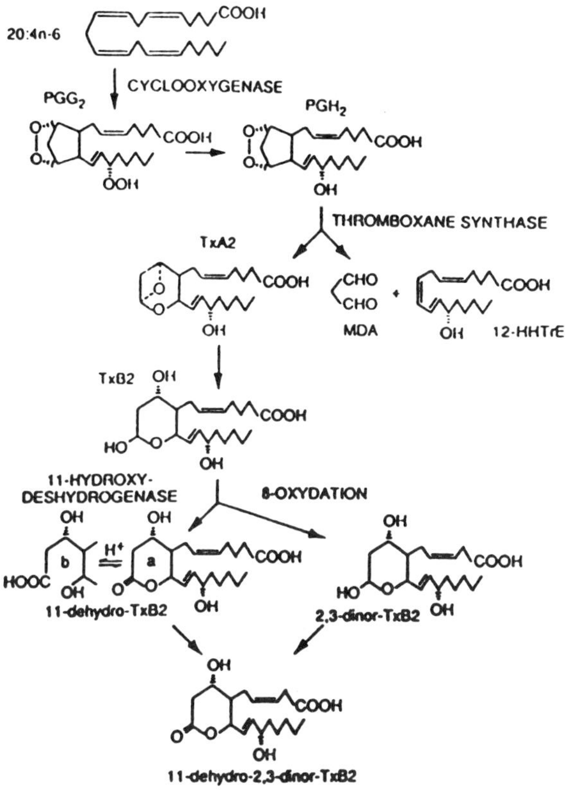

Figure 1. Thromboxane synthesis and metabolism. Arachidonic acid (20 :4n-6) is di-oxygenated by cyclooxygenase into prostaglandin endoperoxides PGG_2 and PGH_2. The platelet dismutase, thromboxane synthase leads to the formation of thromboxane A_2 (TxA_2) and malondialdehyde (MDA) plus 12-hydroxy-heptatrienoic acid (12-HHTrE). In biological fluid, the unstable compound TxA_2 is rapidly degraded into thromboxane B_2 (TxB_2). The last is then metabolised through two major pathways. The first is by ß-oxidation, leading to 2,3-dinor-TxB_2, or secondly by dehydrogenation into 11-dehydro-TxB_2 (a, lactone form ; b, diacid or open form). A combination of these two pathways leads to the formation of 11-dehydro-2,3-dinor-TxB_2. These three major metabolites found in urine are representative of the total body thromboxane synthesis. Variations of 11-dehydro-TxB_2 levels are more pronounced and they follow thromboxane synthesis in pathological states when platelets are activated.

immunoassays that now have better specificity and recently a more rapid and direct detection of 11-dHTxB$_2$ has been described.[76]

The following method can be done easily at a low cost of equipment and other materials. Urine or plasma samples (1-2 ml) are combined with 75 Bq (6 TBq/mmol) of the tritiated prostanoid to be evaluated and then acidified to pH 3. The bulk of urinary or plasma prostanoids are extracted on reversed phase columns (for example 300-500 mg of octadecyl or ethyl phases, SepPak cartridges from Waters) with a slight modification of Powell's method[77]. Columns are prewashed with ethanol and water, 5 ml each. The samples are loaded and then the columns are washed with 15% ethanol in water and isooctane (5 to 10 ml each). The prostanoids are eluted with 7 ml of ethyl acetate/dichloromethane (75/25). After evaporation of the organic solvents, the concentrated samples are chromatographied on a silicagel G 60 (Merck). The thin layer plates are developed in the organic phase of ethyl acetate/isooctane/acetic acid/H_2O (130 : 30 : 20 : 100, V/V). The metabolites 2,3-dinor-TxB_2 and 11-dHTxB_2 are resolved at an Rf value of 0.40 and 0.69 respectively. Other metabolites such as those of prostacyclin, 6-Oxo-PGF1a and 2,3-dinor-6-Oxo-PGF1α have Rf values of 0.26 and 0.52 respectively. [78] Gel fractions corresponding to comigrating standards (10 μg, visualized by phosphomolybdic acid spray at 10% in methanol and heating at 110°C) are scraped, prostanoids are eluted from the gel with acetonitril/water (9 :1) and resuspended in the buffer used for RIA [79] or EIA [80] after drying.

C . NORMAL VALUES

Platelet activity and TxA_2 formation rise during the neonatal period, decrease after birth, and increase with age. On the contrary excretion rates corrected for body surface show very little variation over different age and sex groups.[81]

The excretion of TxB_2-M increases during pregnancy.[82,83]

Levels of TxB_2-M in normal subjects are higher in men than in women.[84]

Urinary TxB_2-M metabolite levels are not changed by physical exercise.[85,86]

Diet may influence TxA_2 synthesis because urinary 11-dHTxB_2 is diminished after fish-oil intake.[87]

Diurnal variations of 2,3-dinor-TxB_2 measurements were reported by Vesterqvist, but this result was not encountered by others.[88] The quantities of TxB_2-M and other prostanoids in urine are not found to be correlated with their concentration, but they are well correlated to creatinine levels. Results are expressed as daily production from the collection of urine over a 24 hour period. Three hour collections expressed as a ratio of prostanoid to creatinine quantities have also been found to be accurate.[89] Results are sometimes expressed as rate/hour/body surface.[81] Values found in the literature varied from 80 to 1500 ng/g of creatinine for 2,3-dinor-TxB_2 and from 200 to 3500 ng/g of creatinine for 11-dHTxB_2.

D . RESULTS IN CASES WITH RISK FACTORS

The level of TxB_2-M in urine for smokers is significantly higher than that of non-smokers,[90] but smokers have a higher increase of 2,3-dinor-TxB_2 than that of 11-dHTxB_2 when compared to the increases found in cardiovascular disorders. Thus nicotine might also inhibit the enzymatic formation of 11-dHTxB_2.

Age, hypercholesterolemia and atherosclerosis are also risk factors to platelet activation in vivo and to consequently develop carotid atherosclerosis. All of these are correlated to an enhanced excretion of 11-dHTxB_2.[91] It is possible that oestrogen therapy might reduce the TxB_2-M increase found in atherosclerosis.[92]

Children with congenital heart disease and a high pulmonary blood flow have an enhanced production of TxB_2-M.[93]

E . RESULTS IN PATHOLOGICAL STATES

The aetiological role of TxA_2 formation by activated-platelets in vivo has been well documented in many pathological states. This is summarized in the following list [Table II].

Cardiac catheterization, coronary angioplasty, synthetic arterial grafts, artificial heart and extracorporeal circulation have all been found to activate platelets and enhance TxA_2 synthesis.[109,76,85]

The level of TxB_2-M in normal subjects was found to be higher in men than in women, but the difference in level has been described to be reversed in patients undergoing a myocardial infarction.[67]

Overall, level determinations of 11-dHTxB_2 thromboxane metabolites in pathological states appear to be the best complementary tool for the diagnosis of an in vivo platelet activation.

Table II - In vivo thromboxane metabolites in pathological states

Increased production	Reference(s)
allograph rejection	94
atherosclerotic vascular disease	70
coronary disease	95,96
homocysteinuria	82
hypercholesterolemia (IIa)	97
ischemic stroke	98
myocardial infarction	82,67
pulmonary embolism	99
pulmonary hypertension	100
reocclusion after thombolysis	101
sickle cell disease	102,103
systemic lupus erythamatosus	104
venous thrombosis	105,98
Variable or not significant differences :	
diabetes mellitus	106
hypertension	82,107
glucocorticoids	108

In order to give an example of urinary 11-dHTxB$_2$ amounts which are representative of the literature, we can quote Lorenz et al[99] who found ranges of 231-1141 in controls, 680-1540 in heavy smokers and 2370-13350 ng/g of creatinine in venous thrombosis or pulmonary embolism. For plasma values, Catella et al[70] found 11-dHTxB$_2$ amounts to be in the range 1-50 pg/ml.

In spite of the fact that the urinary measurement of 11-dHTxB$_2$ is a non-invasive method, it appears to be better than blood evaluations in a clinical environment because conversion of TxB$_2$ into 11-dHTxB$_2$ (non-enzymatically ?) will occur if blood samples are not immediately treated with indomethacin, centrifuged at a low temperature, and then the plasma frozen. When these basic precautions of blood collection can be performed with high quality and reproducibility, circulating blood determinations can be more sensitive than urinary excretion[110] in the case of time-dependent phenomenon studies.

III. MEASUREMENTS OF CHANGES IN PLATELET MEMBRANE GLYCOPROTEINS

Upon stimulation with weak agonists such as ADP and epinephrine the platelet membrane glycoprotein IIb-IIIa complex undergoes a conformational change and converts to a functional fibrinogen receptor. Stimulation with strong agonists such as thrombin, collagen, or the binding of fibrinogen to the activated glycoprotein IIb-IIIa complex, leads to platelet degranulation. Alpha granules, dense bodies and lysosomes migrate to the platelet surface, fuse with the plasma membrane and release their contents. In addition, neo-antigens derived from the membrane of these organites become exposed on the platelet surface. Some examples are P-selectin from the alpha granule membrane, CD 63, LAMP-1 from the lysosomal membrane and a glycoprotein of apparent molecular weight 40 KDa from the dense bodies membrane. In addition, after thrombin stimulation, or other agonists such as ADP, plasma membrane glycoprotein Ib-IX complexes go into the channels of the surface-connected canalicular system.

A. MONOCLONAL ANTIBODIES DETECTING PLATELET ACTIVATION

The use of specific monoclonal antibodies exposed on the surface of activated platelets, coupled with the technique of flow cytometry offers an accurate and quantitative method for detecting small subpopulations of activated platelets ex vivo. Several monoclonal antibodies have been described that recognize antigenic determinants on the platelet surface only after platelet activation. Some monoclonal antibodies detect an activation of the glycoprotein IIb-IIIa complex. For example, PAC_1 is an IgM antibody that binds only to the activated form of the glycoprotein IIb-IIIa complex. The complex has between 10,000 and 15,000 binding sites after ADP stimulation and between 20,000 and 25,000 after thrombin activation. PAC_1 inhibits platelet aggregation and the binding of fibrinogen in a competitive manner. PM1-1 and LIBS-1 (ligand induced binding sites) recognize two distinct epitopes, respectively on glycoprotein IIb and IIIa. They are expressed only after the binding of a ligand containing the Arg-Gly-Asp sequence peptide. Other monoclonal antibodies such as 9F9 normally recognize epitopes expressed on ligands, or for fibrinogen only after it binds to the glycoprotein IIb-IIIa complex (receptor-induced binding sites). Moreover, several monoclonal antibodies are able to detect the expression of P-selectin, CD_3, LAMP, thrombospondin on the plasma membrane.

B. FLOW CYTOMETRY TECHNIQUES

The flow cytometric measurement of changes in platelet surface membrane is a widely used method for assessing the status of platelet activation. Flow cytometry on diluted whole blood samples has some advantages over using fixed, washed platelet methods. It is rapid and avoids manipulations that might introduce artefactual activation of platelets, as for example during centrifugation or separation procedures.

Blood is obtained from an antecubital vein through a 19-gauge butterfly needle with either a light tourniquet or no tourniquet. The first 2 ml of blood are discarded, and then 4.5 ml of blood are placed into a plastic tube containing 0.5 ml of 3.8 % sodium citrate or acid-citrate dextrose (85 mM/L trisodium citrate, 71 mM/L citric acid, 111 mM/L dextrose, pH 4.5). Blood can be drawn on a sodium citrate Vacutainer (Becton-Dickinson, Rutherford, NJ). Within 3 minutes after collection, 5 μl of whole blood are added to polystyrene tubes containing 40 μl of isotonic HEPES buffer and antibodies. When studying whole blood, monoclonal rather than polyclonal antibodies are preferred to minimize non-specific antibody binding. A two-color technique is usually performed and platelets are discriminated from red and white blood cells by using an activation-independent platelet-specific antibody which specifically recognizes an epitope on the platelet surface. This antibody can be a biotinylated antibody directed against GP Ib. The flow cytometer threshold is set to detect phycoerythrin-positive particles, and platelets are stained simultaneously with a FITC-conjugated activation-dependent antibody to assess platelet activation. Aliquots of blood are placed immediately into tubes containing isotonic HEPES buffer, a saturating concentration of biotin-AP_1 (anti-Ib) and one of the following FITC-labeled monoclonal antibody. The tubes are incubated without stirring for 15 minutes in the dark at room temperature. Phycoerythrin-streptavidin is added and the reaction is stopped after 10 min by adding a buffer.[111]

An antibody directed against any abundant platelet surface protein can be used to discriminate platelets. For example, Michelson used FITC-anti IIIb (OKM5) to study the downregulation of GP Ib-IX complexes. Diluted whole blood is aliquoted into a tube containing a saturating concentration of biotinylated test antibody and incubated for 15 min at 22°C. Then a saturating concentration of FITC-conjugated OKM5 is added and incubated 15 min with phycoerythrin-streptavidin. Samples are incubated for 30 min at 22°C with an equal volume of 2 % formaldehyde in Tyrode's buffer.[112]

The flow cytometer is calibrated with standard fluorescent microbeads or fixed chicken red blood cells. Fluorescence and scattered light data are acquired in a logarithmic mode. Fluorescein fluorescence is detected using a 530/30 band pass filter, and phycoerythrin fluorescence using a 585/42 filter. Blood samples are passed through the laser beam at a flow rate not exceeding 2000 cells per second.

Platelets in the diluted whole blood sample are identified by characteristic forward and orthogonal light scattering. The fluorescence of positive cells are detected with an activation-independent antibody. Acquisition is gated to include only the particles distinctively positive with an activation-independent platelet specific antibody. Binding of fluorescent antibodies to platelets is expressed either as the mean fluorescent intensity of the particle in arbitrary fluorescence units, or as the number of bound antibody molecules per particle. The binding of the antibody as determined by flow cytometry, is highly correlated with the binding data determined by a standard ^{125}I-antibody binding assay. The results are expressed as the percentage of particles positive for a specific antibody. The measurement of background binding is obtained from parrallel samples with purified fluorescent mouse IgG or IgM, which is then subtracted from each test sample.

The lower limit of detection of antibody binding by flow cytometry is approximately 500 bound molecules per platelet.

There are several advantages in studying activated platelets by whole blood flow cytometry. Only microliter volumes of blood are required and platelet subpopulations that are heterogeneous in their platelet response to stimulation can be detected. Studies have shown that as little as 0.8 % of activated platelets present in a platelet sample can be detected by flow cytometry.[111]

C. RESULTS IN PATHOLOGICAL STATES

Some studies have shown that during cardiopulmonary bypass there is a decrease in the platelet surface glycoprotein IIb-IIIa complex[113]. Abrams et al reported that there was an increase in the binding of PAC-1 directed against the fibrinogen binding site, as well as the binding of 9F9 directed against platelet-bound fibrinogen. Platelet surface expression of P-selectin was either increased or normal. Others investigators have studied the effects of cardiopulmonary bypass on the binding of monoclonal antibodies directed against granule antigens that are only present on the platelet surface after degranulation (GMP-140). They have found a modest or inconsistant increase during cardiopulmonary bypass and the overall P-selectin expression on the surface of platelets is minimal.[114,115] However, cardiopulmonary bypass induces an increase in plasma ß-thromboglobulin and platelet factor 4.[46] This data suggests that plasma ß-thromboglobulin originates either from degranulated platelets that are cleared from the circulation, or from platelets adhering to synthetic surfaces. This might also reflect an in vitro degranulation.

Some patients have shown that after percutaneous transluminal angioplasty, platelets in coronary sinus blood show an increase in the binding of both PAC-1 and LIBS 1.[117] The binding of 9F9 directed against platelet-bound fibrinogen is lower than the binding of PAC-1 and LIBS 1. It is possible that 9F9 may only recognize a proportion of activated platelets which have irreversibly bound to fibrinogen. The expression of P-selectin on the platelet membrane is detected less often than the expression of the activated glycoprotein IIb-IIIa complex.[117] In peripheral venous blood, P-selectin positive platelets are inconsistantly detectable.[118] Interestingly, the highest levels of P-selectin expression are observed in patients who have developed an acute vascular thrombosis within 24 hours.[119]

Flow cytometry has also been used for the detection of circulating activated platelets in a number of clinical situations such as diabetes mellitus,[120] peripheral vascular disease,[121] cerebral ischemia,[122] homozygous beta thalassemic patients,[123] essential thrombocythemia and myeloproliferative disorders.[124]

D. GENERAL CONSIDERATIONS

The main question concerning flow cytometric assays is the sensitivity level. The limit of detection for the assay appears to be 0.8 % of activated platelets in a blood sample.[111] The assay can easily detect activated platelets emerging from a bleeding time incision.[111] It is not clear how many activated platelets are formed in vivo and enter the general circulation in different clinical situations. Using an anti-P selectin antibody in a baboon model of thrombosis Palabrica et al[125] showed that activated platelets and not resting platelets, are incorporated into thrombi at sites of vascular injury. It is also not precisely known how long activated platelets circulate. Following in vitro spontaneous activation, infused platelets have a shortened survival time in circulation.[126] It is also possible that some changes in the platelet membrane glycoprotein are transient. Binding of fibrinogen to the glycoprotein IIb-IIIa complex is initially reversible in vitro.

Alternatively, redistribution or endocytosis of the glycoprotein IIb-IIIa complex, glycoprotein Ib-IX complex and P-selectin may occur. Therefore, it is recommended to use a panel of activation-dependent antibodies for the detection of different platelet activation states. Based on the studies performed up to date, it can be stated that flow cytometric assays are useful in characterizing the role of platelets in vascular thrombosis. The absence of standardization from one laboratory to another is a major limitation.

REFERENCES

1. **Van Oost, B. A., Timmermans, A. P. M. and Sixma, J. J.**, Evidence that platelet density depends on the alpha granule content in platelets. *Blood*, 63, 482, 1984.
2. **Wu, K.K. and Hoak J. C.,** A new method for the quantitative detection of platelet aggregation in patients with arterial insufficiency. *Lancet*, II, 924, 1974.

3. **Harker, L. A. and Slichter, S. J.** Platelet and fibrinogen consumption in man. *N. Engl. J. Med.*, 287, 999, 1972.

4. **Minar, E. and Ehringer, H.**, Reproducibility of platelet survival time measurements in patients with peripheral arterial occlusive disease. *Thromb. Res.*, 48, 73, 1987.

5. **Steele, P. P., Weily, H. S., Davies, H., Pappas, G. and Genton, E.**, Platelet survival following aortic valve replacement. *Circulation*, 51, 358, 1975.

6. **Zucker, M. B., Rifkin, P. L., Friedberg, N. M. and Coller, B. S.**, Mechanisms of platelet function as revealed by the retention of platelets in glass bead columns. *Ann. N. Y. Acad. Sci.*, 201, 138, 1972.

7. **Fox, S. C., Burgess-Wilson, M., Heptinstall, S. and Mitchell, J. R. A.**, Platelet aggregation in whole blood determined using the ultra-Flo 100 platelet counter. *Thromb. Haemost.*, 48, 327, 1982.

8. **Breddin, K., Grun, H., Krywanek, H. J. and Schremmer, W. P.**, On the measurement of spontaneous platelet aggregation. The platelet aggregation test III. Methods and first clinical results. *Thromb. Haemost.*, 35, 669, 1976.

9. **Uchiyama, S., Yamakaki, M. and Maruyama, S.**, Shear-induced platelet aggregation in cerebral ischemia. *Stroke*, 25, 1547, 1994.

10. **Mandal, S., Sarode, R., Dash, S. and Dash, R. S.**, Hyperaggregation of platelets detected by whole blood platelet aggregometry in newly diagnosed non insulin-dependent diabetes mellitus. *Am. J. Clin. Pathol.*, 100, 103, 1993.

11. **Meade, T. W., Vickers, M. V., Thompson, S. G. and Stirring, Y.**, Epidemiological characteristics of platelet aggregability. *Br. Med. J.*, 290, 428, 1985.

12. **Kaplan, K. L. and Owen, J.**, Radioimmunoassays of platelet alpha-granule proteins, in *Measurements of platelet function*, Harker, L. A. and Zimmerman, T. S., Eds, Churchill Livingstone, Edinburgh, 1983, 115, 125.

13. **De Boer, A.C., Han, P. Turpie, A.G.G., Butt, R., Zielinski, A., and Genton, E.**, Plasma and urine beta-thromboglobulin concentration in patients with deep vein thrombosis. *Blood*, 58, 693, 1981.

14. **Van Oost, B. A., Veldhuyzen, B., Timmermans, A. P. M. and Sixma, J. J.**, Increased urinary beta-thromboglobulin excretion in diabetes assayed with a modified RIA kit-technique. *Thromb. Haemost.*, 49, 18, 1983.

15. **Dawes, J., Clemetson, K. J., Gogstad, G. O., McGregor, J. L., Clezardin, P., Prowse, C. V. and Pepper, D. S.**, A radioimmunoassay for thrombospondin, used in a comparative study of the thrombospondin, beta-thromboglobulin and platelet factor 4 in healthy volunteers. *Thromb. Res.*, 29, 569, 1983.

16. **Ffrench, P., McGregor, J. L., Berruyer, M., Belleville, J., Touboul, P., Dawes, J. and Dechavanne, M.**, Comparative evaluation of plasma thrombospondin, beta-thromboglobulin and platelet factor 4 in acute myocardial infarction. *Thromb. Res.*, 39, 619, 1985.

17. **Chong, B.H., Murray, B., Berndt, M. C., Dunlop, L. C., Brighton, T.**, and Chesterman, C. N. Plasma P-selectin is increased in thrombotic consumptive platelet disorders. *Blood*, 83, 1535, 1994.

18. **Beer, J. H., Bücki, L. and Steiner, B.**, Glycocalicin : a new assay. The normal plasma levels and its potential usefulness in selected diseases. *Blood*, 83, 691, 1994.

19. **Holmsen, H., Molsen, I. and Bernhardsen, A.**, Micro-determination of adenosine diphosphate and adenosine triphosphate in plasma with firefly luciferase system. *Anal. Biochem.*, 17, 456, 1966.

20. **Barradas, M. A., Gill, D. S., Fonseca V. A., Mikhailidis, D. P. and Dandon, A.**, Intraplatelet serotonin in patients with diabetes mellitus and peripheral vascular disease. *Eur. J. Clin. Invest.*, 18, 399, 1988.

21. **Drummond, A. H. and Gordon, J. L.**, Rapid sensitive microassay for platelet 5HT. *Thromb. Diath. Haemorrh.*, 31, 366, 1974.

22. **Patrono, C., Ciabattoni, G., Patrignani, P., Filabozzi, P., Pinca, E., Satta, M. A., Van Dorne, D., Cinotti, A., Pugliese, F., Pierucci, A. and Simonetti, B. M.**, Evidence for a renal origin of urinary thromboxane B_2 in health and diseases, in *Advances in Prostaglandin, Thromboxane and Leukotriene Research*, Samuelson, B., Paoletti, R. and Ramwell P, Eds, New York, Raven Press, 1983, 493.

23. **Shattil, S. J., Hoxie, J. A., Cunningham, M. and Brass, L. F.**, Changes in the platelet membrane glycoprotein IIb-IIIa complex during platelet activation. *J. Biol. Chem.*, 260, 11107, 1985.

24. **Warkentin, T. E., Powling, M. J., Hardisty, R. M.**, Measurement of fibrinogen binding to platelets in whole blood by flow cytometry : a micro-method for the detection of platelet activation. *Br. J. Haematol.*, 76, 387, 1990.

25. **Zamarron, C., Ginsberg, M. H. and Plow, E. F.**, Receptor-induced binding sites (RIBS) are exposed in fibrinogen as a consequence of its interaction with platelets. *Blood*, 74, 208a, 1989.

26. **Zamarron, C., Ginsberg, M. H. and Plow, E. F.**, Monoclonal antibodies specific for a conformationally altered state of fibrinogen. *Thromb. Haemost.*, 64, 41, 1990.

27. **Frelinger, A. L., Cohen, I., Plow, E. F., Smith, M. A., Roberts, J., Lam, S. C. T., Ginsberg, M. H.**, Selective inhibition of integrin function by antibodies specific for ligand-occupied receptor conformers. *J. Biol. Chem.*, 265, 6346, 1990.

28. **Michelson, A. D. and Barnard, M. R.**, Thrombin induced changes in platelet membrane glycoprotein Ib-IX and IIb-IIIa complex. *Blood*, 70, 1673, 1987.

29. **McEver, R. P. and Martin, M. N.**, A monoclonal antibody to a membrane glycoprotein binds only to activated platelets. *J. Biol. Chem.*, 259, 9799, 1984.

30. **Febbraio, M. and Silverstein, R. L.**, Identification and characterization of LAMP-1 as an activation-dependent platelet surface glycoprotein. *J. Biol. Chem.*, 265, 18531, 1990.

31. **Nieuwenhuis, H. K., Van Oosterhout, J. J. G., Rozemuller, E., Van Ikwaarden, F. and Sixma, J. J.**, Studies with a monoclonal antibody against activated platelets : evidence that a secreted 53,000 molecular weight lysosome-like granule protein is exposed on the surface of activated platelets in the circulation. *Blood*, 838, 845, 1987.

32. **Gerrard, J. M., Lindt, D., Sims, P. J., Wiedmer, T., Fugate, D., McMillan, E., Roberts, C. and Israel, S. J.**, Identification of a platelet dense granule membrane protein that is deficient in a patient with the Hermansky-Puldak syndrome. *Blood*, 77, 101, 1991.

33. **Aiken, M. L., Ginsberg, M. H. and Plow, E. F.**, Mechanisms for expression of thrombospondin on the platelet cell surface. *Semin. Thromb. Haemost.*, 13, 307, 1993.

34. **Boukerche, H. and Mc Gregor, J.L.**, Characterization of an anti-thrombospondin monoclonal antibody (P8) that inhibits human platelet functions. *Eur. J. Biochem.*, 171, 383, 1988.

35. **Sims, P. J., Wiedmer, T., Esmon, C. T., Weiss, H. J., Shattil, S. J.,** Assembly of the platelet prothrombinase complex is linked to vesiculation of the platelet plasma membrane. Studies in Scott syndrome : an isolated defect in platelet procoagulant activity. *J. Biol. Chem.*, 264, 17049, 1989.

36. **George, J. N., Pickett, E. B., Saucerman, S., McEver, R. P., Kunicki, T. J., Kieffer, N. and Newman, P. J.,** Platelet surface glycoproteins : studies on resting and activated platelets and platelet membrane microparticles in normal subjects and observations in patients during adult respiratory distress syndrome and cardiac surgery. *J. Clin. Invest.*, 78, 340, 1986.

37. **Ludlam, C. A.,** Evidence for the platelet specificity of ß-thromboglobulin and studies on its plasma concentration in healthy individuals. *Br. J. Haematol.*, 41, 271, 1979.

38. **Prowse, C. V., Pepper, D. and Dawes, J.,** Prevention of the platelet alpha-granule release reaction by membrane-active drugs. *Thromb. Res.*, 25, 219, 1982.

39. **Rasi, V.,** Beta-thromboglobulin in plasma : false high values caused by platelet enrichment of the top layer of plasma during centrifugation. *Thromb. Res.*, 15, 543, 1979.

40. **Berruyer, M., Ville, D., Ffrench, P., Trzeciak, M. C. and Dechavanne, M.,** Dosage immunoenzymologique de la beta-thromboglobuline et du facteur plaquettaire 4 : corrélation avec un dosage radio-immunologique. *Int. Sci. Biol.*, 13, 187, 1987.

41. **Kaplan, K. L. and Owen, J.,** Plasma levels of beta-thromboglobulin and platelet factor 4 as indices of platelet activation in vivo. *Blood*, 57, 199, 1981.

42. **Kerry P. J. and Curtis, A. D.,** Standardization of beta-thromboglobulin, and platelet factor 4 : a collaborative study to establish international standards for ß-TG and PF4. *Thromb. Haemost.*, 52, 236, 1984.

43. **Dawes, J., Smith, R. C. and Pepper, D. S.,** The release, distribution and clearence of human beta-thromboglobulin and platelet factor 4. *Thromb. Res.*, 12, 851, 1978.

44. **Zahavi, J., Jones, N. A. G., Leyton, J., Dubiel, M. and Kakkar, V.V.,** Enhanced in vivo platelet « release reaction » in old healthy individuals. *Thromb. Res.*, 17, 329, 1980.

45. **Depperman, D., Andrassy, K., Selig, H., Ritz, E. and Post, D.,** ß-thromboglobulin is elevated in renal failure without thrombosis. *Thromb. Res.*, 17, 63, 1980.

46. **Cella, G., Vittadello, O., Gallucci, V. and Girolami, A.,** The release of beta-thromboglobulin and platelet factor 4 during extracorporeal circulation for open heart surgery. *Eur. J. Clin. Invest.*, 11, 165, 1981.

47. **Gavaghan, T. P., Hickie, J. B., Krilis, S. A., Baron, D. W., Gebski, V., Low, J. and Chesterman, C. N.,** Increased plasma beta-thromboglobulin in patients with coronary artery vein graft occlusion : response to low dose aspirin. *J. Am. Coll. Cardiol.*, 15, 1250, 1990.

48. **White, G. C., Marouf, A. A.,** Platelet factor 4 levels in patients with coronary artery disease. *J. Lab. Clin. Med.*, 97, 369, 1981.

49. **Nichols, A. B., Owen, J., Kaplan, K. L., Sciacca, R. R., Cannon, P. J. and Nossel, H. L.,** Fibrinopeptide A, platelet factor 4 and beta-thromboglobulin levels in coronary heart disease. *Blood*, 60, 650, 1982.

50. **Preston, F. E., Ward, J. D., Marcola, B. H., Porter, N. R., Timperley, W. R. and O'Malley, B. C.,** Elevated beta-thromboglobulin levels and circulating platelet aggregates in diabetic micro-angiopathy. *Lancet*, 1, 238, 1978.

51. **Fritschi, J., Christe, M., Lammle, B., Marbet, G. A., Berger, W. and Duckert, F.,** Platelet aggregation, beta-thromboglobulin and platelet factor 4 in diabetes mellitus and in patients with vasculopathy. *Thromb. Haemost.*, 52, 236, 1984.

52. **Zahavi, J. and Zahavi, M.,** Platelet function in type I diabetes mellitus. *N. Engl. J. Med.*, 319, 166, 1989.

53. **Voisin, P., Rousselle, D., Drouin, P. and Stoltz, J. F.,** Beta-thromboglobulin levels in diabetes mellitus : influence of degenerative lesions and glycemic regulation using an artificial pancreas. *Thromb. Res.*, 30, 245, 1983.

54. **Ireland, H., Lane, D. A., Wolff, S. and Foadi, M.,** In vivo platelet release in myeloproliferative disorders. *Thromb. Haemost.*, 48, 41, 1982.

55. **Rueda, F., Pinol, F., Marti, G. and Pujol-Moix, N.,** Abnormal levels of platelet-specific proteins and mitogenic activity in myeloproliferative disease. *Acta Haematol.*, 85, 12, 1991.

56. **Bellucci, S., Ignatova, E., Jaillet, N. and Boffa, M. C.,** Platelet hyperactivation in patients with essential thrombocythemia is not associated with vascular endothelial cell damage as judged by the level of plasma thrombomodulin, protein S, PAI-1, t-PA and vWF. *Thromb. Haemost.*, 70, 736, 1993.

57. **Adamides, S., Konstantopoulos, K., Toumbis, M., Douratsos, D., Travlou, A. and Kasfiki, A.,** A study of beta-thromboglobulin and platelet factor 4 plasma levels in steady state sickle cell patients. *Blood*, 61, 245, 1990.

58. **Han, P., Turpie, A. G. and Genton, E.,** Plasma beta-thromboglobulin : differentiation between intravascular and extravascular platelet destruction. *Blood*, 54, 1192, 1979.

59. **Rasi, V., Ikkala, E. and Valtonen, V.,** Plasma beta-thromboglobulin in severe infection. *Thromb. Res.*, 26, 267, 1982.

60. **Roth, G. and Calverley, D. C.,** Aspirin, platelets, and thrombosis : theory and practice. *Blood*, 83, 885, 1994.

61. **Grandström, E. and Kumlin, K.,** Assay of thromboxane production in biological systems : reliability of TxB_2 versus 11-dehydro-TxB_2 for measurement. *Prostagland. Thromb. Leuk. Res.*, 17, 587, 1985.

62. **Catella, F., Healy, D., Lawson, J.A. and FitzGerald, G.A.,** 11-dehydrothomboxane B_2: a quantitative index of thromboxane A_2 formation in the human circulation. *Proc. Natl. Acad. Sci. USA*, 83, 5861, 1986.

63. **Chiabrando, C., Rivoltella, L., Martelli, L., Valzacchi, S. and Fanelli, R.,** Urinary excretion of thromboxane and prostacyclin metabolites during chronic low-dose aspirin - evidence for an extrarenal origin of urinary thromboxane B_2 and 6-Keto-Prostaglandin F_1 alpha in healthy subjects. *Biochim. Biophys. Acta*, 1133, 247, 1992.

64. **Roberts, L. J., Sweetman, B. J. and Oates, J. A.,** Metabolism of thromboxane B_2 in man. Identification of twenty urinary metabolites. *J. Biol. Chem.*, 256, 8384, 1981.

65. **Reinke, M.,** Monitoring thromboxane in Body Fluids - A specific ELISA for 11-dehydrothromboxane B_2 using a monoclonal antibody. *Am. J. Physiol.*, 262, 658, 1992.

66. **Takasaki, W., Nakagawa, A., Asai, F., Ushiyama, S., Sugidachi, A., Matsuda, K., Oshima, T. and Tanaka, Y.,** Superiority of plasma 11-dehydro-TXB_2 to TXB_2 as an index of invivo TX formation in rabbits after dosing of CS-518, a TX synthase inhibitor. *Thromb. Res.*, 71, 69, 1993.

67. **Foegh, M. L., Zhao, Y., Madren, L., Rolnick, M., Stair, T.O., Huang, K. S. and Ramwell, P. W.,** Urinary thromboxane A_2 metabolites in patients presenting in the emergency room with acute chest pain. *J. Intern. Med.,* 235, 153, 1994.

68. **Westlung, P., Granström, E., Kumlin, M. and Nordenström, A.,** Identification of 11-dehydro-TxB$_2$ as a suitable parameter for monitoring thromboxane production in the human. *Prostaglandins,* 31, 929, 1986.

69. **Schweer, H., Meese, C. O., Fürst, O., Kühl, P. G. and Seyberth, H. W.,** Tandem mass spectrometric determination of 11-dehydrothromboxane B$_2$, an index metabolite of thromboxane B$_2$ in plasma and urine. *Anal. Biochem.,* 164, 156, 1987.

70. **Catella, F. and FitzGerald, G.A.,** Paired analysis of urinary thromboxane B$_2$ metabolites in humans. *Thromb. Res.,* 47, 647, 1987.

71. **Lawson, J. A., Patrono, C., Ciabattoni, G. and FitzGerald, G. A.,** Long-lived enzymatic metabolites of thromboxane B$_2$ in the human circulation. *Anal. Biochem.,* 155, 198, 1986.

72. **Patrono, G., Ciabattoni, G. and C., Davi.,** Thromboxane biosynthesis in cardiovascular disease. *Stroke,* 21, 130, 1990.

73. **Fisher, S.,** Analysis of eicosanoid formation in humans by mass spectrometry. *Advan. Lipid Res.,* 23, 199, 1989.

74. **Tsikas, D., Fauler, J., Bracht, S., Brunner, G. and Frolich, J. C.,** Analysis of leukotrienes, prostaglandins, thromboxane-B$_2$ and their metabolites by capillary isotachophoresis. *Electrophoresis,* 14, 664, 1993.

75. **Koski, I. J., Jansson, B. A., Markides, K. E. and Lee, M. L.,** Analysis of prostaglandins in aqueous solutions by supercritical fluid extraction and chromatography. *J. Pharmaceut. Biomed. Anal.,* 9, 281, 1991.

76. **Djurup, R., Chiabrando, C., Jorres, A., Fanelli, R., Foegh, M., Soerensen, H.U. and Joergensen, P. N.,** Rapid, direct enzyme immunoassay of 11-Keto-Thromboxane B$_2$, in urine, validated by immunoaffinity gas chromatography mass spectrometry. *Clin. Chem.,* 39, 2470, 1993.

77. **Powell, W. S.,** Rapid extraction of oxygenated metabolites of arachidonic acid from biological samples using octadecylsilyl silica. *Prostaglandins,* 20, 947, 1980.

78. **Bordet, J. C., de Lorgeril, M., Durbin, S., Boissonnat, P., Renaud, S., Dureau, G. and Dechavanne, M.** ,Systemic but not renal production of prostacyclin is highly reduced in cyclosporin-treated heart transplant recipients. *Am. J. Cardiol.* 72, 486, 1993.

79. **Dray, F., Charbonnel, B. and Maclouf, J.,** Radioimmunoassay of prostaglandin F_{2a}, E_1 and E_2 in human plasma. *Eur. J. Clin. Invest.,* 5, 311, 1975.

80. **Pradelles, P., Grassi, J. and Maclouf, J.,** Enzyme immunoassays using acetylcholinesterase as label : an alternative to radioimmunoassay. *Anal. Chem.,* 57, 1170, 1985.

81. **Leonhardt, A., Busch, C., Schweer, H. and Seyberth, H. W.,** Reference intervals and developmental changes in urinary prostanoid excretion in healthy newborns, infants and children. *Acta Paediat.,* 81, 191, 1992.

82. **Vesterqvist, O. and Gréen, K.,** Urinary excretion of 2,3-dinor-thromboxane B$_2$ in man under normal conditions, following drugs and during some pathological conditions. *Prostaglandins,* 27, 627, 1984.

83. **Wennmalm, A., Benthin, G., Caidahl, K., Granström, E. F., Lanne, B., Persson, L., Petersson, A. S. and Winell, S.** Non-invasive assessment of the cardiovascular eicosanoids, thromboxane-A$_2$ and prostacyclin, in randomly sampled males, with special reference to the influence of inheritance and environmental factors. *Clin. Sci.,* 79, 639, 1990.

84. **Chiba, S., Abe, K., Kudo, K., Omata, K., Yasujima, M., Sato, K., Seino, M., Imai, Y., Sato, M.and Yoshinaga, K.,** Sex and age-related differences in the urinary extraction of TxB$_2$ in normal human subjects : a possible pathophysiological role of TxA$_2$ in the aged kidney. *Prostagland. Leuk. Med.,* 16, 347, 1984.

85. **Vesterqvist, O.,** Measurements of the in vivo synthesis of thromboxane and prostacyclin in humans. *Scand. J. Clin. Lab. Invest.,* 48, 401, 1988.

86. **Wennmalm, A. and Fitzgerald, G. A.,** Excretion of prostacyclin and thromboxane A$_2$ metabolites during leg exercise in humans. *Am. J. Physiol.,* 255, H15, 1988.

87. **Ferretti, A., Flanagan, V. P. and Maida, E.J.** GC/MS/MS quantification of 11-dehydrothromboxane-B2 in human urine. *Prostagland. Leuk. Essent. Fatty,* 46, 271, 1992.

88. **Vesterqvist, O., Gréen, K., Lincoln, F. H. and Sebek, O. K.,** Development of a GC-MS method for quantitation of 2,3-dinor-TxB$_2$ and determinations of the daily urinary excretion rates in healthy humans. *Thromb. Res.,* 33, 39, 1983.

89. **Wennmalm, A., Benthin, G., Grandström, E. F., Persson, L. and Winell, S.,** 2,3-dinor metabolites of thromboxane A$_2$ and prostacyclin in urine from healthy subjects : diurnal variation and relation to 24 h excretion. *Clin. Sci.,* 83, 461, 1992.

90. **Uedelhoven, W. M., Rutzel, A., Meese, C. O. and Weber, P. C.,** Smoking alters thromboxane metabolism in man. *Biochim. Biophys. Acta,* 1081, 197, 1991.

91. **Uyama, O., Matsui, Y., Shimizu, S., Michishita, H. and Sugita, M.,** Risk factors for carotid atherosclerosis and platelet activation. *Jpn. Circ. J.,* 58, 409, 1994.

92. **Fogelberg, M., Vesterqvist, O., Diczfalusy, U. and Henriksson, P.,** Experimental atherosclerosis - effects of oestrogen and atherosclerosis on thromboxane and prostacyclin formation. *Eur. J. Clin. Invest.,* 20, 105, 1990.

93. **Adatia, I., Barrow, S.E., Stratton, P.D., Miallallen, V.M., Ritter, J.M. and Haworth, S.G.,** Thromboxane A$_2$ and prostacyclin biosynthesis in children and adolescents with pulmonary vascular disease. *Circulation,* 88, 2117, 1993.

94. **Johnson, B. F., Wiley, K. N., Greaves, M., Preston, F. E., Fox, M. and Raftery, A. T.,** Urinary thromboxane and 6-keto-prostaglandin F$_1$ alpha are early markers of acute rejection in experimental pancreas transplantation. *Transplantation,* 58, 18, 1994.

95. **Fitzgerald, D. J., Roy, L., Catella, F. and Fitzgerald, G. A.,** Platelet activation in unstable coronary disease. *N. Engl. J. Med.,* 315, 983, 1986.

96. **Lorenz, R., Uedelhoven, W., Fisher, S., Ruetzel, A. and Weber, P. C.,** A critical evaluation of urinary immunoreactive thromboxane : feasibility of its determination as a potential vascular risk factor. *Biochim. Biophys. Acta,* 993, 259, 1989.

97. **Davi, G., Averna, M., Catalano, I., Bargallo, C., Ganci, A., Notarbartolo, A., Ciabattoni, G. and Patronno, C.,** Increased thromboxane biosynthesis in type IIa hypercholesterolemia. *Circulation,* 85, 1792, 1992.

98. **Satoh, K., Imaizumi, T., Yoshida, H., Hiramoto, M., Konta, A. and Takamatsu, S.,** Plasma 11-dehydrothromboxane-B$_2$ - A reliable indicator of platelet hyperfunction in patients with ischemic stroke. *Acta Neurol. Scand.,* 83, 99, 1991.

99. **Lorenz, R., Helmer, P., Uedelhoven, W., Zimmer, B. and Weber, P. C.,** A new method using simple solid phase

extraction for the rapid gas-chromatographic mass-spectrometric determination of 11-dehydro-thromboxane B_2 in urine. *Prostaglandins*, 38, 157, 1989.

100. **Christman, B.W., Mcpherson, C.D., Newman, J.H., King, G.A., Bernard, G.R., Groves, B.M. and Loyd, J.E.,** An imbalance between the excretion of thromboxane and prostacyclin metabolites in pulmonary hypertension. *N. Engl. J. Med.*, 327, 70, 1992.

101. **Fitzgerald, D. J., Catella, F., Roy, L. and Fitzgerald, G. A.,** Marked platelet activation in vivo after intravenous streptokinase in patients with acute myocardial infarction. *Circulation*, 77, 142, 1990.

102. **Foulon, I., Bachir, D., Galacteros, F. and Maclouf, J.,** Increased in vivo production of thromboxane in patients with sickle cell disease is accompanied by an impairment of platelet functions to the thromboxane A_2 agonist U46619. *Arterioscler. Thromb.*, 13, 421, 1993.

103. **Kurantsinmills, J., Ibe, B.O., Natta, C.L., Raj, J. U., Siegel, R. S. and Lessin, L.S.,** Elevated urinary levels of thromboxane and prostacyclin metabolites in sickle cell disease reflects activated platelets in the circulation. *Br. J. Haematol.*, 87, 580, 1994.

104. **Martinuzzo, M. E., Maclouf, J., Carreras, L. O. and Levy-Toledano, S.,** Antiphospholipid antibodies enhance thrombin-induced platelet activation and thromboxane formation. *Thromb. Haemost.*, 70, 667, 1993.

105. **Vesterqvist, O., Gréen, K. and Johnsson, H.** , Thromboxane and prostacyclin formation in patients with deep vein thrombosis. *Thromb. Res.*, 45, 393, 1987.

106. **Gréen, K., Vesterqvist, O. and Grill, V.,** Urinary metabolites of thromboxanes and prostacyclin in diabetes mellitus. *Acta Endocrinol.*, 118, 301, 1988.

107. **Lemne, C., Vesterqvist, O., Egberg, N., Green, K., Jogestrand, T. and Defaire, U.,** Platelet activation and prostacyclin release in essential hypertension. *Prostaglandins*, 44, 219, 1992.

108. **Duval, D. and Freyss-Beguin, M.,** Glucocorticoids and prostaglandin synthesis : we cannot see the wood for the trees. *Prostagland. Leuk. Essent. Fatty*, 45, 85, 1992.

109. **Ciabattoni, G., Ujang, S., Sritara, P., Andreotti, F., Davies, G., Simonetti, B.M., Patrono, C. and Maseri, A.,** Aspirin, but not heparin, suppresses the transient increase in thromboxane biosynthesis associated with cardiac catheterization or coronary angioplasty. *J. Am. Coll. Cardiol.*, 21, 1377, 1993.

110. **Uematsu, T., Takasaki, W., Kosuge, K., Wada, K., Matsuno., H., Tanaka, Y., Yamamura, N. and Nakashima, M.**, Changes in plasma and urinary 11-dehydrothromboxane-B2 in healthy subjects produced by oral CS-518, a novel thromboxane synthase inhibitor. *Eur. J. Clin. Pharmacol.*, 45, 283, 1993.

111. **Shattil, S. J., Cunningham, M., and Hoxie, J. A.,** Detection of activated platelets in whole blood using activation dependent monoclonal antibodies and flow cytometry. *Blood*, 70, 307, 1987.

112. **Michelson, A. D., Ellis, P. A., Barnard, M. R., Matic, G. B., Viles, A. F. and Kestin, A. S.,** Down regulation of the platelet surface glycoprotein Ib-IX in whole blood stimulated by thrombin, ADP or an in vivo wound. *Blood*, 77, 770, 1991.

113. **Dechavanne, M., Ffrench, M., Pages, J., Ffrench, P., Boukerche, H., Bryon, P.A., McGregor, J.L.,** Significant reduction in the binding of a monoclonal antibody (LYP 18) directed against the IIb/IIIa glycoprotein complex to platelets of patients having undergone extracorporeal circulation. *Thromb. Haemost.*, 57, 106, 1987.

114. **Rinder, C. S., Mathew, J. P., Rinder, H. M., Bonan, J., Ault, K. A. and Smith, B. R.,** Modulation of platelet surface adhesion receptors during cardiopulmonary bypass. *Anesthesiology*, 75, 563, 1991.

115. **Kestin, A. S., Valeri, C. R., Khuri, S. F., Loscalzo, J., Ellis, P. A., McGregor, H., Birjiniuk, V., Ouimet H., Pasche, B., Benoit, S. E., Rodino, L. J., Barnard, M. R. and Michelson, A. D.,** The platelet function defect of cardiopulmonary bypass. *Blood*, 82, 107, 1993.

116. **Abrams, C. S., Ellison, N. , Budzynski A. Z. and Shattil, S. J.,** Direct detection of activated platelets and platelet-derived microparticles in humans. *Blood*, 75, 128, 1990.

117. **Scharf, R. E., Tomer, A., Marzec, U. M., Teirstein, P. S., Ruggieri, Z. M. and Harker, L. A.,** Activation of platelets in blood perfusing angioplasty damaged coronary arteries. Flow cytometry detection. *Arterioscler. Thromb.*, 12, 1475, 1992.

118. **Nurden, A.T., Lacaze, D., Macchi, L., Pintigny, D., Durrieu, C., Besse, P., Sanchez, G., Chevaleyre, J., Ferrer, A. M., Vezon, G., Hourdille, P.** , Platelet activation in two different clinical conditions. Patients with severe burns and after angioplasty in coronary artery disease (abstract). *Thromb. Haemost.*, 65, 679, 1991.

119. **Palabrica, T. M., Smith, J. J., Aronovitz, M. J., Kimmelstiel, D., Golden, J. S., Scott, D., Haik, B. J., Salem, D. N. and Konstam, M. A.** Flow cytometric analysis of platelet PADGEM expression during percutaneous transluminal coronary angioplasty (abstract). *Circulation*, 82, 655, 1990.

120. **Tschöpe, D., Esser, J., Schwippert, B., Rösen, P., Kehrel, B., Nieuwenhuis, H. K. and Gries, F. A.** Large platelets circulate in an activated state in diabetes mellitus. *Semin. Thromb. Haemostasis*, 17, 433, 1991.

121. **Ejim, O. S., Powling, M. J., Dandona, P., Kernoff, P. B. and Goodall, A. H.,** A flow cytometric analysis of fibronectin binding to platelets from patients with peripheral vascular disease. *Thromb. Res.*, 58, 519, 1990.

122. **Legrand, C., Bellucci, S., Edelman, L. and Tobelem, G.,** Platelet thrombospondin and glycoprotein abnormalities in patients with essential thrombocythemia : effect of a-interferon treatment. *Am. J. Hematol.*, 38, 307, 1991.

123. **Del Principe, D., Menichelli, A., Di Giulio, S., De Matteis, W., Cianciulli, P. and Papa, G.,** PADGEM/GMP-140 expression on platelet membranes from homozygous beta thalassemic patients. *Br. J. Haematol.*, 84, 111, 1993.

124. **Wehmeier, A., Tschope, D., Esser, J., Menzel, C., Nieuwenhuis, H. K. and Schneider, W.** Circulating activated platelets in myeloproliferative disorders. *Thromb. Res.*, 61, 271, 1991.

125. **Palabrica, T. M., Furie, B. C., Konstam, M. A., Aronovitz, M. J., Connoly, R., Brockway, B. A., Ramberg, K. L. and Furie, B.,** Thrombus imaging in a primate model with antibodies specific for an external membrane protein of activated platelets. *Proc. Natl. Acad. Sci. USA*, 86, 1036, 1989.

126. **Rinder, H. M., Murphy, M., Mitchell, J. G., Stocks, J., Ault, K. A. and Killman, R. S.,** Progressive platelet activation with storage : evidence for shortened survival of activated platelets after transfusion. *Transfusion*, 31, 409, 1991.

VON WILLEBRAND FACTOR IN THROMBOTIC DISORDERS

J. Seghatchian*, A.A. Halle, T. McKiernan**, S. Johnson**,
S. Farid*** and H. Messmore, Jr.*****
* North London Blood Transfusion Centre, London
** Loyola University Stritch, School of Medicine
*** Hines Veterans Affairs Hospital

I. INTRODUCTION

Arterial thrombosis secondary to atherosclerosis is a leading health problem of middle aged and elderly adults. It results in serious disability and/or death due to stroke, myocardial ischemia and ischemia of other organs and extremities. There is evidence to suggest that vWF promotes atherosclerosis, arterial thrombosis and probably post angioplasty re-stenosis. Thus, the studies of the biochemistry, physiology, pathophysiology and genetics of this molecule that were initially prompted by efforts to diagnose and treat von Willebrand disease have now been applied to the study of arterial thrombotic disorders. Studies of the normal physiology have been continuously expanded over the past twenty years and information on the blood levels and the composition of this molecule in a variety of disease states has been documented[1-12]. In this review, selected studies that have helped clarify the role of vWF in normal physiology as well as in the pathophysiology of thrombosis and re-stenosis will be discussed. Strategies to modulate the normal functions of this molecule in order to reduce the likelihood of thrombosis occurring or to slow its progression will be reviewed as well.

II. NORMAL PHYSIOLOGY

Von Willebrand factor is a very large multimeric molecule synthesized in endothelial cells and megakaryocytes. It functions as a carrier for factor VIII and as a bridge between the platelet and the subendothelium or collagen of the vascular wall at sites of injury.[8] The platelet thus is able to adhere to the site of injury and undergo further activation, releasing its dense and alpha granule contents which include platelet vWF. Circulating vWF does not bind to its receptor, platelet glycoprotein 1b (GP1b) except when high shear rate occurs (>800 sec^{-1}) which is always in the arterial circulation and is near the endothelial surface[13]. When binding by a specific domain of the sub-unit of vWF to GP 1b occurs, the platelet is activated, intraplatelet calcium levels rise and glycoproteins IIb and IIIa are expressed upon the release of ADP from the platelet dense granules. Another domain of the vWF binds to the GPIIb-IIIa receptor. By way of interplatelet cross linking the platelets can be bound to each other by vWF. At the same time the vWF molecule is able to bind to collagen at the site of vascular injury via it is specific collagen binding domain peptides.[14] There is a specific heparin binding which may be significant in terms of binding of the molecule to glycosaminoglycans in the subendothelial matrix.[12] Ristocetin induces changes in the vWF molecule by altering its electrical charge. These changes facilitate its binding to GP1b.

The vWF is stored in Weibel Palade bodies in endothelial cells and can be released by a variety of stimuli as determined from in vitro studies. Any noxious stimulus may be capable of causing release as well as the stimulation of synthesis by endothelial cells.[15] It is an acute phase reactant, and when the level increases, the level of factor VIII rises as well, and when its levels are low due to impaired production as in von Willebrand disease, the factor VIII levels are low.[16] The levels in females vary with the menstrual cycle, lower levels occurring at the time of menses. The levels rise to several fold normal during pregnancy. The levels of vWF are stimulated to rise by 1-desamino 8-D-arginine vasopressin (DDAVP) (desmopressin).[17,19]

III. vWF IN VARIOUS DISEASE STATES

The blood level and molecular structure of vWF in hereditary disorders such as von Willebrand's disease will not be discussed. The multimer patterns are altered in a variety of acquired diseases associated with elevated blood levels of vWF. This is readily demonstrable by comparing the crossed immunoelectrophoresis pattern of patient vWF with the normal pattern. Changes in the relative amount of high molecular weight multimers with respect to lower molecular weight multimers results in slow versus fast migrating molecules in the electrophoresis gel.[6,7] More precise multimer distribution patterns can be demonstrated by specific multimer assays utilizing electrophoresis and radioactive or enzyme linked antibodies.[9,13,14,18]

It has been shown that the syndromes of TTP and HUS are associated with increased levels of "unusually" high molecular weight multimers, but the precise role these play in the process of thrombosis of arterioles in these syndromes is not clear.[9] It is generally believed that the higher molecular weight multimers are more effective in promoting hemostasis than the lower molecular weight multimers. Whether one can correlate the level of higher molecular weight multimers with thrombosis in atherosclerosis is unknown. It has been shown that increased vWF levels represent a risk factor for arteriosclerosis and thrombosis, and that acute re-occlusion following coronary artery angioplasty is more likely to occur in patients with high levels of vWF prior to the angioplasty procedure.[20,21] Anecdotal cases of acute myocardial infarction and death following the administration of DDAVP for uremic bleeding have been reported.[17] There has been a reported association of elevated factor VIIIC as well as of vWF in patients with ischemic heart disease, particularly in those who have had fatal outcomes.[20] A correction for the ABO blood group of the patient had to be made based on the fact that normally the non-O blood groups have higher levels of vWF than those with group O.[11,19]

In some disorders, there appears to be an increase of smaller multimers. This has been observed in the presence of a fibrinolytic process occurring, either endogenously or by thrombolytic therapy.[12] This may occur endogenously in uremia as well due to enzymatic degradation of the molecule after its release from endothelial cells.[4,7] Hemophiliacs with liver disease have been reported to have this problem as well.[4]

IV. ANIMAL MODELS

The von Willebrand disease pig has been an extremely useful model to study the role of vWF in thrombosis and in atherosclerosis.[23] It has been possible with this model to show that occlusive coronary thrombosis is a vWF dependent process, and that with high grade stenosis thrombosis does not occur in von Willebrand disease pigs.[4,25] Ruptured atherosclerotic plaques also do not thrombose in this model. It has also been shown that the likelihood of atherosclerosis is less in pigs with vWF deficiency as compared with pigs who are normal when both groups have been placed under long term observation (4 years on a normal diet).[26-30] When pigs are given anti-vWF antibodies and are subjected to both vascular injury and stenosis, they do not develop vascular occlusion as compared with pigs who did not receive anti-vWF anti-body.[31,32]

V. THERAPEUTIC MODULATION OF vWF

By lowering the level or by impairing the function of vWF, it should be possible to reduce the likelihood of arterial thrombosis whenever there is vascular injury, or when plaque rupture or severe stenosis occurs in atherosclerosis. Since vWF is an acute phase reactant,[16] it is possible that the elevated levels seen in elderly populations are due to atherosclerosis itself since macrophage activation is occurring in the vascular wall with release of cytokines. It is also likely that the elevated vWF in some of the elderly is due to arthritis since the association of arthritis and elevated vWF has been reported.[33]

The use of antiinflammatory drugs of the non-steroidal or steroidal type might lower vWF levels. Heparin binds to vWF and it impairs platelet-vWF interaction, by binding to the GP1b binding domain when the heparin molecule is of sufficient length, or it could be via binding of heparin to GP1b on the platelet.[14,34,35] Both these mechanisms are known to occur with standard heparin, but only to a minor degree with low molecular weight heparin.[36] It has been postulated that the prolonged bleeding time seen with high dose standard heparin is due to interference with vWF function.[35] Heparin interferes with the ristocetin cofactor assay for vWF.[34] Low affinity heparin interferes with vWF function by the same mechanism,[34,35] and it has been shown to be antithrombotic in an animal model of thrombosis, possibly by its interference with vWF function.[36] Some unique chemicals such as aurintricarboxylic acid inhibit the binding of vWF to platelet GP1b and inhibit platelet retention and thrombus formation in vivo.[37]

A number of investigators have produced monoclonal antibodies to various domains of the vWF and have in animal models been able to modulate arterial thrombosis utilizing these antibodies.[31,32,38] In similar models it has been possible to utilize peptides that interfere with platelet-vWF interaction. Plasmapheresis has been an effective treatment for TTP and HUS, possibly by removing vWF from the circulation.[9] This concept has not been applied to unstable angina,[5,39] where it might be effective but its safety in such patients would be in doubt

Thrombolytic therapy lowers the functional level of vWF and therefore could be useful in preventing vascular occlusion from occurring in unstable angina.[22] The benefit seen with antiplatelet agents might in part be due to decreased release of platelet vWF at sites of platelet adherence to injured endothelium.[13]

Continued investigation of the functions of vWF and the pathophysiology of vascular occlusive events will undoubtedly lead to newer approaches to thrombosis in the arterial circulation by modulation of von Willebrand factor levels or functions.

VI. CONCLUSION

There is little doubt that von Willebrand factor plays an important role in arterial vascular occlusion. While it does appear to be a risk factor for atherosclerosis in an animal model, its role in the pathogenesis of atherosclerosis in the human is not clear. The blood level is increased in patients at increased risk for atherosclerosis and arterial thrombosis. This may be due to the fact that it is an acute phase reactant and that it causes no adverse events such as thrombosis unless there is endothelial injury, plaque rupture or severe arterial stenosis. It may be possible to prevent thrombosis in some acute coronary or carotid artery syndromes by lowering the blood level or by interfering with the function of vWF. Heparin, low affinity domains and peptides synthesized to mimic those domains have each shown some promise as drugs to modulate the function of vWF.

REFERENCES

1. **Folsom AR, Wu KK, Shahar E.** Association of hemostatic variables with prevalent cardiovascular disease and asymptomatic carotid artery atherosclerosis. *Arterioscl Thromb.* 13: 1829, 1993.
2. **Jansson J-H, Nillson TK, Johnson O.** von Willebrand factor in plasma: A novel risk factor for recurrent myocardial infarction and death. *Br Heart J* 66: 351, 1991.

3.   **Andreotti F, Roncaglioni MC, Hackett DR, et al.** Early coronary reperfusion blunts the procoagulant response of plasminogen activator inhibitor - 1 and von Willebrand factor in acute myocardial infarction.*JACC* 16: 1553, 1990.

4.   **Greeno E, Boelsen R, Chase B, et al.** von Willebrand factor proteolysis as an additional hemostatic defect in hemophilia patients with liver disease. *Blood* 81 (Suppl 1): 198a (abst 778), 1994.

5.   **Mossard JM, Wiesel ML, Casenave JP, et al.** Relations entre augmentation du facteur de Willebrande plasmatique, infarctus du myocarde aigu, angor instable et thrombose coronaire. *Arch Mal Coeur* 82: 1813, 1989.

6.   **Lombardi R, Mannucci PM, Seghatchian MJ, Garcia VV, Coppola R.** Alterations of factor VIII von Willebrand factor in clinical conditions associated with an increase in its plasma concentration. *Br J Haematol* 49: 61, 1981.

7.   **Winter M, Seghatchian MJ, Cameron JS.** An abnormal factor VIII molecule in uraemia. *Lancet* 1: 1112, 1983 (letter).

8.   **Meyer D, Pietu G, Fressinaud E.** von Willebrand factor: Structure and function.*Mayo Clin Proc* 66: 516, 1991.

9.   **Moake JL, McPherson PD.** Abnormalities of von Willebrand factor multimers in thrombotic thrombocytopenic purpura and the hemolytic uremic syndrome. *AM J Med* 87: 3-21N, 1989.

10. **Upshaw JD.** Congenital deficiency of a factor in normal plasma that reverses mircoangiopathic hemolysis and thrombocytopenia. *N Eng J Med* 298: 1350, 1978.

11. **Meade TW, Cooper JA, Stirling Y.** Factor VIII, ABO blood group and the incidence of ischemic heart disease. *Br J Haematol* 88: 601, 1994.

12. **Fujimura Y, Titani K, Holland LZ, et al.** A heparin binding domain of human von Willebrand factor. *J Biol Chem* 262: 1374, 1987.

13. **Moake JL, Turner NA, Stathopoulos NA, et al.**Shear induced platelet aggregation can be mediated by vWF released from platelets as well as by exogenous large or unusually large vWF multimers, requires adenosine diphosphate and is resistant to aspirin. *Blood* 71: 1366, 1988.

14. **Ruggeri ZM.** Structure and function of von Willebrand factor: Relationship to von Willebrand's disease. *Mayo Clin Proc* 66: 847, 1991.

15. **Blann AD.** von Willebrand factor as a marker of injury to the endothelium in inflammatory vascular disease. *J Rheum* 20: 1469, 1993.

16. **Pottinger BE, Read RC, Paleolog EM, et al.**von Willebrand factor is an acute phase reactant in man. *Thromb Res* 53: 387- 394, 1989.

17. **Mannucci PM, Carsson S, Harris AS.** Desmopressin, surgery and thrombosis. *Thromb Haemostas* 71: 154, 1994 (letter).

18. **Triplett DA.** Laboratory diagnosis of von Willebrand's disease. *Mayo Clin Proc* 66: 832, 1991.

19. **Bloom AL.**von Willebrand factor: Clinical features of inherited and acquired disorders.*Mayo Clin Proc* 66: 743, 1991.

20. **Jansson J-H, Torbjorn KN, Johnson O.** von Willebrand factor in plasma: a novel risk factor for recurrent myocardial infarction and death. *Br Heart J* 66: 351-°356, 1991.

21. **Halle AA, Johnson S, McKiernan T, et al.** The importance of von Willebrand factor in post-PTCA acute thrombotic complications. Submitted for publication.

22. **Federici A, Berowitz S, Zimmerman T, Mannucci P.** Proteolysis of von Willebrand factor after thrombolytic therapy in patients with acute myocardial infarction. *Blood* 79: 38, 1992.

23. **Brinkhous KM, Reddick RL, Read MS, et al.** von Willebrand factor and animal models: contributions to gene therapy, thrombocytopenic purpura and coronary artery thrombosis. *Mayo Clin Proc* 66: 733, 1991.

24. **Nichols TC, Bellinger DA, Johnson AJ, et al.** von Willebrand's disease prevents occlusive thrombosis in stenosed and injured porcine coronary arteries. *Circ Res* 59: 15, 1986.

25. **Nichols TC, Bellinger DA, Tate D, et al.** von Willebrand factor and occlusive arterial thrombosis. A study in normal and von Willebrand disease pigs with diet-induced hypercholesterolemia and atherosclerosis. *Arteriosclerosis* 10: 449, 1990.

26. **Badimon L, Badimon JJ, Turitto VT, et al.** Platelet thrombus formation on collagen type 1. A model of deep vessel injury - influence of blood rheology, von Willebrand factor and blood coagulation. *Circulation* 78: 1431, 1988.

27. **Badimon L, Badimon JJ, Turitto VT, et al.** Platelet deposition in von Willebrand factor deficient vessel wall. *J Lab Clin Med* 110: 634, 1987.

28. **Badimon L, Badimon JJ.** Mechanism of arterial thrombosis in non-parallel streamlines: platelet thrombi grow at the apex of stenotic severely injured vessel wall. Experimental study in the pig model. *J Clin Invest* 84: 1143, 1989.

29. **Fuster V, Badimon L, Badimon JJ, et al.** The porcine model for understanding of thrombogenesis and atherogenesis. *Mayo Clin Proc* 66: 818, 1991.

30. **Fuster V, Badimon L, Rosemark J, et al.** Spontaneous and diet-induced coronary atherosclerosis in normal swine and swine with von Willebrand's disease. *Arteriosclerosis* 5: 67, 1985.

31. **Bowie EJW, Fass DN, Katzmann JA.** Functional studies of Willebrand factor using monoclinal antibodies. *Blood* 62: 146, 1983.

32. **Badimon L, Badimon J, Ruggeri Z, et al.** A peptide-specific monoclinal antibody that inhibits von Willebrand factor binding to GPIIb-IIIa (152 B6) inhibits platelet deposition to human atherosclerotic vessel wall. *Circulation* 80 (suppl 2): 24, 1989.

33. **Barin AD.** Association of von Willebrand factor with age, sex and other risk factors for atherosclerosis. *Thromb Haemostas* 71: 528, 1994.

34. **Messmore H, Griffin B, Koza M, et al.** Interaction of heparinoids with platelets: Comparison with heparin and low molecular weight heparins. *Sem Thromb Haemostas* 17 (suppl 1): 57, 1991.

35. **Sobel M, McNeil P, Carlson P, et al.** Heparin inhibition of von Willebrand factor-dependent platelet function in vitro and in vivo. *J Clin Invest* 87: 1787, 1991.

36. **Baruch D, Ajzenberg N, Denis C, et al.** Binding of heparin fractions to von Willebrand factor: Effect of molecular weight and affinity for antithrombin III. *Thromb Haemostas* 71: 141, 1994.

37. **Kawaskai T, Kaku S, Kohinata T.** Inhibition by aurintricarboxylic acid of von Willebrand factor binding to platelet GP1b platelet retention and thrombus formation in vivo. *Am J Hematol* 47: 6, 1994.

38. **Cadroy Y, Kelly A, Marzec U, et al.** Comparison of the antihemostatic and antithrombotic effects of monoclonal antibodies against von Willebrand factor and platelet glycoprotein IIB-IIIa. **Circulation** 80 (Suppl 2): 24, 1989.

39. **Berglund V, Wallentin L.** Influence in platelet function by heparin in men with unstable coronary artery disease. *Thrombos Haemostas* 66: 648, 1991.

CRITICAL EVALUATION OF FIBRINOGEN ASSAYS

M.P.M. de Maat, F. Haverkate
Gaubius Laboratory TNO-PG, Leiden

I. INTRODUCTION

Fibrinogen is a soluble plasma glycoprotein that is present in normal human plasma at a concentration of 2-4 g/L. In pathological states clottable fibrinogen can fluctuate from approximately 0 to above 10 g/L. It is composed of two pairs of three polypeptide chains (Aα, Bβ and γ) that are interconnected by disulphide bridges. The aminoterminal segments of the six chains form a central domain from which the fibrinopeptides A and B protrude[1]. During clotting thrombin cleaves off the fibrinopeptides A from the Aα chains which leads to a conformational change of the molecule and, via intermediate stages, eventually leads to polymerization into the insoluble fibrin fibres. Somewhat delayed also the fibrinopeptides B from the Bβ-chains are cleaved off, which initiates the lateral polymerization of the fibrin fibres. The fibrin network is normally constructed of fibres that are about 1 μm in diameter, corresponding to a width of several hundred molecules. Only 0.3% of the mass of a blood clot is made up of fibrin, about 80% of the volume is liquid and the remainder includes blood elements like platelets and red and white blood cells.

Fibrinogen concentrations are subject to considerable biological variation. Fibrinogen is one of the major acute phase reactant proteins, and increased hepatic synthesis occurs as a physiological response to inflammation and tissue necrosis[2]. Altered protein catabolism due to intravascular consumption may also influence circulating plasma concentrations. The plasma fibrinogen concentration rises 5-7% per ten years of age[3-6], and a gender difference is described in both young and old groups[3,5]. Fibrinogen levels are also correlated with smoking (overview: 7), body weight[4,6] and degree of coronary stenosis[6,8-12]. In women, the fibrinogen levels rise after menopause. The effects of hormone replacement therapy are inconsistent[13]. The plasma fibrinogen level is increased in users of combined oral contraceptives[14] and during pregnancy[15].

At least three molecular forms of fibrinogen have been identified in plasma[16-23]. Fibrinogen is synthesized in the high molecular weight form (HMW), with two intact carboxyl ends of the α-chain. In plasma two groups of degraded forms of fibrinogen can be distinguished. One group has one degraded Aα-chain carboxyl end and is called the low molecular weight (LMW) form, in the other form both Aα-chains are degraded and this is called the LMW' form. In a normal, average plasma 70% of fibrinogen is HMW, 26% is LMW and only 4% is LMW'. The LMW and LMW' forms are heterogenous due to the different length of their constituent Aα-chain. The enzymes responsible for the degradation have not yet been identified[24].

There are indications of a pathological significance of the occurrence of relatively high levels of HMW fibrinogen. Treatment of patients with acute myocardial infarction (AMI) with streptokinase results in a radical consumption of their fibrinogen. Fibrinogen is then newly synthesized in the HMW form[25] which has an increased clotting capacity. This procoagulant tendency might explain the observation that in patients with the highest HMW-fibrinogen levels more reinfarctions are observed. For the management of AMI patients it is therefore advisable to measure fibrinogen levels with a method that is more sensitive to HMW fibrinogen than to the other fibrinogen forms, because such an assay may give the best estimation of the thrombotic risk. Promising methods for this purpose are in development and will be discussed. A prethrombotic state due to increased HMW-fibrinogen also rapidly develops after hip surgery; after MI not treated with streptokinase; or after any major trauma, where much HMW-fibrinogen is synthesized while the LMW only increases much later[26].

Usually plasma fibrinogen levels are measured in the management of consumptive coagulopathies. During the last decade fibrinogen levels have been studied in other diseases. An association between fibrinogen levels and the severity of atherosclerosis has been repeatedly observed[8-12,27]. Also, the results of the Northwick Park Heart Study[28] and several other studies in healthy populations[6,29-35] have shown that elevated plasma fibrinogen levels are associated with an increased risk for ischaemic heart disease (IHD). Although methods for fibrinogen quantification differ from study to study, a significant association between plasma fibrinogen levels and risk for cardiac events was found in all of them.

There are several different principles on which the measurement of fibrinogen can be based[36,37]. First, there are the clotting rate assays, that give a functional fibrinogen level. The second group of assays measures the amount of protein that can be clotted with thrombin. Furthermore, there are the methods based on heat- and salt precipitation of fibrinogen. Finally there are the immunological methods for which there is growing interest since the introduction of specific monoclonal antibodies.

Each of these methods will be susceptible in its own way to sources of variation. The expression of the three forms of fibrinogen mentioned above is likely to be different in clotting assays, because the thrombin clotting times of the three fibrinogen forms differ[18,21,22,38]. The different fibrinogen forms also produce clots with a different fibre structure[38], which might influence methods where the end point depends on the clot structure (Ellis and Stransky, Prothrombin Time-derived (discussed later)). In this paper, we will focus on the currently used methods to determine fibrinogen, and on the methodological aspects including specificity, sensitivity, interfering substances and calibration.

II. CLOTTING RATE BASED ASSAYS

The assays that are most often used in a routine laboratory are based on measuring the time it takes to clot plasma after the addition of excess thrombin[39]. The concentration of fibrinogen is expressed as a function of the clotting time. By applying different dilutions of the plasma, it is possible to measure fibrinogen levels between 0.5 and 10 g/L. It is also possible to use snake venom (Arvin) or reptilase in clotting rate assays instead of thrombin. The latter enzymes function more specifically than thrombin because they will only split off the fibrinopeptide A[40].

It has to be remembered that this method yields a functional fibrinogen level, and not an absolute concentration of fibrinogen. As will be discussed below, the fibrinogen levels found with this method are influenced by forms of fibrinogen that have an altered fibrinogen clotting rate.

An additional point of importance is that the effect of certain factors (such as the degradation products of fibrin and fibrinogen (FDP); heparin) on the clotting rate assays may be different from the effect they have on the clotting rate *in vivo*.

A. FACTORS INFLUENCING THE CLOTTING TIME

Fibrin degradation products (FDP) have a strong anticoagulant effect and affect the polymerisation times of fibrinogen solutions. This effect is most pronounced for fragments X and Y[41], but fragment D also has anticlotting properties[42]. Increased FDP levels are therefore expected to delay clotting in clotting rate based assays and as a consequence yield spuriously low fibrinogen levels. However, no effect of FDP (< 190 μg/mL) on the Clauss assay was found in samples containing normal fibrinogen levels. Only in samples with fibrinogen levels below 1 g/L did the high FDP levels interfere[43,44]. This might be explained by a difference in the type of FDP in that situation[45,46]. Increased fibrin monomer levels in the patient are expected to cause spuriously high levels through reduction of the clotting time.

Also, an alteration in the distribution of the three fibrinogen forms (HMW, LMW and LMW') in plasma may affect the Clauss assay. The LMW and LMW' forms have a prolonged thrombin clotting time[16,18,22] and therefore changes in the ratio of the three fibrinogen forms will affect the thrombin clotting time and result in different values without differences in molar concentrations. The time required for the transformation from HMW- and LMW-fibrinogen to fibrin by thrombin is similar, but the rate of polymerization is reduced for LMW compared to HMW and is even lower for LMW'. Also, the different heights of the polymerization curves indicate different fibril length and thickness. Clots from HMW fibrin have thicker and shorter fibrils than those from LMW fibrin [38]. A more compact clot has a higher turbidity and firmness than a looser clot and this influences the turbidimetric and mechanical end point measurements.

Newly synthesized fibrinogen is more phosphorylated, particularly in fibrinopeptide A at serine 3, than normal fibrinogen[25,47,48]. The fibrinogen found after streptokinase treatment has 66% of the possible sites phosphorylated whereas normal fibrinogen has only 30%[25]. Reports on the effect of phosphorylation on clotting are conflicting. Witt et al[47] find no effect, but both Hanna et al[48] and Reganon et al[23] describe that phosphorylation increases the release of FPA, which they ascribe to an enhanced binding of thrombin to the phosphorylated fibrinogen. If indeed phosphorylated fibrinogen clots faster, this further emphasizes that not all forms of fibrinogen show the same clotting behaviour.

Another component that influences the clotting rate assay is heparin, which in patients' plasma (concentrations 0.03 - 3 IU/mL) gives apparent increases up to 20% of the estimated plasma fibrinogen level in the Clauss assay[44]. This artefact might hinder the use of the fibrinogen level to predict the thrombotic risk. Polybrene (1,5-dimethyl-1,5-diazaundeca-methylene polymethobromide) can be used to neutralize heparin in the sample[49].

Little is known about the disturbance by lipids in the clotting rate assay. No effect was found when plasma from healthy volunteers was supplemented with plasma with increasing levels of β-lipoprotein[50]. In assays based on a turbidimetric end point, lipemic and haemolytic plasmas may disturb the measurements.

In patients with cirrhosis of the liver, the fibrinogen molecules have an increased sialic acid content. This causes prolonged clotting times with thrombin[51,52]. After removing the sialic acid from the fibrinogen molecules with neuraminidase, the clotting times normalize. It has been reported that during inflammation the glycosylation of the acute phase proteins is altered[53,54]. As fibrinogen is an acute phase protein, this may result in defective functional fibrinogen levels[55] in patients with an increased inflammatory status.

One freezing-thawing step does not give levels different from those found in fresh plasma[56].

B. PRECISION

In a quality control study performed in 18 different laboratories, the Clauss method was the most accurate haemostatic assay[57], reporting a coefficient of variation (CV) of 3.3% between duplicate measurements in the same series, a between day CV of 4.7% and a between centres CV of 5.3%.

C. USE AS ROUTINE ASSAY

The clotting rate based methods are the most frequently used in routine laboratories, because they measure the functional fibrinogen levels and also because they are fast, cheap and have little variation[58].

A major problem, especially in the assessment of thrombotic risk, is the discrepancy between the different laboratories. This will be discussed below.

D. COMMENTS

In clotting rate assays the velocity of the fibrinogen to fibrin conversion can be enhanced by the presence of dextran and calcium chloride. Dextran increases the turbidity of the fibrin polymer at subnormal plasma concentrations of fibrinogen[49].

Calcium ions are not essential for fibrinopeptide release nor for polymerisation of fibrin monomers, but they greatly accelerate the aggregation of soluble fibrin monomer[59,60]. Calcium also makes fibrinogen more resistant to thermal and acid denaturation, and to digestion by plasmin[61].

III. CLOTTABLE PROTEIN BASED ASSAYS

A. ASSAYS BASED ON CLOT MASS MEASUREMENT

Methods that determine the amount of clottable protein use the unique property of fibrinogen that it becomes a clot after the addition of thrombin. After *complete* clotting of the fibrinogen, the non-clottable proteins trapped in the fibrin network must be washed out before the weight and protein content of the clot is used as a measure of the fibrinogen content of the plasma sample.

The methods are time-consuming, because both complete clotting and thorough washing out of the non-clottable proteins take time.

Compared to the clotting rate method, measurement of clottable protein is more representative of the molar concentration of fibrinogen, because fibrinogen forms with prolonged clotting times are also measured.

B. INTERFERING FACTORS

Arnesen et al[62] found only a minor increase of up to 1 g/L early FDP in the measured amount of total clottable protein. This is confusing, because the fragment X is an early FDP that still has clotting capacity. Hoffmann et al[46] describe a marked increase of the apparent fibrinogen levels when ± 2.5 g/L fragment X is added to pooled plasma, a small increase when fragment Y is added and no effect from fragments D and E. These concentrations are only obtained after thrombolytic therapy. Interference by heparin, haemolytic plasma or increased sialic acid content of fibrinogen has never been described and is unlikely.

Fat is trapped in the fibrin clot formed from blood collected during alimentary lipemia. The error in the determination of fibrinogen, due to trapped fat, is small provided correction is made for "extraneous absorption"[63,64]. Lipid containing plasmas that have been lyophilized cannot be used in a gravimetric assay, because clotting is disturbed by the lipids. We observed this repeatedly with this method, but not with other fibrinogen assays. One freezing-thawing step of the plasma yields the same levels as in fresh plasma[57].

C. PRECISION

The total clottable protein methods have a 4.6% variation in duplicate measurements[65]. The method is less accurate with low fibrinogen levels, because weak clots are formed that are difficult to handle.

D. USE IN ROUTINE ASSAYS

This assay is hardly ever used in a routine laboratory, because it is very labour-intensive. However, two epidemiological studies, the Northwick Park Heart Study[28] and the Framingham Study[29] employed this method.

E. COMMENTS

Originally, the final step was drying the clot and weighing it (gravimetric assay)[66], as in the Northwick Park Heart Study[28]. Alternatively, the fibrin clot can be dissolved in urea and the protein content is then calculated from the absorbance at 279 nm[63]. To correct for non-protein contamination, such as lipids, the absorbance at 315 nm was subtracted from the absorbance at 279 nm[64]. Astrup et al[67] dissolved the clot in 2.5 N NaOH in a boiling water bath and then measured the protein content with sodium carbonate and phenol reagent, obtained thereby a variance of less than 1%. Ratnoff and Menzie [68] dissolved the clot in 1 N NaOH and measured the protein with the Biuret test.

IV. ASSAYS BASED ON CHANGE IN TURBIDITY

The Ellis and Stransky method[69] is also based on complete clotting of fibrinogen by thrombin, but the quantitation is based on the increase in opacity (turbidity) at 470 nm, due to the formation of fibrin. This method gives additional information on kinetics of fibrin formation and fibrinolysis which can be obtained from the continuous monitoring of the absorbance.

Nowadays, many laboratories use automatic coagulometers. These machines often derive the fibrinogen levels from the prothrombin time (PT)[70,71]. This method is usually called the nephelometric method and it is based on the Ellis and Stransky method because it measures increased optical density after clotting. It yields good results when the prothrombin time is relatively normal [49,70,71].

A. PRECISION
The Ellis and Stransky method has a 5.6% variation between duplicate measurements[65]. The PT derived fibrinogen assay gives a same day CV of 5.6% and a different day CV of 6.5%[49].

B. USE AS ROUTINE ASSAY
Measurement of PT-derived fibrinogen levels is used frequently nowadays, because this assay can be performed on automatic coagulatometers. Because this test can be performed in combination with the PT, it is relatively cheap.

C. COMMENTS
Changes in the fibrin clot structure will affect the turbidity of the clot. Because the different molecular weight forms of fibrinogen and the degree of phosphorylation of fibrinogen affect clot structure, these factors influence the measurement of fibrinogen with this method. The presence of calcium during clot formation also modifies the clot structure[72].

The effects of lipids on turbidity and thereby on the PT-derived measurement can be corrected for with the newest apparatus. In patients on oral anticoagulants, results do not significantly differ from those in the Clauss assay[71]. Bilirubin (<15 mg/dL) and haemoglobin (<150 mg/dL) have no disturbing effects[70,72]. An effect of the clottable, early FDP has not yet been described, but is theoretically expected.

Unless clot formation is complete, spuriously low levels are obtained. This might be a problem in patients receiving heparin; therefore it is usually neutralized with polybrene[69]. One freezing-thawing step does not alter the measured fibrinogen levels[57].

V. PRECIPITABLE PROTEIN BASED ASSAYS

Fibrinogen can be precipitated by heating[65,73] or with salt[74-76]. These methods determine both the clottable and the non-clottable fibrinogen.

The heat precipitation method measures the amount of protein that precipitates at 56°C. It is very sensitive to assay conditions. An increase in the temperature of 1°C leads to a 12% error due to co-precipitation of other proteins. The assay is also sensitive to the pH in the system.

Sulphite[74,76] and ammonium sulphate[75] have been used in quantitative assays because they specifically precipitate fibrinogen. Other salts have the disadvantage that they co-precipitate many other proteins. The best results are obtained with sodium sulphite because it cleaves the disulphide bonds of fibrinogen specifically and accurately[76].

A. PRECISION
If the assay conditions are well controlled the heat precipitation method gives coefficients of variation of 3.9%, precipitation with sodium sulphite 7.1% and precipitation with ammonium

sulphate 5.4%[65]. Because of the many possible technical errors and interferences, these methods are generally considered unreliable[65].

B . USE IN ROUTINE ASSAYS

As the precipitation methods are prone to errors they are not routinely used.

C . COMMENTS

Low levels of fibrin monomers (< 0.1 g/L) do not influence the precipitation of fibrinogen by heat or by salt. Lipids in the sample do not influence the turbidimetric measurement when sufficient care is taken of the cooling procedure in the heat precipitation method[73].

If the assay conditions are well controlled the heat precipitation method is not influenced by moderate haemolysis, heparin, fibrin monomers, hyperlipemia and bilirubin[73]. There is however an effect of early fibrin(ogen) degradation products (X and Y), but not of D and E[36], if they are present in large amounts (>15% of the fibrinogen level).

VI. IMMUNOLOGICAL ASSAYS

Immunological methods measure the fibrinogen related antigens, rather than the amount of fibrin that can be formed. They include immuno-precipitation methods like radial immunodiffusion (RID)[77] or rocket immuno electrophoresis[78] where polyclonal antibodies are applied. These precipitation assays need polyclonal antibodies, which unfortunately crossreact with fibrin degradation products, fibrinogen degradation products and soluble fibrin. The enzyme immune assays (EIA) can use either polyclonal or specific monoclonal antibodies (e.g. specific to HMW+LMW fibrinogen[79]). The use of fibrinogen-specific monoclonal antibodies specifically determines fibrinogen and gives an assay system that has a lower detection limit than clotting rate or total clottable protein methods. The disadvantage of EIAs is that they are more time-consuming than clotting rate assays, although for instance the recently developed HMW+LMW fibrinogen EIA[79] takes less than 1 hour (apart from sample preparation time).

The specificity of the monoclonal antibodies used in the HMW+LMW fibrinogen assay has the advantage of measuring specifically those molecular weight forms of fibrinogen that have the highest clottability and therefore are possibly associated with the highest thrombotic risk.

A . INTERFERING FACTORS

It depends on the specificity of the antibody[80] whether FDP are measured in immunological assays. Usually, polyclonal antibodies crossreact with FDP, but the FDP levels have to be very high to noticeably influence the fibrinogen levels. In patients treated with streptokinase, apparently normal fibrinogen levels are found in radial immunodiffusion assays due to the high level of FDP. The clotting rate and total clottable protein assays would suggest a marked reduction in fibrinogen in these patients[46].

The influence of the different forms of fibrinogen also depends on the specificity of the antibody. The recently developed HMW+LMW fibrinogen EIA[79] uses antibodies that do not detect the LMW' form of fibrinogen. Most polyclonal antibodies are not expected to react differently to the three fibrinogen forms. However, as stated above they will cross-react with FDP.

Effects of lipids, heparin, haemolysis, phosphorylation and sialic acid on the measurement have not been reported, but are unlikely. One step of freezing-thawing does not influence the RID assay[56]. In the rocket immuno-electrophoresis the addition of EDTA is required.

B . PRECISION

When RID is performed on blood plasma that has been collected in heparin, the fibrinogen levels will be 10.7% higher than in sodium citrate plasma, whereas the concentrations in EDTA plasma are 10.3% higher than the heparin plasma[81]. This difference may partly be due to the dilution effect of plasma in citrate. Heparin is known to inhibit the formation of antigen-antibody complexes in immunoassays.

The same day CV of the HMW+LMW EIA was between 3% and 7%, depending on the plasma dilution used, the different day CV was between 2.8% and 7.7%[79].

C . USE AS ROUTINE ASSAY

The traditional immunological methods were very time-consuming, a radial immunodiffusion assay takes three days. In most routine laboratories the immunological methods are mainly used when the presence of dysfibrinogenaemia is suspected.

The earlier EIAs took one day because they used relatively long incubation periods. The new HMW+LMW fibrinogen EIA only takes one hour, from the first incubation to the end of the staining reaction[79], which makes it suitable for routine use.

VII. COMPARISON BETWEEN METHODS AND BETWEEN LABORATORIES

A . STANDARDS

To identify an increased fibrinogen level as a potential cardiovascular risk factor, it is essential that a correct standard is used. Furlan[82] reported that there were giant differences between the indicated levels of commercial fibrinogen standards and the actual levels. To overcome the problem of differences between standards, it is desirable to establish the potency of a standard after a collaborative study, by agreement with the participants. For a long term reference standard the stability has to be checked. An international standard for fibrinogen is now available[64].

B . COMPARISON BETWEEN THE DIFFERENT METHODS

In various studies the available fibrinogen assay methods have been compared. In general, there is good correlation between different methods when rank order is considered (i.e. high levels with one method yield high levels in another and, similarly, for intermediate or low levels[73,83]. There is also a high degree of consistency in different studies of the association between fibrinogen levels on the one hand and physiological factors (e.g. smoking, age, body mass index (BMI)) and risk of arterial disease on the other.

One study compared the clotting rate[39], clottable protein (PT-derived) and immunological (RID) methods in plasma samples from healthy individuals and patients with acute pneumonia and postoperative patients with increased fibrinogen levels[57]. Palareti et al[57] found large discrepancies between the results obtained with the same samples applying different methods when they used the standard included in the different test kits. When they calibrated all methods to the same reference, there was satisfactory agreement, i.e. in the relation between different methods and the average of the methods. The most accurate is the Clauss method, but all methods had an inaccuracy below 8%. Although agreement in the group as a whole was acceptable, differences in agreement between the healthy individuals and the patients was not studied. Less agreement might be observed in patients with increased levels of HMW- and phosphorylated fibrinogen.

In another study Exner et al[65] compared the Clauss method, total clottable fibrinogen (protein and clot opacity), salt ((NH_4)$_2SO_4$ and Na_2SO_3) and heat precipitation methods to measure the plasma fibrinogen levels in patients with various diseases, e.g. consumptive coagulopathy and hepatic cirrhosis. The correlation of the total clottable protein level with the other methods was satisfactory (>0.91), but the results of salt precipitation methods were inaccurate at low levels (below 1 g/L) and gave spuriously high values in jaundiced samples. The Clauss method had the best reproducibility.

C . COMPARISON BETWEEN LABORATORIES

The differences between laboratories are much larger than those between different methods in one laboratory. In 1993, the results of the College of American Pathologists (CAP) Proficiency Testing Program in 2250 laboratories from 1988 to 1991 were published[84]. Poor interlaboratory reproducibility was described. The authors ascribe this to both instrument and reagent variables. The absence of an international standard for plasma fibrinogen was believed to be the major reason for the reagent variation.

In the European Concerted Action on Thrombosis (ECAT) project the patients' plasma samples were not analyzed centrally and therefore the study included a quality control programme. The CV between the 16 participating European laboratories was assessed as 5.3% for the Clauss assay, which is only slightly higher than the mean different day CV of 4.7%[57]. These variation levels remained constant after five quality assessment exercises[85].

VIII. PHYSIOLOGICAL VARIATION

We have recently reported a longitudinal study of healthy volunteers[86] which found that the longitudinal variation for fibrinogen within an individual (physiological + methodological variation) was 18%. Because the methodological variation was very small, its effect on this within-individual variation was negligible. Similar within-individual variations have been described in healthy volunteers by Thompson[87] and Marckmann[88]. Because the variations within individuals are comparable to the variation between individuals, it will be necessary in order to classify groups with different thrombotic risks to study large groups or to calculate habitual levels from multiple samples.

A . PATHOLOGY

An overview of fibrinogen levels in different diseases and of acquired dysfibrinogen is given by Dang et al[55]. Hereditary dysfibrinogenemia may yield decreased levels with functional fibrinogen assays and normal or slightly decreased levels of fibrinogen with immunological assays. Most of these dysfibrinogens are either asymptomatic or cause a bleeding tendency. However, several families have now been identified in which the dysfibrinogen yields apparently low levels in functional assays in association with thrombophilia (overview: 89).

In epidemiological studies for haemostatic indicators of cardiovascular risk, the gravimetric assay[28,31,33,90], clotting assays[32,35,91,92] and immunologic assays[30,33,34] work equally well.

IX. CONCLUSION

In this paper we have described the major categories of assays. The clotting rate assays give a functional fibrinogen level, are reproducible, fast, cheap and, in normal circumstances, not very easily affected by disturbing factors. The tests can be used in automatic coagulometers with turbidimetric end point assessment. The clottable protein assays also give fibrinogen levels based on the clotting capacity, but prolonged clotting is not detected by these tests. The advantage of the Ellis and Stransky derived methods is that they can easily be used in automatic coagulometers in combination with the prothrombin time.

A promising development in immunological methods is the introduction of the EIA that uses monoclonal antibodies specific for the HMW and LMW forms of fibrinogen. As these are the most clottable forms, this assay may eventually be valuable to assess thrombotic risk.

When using plasma fibrinogen levels to determine thrombotic risk, it is very important to have 1) a reliable method and 2) a good standard. When such a standard is used, the different methods give comparable results in healthy volunteers. Good comparability is also described for patients, but the evidence is less convincing. An international reference for fibrinogen is now available.

The value of the different assays to estimate thrombotic risk has not yet been described. Therefore, epidemiological studies are needed in which the value of fibrinogen as risk indicator is compared with different assays, to establish a standardized fibrinogen method.

REFERENCES

1   **Doolittle RF.** Fibrinogen and Fibrin. In: Haemostasis and Thrombosis. Bloom AL, Forbes CD, Thomas DP and Tuddenham EGD (Eds), 3th ed, Churchill Livingstone, Edinburgh, 1993, pp 491.

2   **Kusher I.** The phenomenon of the acute phase response. *Ann N Y Acad Sci* 1982;389:39.

3   **Meade TW, Chakrabarti R, Haines AP, North WR, Stirling Y.** Characteristics affecting fibrinolytic activity and plasma fibrinogen concentrations. *Br Med J*;1;153,1979.

4   **Balleisen L, Bailey J, Epping PH, Schulte H, van de Loo J.** Epidemiological study on factor VII, factor VIII and fibrinogen in an industrial population: I. Baseline data on the relation to age, gender, body weight, smoking, alcohol, pill-using, and menopause. *Thromb Haemost*;54:475, 1985.

5   **Siegert G, Bergmann S, Jaross W.** Influence of age, gender and lipoprotein metabolism parameters on the activity of the plasminogen activator inhibitor and the fibrinogen concentration. *Fibrinolysis*;6(suppl 3):47, 1992.

6   **ECAT Angina Pectoris Study Group.** ECAT Angina Pectoris Study: baseline associations of haemostatic factors with extent of coronary arteriosclerosis and other coronary risk factors in 3000 patients with angina pectoris undergoing coronary angiography. *Eur Heart J*;14:8-17, 1993.

7   **Ernst E.** Fibrinogen, smoking and cardiovascular risk. *J Smoking-Related Dis*;4:37, 1993.

8   **Fulton RM, Duckett K.** Plasma fibrinogen and thromboembolism after myocardial infarction. *Lancet* 1976;ii:1161.

9   **Lowe GDO, Drummond MM, Lorimer AR, Hutton I, Forbes CD, Prentice CR, Barbenel JC.** Relation between extent of coronary artery disease and blood viscosity. *Br Med J*;281:673, 1980.

10   **Handa K, Kono S, Saku K, Sasaki J, Kawano T, Sasaki Y, Hiroki T, Arakawa K.** Plasma fibrinogen levels as independent indicator of severity of coronary atherosclerosis. *Atherosclerosis*;77:209, 1989.

11   **Broadhurst P, Kelleher C, Hughes L, Imeson JD, Raftery EB.** Fibrinogen, factor VII clotting activity and coronary artery disease severity. *Atherosclerosis*;85:169, 1990.

12   **Cattaneo M, Mannucci PM.** Predictive value of coagulation tests in arterial thrombosis. *Res Clin Lab* 1990;20:167.

13   **Lee AJ, Lowe GDO, Smith WCA, Tunstall-Pedoe H.** Plasma fibrinogen in women: relationship with oral contraception, the menopause and hormone replacement therapy. *Br J Haematol*;83:616, 1993.

14   **Cohen H, Mackie IJ, Walshe K, Gillmer MDG, Machin SJ.** A comparison of the effects of two triphasic oral contraceptives on haemostasis. *Br J Haematol*;69:259, 1988.

15   **Inglis TCN, Stuart J, George AJ, Davies AJ.** Haemostatic and rheological changes in normal pregnancy and pre-eclampsia. *Br J Haematol*;50:461, 1982.

16   **Mosesson MW, Alkaersig N, Sweet B, Sherry S.** Human fibrinogen of relatively high solubility. Comparative biophysical, biochemical, and biological studies with fibrinogen of lower solubility. *Biochemistry*;6:3279, 1967.

17   **Mosesson MW, Finlayson JS, Umfleet RA, Galanakis D.** Human fibrinogen heterogeneities. I. Structural and related studies of plasma fibrinogens which are high solubility catabolic intermediates. *J Biol Chem*;247:5210, 1972.

18   **Lipinska I, Lipinski B, Gurewich V.** Fibrinogen heterogeneity in human plasma. Electrophoretic demonstration and characterization of two major fibrinogen components. *J Lab Clin Med* 84:509, 1974.

19   **Weinstein MJ, Deykin D.** Low solubility fibrinogen examined by two-dimensional sodium dodecyl sulfate gel electrophoresis and isoelectric focusing. *Thromb Res*;13:361, 1978.

20   **Galanakis DK, Mosesson MW, Stathakis NE.** Human fibrinogen heterogeneities: distribution and characteristics of Aα-chain origin. *J Lab Clin Med*;92:376, 1978.

21   **Phillips HM.** Isolation of size homogeneous preparations of high molecular weight and low molecular weight fibrinogens. *Can J Biochem*;59:332, 1981.

22   **Holm B, Nilsen DWT, Kierulf P, Godal HC.** Purification and characterization of 3 fibrinogens with different molecular weights obtained from normal human plasma. *Thromb Res* 1985;37:165-176.

23   **Regañon E, Vila V, Aznar J, Laiz B.** Human fibrinogen heterogeneity. A study of limited fibrinogen degradation. *Clin Chim Acta*;184:7, 1989.

24   **Nakashima A, Sasaki S, Miyazaki K, Miyata T, Iwanaga S.** Human fibrinogen heterogeneity: the COOH-terminal residues of defective Aα chains of fibrinogen II. *Blood Coag Fibrinol*;3:361, 1992.

25   **Regañon E, Vila V, Aznar J, Lacueva V, Martinez V, Ruano M.** Studies on the functionality of newly synthesized fibrinogen after treatment of acute myocardial infarction with streptokinase, increase in the rate of fibrinopeptide release. *Thromb Haemost*;70:978, 1993.

26   **Holm B, Godal HC.** Quantitation of the three normally occurring plasma fibrinogens in health and during socalled "acute phase" by SDS electrophoresis of fibrin obtained from EDTA-plasma. *Thromb Res*;35:279, 1984.

27   **Haines AP, Howarth D, North WRS, et al.** Haemostatic variables and the outcome of myocardial infarction. *Thromb Haemostas*;50:800, 1983.

28   **Meade TW, Brozovic M, Haines AP, Imenson JD, Mellows S, Miller GJ, North MRS, Stirling Y, Thompson SG.** Haemostatic function and ischaemic heart disease: Principal results of the Northwick Park Heart Study. *Lancet* ; 2 : 533, 1986.

29   **Kannel WB, Wolf PA, Castelli WP, D'Agostino RBD.** Fibrinogen and risk of cardiovascular disease: The Framingham Study. *JAMA*;258:1183, 1987.

30   **Stone MC, Thorp JM.** Plasma fibrinogen - a major risk factor. *J R Coll Gen Pract*;12:565, 1985.

31   **Wilhelmsen L, Svärdsudd K, Korsan-Bengtsen K, Larsson B, Welin L, Tibblin G.** Fibrinogen as a risk factor for stroke and myocardial infarction. *N Engl J Med*;311:501, 1984.

32   **Heinrich J, Balleisen L, Schulte H, Assmann G, van de Loo J.** Fibrinogen and factor VII in the prediction of coronary risk. Results from the PROCAM Study in healthy men. *Arterioscler Thromb*;14:54, 1994.

33   **Yarnell JWG, Baker IA, Sweetnam PM, Bainton D, O'Brien JR, Whitehead PJ, Elwood PC**. Fibrinogen, viscosity, and white blood cell count are major risk factors for ischemic heart disease. The Caerphilly and Speedwell Collaborative Heart Disease Studies. *Circulation*;83:836, 1991.

34   **Cremer P, Nagel D, Labrot B, Mann H, Muche R, Elster H, Seidel D**. Lipoprotein Lp(a) as predictor of myocardial infarction in comparison to fibrinogen, LDL cholesterol and other risk factors: results from the prospective Göttingen Risk Incidence and Prevalence Study (GRIPS). *Eur J Clin Invest*;24:444, 1994.

35   **Haverkate F**. Thrombosis and disabilities. In: Advances of Medical Biology, Baya C (Ed), vol 3, IOS Press, Amsterdam, Oxford, Washington, Tokyo, 1994, pp 81.

36   **Rampling MW, Gaffney PJ**. Measurement of fibrinogen in plasma. In: Progress Chemical Fibrinolysis and Thrombosis, Davidson JF, Samama MM, Desnoyres PC (Eds), vol 2, Raven Press New York, pp 91, 1976.

37   **Shaw TW**. Assays for fibrinogen and its derivatives. *CRC Crit for Clin Lab Sci*;8:145, 1977.

38   **Holm B, Brosstad F, Kierulf P, Godal HC**. Polymerization properties of two normally circulating fibrinogens, HMW and LMW. Evidence that the COOH-terminal end of the a-chain is of importance for fibrin polymerization. *Thromb Res*;39:595, 1985.

39   **Von Clauss A**. Gerinnungsphysiologische Schnellmethode zur Bestimmung des Fibrinogens. *Acta Haematol*;17:237, 1957.

40   **Bell WR, Bolton G, Pitney WR**. The effect of Arvin on blood coagulation factors. *Br J Haematol*;15:589, 1968.

41   **Nieuwenhuizen W, Gravesen M**. Anticoagulant and calcium-binding properties of high molecular weight derivatives of human fibrinogen, produced by plasmin (fragments X). *Biochim Biophys Acta*;668:81, 1981.

42   **Haverkate F, Timan G, Nieuwenhuizen W**. Anticlotting properties of fragments D from human fibrinogen and fibrin. *Eur J Clin Invest*;9:253, 1979.

43   **Alving BM, Bell WR**. Methods for correcting inhibitory effects of fibrinogen degradation products in fibrinogen determinations. *Thromb Res*;9:1, 1976.

44   **Jespersen J, Sidelmann J**. A study of the conditions and accuracy of the thrombin time assay of plasma fibrinogen. *Acta Haematol*;67:2, 1982.

45   **Oethinger M, Tanswell P, Hoegee-de Nobel E, Nieuwenhuizen W, Seifried E**. Verlauf von zirkulierendem Fibrinogen beim akuten Myokardinfarkt unter thrombolytischer Therapie mit rt-PA. *Lab Med*;18:62, 1994.

46   **Hoffmann JJML, Vijgen M, Nieuwenhuizen W**. Comparison of the specificity of four fibrinogen assays during thrombolytic therapy. *Fibrinolysis*;4(suppl 2):121, 1988.

47   **Witt I, Hasler K**. Influence of organically bound phosphorus in fetal and adult fibrinogen on the kinetics of interaction between thrombin and fibrinogen. *Biochim Biophys Acta*;271:357:362, 1972.

48   **Hanna I, Scheraga HA, Francis CW, Marder VJ**. Comparison of various human fibrinogens and a derivative thereof by a study of the kinetics of release of fibrinopeptides. *Biochemistry*;23:4681, 1984.

49   **Siefring GE, Friabov DK, Wehrly JA**. Development and analytical performance of a functional assay for fibrinogen on the Du Pont aca^{TM} Analyzer. *Clin Chem*;29:614, 1983.

50   **Stevens DA, Sanfelippo MN**. Evaluation of three methods for plasma fibrinogen determination. *Am J Clin Pathol* ;60:182, 1973.

51   **Martinez J, MacDonald KA, Palascak JE**. The role of sialic acid in the dysfibrinogenemia associated with liver disease: distribution of sialic acid on the constituent chains. *Blood*;61:1196, 1983.

52   **Chang CV, Shin CK, Bell WR, Nagaswami C, Weisel JW**. Fibrinogen sialic acid residues are low affinity calcium-binding sites that influence fibrin assembly. *J Biol Chem*;264:15104, 1989.

53   **Bories PN, Feger J, Benbernou N, Rouzeau J-D, Agneray J, Durand G**. Prevalence of tri- and tetraantennary glycans of human α_1-acid glycoprotein in release of macrophage inhibitor of interleukin-1 activity. *Inflammation* ;14:315, 1990.

54   **LeJeune P-J, Mallet B, Farnarier C, Kaplanski S**. Changes in serum level and affinity for Conavalin A of human α_1-protease inhibitor in severe burn patients: relationship to natural killer activity. *Biochim Biophys Acta*;990:122, 1989.

55   **Dang CV, Bell WR**. The normal and morbid biology of fibrinogen. *Am J Med*;87:567, 1989.

56   **Palareti G, Maccaferri M, Manotti C, et al**. Fibrinogen Assays:a Collaborative Study of Six Different Methods. *Clin Chem*;37:714, 1991.

57   **Thompson SG, Duckert F, Haverkate F, Thomson JM, + 20 participating ECAT centres**. The measurement of haemostatic factors in 16 European laboratories: quality assessment for the multicentre ECAT Angina Pectoris Study. Report from the European Concerted Action on Thrombosis and Disabilities (ECAT). *Thromb Haemostas*;61:301, 1989.

58   **ECAT Assay Procedures**. A manual of laboratory techniques. Jespersen J, Bertina RM, Haverkate F (Eds), Kluwer Academic Publishers, Dordrecht, Boston, London: 1992, 230 pp.

59   **Ratnoff OD, Potts AM**. The accelerating effect of calcium and other cations on the conversion of fibrinogen to fibrin. *J Clin Invest*;33:206, 1954.

60   **Rosenfeld G, Janszky B**. The accelerating effect of calcium on the fibrinogen-fibrin transformation. *Science*;116:36, 1952.

61   **Haverkate F, Timan G**. Protective effect of calcium in the plasmin degradation of fibrinogen and fibrin fragments D. *Thromb Res*;10:803, 1977.

62   **Arnesen H**. Quantitation of plasma fibrinogen in the presence of fibrinogen degradation products. *Scand J Haem*;11:204, 1973.

63   **Jacobsson K**. Studies in the determination of fibrinogen in human blood plasma. *Scand J Clin Lab Invest*;7 (suppl 14):1, 1955.

64   **Gaffney PJ, Wong MY**. Collaborative study of a proposed international standard for plasma fibrinogen measurement. *Thromb. Haemostas.*;68:428, 1992.

65   **Exner T, Burridge J, Power P, Rickard KA**. An evaluation of currently available methods for plasma fibrinogen. *Am J Clin Pathol*;71:521, 1979.

66   **Gram HC**. A new method for the determination of the fibrin percentage in blood and plasma. *J Biol Chem*;49:279, 1921.

67   **Astrup T, Brakman P, Nissen U**. The estimation of fibrinogen: a revision. *Scand J Clin Lab Invest*;17:57, 1965.

68   **Ratnoff O, Menzie C**. A new method for the determination of fibrinogen in small samples of plasma. *J Lab Clin Med*;37:316, 1951.

69   **Ellis BC, Stransky A**. A quick and accurate method for the determination of fibrinogen in plasma. *Scand J Lab Clin Med*;58:477, 1961.

70   **Natelson EA, Dooley DF**. Rapid determination of fibrinogen by thrombokinetics. *Am J Clin Pathol*;61:828, 1974.

71   **Rossi E, Mondonico P, Lombardi A, Preda L**. Method for the determination of functional (clottable) fibrinogen by the new family of ACL coagulometers. *Thromb Res*;52:453, 1988.

72   **Nair CH, Azhar A, Dhall DP**. Studies on fibrin network structure in human plasma. Part one: methods for clinical application. *Thromb Res*;64:455, 1991.

73   **Desvignes P, Bonnet P**. Direct determination of plasma fibrinogen levels by heat precipitation. A comparison of the technique against thrombin clottable fibrinogen with spectrophotometry and radial immuno-diffusion. *Clin Chim Acta* ;110:9, 1981.

74   **Goodwin JF**. Estimation of plasma fibrinogen, using sodium sulfite fractionation. *Am J Clin Pathol*;35:227, 1961.

75   **Parfentjer JA, Johnson ML, Clifton EE**. The determination of plasma fibrinogen by turbidity with ammonium sulfate. *Arch Biochem Biophys*;46:470, 1953.

76   **Rampling MW, Gaffney PJ**. The sulphite precipitation method for fibrinogen measurement. Its use on small samples in the presence of fibrinogen degradation products. *Clin Chim Acta*;67:43, 1976.

77   **Mancini G, Carbonaro O, Heremans JP**. Immunochemical quantitation of antigens by single radial immunodiffusion. *Immunochemistry*;2:235, 1965.

78   **Laurell CB**. Quantitative estimations of proteins by electrophoresis in agarose gel containing antibodies. *Anal Biochem*;15:57, 1966.

79   **Hoegee-de Nobel E, Voskuilen M, Briet E, Brommer EJP, Nieuwenhuizen** W. A monoclonal antibody-based quantitative enzyme immunoassay for the determination of plasma fibrinogen concentrations. *Thromb Haemostas*;60:415, 1988.

80   **Beller FK, Maki M**. Properties of Fibrinogenolysis and Fibrinolysis products in immune assays. *Thromb Diath Haemorrh*;18:114, 1967.

81   **Gleeson M, Kinlay S**. Choice of anticoagulant affects measurement of plasma fibrinogen. *Clin Chem* 1993;39:1754.

82   **Furlan M, Felix R, Escher N, Laemmle B**. How high is the true fibrinogen content of fibrinogen standards? *Thromb. Res.*;56:583, 1989.

83   **Knapp ML, Feher MD, Carey H, Mayne PD**. Comparison of an immunochemical assay for plasma fibrinogen and a turbidimetric thrombin clotting technique to discriminate hyperlipidaemic patients from healthy controls. *J Clin Pathol*;43:508, 1990.

84   **Bovill EG, McDonagh J, Triplett DA, Arkin CF, Brandt JT, Hayes TE, Kaczmarek E, Long T, Rock WA.** Performance characteristics of fibrinogen assays: Results of the College of American Pathologists Proficiency Testing Program 1988-1991. *Arch. Pathol. Lab. Med.*;117:58, 1993.

85   **Thompson SG, Calori G, Thomson JM, Haverkate F, Duckert F.** The impact of sequential quality assessment exercises on laboratory performance: the multicentre ECAT Angina Pectoris Study. Report from the European Concerted Action on Thrombosis and Disabilities (ECAT). *Thromb Haemostas*;65:159, 1991.

86   **de Maat MPM, Bart de ACW, Hennis BC, Kluft C**. Longitudinal variation in plasma levels of fibrinogen, plasminogen activator inhibitor (PAI) activity, C-reactive protein and histidine-rich glycoprotein. Submitted.

87   **Thompson SG, Martin JC, Meade TW**. Sources of variability in coagulation factor assays. *Thromb Haemost*;58:1073, 1987.

88   **Marckmann P. Sandström B, Jespersen J**. The variability of and associations between measures of blood coagulation, fibrinolysis and blood lipids. *Atherosclerosis*;96:235, 1992.

89   **Koopman JL and Haverkate F**. Hereditary variants of human fibrinogens. In: Haemostasis and Thrombosis, Bloom AL, Forbes CD, Thomas DP, Tuddenham EGD (Eds), 3th ed, Churchill Livingstone, London, 1992, pp 515.

90   **Møller L, Kristensen TS**. Fibrinogen and associations with risk factors for cardiovascular disease. *Fibrinolysis*;4(suppl 2):56, 1990.

91   **Folsom AR, Wu KK, Shahar E, Davis CE**. Association of hemostatic variables with prevalent cardiovascular disease and asymptomatic carotid artery atherosclerosis. *Arterioscler Thromb*;13:1829, 1993.

92   **Cortellaro M, Boschetti C, Cofrancesco E, Zanussi C, Catalano M, de Gaetano G, Gabrielli L, Lombardi B, Specchia G, Tavazzi L, Tremoli E, Della Volpe A, Polli E, and the PLAT study group.** The PLAT Study: a multidisciplinary study of hemostatic function and conventional risk factors in vascular disease patients. *Atherosclerosis*;90:109, 1991.

FIBRINOLYSIS AND THE HYPERCOAGULABLE STATE

P.J. Gaffney
National Institute for Biological Standards and Controls, Hertfordshire

I. INTRODUCTION

Disseminated intravascular coagulation (DIC), the hypercoagulable state, and the prethrombotic state are three terminologies which may relate to each other in mechanistic terms but conjure up distinct clinical scenarios. A hypercoagulable state is not clearly comparable with a prethrombotic state. Our understanding of DIC is that the coagulation system has become activated systemically (eg by shock etc) and it can be argued that there is a disseminated state of hypercoagulability. It is not clear whether we can relate the hypercoagulable state with a prethrombotic condition. Most studies that try to relate these two concepts have been in venous disease. The notion that a systemic condition in flowing blood can predict arterial thrombosis such as myocardial infarction, while an earnestly desired ambition, seems to elude us completely. This chapter concentrates on venous thrombosis and the relevance of fibrinolytic activity to its occurrence. Patients with a presumed hypercoagulable state have been divided[1] into two broad categories. The first group consists of inherited thrombotic disorders or primary hypercoagulable states which involve a specific defect in one of the major anticoagulant mechanisms eg heparin, antithrombin, protein C, thrombomodulin and protein S, plasminogen, plasminogen activator and dysfibrinogenemia (reviewed by Lijnen and Collen[2]). Secondary hypercoagulable states are generally acquired disorders in patients with an underlying systemic disease or condition such as malignancy, pregnancy, use of oral contraceptives, hyperlipidemia, diabetes mellitus, or abnormalities of the vasculature or rheology. The relationship between the acquired hypercoagulable state and the fibrinolytic system will be discussed.

The major hazard to man's survival is bleeding rather than thrombosis and thus the coagulation system is constantly poised for clotting. The major direct control mechanisms on the thrombin mediated hypercoagulable state involve the protein C-protein S system, thrombomodulin and antithrombin. Fibrinolysis is stimulated by the formation of fibrin[3] and the notion[4] that fibrin orchestrates its own destruction by generating plasmin proximate to forming fibrin is generally accepted. This secondary fibrinolysis associated with fibrin formation will be the main theme of this review. Changes in the fibrinolytic system during the hypercoagulable state will be described and an effort made to delineate which are of value in diagnosis.

II. FIBRIN AND FIBRINOLYSIS

As fibrin forms in blood it binds a large number of the components of haemostasis[5]. The major activator of the fibrinolytic system, tissue plasminogen activator (t-PA), binds avidly to forming fibrin while plasminogen also binds. The two major inhibitors of fibrinolysis, α_2-antiplasmin (AP) and plasminogen activator inhibitor-1 (PAI-1), also bind to fibrin. While many other components of haemostasis bind to forming fibrin, their role in its fate is not clear, thus only those components for which we can rationalise a role in survival or destruction of fibrin will be discussed. Furthermore, not only does t-PA bind to forming fibrin but its role as a plasminogen activator is considerably enhanced while the natural form of plasminogen, namely the glu-form, is converted to the more activatable lys-form following binding to fibrin. Figure 1 shows the interaction between the coagulation system resulting in the formation of fibrin and the response of the fibrinolytic system.

Fibrinolysis and the Hypercoagulable State

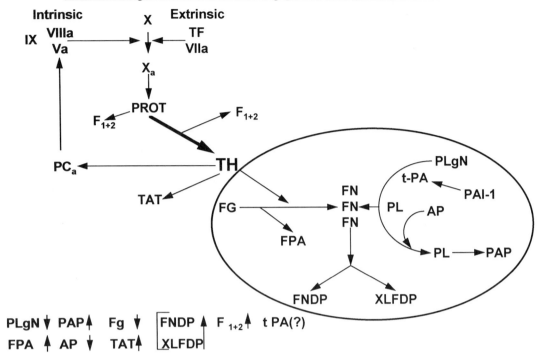

Figure 1: This shows some of the essential components of the coagulation system leading to thrombin (TH). Some of the major components of both the intrinsic and extrinsic pathways are shown. The response of the fibrinolytic system is also depicted showing the thrombin-mediated conversion of fibrinogen (Fg) to fibrin (FN-FN-FN). This in turn provokes the interaction of tissue plasminogen activator (t-PA) with plasminogen (PLgN) on the surface of the forming fibrin. Fibrin is digested by plasmin (PL). The digested fibrin generates both crosslinked and non-crosslinked fibrin degradation products (FNDP, XLFDP). The released plasmin forms a plasmin-antiplasmin (PAP) complex. Other details and identities are discussed in the text.

Overt fibrinolysis in the circulation in the presence of fibrin is best studied during thrombin-induced disseminated intravascular coagulation (DIC) or during the more controlled clinical condition related to Ancrod-induced defibrination[6]. Both these conditions involve the generation of large amounts of systemic fibrin. Thrombin has, amongst its numerous activities, those which involve platelet aggregation, factor XIII activation and the activation of protein C. Fibrin binds a number of components of the fibrinolytic and coagulation systems to its network. The binding of these components presumably influences whether the fibrin survives and takes part in thrombus organisation or is degraded by plasmin to fibrin degradation products (FnDP). The two major prolysis components involved in this latter process are plasminogen and its activator, t-PA, while the inhibitors of the process are plasminogen activator inhibitor-1 (PAI-1), and α_2-antiplasmin (AP). Plasminogen and t-PA react optimally on the surface of fibrin polymers. T-PA has a high affinity for fibrin[7] while plasminogen binds to fibrin, this latter binding being enhanced by partial degradation[8]. During this process of orchestration of the fibrinolytic system by the forming fibrin AP also binds and is crosslinked to the chains of fibrin. During most episodes of DIC the bound AP does not overtly inhibit lysis of circulating fibrin or local fibrin deposits. It is unclear whether the role of AP is different in the microcirculation where organ damage due to thrombosis can occur during DIC. It would seem most reasonable to assume that in the circulation AP only plays a role in neutralising free plasmin and the binding of AP to fibrin may represent a neutralisation of the inhibitor and may even allow more rapid destruction of the forming fibrin[9]. Thus it would seem that in the circulation the mechanisms which enhance fibrin destruction are favoured with large reserves of AP available to neutralise any plasmin which 'escapes' from the lysing fibrin clot[10]. The other inhibitor, PAI-1, seems to play no overt role in neutralising the activity of t-PA/plasminogen in the circulation[11]. FnDP also inhibits fibrin formation and platelet aggregation ; thus the enhanced and active fibrinolytic system not only protects the vasculature from fibrin deposition but also prevents the further generation of thrombi. In the circulation it would seem that only small amounts of APC are found in the absence of thrombomodulin and the interaction of PC inhibitors, PC-1 and α_1-antitrypsin probably fully control the residual APC pathway. Figure 1 makes it clear that during systemic (or possibly local) episodes of hypercoagulability a number of markers can be of value. The formation of thrombin (TH) is usually indicated by elevated levels of prothrombin (PROT) fragments 1 and 2 (F_{1+2}) while an increased thrombin-antithrombin (TAT) complex gives a similar indication of prothrombin activation. The response of the fibrinolytic system is accompanied by a reduction in fibrinogen (FG) and an increase in fibrinopeptide A (FPA) and soluble fibrin (FN-FN-FN). The formation of a plasmin-antiplasmin (PAP) complex indicates the formation of plasmin due to fibrin-stimulated activation of tissue plasminogen activator (t-PA) with resultant increase in fibrin degradation products (FNDP, XLFDP). A corresponding consumption of plasminogen (PLgN) will also occur. Of these markers of the hypercoagulable state the most reliable and easily measurable entities are F_{1+2}, TAT, FNDP (XLFDP) eg D dimer and soluble fibrin. While this view of the interaction of enzymes/inhibitors in the presence of forming fibrin may explain how fibrinolysis protects against unnecessary fibrin formation in the circulation, it is probably an inadequate explanation of the fibrinolytic events which occur at the vessel wall or in a haemostatic plug. It is emphasised that although the same fibrinolytic components are involved, we will present an argument that certain cellular environments tip the delicate balance of coagulation and fibrinolysis in favour of clot stability and the containment of blood flow.

III. FIBRINOGEN/FIBRIN FRAGMENTS

The structure and shape of fibrinogen dictate the sequence of degradative reactions by which plasmin attacks the molecule. Despite the fact that plasmin has a general hydrolytic affinity for most arginines and lysines, only a limited number are available in fibrinogen because it contains three major disulphide-rich inaccessible core regions. The carboxy terminal (40,000 MW) of the two A-alpha chains of fibrinogen are first digested by plasmin, followed by segregation of one disulphide-rich region of the molecule known as fragment D. As shown in Figure 2, there is a consensus that the digestion of fibrinogen to its plasmin-resistant core fragments D and E takes place through an asymmetric sequence which involves the generation of an intermediate fragment called Y, which subsequently degrades to its two core fragments, D and E. This sequence of degradation reactions has been reviewed elsewhere[12] and Figure 2 demonstrates that a number of new epitopes are generated during the degradation sequence.

Domainally-directed fragmentation of fibrinogen by plasmin

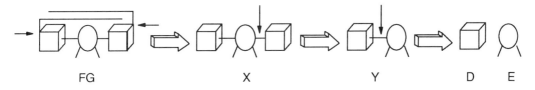

FG   X   Y   D   E

Figure 2: A domainal perspective of the plasmin-mediated conversion of fibrinogen to its fragments D and E showing the intermediate fragments X and Y. The major plasmin digestion takes place at the C-terminals of the Aα chains, the N-terminals of the Bβ chains and the coiled coil peptide sequences joining the plasmin-resistant domains D and E. This domainally-directed digestion determines the structure of the fragments generated by plasmin from both fibrinogen and fibrin (reproduced from Gaffney et al,[41])

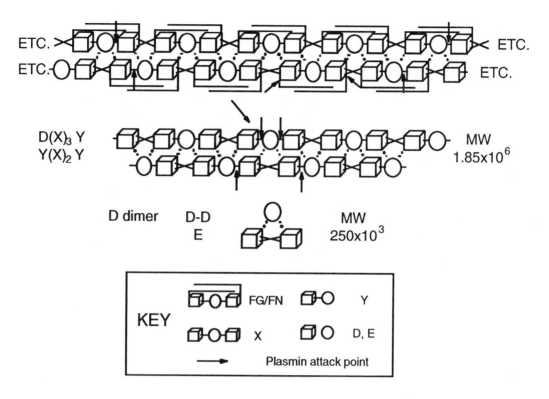

Figure 3: Domainally-directed fragmentation of cross-linked fibrin (XL-FN) : an example of typical cross-linked fragments. The top of the figure depicts the half-stagger two-chain structure of fibrin, showing cross-links between the D domains of adjacent fibrin subunits. The action of plasmin generates various molecular weight structures, all having various X, Y, D, E domains associated by the γ-chain cross-links in the originating fibrin. This figure shows only a typical intermediate fraction (MW = 2 x 10⁶) and the terminal cross linked fragment D dimer-E. Lysis by plasmin of only COOH-Aα regions and the coiled coil sequences between the D and E domains dominates the sequence of lytic events (reproduced from Gaffney et al,[41])

Monoclonal antibodies to some of these new structures have been developed[13,14]. The interaction of thrombin with fibrinogen generates a half-stagger polymeric fibrin (Figure 3) which becomes crosslinked rather rapidly between the gamma chains of adjacent fibrin subunits and later between the alpha chains of these subunits (for review see ref 15). When crosslinked fibrin is digested by plasmin the same domainal fragmentation takes place as shown in Figure 2 for fibrinogen. Thus it is not surprising that in crosslinked fibrin digests there is a large variety of X, Y, D and E structural combinations held together by Factor XIII mediated gamma chain crosslinks from the originating crosslinked fibrin. Figure 3 is an attempt to domainally characterise some of this heterogeneous group. A general formula for all these crosslinked fragments is given as :

$$(Y \text{ or } D - X_n - Y \text{ or } D)_2$$

Regardless of the uncertainties expressed above concerning the roles of various components in systemic fibrinolysis, it is clear that an adequate fibrinolytic system can degrade significant quantities of fibrin in the circulation. This degradation is significantly influenced by the balance of activators (such as t-PA) and inhibitors (PAI-1 and α_2-AP) in the blood. There is increasing evidence that most of the fibrin formed in blood is crosslinked via the γ-chains and the subsequent fibrin degradation products (FnDP) are mostly crosslinked. Thus crosslinked FnDP as measured by assays specific for D dimer[16] and X-oligomer[17] indicates the prior formation of crosslinked fibrin in the blood, the presence of which is one understandable definition of the hypercoagulable state. It can be concluded that enhanced level of FnDP is a reliable marker of the hypercoagulable state.

While a prior disposition to the hypercoagulable state may exist *in vivo* it is known that there is no expression of fibrinolytic activity until fibrin is generated[3]. The behaviour of clotted blood or plasma differs enormously depending on the presence of inhibitors and whether the clot is found *in vivo* or *in vitro*. Table I shows the behaviour of clots formed under a variety of circumstances and highlights the role the vessel wall may play in the degradation of fibrin clots *in vivo* in flowing blood. The euglobulin fraction of human plasma, following clotting, will lyse in a finite time. This time is called the euglobulin clot lysis time (ECLT) and has been traditionally regarded as a measure of the fibrinolytic potential of blood. Since no AP and about 80% of the PAI-1 is present in the euglobulin fraction the role of PAI-1 in neutralising t-PA in the presence of fibrin can be questioned. Indeed data from Paramo et al[11] suggests that the level of PAI-1 may be irrelevant to the fibrinolytic effect in the circulation. The clot derived from whole plasma (Table I) is stable indefinitely and this must be due to the presence of α_2-antiplasmin. The fact that *in vivo* defibrination during DIC is accompanied by avid fibrin lysis suggests that AP does not effectively inhibit the activity of plasmin, presumably on the surface of the forming fibrin.

Table I : Behaviour of fibrin clots *in vivo* and *in vitro*

	Whole Blood Clot	Plasma Clot	Euglobulin Clot	In Vivo Clot
Lysis Time	Inf	Inf	50-200 min	v. rapid
α_2-AP	+	+	-	+
PAI-1	+	+	+	+
t-PA	+	+	+	++ (?)

It is difficult to know whether the fibrinolytic system in the healthy circulation is dormant or sporadically active. Certain stimuli (exercise, DDAVP etc) elevate fibrinolytic potential by increasing the level of plasma t-PA ; however no other effect is obvious. No activation of plasminogen occurs with the concomitant lack of formation of the plasmin/α_2-antiplasmin (PAP) complex. These effects only occur following the formation of fibrin[3]. However, resting plasma contains significant levels of the crosslinked fibrin degradation products, X-oligomer and D-dimer[18,19] which it is assumed comes from the digestion of crosslinked (probably soluble) fibrin. Whether this fibrin forms systemically or at some local juncture in the circulation is not known ; however that fibrin formation and lysis is an ongoing phenomenon in the healthy circulation is now accepted. Understanding these physiological mechanism(s) of fibrinolysis will allow us to manipulate the system and to respond therapeutically during various pathological expressions of fibrinolytic imbalance.

The most tangible evidence of ongoing fibrinolysis in blood during the hypercoagulable state is the generation of fibrin degradation products. The formation and lysis of fibrin in the circulation is a dynamic process which is depicted in Figure 4. If we assume that fibrin formation is relevant to thrombosis and that fibrinolytic activity is promoted by the presence of fibrin, then the measurement of levels of FDP in blood may be valuable in either predicting the onset or monitoring the progress of a fibrin-based thrombotic event. In the past, FDP measurements have been performed in serum (for review see ref 20) but the availability of monoclonal antibodies (mabs) to specific crosslinked FDP has allowed direct FDP assays in plasma. Using these mabs, Gaffney & Perry (21) demonstrated that thrombin-generated serum samples contain in excess of 1,000 ng/ml of crosslinked FDP while the originating plasma contained only about 40 ng/ml. Most serum FDP assays using polyclonal antibodies therefore measure an artefactual background level in excess of 1 µg/ml ; indeed most commercial serum FDP assay kits do not measure below 2 µg/ml.

DIC PLASMA FRACTIONS
Fibrinopeptide-A and X-Oligomer

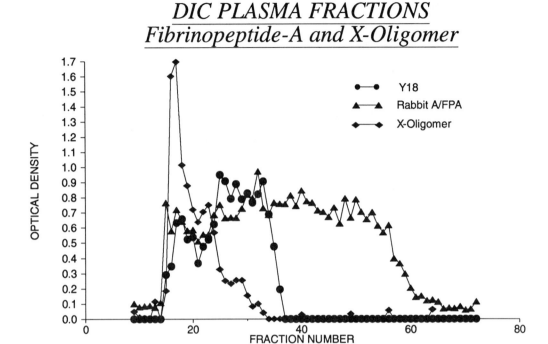

Figure 4: Fibrinopeptide A and X-oligomer in plasma from patients with disseminated intravascular coagulation (DIC). The elution profile shown is from a gel exclusion column Biogel A-15. The elution fractions were monitored using three specific antibodies. The major FDP peak eluted at the void volume ($=2 \times 10^6$ Daltons) and crossreacted with the X-oligomer mab (NIBn-123) ; this same fraction crossreacted with antibodies to fibrinopeptide A (A/FPA) and with an antibody (Y18) to fragments which contain FPA. A variety of other fractions reacted with Y18 while crossreactivity with A/FPA persisted to near the total exclusion volume of the column (reproduced from Gaffney and Longstaff[4]).

Ultimately, antibodies may be developed which have specificity for each component within the heterogeneous group of crosslinked fibrin degradation products (XL-FnDP) two of which are shown in Figure 3. Currently, efforts to generate monoclonal antibodies have been guided by a negative reaction with fibrinogen and a positive reaction with one or other of a rather mixed group of FDP's found in plasma. The most common example is that of D dimer, which for many years has been regarded as a potentially valuable marker of *in vivo* fibrin formation and degradation[22]. The first such assay was developed by Rylatt et al[19] and involved the use of a D dimer-specific mab (coded DD3B6) as a catcher antibody on a polyvinyl 96-well plate and the tagging of the immunologically-immobilized D dimer fraction with a pan-specific mab. Using a two-site ELISA system this assay can detect various crosslinked FDP fractions which include D dimer structures, crosslinked Y-D and the heterogeneous X-oligomer fraction. This D dimer assay has demonstrated a mean concentration of D dimer-like fragments in normal plasma of 75 ng/ml, with an upper limit of about 140 ng/ml. Elevated concentrations of D dimer were observed in the plasma of patients with pulmonary embolism (PE), deep vein thrombosis (DVT), arterial thrombo-embolism and DIC[16,23]. Another similar assay[17] involves a two-site ELISA system using IgM mabs (NIBn 52) coated on PVC 96-well plates as a catcher and horseradish peroxidase HRP-labelled NIBn 178 as the tag antibody. This assay system has high specificity for the X-oligomer fraction, while no reaction is observed with fibrinogen, D dimer or NXL-FDP. Using this assay in conjunction with a lyophilized X-oligomer standard, Gaffney et al[18] have shown that patients with PE, DVT, myocardial infarction (MI) and peripheral vascular disease (PVD) had elevated levels of X-oligomer. The same assay has indicated that individuals following MI have consistently elevated levels[24]. Normal plasma contained levels of 10-200 ng/ml. The assay was reproducible in samples which had been snapfrozen and thawed many times. Two mabs with specific affinity for X-oligomer have been developed. Each is directed toward a different conformational epitope on the complex X-oligomer structure[17].

It can be argued (see Figure 1) that the production of fibrin in the circulation is a prerequisite for the activation of plasminogen and thus the formation of NXL- and XL-FDP ; however, the third assay system to be described here has been developed to allow the assessment of the total FDP fraction and the subfractions derived from both fibrinogen (FgDP)[25] and XL-fibrin (FnDP)[26]. Mabs specific for the E domain of fibrinogen (FDP 14) have been used to immobilize the total FDP (TDP) in plasma, and the fibrinogen and fibrin-derived FDP fractions can be individually identified using, respectively, an HRP-labelled mab for fibrinopeptide A-containing fragments (Y-18) and an HRP-labelled mab for crosslinked FDP (DD-13). Should only the TDP level in plasma be required, then the second antibody used was a polyclonal to FDP. Whether primary fibrinogen digestion in the circulation is a frequent event is questionable. However, using the specific assay for FgDP it has been surprisingly demonstrated that high levels exist in plasma during arvin induced defibrination[6]. Whether this plasma FgDP fraction originates from circulating fibrinogen, from fibrinogen bound to fibrin in the circulation or from a form of fibrin which retains one FPA is unknown ; however the latter seems most probable. This opinion depends on recent data obtained using a variety of mabs to monitor DIC plasma fractions from a Biogel A-15 column. Figure 4 shows the data and indicates that, using specific antibodies to FPA, FPA-containing FDP (Y18) and X-oligomer, DIC-plasma contains crosslinked FDP fraction of molecular weight > 2 X 10^6 daltons and containing high levels of FPA. Similar data have been obtained by Gron et al[27] during their study of the plasma of fibrinaemic patients. Other data (not shown) indicate that normal and pathological plasma display this type of FDP. These findings suggest that crosslinked polymerised protofibrils of the empirical formula $(A\alpha/\alpha\ B\beta_2\ \gamma_2)_n$ are digested during DIC episodes generating FDP. These have been erroneously classified as FgDP while they are actually FnDP still containing a residual FPA. Thus, the ratio of so-called FgDP and FnDP may be of value in delineating the severity of DIC and the prediction of vascular and organ damage.

While the above description has concentrated on assays of plasmin-mediated fibrinogen/fibrin degradation products, there is also interest in monitoring fibrin formation *in vivo* as a marker of the hypercoagulable or prethrombotic state. While Nossel et al[28] suggested FPA as a reliable marker, subsequent commercial assays never satisfied the demands of routine laboratory practice. An alternative approach involves the measurement of soluble fibrin with specific mabs to sequences exposed at the NH$_2$ terminus of the α chain of fibrin following the removal of FPA. These soluble forms of fibrin are complexed with fibrinogen in the circulation. Scheefers-Borchel[29] have developed one such assay while Nieuwenhuizen and colleagues[30] have reported a similar assay using an ELISA system which uses mabs to an epitope on the Aα chain (148-160) and to a carboxy terminal sequence of the same chain. The robustness of these assays has yet to be demonstrated in kits under routine laboratory conditions. Another assay has been developed which depends on the rate enhancing effect of plasma fibrin on plasminogen activation by t-PA[31]. This is now available as a commercial kit for the measurement of soluble fibrin complexes.

IV. SPECULATIVE CONTACTS BETWEEN COAGULATION AND FIBRINOLYSIS

Thrombin generation seems to be an essential control feature of the hypercoagulable state. It is worthwhile to consider some of the control features of thrombin generation to some components on the fibrinolytic system. While it is accepted that the vessel wall has an essentially anticoagulant effect due to thrombomodulin[32] (especially in the microvasculature) it also has other activities which may impinge on the fibrinolytic response to, firstly, thrombin generation and subsequently, fibrin formation. Thrombin activates protein C to form activated protein C (APC) which cleaves both Factors V a and VIII a, thus curtailing the generation of thrombin via both the so-called intrinsic and extrinsic coagulation cascades. The clinical relevance of these reactions and the strategic importance of APC has been demonstrated by the description of a condition known as activated Protein C resistance which highly disposes to thrombosis[33]. The influence of the vessel wall and haemostatic plug formation on these reactions is briefly discussed below.

A. FIBRINOLYSIS AT THE VESSEL WALL

Vessel endothelium is in direct contact with flowing blood. Blood contains a variety of cells, including the potentially thrombogenic platelets. The cellular components of blood make up about 50% of its volume. While we will deal here with the role of the endothelial cells in human fibrinolysis, a true perspective on human fibrinolysis also requires an understanding of the biology of fibrinolytic activity on the surfaces of these circulating cell types.

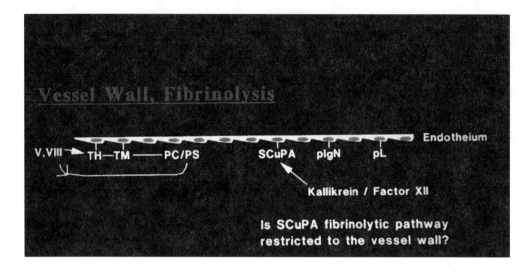

Figure 5: A schematic view of some anticoagulant features of the vessel wall. The thrombomodulin (TM) enhancing effect on thrombin (TH) activation of the PC/PS complex to activated protein C (APC) and the subsequent quenching of the factor V/VIII driven coagulant pathway is shown to be vessel wall directed. The proposition that single chain urinary type plasminogen activator (SCuPA) may play a role in plasminogen (PLgN) → plasmin (PL) conversion at the vessel wall is proposed. This latter pathway may be mediated via the kallikrein/factor XII pathway.

Two pathways which may relate to fibrinolysis at the vessel wall are the protein C and prourokinase pathways. While the major fibrin-related fibrinolytic pathway which protects against fibrin deposition is still relevant, the endothelium influences the outcome of fibrin deposition. Thrombomodulin (TM) in endothelial cells combines with thrombin and enhances the activation of the protein C-S complex by thrombin (Figure 5) to such an extent that the generation of thrombin is strictly controlled by the activated protein C (APC) destruction of both factors V and VIII. On binding to TM, thrombin loses its ability to clot fibrinogen and to activate factors V, VIII and XIII and platelets (review in ref 32). This anti-thrombotic pathway is unique to the vessel wall, TM being a unique component of the endothelium. Another pathway operative at the vessel wall (Figure 5) involves the binding of both single chain and two chain urokinase together with plasminogen to unique receptors on the endothelium[34,35]. This would allow the generation of plasmin via the prourokinase pathway, neutralising the possibility of fibrin degradation. This plasmin may also be less prone to inhibition by the circulating α_2-antiplasmin[35]. As long as the vessel wall has undamaged endothelium, both antithrombotic and profibrinolytic mechanisms are operative on its surface. This situation may change dramatically when the endothelium is damaged and a procoagulant subendothelium allows platelet deposition and subsequent thrombosis. Indeed, the physiology of this latter situation may not differ greatly from that observed when the vasculature is ruptured during an episode of bleeding. Platelets and ill-understood elements of vasoconstriction would then come into play.

B. FIBRINOLYSIS AND HAEMOSTATIC PLUG FORMATION

The main evolutionary intention of the haemostatic mechanism in man and other animals is to prevent haemorrhage at a site of rupture of the vasculature. This mechanism is essential for day to day survival. Here we present a hypothesis that blood platelets combined with vasoconstriction, procoagulant enhancement and neutralisation of fibrinolysis all play a part in maintaining the stability of the haemostatic plug (Figure 6). While it has been proposed[36] that PAI-1 released from platelets by thrombin stimulation in the presence of APC is prevented from interacting with t-PA, thus enhancing clot lysis, an alternative view may be taken[37]. This view suggests that PAI-1 released from platelets in the haemostatic plug inhibits protein C, enhancing further production of thrombin and strengthening the platelet-rich clot. This proposal would support the recognised procoagulant function of activated platelets. It is, of course, possible that because of the excess PAI-1 present fibrinolysis may also be inhibited. While we have presented a case that protein C is anticoagulant and profibrinolytic at the vessel wall, in a platelet-rich haemostatic plug or extensive thrombus this activity could be neutralised by the large quantity of PAI-1. A further procoagulant influence in the haemostatic plug may be the neutralisation of the cofactor protein S by thrombin, thus neutralising the inhibiting effect of PC on the coagulation system. It seems[38] that both thrombin and the platelet surface may regulate the activity of protein S enhancing clotting in the platelet-rich plug. The high affinity of both protein S and C for endothelial cells may be an important expression of anticoagulation at the vessel wall[39]. The stabilising crosslinked fibrin in the platelet rich haemostatic plug is probably organised after initial aggregation of the platelets ; this fibrin would then be protected from lysis by both procoagulant and antifibrinolytic forces generated on the platelets and other cell surfaces.

While there are many conditions present in a haemostatic plug which remain unknown, a simplistic approach to the paramount need for effective haemostasis must involve the surface biology of the platelet. The presence of other cells in the haemostatic plug suggests that cell surface-related tissue factor with its interdependence on protein S and possibly protein C[40] may play an important procoagulant role, thus ensuring freedom from haemorrhage.

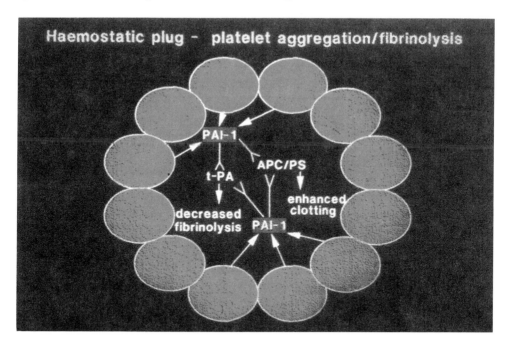

Figure 6: In this scheme it is proposed that plasminogen activator inhibitor-1 (PAI-1) may play a role in stabilising haemostatic plugs via the neutralisation of the anticoagulant effect of the activated protein C (APC)/Protein S (PS) system causing a quenching of the generation of thrombin. The PAI-1 could also act in its more expected manner in neutralising the activation of the fibrinolytic system. It is suggested that platelets play a major role in wound sealant stability

V. CONCLUDING REMARKS

Activation of the fibrinolytic system in response to the hypercoagulable state is classically demonstrated during DIC. The major markers of such activation have been discussed above. There is little doubt that the assay of XL-FDP (notably D dimer) in plasma is a valuable marker of an advanced state of hypercoagulability, whether transient, transient/local, disseminated, or otherwise. The extensive use of mab-specific XL-FDP assays in many laboratories will be the final arbiter of the value of these assays in evaluating the role of activated coagulation/fibrinolysis in health and disease. While there is a change in the levels of the components (enzymes and inhibitors) of fibrinolysis during the hypercoagulable state, it is still not clear that measuring any one component of this complex system of fibrinolysis is of value during an assessment of an acquired secondary hypercoagulable state. A global assay which measures plasma fibrinolytic potential may be of some value and such assays are currently under assessment.

REFERENCES

1. **Schafer, A.**, The hypercoagulable states, *Ann. Int. Med.*, 102, 814, 1985.
2. **Lijnen, H. R., Collen, D.**, Congenital and acquired deficiencies of components of the fibrinolytic system and their relation to bleeding or thrombosis, *Fibrinolysis*, 3, 67, 1989.
3   **Marsh, N. A., Gaffney, P. J.**, Exercise induced fibrinolysis - fact or fiction?, *Thromb. Haemostasis*, 48, 201, 1982.
4. **Gaffney, P. J., Longstaff, C.**, Fibrinolysis, in Haemostasis and Thrombosis. Bloom, A. L., Thomas, D. P., Eds., Churchill Livingstone, Edinburgh, 1994, 549.
5. **Gaffney, P. J., Templeman, J., Mahmoud, M., Joe, F.**, Fibrin formation : the influence of plasminogen, thrombin and calcium, 7th Int. Cong. Thromb., Valencia, Spain, October 1982 (abstract).
6. **Prentice, C. R. M., Hampton, K. K., Grant, P. J., et al**, The effect of therapeutic ancrod defibrinogenation on circulating components of fibrinolysis, *Br. J. Haematol.*, 83, 276, 1993.
7. **Collen, D.**, Regulation of fibrinolysis - recent developments, in Haemophilia and Haemostasis. A R Liss, New York, 1981, 221.
8. **Tran-Thang, C., Kruithof, E. K. O., Bachmann, F.**, Tissue-type plasminogen activator increases the binding of glu-plasminogen to clots, *J. Clin. Invest.*, 74, 2009, 1984.
9. **Takada, A., Urano, T., Takada, Y.**, The regulation of the activation of the fibrinolytic system, Adv. *Exp. Med. Biol.*, 281, 209, 1990.
10. **Wiman, B., Collen, D.**, Molecular mechanisms of physiological fibrinolysis, *Nature*, 272, 549, 1978.
11. **Paramo, J. A., Gascoine, P. S., Pring, J. B., Gaffney, P. J.**, The relative inhibition by α_2-antiplasmin and plasminogen activator inhibitor-1 of clot lysis *in vitro*, *Fibrinolysis*, 4, 169, 1990.
12. **Francis, C. S., Marder, V. J.**, A molecular model of plasmic degradation of crosslinked fibrin, *Sem. Thromb. Haemost.*, 8, 25, 1981.
13. **Plow, E. F., Edgington, T. S.**, Surface markers of fibrinogen and its physiological derivatives revealed by antibody probes, *Sem. Thromb. Haemost.*, 8, 35, 1982.
14. **Kudryk, B., Grossman, Z. D., McAfee, J. G., Rosebrough, S. F.**, Monoclonal antibodies as probes for fibrin(ogen) proteolysis, in Monoclonal Antibodies in Immunoscintigraphy. Chatal, J.-F., Ed., C.R.C. Press, Boca Raton, U.S.A., 1989, Ch. 19, 365.
15. **Curtis, C. G.**, Plasma factor XIII, in : Haemostasis and Thrombosis. Bloom, A. L., Thomas, D. P., Eds., Churchill Livingstone, Edinburgh 1987, 216.
16. **Whitaker, A. N., Elms, M., Masci, P. P., Bundesen, P. G., Rylatt, D. B., Webber, A. J., Bunce, I.**, Measurement of crosslinked fibrin derivatives in plasma : an immunoassay using monoclonal antibodies, *J. Clin. Path.*, 37, 882, 1984.
17. **Gaffney, P. J., Creighton, L. J., Perry, M. J., Callus, M., Thorpe, R., Spitz, M.**, Monoclonal antibodies to crosslinked fibrin degradation products (XL-FDP) I : Characterisation and preliminary evaluation in plasma, *Br. J. Haematol.*, 68, 83, 1988.
18. **Gaffney, P. J., Creighton, L. J., Callus, M., Thorpe, R.**, Monoclonal antibodies to crosslinked fibrin degradation products (XL-FDP) II : Evaluation in a variety of clinical conditions, *Br. J. Haematol.*, 68, 91, 1988.
19. **Rylatt, D. B., Blake, A. S., Cottis, L. E., Massingham, D. A., Fletcher, W. A., Masci, P. P., Whitaker, A. N., Elms, M., Bunce, I., Webber, A. J., Wyatt, D., Bundesen, P. G.**, An immunoassay for human D-dimer using monoclonal antibodies, *Thromb. Res.*, 31, 767, 1983.
20. **Donati, M. B.**, Assays for fibrinogen-fibrin degradation products in biological fluids : some methodological aspects, *Thromb. Haemostasis*, 34, 652, 1975.
21. **Gaffney, P. J., Perry, M. J.**, Unreliability of current serum fibrin degradation product (FDP) assays, *Thromb. Haemostasis*, 53, 301, 1985.
22. **Gaffney, P. J.**, FDP, Lancet, 2, 1422 (letter), 1972.
23. **Elms, M., Bunce, I. H., Bundesen, P. G., Rylatt, D. B., Webber, A. J., Masci, P. P., Whitaker, A. N.**, Measurement of crosslinked fibrin degradation products - an immunoassay using monoclonal antibodies, *Thromb. Haemostasis*, 50, 591, 1983.
24. **Rogers, S., Sweetman, P. M., Perry, M. J., Gaffney, P. J.**, Plasma levels of fibrin fragments in men with myocardial infarction, *Thromb. Res.*, 43, 389, 1985.
25. **Koppert, P. W., Kuipers, W., Hoegee-de Nobel, B., Brommer, E. J. P., Koopman, J., Nieuwenhuizen, W.**, A quantitative enzyme immunoassay (EIA) for primary fibrinogenolysis products in plasma, *Thromb. Haemostasis*, 57, 25, 1987.
26. **Koopman, J., Haverkate, F., Koppert, P. W., Nieuwenhuizen, W., Brommer, E. J. P., Van der Werf, W. G. L.**, New immunoassay of fibrin(-ogen) degradation products in plasma using a monoclonal antibody, *J. Lab. Clin. Med.*, 109, 75, 1987.

27. **Gron, B., Bennick, A., Nieuwenhuizen, W., Brosstad, F.**, Normal and fibrinaemic patient plasma contain high molecular weight crosslinked fibrin(ogen) derivatives with intact fibrinopeptide A., *Thromb. Res.* 57, 259, 1990.

28. **Nossel, H., Waser, J., Kaplan, K. L., La Gamma, K. S., Yudelman, L., Canfield, K.**, Sequence of fibrinogen proteolysis and platelet release after intrauterine infusion of hypertonic saline, *J. Clin. Invest.* 64, 1371, 1979.

29. **Scheefers-Borchel, U., Muller-Berghaus, G., Fuhge, P., Eberle, R., Heimburger, N.**, Discrimination between fibrin and fibrinogen by a monoclonal antibody against a synthetic peptide, *Proc. Natl. Acad. Sci. U.S.A.*, 82, 7091, 1985.

30. **Nieuwenhuizen, W., Hoegee-de Nobel, E., Laterveer, R.**, A rapid monoclonal antibody-based enzyme immunoassay (EIA) for the quantitative determination of soluble fibrin in plasma, *Thromb. Haemostasis*, 68, 273, 1992.

31. **Wiman, B., Ranby, M.**, Determination of soluble fibrin in plasma by a rapid and quantitative spectrophotometric assay, *Thromb. Haemostasis*, 55, 189, 1986.

32. **Dahlback, B., Stenflo, J.**, A natural anticoagulant pathway : proteins C, S, C4b-binding protein and thrombomodulin, in *Haemostasis and Thrombosis*. Bloom, A. L., Forbes, C. D., Thomas, D. P., Tuddenham, E. G. D., Eds., Churchill Livingstone, Edinburgh, 1994, 671.

33. **Dahlback, B., Carlsson, M., Svensson, P. J.**, Familial thrombophilia due to a previously unrecognised mechanism characterised by poor anticoagulant response to activated protein C : prediction of a cofactor to activated protein C, *Proc. Natl. Acad. Sci. U.S.A.*, 90. 1004, 1993.

34. **Plow, E. F., Felez, J., Miles, L. A.**, Cellular regulation of fibrinolysis, *Thromb. Haemostasis*, 66 (1), 132, 1991.

35. **Miles, L. A., Plow, E. F.**, Plasminogen receptors : ubiquitous sites for cellular regulation of fibrinolysis, *Fibrinolysis*, 2, 61, 1988.

36. **Sakata, Y., Loskutoff, D. J., Gladson, C. L., Hekman, C. M., Griffin, T. H.**, Mechanism of protein C-dependent clot lysis : role of plasminogen activator inhibitor, *Blood*, 68, 1218, 1986.

37. **Fay, W. P., Owen, W. G.**, Platelet plasminogen activator'inhibitor : purification and characterisation of interaction with plasminogen activators and activated protein C. *Biochemistry*, 28, 5773, 1989.

38. **Mitchell, L., Salem, H.**, Cleavage of protein S by a platelet membrane protease, *J. Clin. Invest.*, 79, 374, 1987.

39. **Esmon, C. T.**, Assembly and function of the protein C anticoagulant pathway on endothelium, in Endothelial cell – biology in health and disease*f*. Simionescu, N., Simionescu, M., Eds., Plenum Press, New York, 1989, 191.

40. **Nemerson, Y.**, Tissue factor and haemostasis, *Blood*, 71, 1, 1988.

41. **Gaffney, P. J., Creighton-Kempsford, L. J., Tymkewycz, P.M.**, Detection of fibrin and its fragments using monoclonal antibodies. Clinical implications*, in Thrombosis and Haemorrhagic Disorders*. Nagy, I., Losanczy, H., Vinazzer, H., Eds., Schmitt and Meyer GmbH, Wurzburg, 1990, 121.

BIOLOGICAL MARKERS OF ACUTE VENOUS THROMBOSIS AND PULMONARY EMBOLISM

H. Bounameaux
Division of Angiology and Haemostasis
Department of Medicine, University Hospital of Geneva, Geneva, Switzerland

I. INTRODUCTION

In the past decade, plasma assays of several markers of activation of plasma coagulation and/or fibrinolysis have been developed and made available for clinical use (Figure 1). They include D-dimer (DD), thrombin-antithrombin III (TAT) complexes, and prothrombin fragment 1+2 (F_{1+2}). DD is a specific degradation product of crosslinked fibrin[1] ; TAT complexes are formed upon inactivation of thrombin by its natural inhibitor, antithrombin III,[2] while F_{1+2} is a peptide which is released from the prothrombin molecule upon cleavage by thrombin.[3] Activation of other coagulation zymogens, such as Factor IX, Factor X or Protein C are also accompanied by the release of "activation peptides" which have proven to be very useful in studying the physiopathology of the plasma coagulation cascade but which have not been used for clinical purposes, so far. The same is true for plasmin induced degradation products of fibrinogen such as fragment $B\beta_{1-42}$ or non-crosslinked fibrin such as fragment $B\beta_{15-42}$, which have been utilized to characterize the effects of plasminogen activators during thrombolytic therapy, as well as for plasmin-alpha$_2$-antiplasmin (PAP) complexes, which result from the inhibition of the enzyme by its natural inhibitor.

In this chapter we will only consider DD, TAT and F_{1+2} as potential aids in the diagnostic approach of deep venous thrombosis (DVT) and pulmonary embolism (PE).

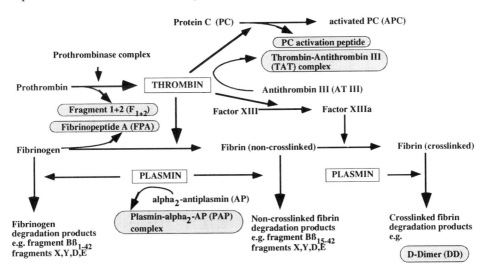

Figure 1 : Activation markers of plasma coagulation and fibrinolysis. Measurement of these markers allows us to better characterize the activation status of these two physiologic systems. Prothrombin fragment 1+2 indicates thrombin formation whilst the presence of TAT complexes, PC activation peptide or FPA are secondary to the action of thrombin. Detection of PAP complexes and fibrin(ogen) degradation products (FDPs) point to a formation and activity of plasmin. The nature of FDPs allows discrimination between a plasmin effect on fibrinogen (fragment $B\beta_{1-42}$), non-crosslinked fibrin (fragment $B\beta_{15-42}$) or crosslinked fibrin (DD).

0-8493-5804-3/96/$0.00+$.50

II. DD AS A DIAGNOSTIC AID IN SUSPECTED VENOUS THROMBOEMBOLISM

A. COMMERCIALLY AVAILABLE ASSAYS

As recently reviewed extensively,[4] several commercial ELISA or latex agglutination tests for DD (Table I) are available for clinical use (Table I). The antibodies used in these tests recognize distinct epitopes. Therefore, direct comparisons of results obtained with different assays are often disappointing. [5] Indeed, the various assays differ in many aspects, including the capture and the tagging antibody, the required sample dilution, the detection limit, and the incubation time. Recently, van Beek et al.[5] performed a systematic comparison of four ELISA assays in 151 plasma samples from patients clinically suspected of pulmonary embolism. These authors reported intra-assay coefficients of variation (CV) in the medium values of 3.5% (assay D, see Table I), 6.3% (assay B), 10.0% (assay C) and even 17.0% (assay A). The inter-assay CV were very similar among the four ELISAs, ranging between 15% and 20% in the medium values. This rather poor reproducibility might account for the only fair correlation (regression coefficients of about 0.60) between the various ELISA assays. On the other hand, the normal values in a reference healthy population differed considerably between the assays. Similarly discordant results were obtained by comparing commercial latex tests.[5] Lastly, results may be expressed both in DD units or in fibrinogen equivalent units (FEU), 1 µg/L FEU being roughly equivalent to 0.5 µg/L of DD units. For the sake of uniformity, all values in this chapter will be expressed in FEU.

Because of the heterogeneity of the assays, the validity of using individual tests has to be carefully assessed in clinical trials. Initially, these trials have to characterize the diagnostic performances of the test against the diagnostic standard. In a further step, the test has to be submitted to real life in so-called management trials.[6] In the latter setting, decision to treat (say anticoagulate) or not to treat is based upon the test's result and patients are followed-up for three to six months in order to assess the safety of the diagnostic approach.

Table I : Characteristics of some Commercial Assays for D-Dimer, TAT and F_{1+2}

Notation	Commercial name	Producer	Capture Ab	Tagging Ab
D-Dimer				
ELISA assays				
A	Dimertest	Agen*	3B6/22	4D2/182
B	Asserachrom DDi	STAGO¶	2F7	polyclonal
C	Fibrinostika FnDP	Organon Teknika	FDP14	FDP DD13
D	D-Dimer micro	Behring	monoclonal	polyclonal
Latex assays				
E	Dimertest I	Agen*	3B6/22	
F	D-dimertest	STAGO¶	2F7	
G	Minutex D-Dimer	Biopool	8D3	
H	FDP-Slidex Direct	Bio-Mérieux	monoclonal	
Thrombin-antithrombin III (TAT) complexes				
ELISA assays				
I	Enzygnost TAT	Behring	anti-human thrombin†	anti-human ATIII†
Prothrombin fragment F_{1+2}				
ELISA assays				
K	Enzygnost F_{1+2}	Behring	polyclonal	anti-human prothrombin†
L	F 1.2	Baxter	monoclonal	N.S.
M	F 1.2	Organon Teknika	monoclonal	N.S.

Ab antibody; *also marketed by MabCo, American Diagnostics, Baxter, Ortho Diagnostics, and Fujirebio; ¶also marketed by Boehringer-Mannheim and American Bioproducts Company, latex from Stago also marketed by Organon Teknika; †from rabbit. N.S. not specified. (Modified and extended after ref. 4).

B. PERFORMANCES OF DD IN PATIENTS CLINICALLY SUSPECTED OF DVT

Diagnosis of DVT is a daily challenge for the clinician because the clinical picture is both nonsensitive and nonspecific. In patients with clinical signs and symptoms, several noninvasive techniques are used, the diagnostic gold standard still being contrast venography, an expensive method and not devoid of hazards.[6] In eleven studies[7-17] totaling more than one thousand three hundred patients clinically suspected of DVT, a population in which the prevalence of DVT was 35%, sensitivity and specificity of DD for the presence of DVT were 96.8% and 35.2%, respectively when using ELISA assays (Table II), and 83.9% and 67.9%, respectively, when using latex assays[7,9,10,14-16,18-21] (Table III). The performances were similar in the trials that used venography or noninvasive tests as diagnostic standard (Table II).

Thus, a DD level found in an ELISA assay below a certain cutoff which slightly differs from one study to another (300-540 µg/L) allows ruling out the diagnosis of DVT. Moreover, in the series reporting the lowest sensitivity (89%),[11] three of the four patients in whom the ELISA result was normal despite a positive venogram had symptoms for more than 60 days, raising the possibility that the venogram may not have represented acute thrombosis in these cases.

On the other hand, a DD concentration above the cutoff cannot be used for positive diagnosis because of the large number of "false-positive" results, especially if the patients tested suffer from a condition which can be associated with fibrin generation. Thus, in 255 patients who were consecutively admitted in general internal medicine wards, the proportion of subjects without clinical suspicion of venous thromboembolism presenting with DD levels below the critical cutoff of 500 µg/L was only 22%.[35] Thus, in spite of its high sensitivity, the usefulness of the test must be questioned in hospitalized patients. Lastly, a pooled analysis of results obtained with latex tests suggests that their sensitivity is not sufficient to allow exclusion of the presence of DVT in clinically suspected patients, although some commercial assays showed good performances in small trials.

Table II : Diagnostic performances of plasma measurement of DD (*ELISA*) in patients clinically suspected of DVT

Study	Assay*	n	n(DVT)	S v	S p	PPV	NPV
Versus venography							
Heaton[7]	A (400)	57	26	100	47	62	100
Rowbotham[8]	A (500)	104	45	100	34	54	100
Ott[9] A (400)		108 39	97	65	61 98		
Bounameaux[10]	B (500)	53	21	95 47	54	94	
Chapman[11]	A (400)	107	35	89 68	57	92	
Mossaz[12]	C (500)	112	64	98 6	58	75	
Weighted average		**541**	**230**	**97.0**	**47.3**	**57.6**	**95.5**
95% CI			(43%)	94.8-99.2	41.8-52.8	52.7-62.5	92.4-98.6
Versus noninvasive diagnosis							
van Bergen[13]	C (540)	239	60	92 20	28	88	
Elias[14]	B (500)	100	45	98 29	53	94	
Boneu[15]	B (500)	116	34	94 51	44	95	
Chang-Liem[16]	B (450)	32	25	100	29	83	100
Heijboer[17]	B (300)	309	70	100	29	29	100
Weighted average		**796**	**234**	**96.6**	**28.5**	**36.3**	**95.4**
95% CI			(29%)	94.4-98.8	24.8-32.2	32.5-40.1	92.2-98.6
Versus all diagnostic methods							
Weighted average		**1337**	**464**	**96.8**	**35.2**	**44.3**	**95.4**
95% CI			(35%)	95.2-98.4	32.0-38.4	41.2-47.4	93.0-97.8

Sv sensitivity (%); Sp specificity (%); PPV positive predictive value (%); NPV negative predictive value (%); n number of patients; n(DVT) number of DVT; 95% CI 95% confidence interval; *after Table I (within brackets cutoff expressed in µg/L of fibrinogen-equivalent units (FEU)).

C.PERFORMANCES OF DD IN PATIENTS CLINICALLY SUSPECTED OF PE

Clinical diagnosis of PE is unreliable and the diagnostic gold standard, pulmonary angiography, is cumbersome, invasive and not without risk. Usually, ventilation/perfusion lung scintigraphy[22] is used for initial screening: normal perfusion virtually rules out PE, thereby avoiding unnecessary anticoagulant treatment,[23,24] whereas a high-probability lung scan pattern is virtually diagnostic of PE.

Unfortunately, the majority of lung scans do not belong to either of these diagnostic categories and are thus inconclusive.[25] In nine studies totaling almost one thousand patients clinically suspected of PE, a collective in which the prevalence of PE was 38%, sensitivity and specificity of DD for the presence of PE were 96.8% and 45.1%, respectively, when using ELISA assays (Table IV) and 92.2% and 54.8%, respectively, when using latex assays (Table III). In the large scale study of Goldhaber et al.[33] which used pulmonary angiography as the diagnostic standard, three patients had an abnormal angiogram and a DD concentration below the cutoff of 500 µg/L, giving a sensitivity of DD of 94% for the presence of PE. However, two of these patients had a prior history of PE, raising the possibility that their angiographic results may not have represented an acute embolic event.

Thus, a DD level found in an ELISA assay below a certain cutoff which slightly differs from one study to another (290-500 µg/L) allows ruling out the diagnosis of PE. Values above the cutoff cannot be used for positive diagnosis because of the low specificity (see above discussion about diagnosis of DVT).

Table III : Diagnostic performances of plasma measurement of DD (*latex* assays) in patients clinically suspected of DVT or PE

Study	Assay*	n	n(DVT/PE)	S v	S p	PPV	NPV
Patients suspected of DVT							
de Boer [18]¶	E (400)	33	21	43	100	100	50
Heaton [7]¶	E (400)	57	26	73	69	63	75
Ott [9]¶	F (NS)	108	39	90	58	55	91
Bounameaux [10]¶	F (500)	53	21	76	87	80	85
Elias [14]	F (500)	100	45	98	22	50	92
Boneu [15]	F (500)	116	34	76	58	43	86
Chang-Liem [16]	F (500)	32	25	96	100	100	87
Lesprit [19]	F (500)	44	22	96	77	81	94
Carter [20]	E (400)	190	36	81	84	55	95
Hansson [21]¶	G (210s)	105	48	94	68	71	93
Weighted average		**838**	**317**	**83.9**	**67.9**	**61.6**	**87.8**
(95% CI)			(38%)	79.9-87.9	63.9-71.9	57.0-66.2	84.6-91.0
Patients suspected of PE							
Rowbotham [30]	E (NS)	145	79	91	88	90	89
Lichey [31]	F (NS)	26	16	81	60	76	67
Harrison [34]	F (500)	64	16	94	58	43	97
van Beek [5]	F (500)	129	56	96	22	48	89
Weighted average		**364**	**167**	**92.2**	**54.8**	**62.9**	**89.3**
(95% CI)			(46%)	88.1-96.3	47.9-61.7	56.9-67.9	83.7-94.9

Sv sensitivity (%); Sp specificity (%); PPV positive predictive value (%); NPV negative predictive value (%); n number of patients; n(DVT) number of DVT; 95% CI 95% confidence interval; NS not stated; *after Table I (within brackets cutoff expressed in µg/L of fibrinogen-equivalent units (FEU) or in s (assay G)). ¶study using contrast venography as diagnostic endpoint. Modified after ref. 4.

D. PERFORMANCES OF DD IN ASYMPTOMATIC PATIENTS AT PARTICULAR RISK OF DVT

Three studies so far have addressed the issue of predicting postoperative DVT and/or screening for this complication after abdominal[36,37] or hip surgery.[38] In a prospective trial of 185 consecutive patients undergoing elective abdominal surgery who were submitted to bilateral ascending venography on the 8th postoperative day, a plasma DD cutoff of 3000 µg/L (as measured by means of assay B, see Table I) was determined by Receiver Operating Characteristics (ROC) curve analysis to discriminate between patients with and without postoperative DVT with a sensitivity and a specificity of 89% and 48%, respectively.[36] Plasma measurement of DD might thus be useful in thromboprophylactic studies for initial screening of patients, a level below 3000 µg/L allowing exclusion of DVT (negative predictive value of 93%) whereas a concentration above the cutoff would require phlebographic confirmation. Similar results were reported in a series of 135 general surgical patients using assay A (see Table I) with a negative predictive value of 89% for postoperative DVT, by using a cutoff of 2400 µg/L on the first postoperative day.[15] Moreover, a preoperative DD level of less than 800 µg/L was associated with the absence of subsequent postoperative DVT with a predictive value of 85%.[37] In a third study[38] in 173 patients undergoing major hip surgery, a preoperative DD concentration below 500 µg/L (measured with assay B) was associated with the absence of postoperative DVT with a predictive value of 96% whilst the cutoff had to be set at 2000 µg/L on the 12th postoperative day to reach a negative predictive value of 95%. In this setting, however, it would be more useful to diagnose DVT rather than to rule it out in a limited number of patients. The use of DD measurement as an initial screening to reduce the number of necessary venograms in thromboprophylactic trials needs to be properly evaluated in specially designed, prospective trials.

Table IV : Diagnostic performances of plasma measurement of DD *(ELISA)* in patients clinically suspected of PE

Study	Endpoint	Assay*n		n(PE)	S v	S p	PPV	NPV
Goldhaber[26]	angiography	A (290)	69	19	89	44	38	92
Bounameaux[27]	lung scan	B (500)	46	10	100	81	59	100
Bounameaux[28]	decision-making	B (500)	170	55	98	39	44	98
Bounameaux[29]	angiography	B (500)	21	10	100	36	59	100
Rowbotham[30]	lung scan	A (500)	145	79	96	46	59	98
Lichey[31]	decision-making	B (1000)	64	43	98	100	100	95
Demers[32]	lung scan	B (300)	90	24	96	52	46	97
Goldhaber[33]	angiography	B (500)	173	45	93	25	30	91
van Beek[5]	scan ± angiography	B¶ (300)	130	57	100	19	49	100
Weighted average			908	342	96.8	45.1	50.2	94.2
95% CI				(38%)	95.0-98.6	40.8-49.4	46.4-54.0	91.2-97.2

Sv sensitivity (%); Sp specificity (%); PPV positive predictive value (%); NPV negative predictive value (%); n number of patients; n(PE) number of PE; 95% CI 95% confidence interval. * after Table I (within brackets cutoff expressed in µg/L of fibrinogen-equivalent units (FEU); ¶ almost identical accuracy with assay A, C and D. Modified after ref. 4.

@ III. TAT AND F_{1+2} AS DIAGNOSTIC AIDS IN SUSPECTED VENOUS THROMBOEMBOLISM

A. COMMERCIALLY AVAILABLE ASSAYS

ELISAs have been made commercially available for thrombin-antithrombin III (TAT) complexes and for prothrombin fragments F_{1+2}. The characteristics of these assays are displayed in Table I. The precision of the ELISA for TAT noted I (see Table I), as described by the within-assay and between-assay coefficients of variation, has been found to be about 4%[2] to 10%.[39] Recently, Tripodi et al.[40] pointed out that two commercial F_{1+2} assays, namely assays K and L according to Table I, correlated poorly (correlation coefficient of only 0.5). Moreover, a discordant classification (normal or abnormal) was noted in 76% of the samples. This could be related to the two standards used, which are qualitatively different, and to the different anticoagulants used in the two test systems.

B. PERFORMANCES OF TAT IN PATIENTS CLINICALLY SUSPECTED OF DVT OR PE

Four studies[15,32,41,42] totaling 463 patients and 127 venous thromboembolic events (prevalence of the disease 27%) evaluated the performances of the plasma measurement of TAT complexes with respect to the presence of DVT or PE (Table V). Of note that none of these studies used the diagnostic gold standard, venography or pulmonary angiography, as diagnostic endpoint. Although it may be questionable to pool data obtained with various cutoffs and clinical diagnoses (DVT or PE), the calculated weighted averages for sensitivity and specificity of the TAT assay are clearly too low to allow their use in the diagnostic approach to venous thromboembolism. In a series of 196 patients undergoing total hip replacement, Hoek et al.[43] reported a significantly higher plasma concentration of TAT complexes in the patients developing postoperative DVT, but no cutoff value showed a satisfactory discriminative power between those who developed DVT and those who did not. On the other hand, Falanga et al.[44] showed that a preoperative TAT concentration below 3.5 µg/L was associated with an increased risk of DVT following surgery for cancer.

Table V : Diagnostic performances of plasma measurement of TAT complexes and prothrombin fragment F_{1+2} *(ELISA* assays) in patients clinically suspected of DVT or PE

Study	Assay* n		n(DVT/PE)	S v	S p	PPV	NPV
TAT ELISA Assay							
Bounameaux [41]	I (4.1)	46	10 (PE)	70	42	25	83
van Bergen [42]	I (5.0)	232	59 (DVT)	37	88	51	80
Boneu [15]	I (3.6)	116	34 (DVT)	64	77	54	84
Demers [32]	I (3.5)	69	24 (PE)	96	51	51	96
Weighted average		**463**	**127(27%)**	**58.3**	**75.3**	**47.1**	**82.7**
(95% CI)				49.3-67.3	70.7-79.9	39.3-54.9	78.5-86.9
F_{1+2} ELISA Assay							
Boneu [15]	K (1.2)	116	34 (DVT)	47	82	52	79

Sv sensitivity (%); Sp specificity (%); PPV positive predictive value (%); NPV negative predictive value (%); n number of patients; n(DVT/PE) number of DVT or PE; 95% CI 95% confidence interval; NS not stated; *after Table I (within brackets cutoff expressed in µg/L of TAT or in nmol/L of F_{1+2}.

C. PERFORMANCES OF F_{1+2} IN PATIENTS CLINICALLY SUSPECTED OF DVT OR PE

To our knowledge, there is only one trial reporting on the performances of the F_{1+2} ELISA assay in patients clinically suspected of DVT.[15] With a sensitivity and a specificity of 47% and 82%, respectively, this test appears to be of no value in the diagnostic approach to venous thromboembolism (Table V).

IV. FROM LABORATORY TO BEDSIDE

The intrinsic performances of a test, such as its sensitivity and specificity, only partly reflect its clinical utility. The population to which the test is applied must also be taken into account: a test which is very useful in a population with a high prevalence of the disease may become totally useless when applied to a group of subjects with a low prevalence of the suspected disease. In daily clinical practice, the prevalence of the disease corresponds to the individual, *a priori* (i.e. before performing the test) clinical probability that the patient has the disease. In a clinical decision-making diagnostic process, the result of the diagnostic test will then be integrated with that information by means of the Bayes' theorem which yields the posterior probability.[45]

Last, after careful assessment of the intrinsic performances of its components, a diagnostic approach should be submitted to real life, which means that it should ideally be tested in the framework of so-called management trials.[6] This kind of trial allows validation of a test (or a combination of tests) under routine conditions which may be at considerable variance with the optimal conditions of a study of test performances. A management study of the utility of plasma DD in the global diagnostic approach to patients with clinically suspected PE is ongoing in our institution according to a decision analysis model which also includes the result of lower limb B-mode venous compression ultrasonography.[46] This test combination theoretically benefits from the high sensitivity of the DD determination for the presence of VTE and the excellent specificity of the lower limb B-mode ultrasound for the presence of DVT, the source of PE. This model predicted that combining plasma DD measurement and lower limb venous B-mode ultrasound imaging would reduce the requirement for pulmonary angiography by one third among patients with inconclusive lung scan and intermediate *a priori* clinical probability of PE.

This prediction was confirmed in a subsequent management trial which was conducted in 355 consecutive outpatients referred to an emergency center during an eighteen-month period.[47] According to the model, PE was diagnosed in 120 patients (34 %) whilst the diagnosis was excluded in the remaining 233 patients who were thus not given anticoagulant treatment. In the subsequent six-month follow-up, 2 patients only (0.9%, 95%CI: 0-2.1%) were diagnosed as having recurrent venous thromboembolism. This very low figure underlines the safety of the management strategy that was proposed by the decision analysis model.

V. CONCLUSIONS AND PERSPECTIVES

Plasma measurement of DD with the ELISA technique has a definite though limited place in the diagnosis of venous thromboembolism. Though the utility of the test is restricted to the exclusion of DVT and/or PE in a few of the patients clinically suspected of these diseases, its integration in a global diagnostic work-up should be considered by clinicians and laboratory physicians. The performances of TAT and F_{1+2} plasma measurement for that particular purpose are definitely lower, probably due to their shorter half-life in plasma and the rapid inhibition of their formation once heparin is administered. In contrast to that, DD will be released from the clot for a longer period of time in response to endogenous fibrinolysis, independently of the anticoagulant treatment.[48]

Further research should aim at developing more rapid DD tests (more sensitive latex assays or more rapid ELISAs or ELISA-derived assays), thereby allowing a widespread use of the test in emergency wards. Standardization and calibration of the various assays should also be attempted.

The last word about the clinical utility of the measurement of the activation markers of coagulation and fibrinolysis has to be derived from well conducted management trials and derived cost-effectiveness analyses. Other potential uses of such measurements include aid in monitoring oral anticoagulant treatment, a promising issue[49,50] which deserves, however, a specific, prospective assessment.

REFERENCES

1. **Kroneman, R., Nieuwenhuizen, W., Knot, E.A.R.** Monoclonal antibody-based plasma assays for fibrin(ogen) and derivatives, and their clinical relevance. *Blood Coag. Fibrinol* ., 1, 91, 1990.
2. **Pelzer, H., Schwarz, A., Heimburger, N.** Determination of human thrombin-antithrombin III complex in plasma with an enzyme-linked immunosorbent assay. *Thromb Haemostas* ., 59, 101, 1988.

3. **Pelzer, H., Stuber, W., Dati, F., Heimburger, N.** New trends in the field of coagulation diagnosis - New possibilities to improve monitoring of antithrombotic therapy. *Folia Haematol .*, 116, 867, 1989.
4. **Bounameaux, H., de Moerloose, P., Perrier, A., Reber, G.** Plasma measurement of D-Dimer as diagnostic aid in suspected venous thromboembolism: an overview. *Thromb Haemostas.*, 71, 1, 1994.
5. **van Beek, E.J.R., van den Ende, B., Berckmans, R.J., van der Heide, Y., Brandjes, D.P.M., Sturk, A., ten Cate, J.W.** A comparative analysis of D-Dimer assays in patients with clinically suspected pulmonary embolism. *Thromb. Haemostas.*, 70, 408, 1993.
6. **Büller, H.R., Lensing, A.W.A., Hirsh, J., ten Cate, J.W.** Deep vein thrombosis: new non-invasive diagnostic tests *Thromb Haemostas.*, 66, 133, 1991.
7. **Heaton, D.C., Billings, J.D., Hickton, C.M.** Assessment of D dimer assays for the diagnosis of deep vein thrombosis. *J. Lab. Clin. Med.*, 110, 588, 1987.
8. **Rowbotham, B.J., Carroll, P., Whitaker, A.N., Bunce, I.H., Cobcroft, R.G., Elms, M.J., Masci, P.P., Bundesen, P.G., Rylatt, D.B., Webber, A.J.** Measurement of crosslinked fibrin derivatives - Use in the diagnosis of venous thrombosis. *Thromb Haemostas.*, 57, 59, 1987.
9. **Ott, P., Astrup, L., Hartving Jensen, R., Nyeland, B., Pedersen, B.** Assessment of D-dimer in plasma: diagnostic value in suspected deep venous thrombosis of the leg. *Acta Med. Scand.*, 224, 263, 1988.
10. **Bounameaux, H., Schneider, P.A., Reber, G., de Moerloose, P., Krahenbuhl, B.** Measurement of plasma D-dimer for diagnosis of deep venous thrombosis. *Am. J. Clin. Pathol .*, 91, 82, 1989.
11. **Chapman, C.S., Akhtar, N., Campbell, S., Miles, K., O'Connor, J., Mitchell, V.E.** The use of D-Dimer assay by enzyme immunoassay and latex agglutination techniques in the diagnosis of deep vein thrombosis. *Clin. Lab. Haemat.*, 12, 37, 1990.
12. **Mossaz, A., Gandrille, S., Vitoux, J.F., Abdoucheli-Baudot, N., Aiach, M., Fiessinger, J.N.** Valeur des D-dimères dans le diagnostic en urgence des thromboses veineuses. *Presse Méd .*, 19, 1055, 1990.
13. **van Bergen, P.F.M.M., Knot, E.A.R., Jonker, J.J.C., de Boer, A.C., de Maat, M.P.M.** Is quantitative determination of fibrin(ogen) degradation products and thrombin-antithrombin III complexes useful to diagnose deep venous thrombosis in outpatients? *Thromb. Haemostas.*, 62, 1043, 1989.
14. **Elias, A., Aillaud, M.F., Roul, C., Villain, Ph., Serradimigni, A., Juhan-Vague, I.** Assessment of D-dimer measurement by ELISA or latex methods in deep vein thrombosis diagnosed by ultrasonic duplex scanning. *Fibrinolysis*, 4, 237, 1990.
15. **Boneu, B., Bes, G., Pelzer, H., Sié, P., Boccalon, H.** D-dimers, thrombin-antithrombin III complexes and prothrombin fragments 1+2: diagnostic value in clinically suspected deep vein thrombosis. *Thromb. Haemostas.*, 65, 28, 1991.
16. **Chang-Liem, G.S., Lustermans, F.A.T., van Wersch, J.W.J.** Comparison of the appropriateness of the latex and Elisa D-dimer determination for the diagnosis of deep venous thrombosis. *Haemostasis*, 21, 106, 1991.
17. **Heijboer, H., Ginsberg, J.S., Büller, H.R., Lensing, A.W.A., Colly, L.P., ten Cate, J.W.** The use of the D-dimer test in combination with non-invasive testing alone for the diagnosis of deep-vein thrombosis. *Thromb. Haemostas .*, 67, 510, 1992.
18. **de Boer, W.A., de Haan, M.A., Huisman, J.W., Klaassen, C.H.L.** D-dimer latex assay as screening method in suspected deep venous thrombosis of the leg. A clinical study and review of the literature. *Neth. J. Med.*, 38, 65, 1991.
19. **Lesprit, P., Gepner, P., Piette, A.M., de Tovar, G., Filiole, M., Didon, D., Chapman, A.** Phlébites profondes des membres inférieurs. Intérêt diagnostique du dosage des D-dimères. *Presse Méd .*, 20, 1927, 1991.
20. **Carter, C.J., Doyle, D.L., Dawson, N., Fowler, S., Devine, D.** Investigations into the clinical utility of latex D-dimer in the diagnosis of deep venous thrombosis. *Thromb. Haemostas .*, 69, 8, 1993.
21. **Hansson, P.O., Eriksson, H., Jagenburg, R., Lukes, P., Risberg, B.** Can laboratory testing improve screening strategies for deep vein thrombosis at an emergency unit? *J. Intern. Med .*, 235, 143, 1994.
22. **Alderson, P.O., Martin, E.C.** Pulmonary embolism: diagnosis with multiple imaging modalities. *Radiology*, 167, 297,1987.
23. **Hull, R.D., Raskob, G.E., Coates, G., Panju, A.A.** Clinical validity of a normal perfusion lung scan in patients with suspected pulmonary embolism. *Chest*, 97, 23, 1990.
24. **Kipper, S.M., Moser, K.M., Kortman, K.E., Ashburn, W.L.** Longterm follow-up of patients with suspected pulmonary embolism and a normal lung scan. *Chest*, 82, 411, 1982.
25. **The PIOPED Investigators.** Value of the ventilation/perfusion scan in acute pulmonary embolism. Results of the prospective investigation of pulmonary embolism diagnosis (PIOPED). *JAMA*, 263, 2753, 1990.
26. **Goldhaber, S.Z., Vaughan, D.E., Tumeh, S.S., Loscalzo, J.** Utility of cross-linked fibrin degradation products in the diagnosis of pulmonary embolism. *Am. Heart J.*, 116, 505, 1989.
27. **Bounameaux, H., Slosman, D., de Moerloose, P., Reber, G.** Diagnostic value of plasma D-dimer in suspected pulmonary embolism. *Lancet*, 2, 628, 1988.
28. **Bounameaux, H., Cirafici, P., de Moerloose, P., Slosman, D., Reber, G., Unger, P.F.** Measurement of D-Dimer in plasma as diagnostic aid in suspected pulmonary embolism. *Lancet*, 337, 196, 1991.
29. **Bounameaux, H., Schneider, P.A., Slosman, D., de Moerloose, P., Reber, G.** Plasma D-dimer in suspected pulmonary embolism: a comparison with pulmonary angiography and ventilation-perfusion scintigraphy. *Blood Coag. Fibrinol.*, 1, 577, 1990.
30. **Rowbotham, B.J., Egerton-Vernon, J., Whitaker, A.N., Elms, M.J., Bunce, I.H.** Plasma cross linked fibrin degradation products in pulmonary embolism. *Thorax*, 45, 684, 1990.
31. **Lichey, J., Reschofski, I., Dissmann, T., Priesnitz, M., Hoffmann, M., Lode, H.** Fibrin degradation product D-dimer in the diagnosis of pulmonary embolism. *Klin. Wschr .*, 69, 522, 1991.
32. **Demers, C., Ginsberg, J.S., Gohnston, M., Brill-Edwards, P., Panju, A.** D-dimer and thrombin-antithrombin III complexes in patients with clinically suspected pulmonary embolism. *Thromb. Haemostas .*, 67, 408, 1992.
33. **Goldhaber, S.Z., Simons, G.R., Elliott, C.G., Haire, W.D., Toltzis, R., Blacklow, S.C., Doolittle, M.H., Weinberg, D.S.** Quantitative plasma D-Dimer levels among patients undergoing pulmonary angiography for suspected pulmonary embolism. *JAMA*, 270, 2819, 1993.
34. **Harrison, K.A., Haire, W.D., Pappas, A.A., Purnell, G.L., Palmer, S., Holdeman, K.P., Fink, L.M., Dalrymple, G.V.** Plasma D-dimer: a useful tool for evaluating suspected pulmonary embolism. *J. Nucl . Med .*, 34, 896, 1993.
35. **Raimondi, P., Bongard, O., de Moerloose, P., Reber, G., Waldvogel, F., Bounameaux, H.** D-Dimer plasma concentration in various clinical conditions: Implication for the use of this test in the diagnostic approach of venous thromboembolism. *Thromb . Res .*, 69, 125, 1993.

36. **Bounameaux, H., Khabiri, E., Huber, O., Schneider, P.A., Didier, D., de Moerloose, P., Reber, G.** Value of liquid crystal contact thermography and plasma level of D-dimer for screening of deep venous thrombosis following general abdominal surgery. *Thromb . Haemostas .*, 67, 603, 1992.

37. **Rowbotham, B.J., Whitaker, A.N., Harrison, J., Murtaugh, P., Reasbeck, P., Bowie, E.J.W.** Measurement of crosslinked fibrin derivatives in patients undergoing abdominal surgery: use in the diagnosis of postoperative venous thrombosis. *Blood Coag. Fibrinol.*, 3, 25, 1992.

38. **Bongard, O., Wicky, J., Peter, R., Simonovska, S., Vogel, J.J., de Moerloose, P., Reber, G., Bounameaux, H.** D-dimer plasma measurement in patients undergoing major hip surgery: use in the prediction and diagnosis of postoperative proximal vein thrombosis. *Thromb. Res.*, 74, 487, 1994.

39. **Hoek, J.A., Sturk, A., ten Cate, J.W., Lamping R.L., Berends, F., Borm, J.J.J.** Laboratory and clinical evaluation of an assay of thrombin-antithrombin III complexes in plasma. *Clin. Chem.*, 34, 2058, 1988.

40. **Tripodi, A., Chantarangkul, V., Bottasso, B., Mannucci, P.M.** Poor comparability of prothrombin fragment 1+2 values measured by two commercial ELISA methods: influence of different anticoagulants and standards. *Thromb. Haemostas .*, 71, 605, 1994.

41. **Bounameaux, H., Slosman, D., de Moerloose, P., Reber, G.** Laboratory diagnosis of pulmonary embolism: value of increased levels of plasma D-dimer and thrombin-antithrombin III complexes. *Biomed. Pharmacother.*, 43, 385, 1989.

42. **van Bergen, P.F.M.M., Knot, E.A.R., Jonker, J.J.C., de Boer, A.C., de Maat, M.P.M.** Is quantitative determination of fibrin(ogen) degradation products and thrombin-antithrombin III complexes useful to diagnose deep venous thrombosis in outpatients? *Thromb. Haemostas.*, 62, 1043, 1989.

43. **Hoek, J.A., Nurmohamed, M.T., ten Cate, J.W., Büller, H.R., Knipscheer, H.C., Hamelynck, K.J., Marti, R.K, Sturk, A.** Thrombin-antithrombin III complexes in the prediction of deep vein thrombosis following total hip replacement. *Thromb. Haemostas.*, 62, 1050, 1989.

44. **Falanga, A., Ofosu, F.A., Cortelazo, S. et al.** Preliminary study to identify cancer patients at high risk of venous thrombosis following major surgery. *Br. J. Haematol.*, 85, 745, 1993.

45. **Sox, H.C., Blatt, M.A., Higgins, M.C., Marton, K.I.** *Medical decision making*, Butterworths, Boston, 1988, 67.

46. **Perrier, A., Bounameaux, H., Morabia, A., de Moerloose, P., Unger, P.F., Slosman, D., Junod, A.F.** Contribution of plasma D-dimer and lower limb venous ultrasound to the diagnosis of pulmonary embolism: a decision analysis. *Am. Heart J.*, 127, 624, 1994.

47. **Perrier, A., Bounameaux, H., Morabia, A., de Moerloose, P., Slosman, D., Didier, D., Unger, P.F., Junod, A.F.** Diagnosis of pulmonary embolism by a decision analysis-based strategy including clinical probability, D-dimer and ultrasonography: a management study. 1994 (submitted).

48. **Estivals, M., Pelzer, H., Sie, P., Pichon, J., Boccalon, H., Boneu, B.** Prothrombin fragment 1+2, thrombin-antithrombin III complexes and D-dimers in acute deep vein thrombosis: effects of heparin treatment. *Br. J. Haematol.*, 78, 421, 1991.

49. **Elias, A., Bonfils, S., Daoud-Elias, M., Gauthier, B., Sie, P., Boccalon, H., Boneu, B.** Influence of long term oral anticoagulants upon prothrombin fragment 1+2, thrombin-antithrombin III complex, and D-dimer levels in patients affected by proximal deep vein thrombosis. *Thromb. Haemostas.*, 69, 302, 1993.

50. **Speiser, W., Mallek, R., Koppensteiner, R., Stümpflen, A, Kapiotis, S., Minar, E., Ehringer, H., Lechner, K.** D-dimer and TAT measurement in patients with deep venous thrombosis: utility in diagnosis and judgement of anticoagulant treatment effectiveness. *Thromb. Haemostas.*, 63, 196, 1990.

ASSESSMENT OF FIBRINOLYSIS IN PATIENTS WITH THROMBOSIS - FROM LABORATORY TO CLINICAL PRACTICE

J. Gram and J. Jespersen
Centralsygehuset, Esbjerg.

I. INTRODUCTION

Since the beginning of the last decade there has been a rapidly growing interest in studying physiological and pathophysiological aspects of the human fibrinolytic system. As a result a number of new assays have become available. Due to the development of new technology, investigations of the fibrinolytic system have become simpler with the advantage that the non-specialized laboratories are now able to determine a number of fibrinolytic quantities. However, it is a general problem that the analytical reliability has not kept up with the technical advance,[1-4] and therefore the increasing number of reports which support an involvement of fibrinolysis in disease have had a limited impact on physicians' clinical work.[5] One of the main reasons this situation has come up is the lack of a general standardization system within the field of fibrinolysis. Although there is a substantial amount of evidence that a significant number of patients with thrombosis are characterized by defects of the fibrinolytic system, the laboratory results, which may deviate considerably from one laboratory to another, have not definitively been used in clinical decision making.

Despite these problems there is a long tradition in the clinical laboratory to measure quantities of the fibrinolytic system. Advance in method development has made it possible to go beyond the traditional clot lysis time measurements. It is our belief that measurements of key quantities in the fibrinolytic system may, in the study of patients with thrombosis, be a piece which can help the clinician to determine optimal care in individual patients.

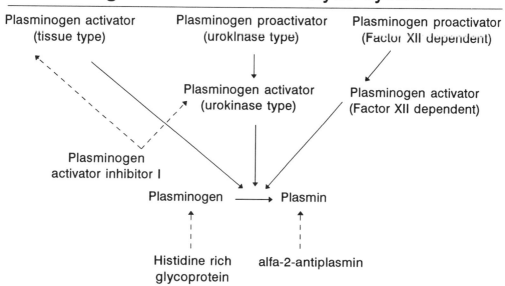

Figure 1. The main activators and inhibitors of the fibrinolytic system. The activation of plasminogen proactivator ; factor XII-dependent, requires acrtivation of factor XII and pro-kallikrein, while activation of plasminogen proactivator, urokinase type might be dependent on the formation of plasmin (for details see text).

0-8493-5804-3/96/$0.00+$.50

II. THE FIBRINOLYTIC SYSTEM AND THE HAEMOSTATIC BALANCE

Astrup proposed that the major role of the fibrinolytic system in the body is to influence the deposition of fibrin following tissue injury in order to regulate the formation of reparative connective tissue[8]. Extending this concept to the regulation of the repair of injuries occurring at the vessel wall it became clear that the proposed concept provided the biochemical and physiological background of the "thrombogenic theory" of arteriosclerosis of Duguid.[8] Later the concept of a dynamic haemostatic balance was introduced.[9]

The main regulatory process of the fibrinolytic system is the activation of plasminogen to plasmin, which may proceed along different pathways (Fig. 1). The activation of the fibrinolytic system in blood involves three different types of plasminogen activator and a variety of inhibitory components (Figs. 1, 2). Quantitation of each of these variables has become possible following progress in the development of new methods of assay.

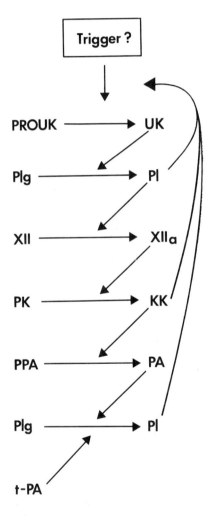

Figure 2. The possible interrelation between activation of the three different pathways of plasminogen activation. Pro-UK: plasminogen proactivator urokinase type; UK: plasminogen activator, urokinase type; PPA: plasminogen proactivator, factor XII-dependent; PA: plasminogen activator, factor XII-dependent; t-PA: plasminogen activator, tissue type; Plg: plasminogen; Pl: plasmin; XII and XIIa: factor $XII_{(\alpha)}$; PK: pro-kallikrein; KK: kallikrein.

Best known is the mechanism of activation of plasminogen by the tissue type plasminogen activator (t-PA) system and its clinical relevance, while the pathways of the plasminogen proactivator systems are only partially elucidated.[10]

t-PA is released into blood from the endothelial cells by mechanisms only partially known. Various stimuli and agents such as stress, exercise, catecholamines, nicotinic acid and vasopressin analogues increase the release of t-PA from the cells. Presence of t-PA in the blood does not immediately result in activation of the fibrinolytic system, because, in the absence of fibrin, t-PA has a very low affinity for plasminogen. However, when an intravascular clot is formed, t-PA and plasminogen bind sequentially to fibrin resulting in the rapid generation of plasmin. This means that physiological fibrinolysis requires fibrin not only as a substrate, - as implied by the terminology -, but also as a stimulatory cofactor (promoter) in plasminogen activation.

Binding of plasminogen to fibrin depends upon the lysine-binding sites of the plasminogen molecule. Histidine-rich glycoprotein is a plasma protein (Fig. 1) that binds to these sites, by decreasing the concentration of free available plasminogen, thereby possibly providing a regulatory mechanism of fibrinolysis.[11]

The solubilization *in vitro* of a fibrin clot is characterized by a sigmoidal pattern, i.e. a lag phase followed by a rapid increase, which slows down approaching completion. During this process the amount of plasminogen bound to fibrin increases, due to the generation of new binding sites in the initial phase of fibrin degradation.[12,13] In this manner the body assures that an optimal amount of plasmin is generated and becomes involved in the early degradation of fibrin. These observations are in accordance with the findings that t-PA present at the time of clotting (thrombus formation) is much more effective than when added to a preformed clot.[14]

Activation of plasminogen by the proactivator systems may be dependent on activated factor-XII, which participates in the initiation of activation together with prekallikrein. This constitutes the so-called contact activation system in which activated factor-XII and kallikrein (themselves only weak activators of plasminogen) initiate activation of an activator precursor to a true plasminogen activator.[15] The other pathway of the proactivator system can be inhibited by anti-urokinase antibodies and is now termed: plasminogen activator/urokinase type pathway. In its native form, it is present in blood as a single chain proenzyme (pro-urokinase - pro-UK). Activation of pro-UK yields a t-PA like activator, which is clot-selective in its action because of its capacity to bind to fibrin.[16] Plasmin is able to activate pro-UK, but it is as yet unknown where the triggering amount of plasmin comes from *in vivo*. Possibly it is generated by activation through t-PA-mediated plasminogen activation,[17,18] as suggested in Fig. 2. This proposed model indicates that the intrinsic system of fibrinolysis may be regarded as an amplification system of t-PA mediated plasminogen activation. The fibrinolytic activity in blood is regulated by inhibitors (Fig. 1) of which the most important are the plasminogen activator inhibitor-1 (PAI-1) and plasmin inhibitor (α_2AP).[10]

Table I : Clinical expression of deviations in coagulation and fibrinolysis

Clinical expression	Coagulation		Fibrinolysis
Thrombosis	↑	and/or	↓
Bleeding	↓	and/or	↑

III. ABNORMALITIES OF FIBRINOLYSIS - CLINICAL ASPECTS

In recent years, clinical experience has shown that the concept of a dynamic haemostatic balance, and the increased knowledge about mechanisms involved in its regulation, can be applied with reasonable success in the elucidation and treatment of cases of bleeding and thrombotic disorders (Table I), which otherwise would have been difficult to explain or to subject to rational treatment. Nature has performed its own experiments in the form of patients with congenital defects of inhibitors or factors of fibrinolysis, and has thereby substantiated the existence not only of a haemostatic balance but also of an antithrombotic potential in patients.

Deviations from normal on balance do not necessarily lead to acute situations of either haemorrhage or thrombosis, but they may cause various forms of subacute disorders resulting from an impaired haemostasis and tissue repair. There is now substantial scientific support for the idea that impaired fibrinolysis is related to the development of atherothrombotic and thromboembolic diseases.

IV. ASSESSMENT QUANTITIES OF THE FIBRINOLYTIC SYSTEM IN THE CLINICAL LABORATORY

For assessment of key quantities of the fibrinolytic system a number of commercial assays have been developed. The principles of these assays are based on those of conventional immunochemical or enzymatic methods. Over the years the robustness of the assays has improved, while precision and accuracy are less satisfactory.[2-5] It is the opinion of the authors that for the study of thrombosis-prone patients global assays such as euglobulin clot lysis time or whole blood clot lysis time produce no significant information for the physician. Instead, well-defined methods which measure single components should be introduced in the laboratory.

Due to the lack of internationally recommended standardization procedures for measurement of fibrinolytic quantities it is important that the laboratory takes action to secure production of results reproducible over a long period of time. It is essential that the laboratory establishes its own reference intervals, and adheres to reliable internal and if possible external (e.g. WHO quality assessment scheme and the ECAT Foundation assessment scheme within the EU) quality control programmes. Finally, the pre-analytical factors should be controlled as thoroughly as possible.

A. PRE-ANALYTICAL FACTORS

For quantities in the fibrinolytic system it is important to minimize the effect of factors which are not directly related to the patient's disease state, because such factors might cause a misclassification of the patients on the basis of laboratory measurements. Thus, it should be considered that some components of the fibrinolytic system are fluctuating during the day,[19-21] may be affected by alcohol intake,[22,23] diet,[24] smoking,[25] exercise and drugs,[26] Also, it is important to note that the concentrations of several fibrinolytic variables are dependent on age.[27] In order to minimize the effect of pre-analytical factors blood samples for measurement of fibrinolytic quantities should, under basal conditions, be obtained from subjects in the morning (8.00-10.00), from subjects after 20 min. rest in the supine position, and that the subjects under study have fasted overnight and refrained from smoking, intake of alcohol, or caffeine-containing beverages.[28] The technique of blood collection, the use of anticoagulants in blood tubes, the kind of tubes, the handling and storage of plasma should adhere strictly to recommended procedures.[28]

B. QUANTITIES TO BE ANALYSED

It is presently impossible to recommend exactly which methods should be used for analysis of the different quantities due to the lack of a general standardization system within the field of fibrinolysis. For clinical studies of the thrombosis-prone patient it is important to adhere to robust methods, which are stable over a long period of time. If commercially available methods are used, preference should be given to manufacturers, who can demonstrate that their methods are precise, accurate and specific and that these properties are essentially unchanged by shift from one batch to another.

Under *basal conditions* the clinical laboratory, which performs investigations of fibrinolysis in the thrombosis-prone patient, should as a minimum make available the following quantities:

- Plasma-plasminogen activator, tissue type (t-PA) measured both by an enzymatic and an immunological procedure

- Plasminogen activator inhibitor 1 (PAI-1) measured both by an enzymatic and an immunologic procedure

- Plasma-plasminogen measured both by an enzymatic and an immunologic procedure

- Plasma-plasmin inhibitor (α_2-AP) measured by an enzymatic procedure

- Plasma-histidine-rich glycoprotein (HRG) measured by an immunologic procedure

- Plasma-fibrin D-dimer measured by an immunologic procedure

Various possible procedures, methodologies and recommended field methods for the above-mentioned quantities have been reviewed elsewhere.[29]

Different procedures such as venous occlusion, exercise, and infusion of 1-Desamino-8-D-Arginin Vasopressin (DDAVP) have been used to study the fibrinolytic system *after stimulation*. The venous occlusion test has been most commonly used. In spite of the reproducibility problems with this procedure it should be preferred in the clinical laboratory, because it is so far the only stimulation test which gives significant clinical information, i.e. it has the capacity to separate patients into "responders" and "non-responders". The preferred conditions under which the venous occlusion should be applied have been described elsewhere.[30]

C. INTERPRETATION OF THE LABORATORY RESULTS

Most of the results from assays of fibrinolytic quantities are produced on an interval scale basis. In spite of precise reporting it may be difficult to interpret the data due to the fact that exact clinical decision limits have hardly been described for any fibrinolytic quantity. Thus, the interpretation of the data of the thrombosis-prone patient is restricted to evaluating whether the patient has excessively abnormal, slightly abnormal, or normal results.

Although *hereditary single factor abnormalities* in the fibrinolytic system are rare, it should be noted that familial thrombosis has been associated with type 1 and type 2 plasminogen deficiency,[31] high plasma levels of HRG,[32,33] and high plasma levels of PAI-1.[34] Also, familial thrombosis has been associated with a defective release of t-PA following the venous occlusion test.[35,36]

In patients with so-called *idiopathic venous thrombosis* it is the experience that abnormalities in the fibrinolytic system to a large extent reflect life style factors. It has been reported that PAI-1 correlates with both body mass index and the serum concentration of triglycerides.[37] Similarly, it should be noticed that a lack of increase in t-PA measured by an enzymatic method after venous occlusion, probably increases the risk of recurrent venous thrombosis in patients with a previous instance of venous thrombosis.[38,39] A lack of an increase in activity of plasminogen activator (non-responder patients) after venous occlusion is caused by either defective release of t-PA or by high basal levels of PAI-1.[40,41]

Single factor abnormalities are unusual in patients with *atherothrombotic diseases*. These patients are typically characterized by combined abnormalities indicating an association with an underlying disease process. Still, such abnormalities may contribute significantly to evolution of atherothrombotic disease, and the measurement of fibrinolytic quantities helps to stratify patients with a previous myocardial infarction to a high or a low risk of thrombosis.[6,42] Patients with atherothrombotic disease and a high risk of myocardial reinfarction are typically characterized by a fibrinolytic profile consisting of high plasma concentrations of t-PA (immunologic procedure), high plasma concentrations of PAI-1 (both immunologic procedure and enzymatic procedure), low plasma concentration of active t-PA (enzymatic procedure), and high plasma concentration of fibrin-D-dimer (immunologic procedure).[43-50]

Assays for assessment of fibrinolytic quantities are in general suitable for risk stratification of patients with thromboembolic and atherothrombotic diseases, but of little use in the diagnosis or exclusion of diagnosis. One exception is assessment of plasma-fibrin D-dimer which in addition to risk stratification might be used to exclude a diagnosis of pulmonary embolism.[51]

V. CONCLUDING REMARKS

A significant number of patients with thrombotic disease are characterized by abnormalities of the fibrinolytic system. Few thrombotic cases can be explained by single factor abnormalities. However, determination of the described fibrinolytic profile may help the physician to stratify such patients to high or low risk groups for rethrombosis, particularly when the fibrinolytic abnormalities are combined with the information from other clinical and paraclinical data.

At present, there is an urgent need for standardization of fibrinolytic assays and a need for research to identify clinical relevant decision limits.

The clinical laboratory dealing with assessment of fibrinolytic quantities should take precautions to control preanalytic, analytic, and post-analytic factors. Here, it is important that laboratory specialists assist the physicians in the interpretation of data.

REFERENCES

1.   **Büttner, J.**, Reference methods as a basis for accurate measuring system, *Eur. J. Clin. Chem. Clin. Biochem.*, 29, 223, 1991.
2.   **Chandler, W. L., Loo, S.-W., Nguyan, S. V., Schmer, G., Stratton, J. R.,** Standardization of measuring plasminogen activator inhibitor activity in human plasma, *Clin. Chem.*, 35, 787, 1989.
3.   **Gram, J., Declerck, P. J., Sidelmann, J., Jespersen, J., Kluft, C.,** Multicentre evaluation of commercial kit methods: plasminogen activator inhibitor activity, *Thromb. Haemost.*, 70, 852, 1993.
4.   **Declerck, P. J., Moreau, H., Jespersen, J., Gram, J., Kluft, C.,** Multicenter evaluation of commercially available methods for the immunological determination of plasminogen activator inhibitor-1 (PAI-1), *Thromb. Haemost.*, 70, 858, 1993.
5.   **Jespersen, J.,** Gaps between the present assay practice in haemostasis and clinical chemistry laboratories, *Fibrinolysis*, 4/Suppl 2, 118, 1990.
6.   **Prins, M. H., Hirsh, J.,** A critical review of the relationship between impaired fibrinolysis and myocardial infarction, *Am. Heart. J.*, 122, 545, 1991.
7.   **Malm, J., Laurell, M., Nilsson, I. M., Dahlbäck, B.,** Thromboembolic disease - critical evaluation of laboratory investigation, *Thromb. Haemost.*, 68, 7, 1992.
8.   **Astrup, T.,** The biological significance of fibrinolysis, *Lancet*, II, 565, 1956.
9.   **Astrup, T.,** The haemostatic balance, *Thromb. Diath. Haemorrh.*, 2, 347, 1958.
10.   **Jespersen, J.,** Pathophysiology and clinical aspects of fibrinolysis and inhibition of coagulation. Experimental and clinical studies with special reference to women on oral contraceptives and selected groups of thrombosis prone patients, *Dan. Med. Bull.*, 35, 1, 1988.
11.   **Lijnen, H. R., Hoylaerts, M., Collen, D.,** Isolation and characterization of a human plasma protein with affinity for the lysine binding sites in plasminogen. Role of the regulation of fibrinolysis and identification as histidine-rich glycoprotein, *J. Biol. Chem.*, 255, 10214, 1980.
12.   **Suenson, E., Lützen, O., Thorsen, S.,** Initial plasmin-degradation of fibrin as the basis of a positive feed-back mechanism in fibrinolysis, *Eur. J. Biochem.*, 140, 513, 1984.
13.   **Tran-Thang, C., Kruithof, E. K. O., Bachmann, F.,** Tissue-type plasminogen activator increases the binding of glu-plasminogen to clots, *J. Clin. Invest.*, 74, 2009, 1984.
14.   **Brommer, E. J. P.,** The level of extrinsic plasminogen activator (t-PA) during clotting as a determinant of the rate of fibrinolysis; inefficiency of activators added afterwards, *Thromb. Res.* 34, 109, 1984.
15.   **Dooijewaard, G., de Jong, Y. F., Jie, A. F. H., Kluft, C.,** The role of kallikrein in the generation of the factor XII-dependent plasminogen activator activity in human plasma, *Thromb. Haemost.*, 54, 268, 1985.
16.   **Binnema, D. J., Dooijewaard, G., van Iersel, J. J. L., Kluft, C.,** Fibrin binding capacity of pro-urokinase (Pro-UK) and urokinase (UK) from plasma, *Fibrinolysis*, Suppl 1, 21, 1986.
17.   **Kluft, C., Jie, A. F. H.,** Interaction between the extrinsic and intrinsic systems of fibrinolysis, in *Progress in Chemical Fibrinolysis and Thrombolysis*, Davidson, J. F., Cepelak, V., Samama, M. M., Desnoyers, P.C., Eds., Churchill Livingstone, New York, 1979, 25.

18. **Jespersen, J.,** The diurnal increase in euglobulin fibrinolytic activity in women using oral contraceptives and in normal women and the generation of intrinsic fibrinolytic activity, *Thromb. Haemost.*, 56, 183, 1986.

19. **Kluft, C., Jie, A. F. H., Rijken D. C., Verheijen J. H.,** Daytime fluctuations in blood of tissue type plasminogen activator (t-PA) and its fast acting inhibitor PAI-1, *Thromb. Haemost.*, 59, 329, 1988.

20. **Grimaudo, V., Hauert, J., Bachmann, F., Kruithof E. K. O.,** Diurnal variation of the fibrinolytic system, *Thromb. Haemost.*, 59, 495, 1988.

21. **Johansen, L. G., Gram, J., Kluft, C., Jespersen, J.,** Chronobiology of coronary risk markers in Greenland Eskimos: a comparative study with Caucasians residing in the same Arctic area, *Chronobiol. Int.*, 8, 352, 1991.

22. **Veenstra, J., Kluft, C., Ockhuizen, T., van der Pol, H., Wedel, M., Schaafsmaa, G.,** Effects of moderate alcohol consumption on platelet function, tissue type plasminogen activator and plasminogen activator inhibitor, *Thromb. Haemost.*, 63, 345, 1990.

23. **Hendriks, H.F.J., Veenstra, J., Wierik, E.J.M.V., Schaafsma, G., Kluft, C.,** Effect of moderate dose of alcohol with evening meal on fibrinolytic factors, *Br. Med. J.*, 308, 1003, 1994.

24. **Marckmann, P., Jespersen, J., Leth, T., Sandström, B.,** Effect of fish diet versus meat diet on blood lipids, coagulation and fibrinolysis, *J. Intern. Med*, 229, 317, 1991.

25. **Allen, R. A., Kluft, C., Brommer, E. J. P.,** The acute effect of smoking on fibrinolysis: increase in the activity level of circulating extrinsic (tissue-type) plasminogen activator, *Eur. J. Clin. Invest.*, 14, 354, 1984.

26. **Prowse, C. V., Cash, J.D.,** Physiologic and pharmacologic enhancement of fibrinolysis, *Semin. Thromb. Hemost.*, 10, 51, 1984.

27. **Jespersen, J., Walker, I.D., Haverkate, F., Lowe, G. D. O.,** Ageing and fibrinolysis - panel discussion, *Fibrinolysis*, 6/Suppl 3, 23, 1992.

28. **Kluft, C., Verheijen, J.,** Leiden fibrinolysis working party: blood collection and handling procedures for assessment of tissue-type plasminogen activator (t-PA) and plasminogen activator inhibitor-1 (PAI-1), *Fibrinolysis*, 4/Suppl 2, 155, 1990.

29. **Jespersen, J., Bertina, R. M., Haverkate, F.,** Eds, *ECAT Assay Procedures. A Manual of Laboratory Techniques. European Concerted Action on Thrombosis and Disabilities of the Commission of the European Communities.* Kluwer Academic Publishers, London, 1992, 1.

30. **Jespersen, J.,** The venous occlusion test in fibrinolysis assays, in *ECAT Assay Procedures. A Manual of Laboratory Techniques. European Concerted Action on Thrombosis and Disabilities of the Commission of the European Communities*, Jespersen, J., Bertina, R.M., Haverkate, F., Eds., Kluwer Academic Publishers, London, 1992, 213.

31. **Dolan, G., Preston, F. E.,** Familial plasminogen deficiency and thromboembolism, *Fibrinolysis*, 2/Suppl 2, 26, 1998.

32. **Engesser, L., Kluft, C., Briët, E., Brommer, E. J. P.** Familial elevation of plasma histidine-rich glycoprotein in a family with thrombophilia, *Br. J. Hematol.*, 67, 355, 1987.

33. **Falkon, L., Gari, M., Montserrat, I., Borrell, M., Fontcuberta, J.,** Familial elevation of plasma histidine-rich glycoprotein. A case associated with recurrent venous thrombosis and high PAI-1 levels, *Thromb. Res.*, 66, 265, 1992.

34. **Jørgensen, M., Bonnevie-Nielsen, V.,** Increased concentration of the fast-acting plasminogen activator inhibitor in plasma, *Br. J. Haematol.*, 65, 175, 1987.

35. **Petäjä, J., Rasi, V., Myllylä, G., Vahtera, E., Hallman, H.,** Familial hypofibrinolysis and venous thrombosis, *Br. J. Haematol.*, 71, 393, 1989.

36. **Petäjä, J., Rasi, V., Vahtera, E., Myllylä, G.,** Familial clustering of defective release of t-PA. *Br. J. Haematol.*, 79, 291, 1991.

37. **Juhan-Vague, I., Thompson, S. G., Jespersen, J.,** Involvement of the hemostatic system in insulin resistance syndrome. A study of 1500 patients with angina pectoris, *Arterioscler. Thromb.*, 13, 1865, 1993.

38. **Korninger, C., Lechner, K., Niessner, H., Gössinger, H., Kundi, M.,** Impaired fibrinolytic capacity predisposes for recurrence of venous thrombosis, *Thromb. Haemost.* 52, 127, 1984.

39. **Juhan-Vague, I., Alessi, M. C., Fossat, C., Valadier, J., Aillaud, M. F., Serradimigni, A.,** Clinical relevance of high PAI-1 level in patients with idiopathic/recurrent deep venous thrombosis, *Fibrinolysis*, 2/Suppl 2, 85, 1988.

40. **Nilsson, I. M., Ljungner, H., Tengborn, L.,** Two different mechanisms in patients with venous thrombosis and defective fibrinolysis: low concentration of plasminogen activator or increased concentration of plasminogen activator inhibitor, *Br. Med. J.*, 290, 1453, 1985.

41. **Grimaudo, V., Bachmann, F., Hauert, J., Christe, M.-A., Kruithof, E. K. O.,** Hypofibrinolysis in patients with a history of idiopathic deep vein thrombosis, *Thromb. Haemost.*, 67, 397, 1992.

42. **Gram, J.,** The haemostatic balance in groups of thrombosis-prone patients. With particular reference to fibrinolysis in patients with myocardial infarction, *Dan. Med. Bull.* 37, 219. 1990.

43. **Gram, J., Jespersen, J., Kluft, C., Rijken, D.,** On the usefulness of fibrinolysis variables in the characterization of a risk group for myocardial infarction, *Acta Med. Scand.*, 221, 149, 1987.

44. **Ridker, P. M., Vaughan, D. E., Stampfer, M. J., Manson, J. E., Hennekens, C. H.,** Endogenous tissue-type plasminogen activator and risk of myocardial infarction, *Lancet*, 1, 1165, 1993.

45. **Hamsten, A., Wiman, B., de Faire, U., Blombäck, M.,** Increased plasma levels of a rapid inhibitor of tissue plasminogen activator in young survivors of myocardial infarction, *N. Engl. J. Med.*, 313, 1557, 1985.

46. **Jespersen, J., Munkvad, S., Gram, J.,** The fibrinolysis and coagulation systems in ischaemic heart disease. - Risk markers and their relation to metabolic dysfunction of the arterial intima, *Dan. Med. Bull.*, 40, 495, 1993.

47. **Lassila, R., Peltonen, S., Lepäntola, M., Saarinen, O., Kauhanen, P., Manninen, V.,** Severity of peripheral atherosclerosis is associated with fibrinogen and degradation of cross-linked fibrin, *Arterioscler. Thromb.*, 13, 1738, 1993.

48. **Gram, J., Jespersen, J.,** A selective depression of tissue plasminogen activator (t-PA) activity in euglobulins characterises a risk group among survivors of acute myocardial infarction, *Thromb. Haemost.*, 57, 137, 1987.

49. **Jespersen, J., Gram, J.,** Fibrinolysis and recurrence of myocardial infarction, *Lancet*, 2, 461, 1987.

50. **Cortellaro, M., Cofrancesco, E., Boschetti, C., et al.,** Increased fibrin turnover and high PAI-1 activity as predictors of ischaemic heart events in atherosclerotic patients, *Arterioscler. Thromb.* 13, 1412, 1993.

51. **Goldhaber, S. Z., Simons, G. R., Elliot, C. G., et al.,** Quantitative plasma D-dimer levels among patients undergoing pulmonary angiography for suspected pulmonary embolism, *JAMA*, 270, 2819, 1993.

DECREASED FIBRINOLYTIC ACTIVITY IN THROMBOTIC DISEASE : AN UPDATE

B. Wiman and A. Hamsten
Karolinska Institute, Stockholm

I. INTRODUCTION

The pathogenic processes involved in thrombotic disease are complicated and may involve multiple disturbances of vessel wall function and blood flow, or alterations of blood composition, leading to changes of viscosity or to an impaired hemostatic balance. The fundamental ideas originally proposed by Virchov still remain relevant.[1] The knowledge of different biochemical risk factors in plasma for the development of thrombotic disease is steadily expanding. The recently described mutation of coagulation factor V, rendering this molecule resistant to activated protein C, has for instance proven to be a common cause of deep vein thrombosis (DVT).[2]

The connection between impaired fibrinolytic function and thrombotic disease has been intensely studied during the past several years, because of the discovery of plasminogen activator inhibitor-1 (PAI-1) in plasma[3,4] and the development of specific assay procedures for PAI-1 and tissue-type plasminogen activator (tPA). Indeed, a decreased fibrinolytic activity is a common finding in patients, both with venous thrombosis and coronary heart disease (CHD).[5-7] However, since prospective epidemiological studies of healthy populations, longitudinal cohort studies of patients with manifest thrombotic disease and genetic studies, which include evaluation of the fibrinolytic system are sparse, it remains to be established whether impaired fibrinolytic function is an etiological factor and a risk factor in the conventional epidemiological context.

In this article we are summarizing some of the recent data on decreased fibrinolytic activity in thrombotic disease. In addition, some aspects of the regulation of the fibrinolytic enzyme system are discussed.

II. MECHANISMS INVOLVED IN REGULATING FIBRINOLYSIS

Both tPA and PAI-1 have important roles in the regulation of fibrinolysis ; tPA is released from endothelial cells lining vessel walls and is quite rapidly cleared from the circulation by uptake in the liver. In conditions where the plasma PAI-1 concentration is increased, the half-life of functional tPA is substantially shortened, causing a decreased fibrinolytic potential. An impaired capacity of the vessel wall to produce, store or release tPA also results in a poor fibrinolytic function.

Plasma levels of both tPA and PAI-1 exhibit circadian variation for unknown reasons ; tPA activity is lowest in the early morning and highest in the afternoon. In contrast, plasma PAI-1 activity peaks in the early morning and then declines to minimum values by the early afternoon.[8-10] The variation in plasma PAI-1 concentration seems to be more pronounced than the corresponding variation in tPA antigen level and is most likely responsible for the decreased fibrinolytic activity found in the early morning. Several studies have demonstrated a correlation between basal plasma levels of tPA antigen and PAI-1. The mechanism for this is unknown, but it seems logical to assume that the increase in tPA antigen concentration is a result of the increase in PAI-1 concentration and not the other way round.

A . STUDIES IN CULTURED CELLS

The mechanisms regulating PAI-1 secretion from various cells into plasma are at present not well understood. It has been shown that endothelial cells are able to increase the PAI-1 production on stimulation with lipopolysaccharide or certain cytokines.[11, 12] Furthermore, it has been demonstrated

0-8493-5804-3/96/$0.00+$.50

that insulin induces a dose-dependent increase of PAI-1 secretion from hepatocytes in culture, whereas no effect of insulin in this respect was obtained on human umbilical vein endothelial cells.[13] Proinsulin may also impair endogenous fibrinolysis by stimulating the secretion of PAI-1 from endothelial cells through an insulin- and insulin-like growth factor-1 (IGF-1) independent pathway.[14] In contrast to insulin, proinsulin increases PAI-1 messenger RNA (mRNA) expression and PAI-1 synthesis concordantly in porcine aortic endothelial cells.[15] Time- and concentration-dependent effects of split products of proinsulin (des31,32 proinsulin and des64,65 proinsulin) on PAI-1 synthesis in HepG2 cells have also been documented, stimulation being at least in part transduced by the insulin receptor and mediated at the level of PAI-1 gene expression.[16] Furthermore, Anfosso et al[17] have demonstrated increased PAI-1 synthesis on insulin stimulation in HepG2 cells after induction of an insulin-resistant state.

Apolipoprotein B-containing lipoprotein particles, especially triglyceride-rich very low density lipoprotein (VLDL) particles and minimally oxidized low density lipoprotein (LDL) particles seem to stimulate the production of PAI-1 in cultured human endothelial cells.[18, 19] VLDL also induces a dose-dependent increase in PAI-1 secretion from hepatocytes.[20] The effect on PAI-1 secretion by VLDL in endothelial cells and hepatocytes in culture appears to be dependent on an interaction with the specific LDL-receptor.[18, 20] In contrast, this is apparently not the case with the effect of LDL particles.[21]

B. ASSOCIATION OF PLASMA PAI-1 WITH CHD RISK FACTORS

Epidemiological data have shown that the plasma concentration of PAI-1 correlates with a number of different metabolic and clinical parameters, such as serum triglyceride concentration, plasma insulin concentration, body mass index and waist-to-hip circumference ratio (for recent reviews see refs 6 and 22). Patients with inflammatory conditions typically also have increased PAI-1 concentration. In addition, hormonal influences need to be considered. Testosterone level has been found to correlate inversely with insulin, high density lipoprotein (HDL) cholesterol and PAI-1 concentrations in men with and without CHD.[23-25]

The nutritional status seems to be connected with the fibrinolytic capacity, primarily because of its effect on plasma PAI-1 levels, which, in turn, might be mediated by lipoproteins or insulin. A negative association exists between the intake of vegetables, fruits, and root vegetables and plasma PAI-1 activity. For the influence of alcohol intake on fibrinolytic function, experimental and epidemiological studies have provided discrepant results.[22] The experimental studies have fairly consistently shown a decrease in blood fibrinolytic activity with alcohol, both immediately and in the longer term, whereas the epidemiological studies have generally shown a positive association between alcohol consumption and fibrinolytic capacity. The short- and long-term effects of cigarette smoking are indicated to be contrary. The immediate effect is an increase in the plasma tPA level. Conversely, endothelial cells seem to produce less tPA activity in habitual smokers.

The positive and fairly strong relation between serum triglycerides and PAI-1 levels in plasma[26-28] is of particular interest, since it raises the possibility that hypertriglyceridemia is connected with a predisposition to thrombosis through a coexisting increase in PAI-1 concentration. Accordingly, diet intervention resulting in reduction of serum triglycerides and weight loss and the lowering of triglycerides by administration of gemfibrozil have been shown to be accompanied by improvement, and even normalization, of fibrinolytic capacity.[29, 30] Mehrabian et al[31] studied the short-term effects of a high complex carbohydrate, low-fat diet in healthy middle-aged individuals. Plasma levels of plasminogen, tPA, and PAI-1 decreased substantially during a 3-week program. Plasma PAI-1 activity correlated strongly with triglyceride concentration, both before and after the intervention. Subjects with high initial PAI-1 values were strikingly responsive, whereas little or no change was noted in those with baseline values within the normal range. However, in all studies of dietary intervention, the lowering of serum triglycerides was associated with weight loss which, in turn, has been connected with reduction of plasma PAI-1 activity and tPA antigen under circumstances in which there was no decrease in triglycerides. Nevertheless, whatever the mechanism might be, dietary intervention can improve fibrinolytic function.

C. ROLE OF INSULIN IN REGULATION OF PLASMA PAI-1 CONCENTRATION

It has been suggested that plasma insulin is the major physiological regulator of PAI-1 activity in plasma and secondary to that of fibrinolytic activity.[32] The mechanism can either be direct or indirect through influences of insulin on plasma triglyceride concentration. In the study of 1484 patients with angina pectoris by the European Concerted Action on Thrombosis and Disabilities (ECAT), a strong correlation was found between plasma insulin and PAI-1 levels.[33] Reducing insulin levels and insulin resistance by exercise, weight loss and medication with metformin also reduces the plasma PAI-1 activity.[32, 34] Indeed, this suggests that plasma PAI-1 elevation should be included as a component of the insulin resistance syndrome, along with hyperinsulinemia, hypertriglyceridemia, hypertension and obesity. However, the relation of hyperinsulinemia to plasma PAI-1 activity elevation appears to be quite complex at the level of our current knowledge. A significant inverse correlation has been noted between insulin sensitivity, measured with the euglycemic clamp technique, and plasma PAI-1 activity. In fact, hyperinsulinemic euglycemic glucose clamp studies in humans suggest that insulin resistance per se, independently of plasma insulin levels, may be associated with elevated plasma PAI-1 activity.[35] Exogenous hyperinsulinemia does not result in significant increases of PAI-1 or in disruption of the circadian variation in PAI-1 activity, in spite of an adequate degree of portal hyperinsulinemia. However, an insulin-mediated regulation of plasma PAI-1 activity might require a longer period to induce an increase in protein synthesis through induction of mRNA.

Specificity problems influencing the insulin measurements by different radioimmunoassays due to cross-reactivity with proinsulin and split proinsulin in the assay procedures might be another confounder in the evaluation of the coupling between insulin and PAI-1 levels.[36]

In conclusion, insulin might be an intermediate risk factor for CHD, exerting many of its effects through modification of other risk factors, including triglyceride-rich lipoproteins and plasma PAI-1 activity. Whether the observed associations of hyperinsulinemia with lipoprotein alterations, impaired fibrinolytic function, and hypertension are related to the amount of circulating insulin or proinsulinlike molecules, to insulin resistance, or to some as yet unknown factor, is uncertain at this stage.

D. PAI-1 POLYMORPHISMS

Variation in the PAI-1 gene, which has been cloned and localized to chromosome 7, seems to be an important factor in determining the levels of PAI-I in plasma. Genotyping of young postinfarction patients and population-based controls for two polymorphisms at the PAI-1 locus revealed an association of plasma PAI-1 activity with both polymorphisms.[37] With the HindIII polymorphism, the 1/1 genotype exhibited higher PAI-1 levels than the 2/2 genotype, within both the patient and control groups. The smaller alleles of an eight-allele dinucleotide repeat polymorphism were also linked to higher plasma PAI-I activity in the patient group. Furthermore, the associations of VLDL and insulin with PAI-1 activity seemed to be genotype-specific. Subjects of the HindIII genotype 1/1 showed a two to three-fold greater increase in plasma PAI-1 with an increase in VLDL triglycerides as compared to individuals with genotype 2/2. Insulin, as reflected by the insulin area under the curve during an oral glucose tolerance test, appeared to influence the PAI-I levels only in 2/2 individuals.

A common single base pair 4/5 guanosine (4G/5G) polymorphism (GACACGTGGGG(G)AGT) in the PAI-I promoter has recently been identified and found to be associated with plasma PAI-1 activity.[38] Individuals who are homozygous for the 4G-allele have higher PAI-1 activity than individuals who are heterozygous or homozygous for the 5G-allele. The 5G-allele contains an additional binding site for a DNA-binding protein found in HepG2 and Hep3B cells. Since the 5G-allele is associated with lower plasma PAI-1 activity levels, it is reasonable to assume that the one base pair insertion in the PAI-1 promoter creates a binding site for a nuclear protein involved in repressing transcription and expression of PAI-1. A further (CA)n dinucleotide repeat polymorphism has also recently been reported in the PAI-1 promoter region.[39] Only two common alleles are present, the less frequent one (allele frequency of 0.01) having an additional CA dinucleotide repeat. The functional significance of this promoter polymorphism in terms of influence on the PAI-1 gene expression is still unknown.

As discussed later in this review, it has been demonstrated that patients suffering myocardial infarction at a young age[36] as well as patients undergoing coronary bypass surgery (unpublished data by Nordenhem, Moor, Blombäck, Rydén, Hamsten and Wiman) are more frequently homozygous for the 4G-allele of the PAI-1 promoter polymorphism than healthy controls. Indeed, this strongly indicates that PAI-1 is an etiologic factor in CHD.

E. INFLUENCE OF LIPOPROTEIN(a) ON FIBRINOLYSIS

Lipoprotein (a), an LDL-like lipoprotein consisting of a unique glyco-protein called apolipoprotein (a) bound to apolipoprotein B, has recently attracted great enthusiasm as a possible link between lipoprotein metabolism and fibrinolytic function. Interest was stimulated by the demonstration of a striking homology between the amino acid sequence of apolipoprotein (a) and the structure of plasminogen.[40] This structural similarity suggested that lipoprotein (a) might mediate a prothrombotic effect by virtue of interfering with some of the physiological functions of plasminogen and prompted in vitro investigations by several groups. Lipoprotein (a) was found to competitively inhibit the binding of plasminogen to fibrin monomer[41,42] and to the plasminogen receptor on endothelial cells, actions that might reduce local fibrinolysis both on blood clots and on cell surfaces[43-45]. Furthermore, lipoprotein (a) has been shown to interfere with the streptokinase-mediated activation of human plasminogen[46] and the tPA-induced lysis of fibrin clots.[41] These experiments have all been performed in a milieu which is quite different from blood. We therefore studied the effect of lipoprotein (a) on activation of plasminogen in unfractionated plasma, by adding tPA and soluble fibrin to plasma and following the appearance of plasmin /α_2-antiplasmin complex (unpublished data by Nordenhem and Wiman). No effect of lipoprotein (a) could be demonstrated on plasminogen activation in this system. Therefore, a clinically important role of lipoprotein (a) for plasminogen activation in vivo seems less likely. An effect on the binding of plasminogen to cellular structures cannot be assessed from these experiments.

III. ASSESSMENT OF IMPAIRED FIBRINOLYTIC FUNCTION IN CONNECTION WITH THROMBOTIC DISEASE

The components of the fibrinolytic system of value to measure when assessing the fibrinolytic function in connection with thrombotic disease are: plasminogen, tPA, PAI-1 and the fibrin fragment D-dimer. Other components of the system, such as α_2-antiplasmin, or components associated with the system, eg histidine-rich glycoprotein or vitronectin, have no place in the routine assessment of fibrinolytic function in connection with thrombotic disease (for a review see ref. no. 6).

Determination of plasminogen should aim at identifying the small number of individuals with dys- or hypoplasminogenemia (also heterozygotes). If the plasminogen concentration is low with a functional method, it should then be checked with an immunochemical method to exclude the presence of dysplasminogenemia.

Measurement of tPA with functional methods requires immediate precautions at the time of blood sampling to prevent inactivation of tPA, eg acidification, or preferably drawing blood into tubes containing, for example, citric acid. Typically, samples are taken both at rest and after some sort of provocation, such as venous stasis or physical exercise. Most often, venous occlusion is used. This is obtained by application of a tourniquet to the upper arm, which is inflated to a blood pressure midway between systolic and diastolic blood pressures for a specified time, normally between 5 to 20 minutes. Venous occlusion for 10 minutes is most frequently used, but it has been claimed that 20 minutes is more accurate, or even that both 10- and 20-minute samples should be taken and evaluated together. If immunochemical methods to assay tPA are used it must be remembered that there is no correlation between tPA activity and antigen in basal plasma samples. At rest, only a few percent of the circulating tPA antigen is functionally active. The remainder is in complex with inhibitors, of which PAI-1 is the predominant. Accordingly, there is generally a fairly strong correlation between basal tPA antigen and PAI-1 levels.[6]

Measurement of PAI-1 activity requires rapid sample handling and quick freezing of the samples, since PAI-1 is a labile molecule. Thawed and refrozen citrated plasma samples must not be used for determination of PAI-1 activity. If PAI-1 antigen is to be measured, precautions must be taken to avoid release of PAI-1 from the platelets (platelet PAI-1 is mostly inactive). Serum samples cannot be used for any of these assays. For fibrin D-dimer analysis, precautions also have to be taken to avoid in vitro effects regarding activation of plasminogen, which may result in falsely increased values (unpublished results by Wiman and Haegerstrand-Björkman).

Generally, the time for blood sampling must be standardized because of the diurnal fluctuation in fibrinolytic activity (both tPA and PAI-1) as previously discussed. Overnight fasting is preferred in the case of morning blood sampling, but a light breakfast without fat and tea or coffee can be permitted. It is to be noted that caffeine-containing beverages should not be allowed during the preceding couple of hours because fibrinolytic activity may be enhanced. Smoking may induce an acute increase in tPA, and subjects should not smoke for at least 1 hour before venipuncture. Evening drinks also may affect next morning plasma PAI-1 activity. Procedures for blood collection and handling have been reviewed by the Leiden Fibrinolysis Working Party[47].

IV. IDIOPATHIC DVT AND IMPAIRED FIBRINOLYTIC FUNCTION

Impaired fibrinolytic function is a very frequently observed biochemical or hemostatic disturbance among patients with idiopathic DVT. Using non-specific assays it was demonstrated long ago that a large proportion of patients with recurrent and phlebographically verified DVT had a decreased fibrinolytic potential measured either as poor fibrinolytic activity in circulating blood after venous occlusion or in vein walls measured histochemically.[48] After the discovery of PAI-1 in plasma and the development of new specific and sensitive assays for tPA and PAI-1 in plasma samples, a large number of studies of fibrinolytic function in DVT have been published. These studies have consistently shown that 30 to 40% of the patients have an impaired fibrinolytic function, mainly due to increased plasma levels of PAI-1, but quite frequently in combination with a decreased capacity to release tPA on venous occlusion.[6] Occasionally, impaired release or production of tPA is the only disturbance detected.

Unfortunately, no prospective studies have been performed on idiopathic DVT using specific assays for the fibrinolytic components. However, using the euglobulin clot lysis time assay, it has been found that a decreased "global" fibrinolytic activity predisposes to recurrent DVT.[49] The Physicians Health Study approached this problem,[50] but since measurement of PAI-1 was not planned from the beginning, suitable plasma samples were lacking. Thus, the PAI-1 antigen levels found were much higher than expected, suggesting release of PAI-1 from platelets during preparation of the samples. Therefore, it is inappropriate to draw any firm conclusions from this study regarding fibrinolytic factors and DVT.

From the clinical data available today, we cannot conclude with certainty that a poor fibrinolytic function is an etiological mechanism in DVT. However, one piece of evidence pointing in this direction is the fact that transgenic mice with an extra human PAI-1 gene and increased plasma PAI-1 concentrations, both in the circulation and in tissues, suffer venous thrombosis shortly after birth.[51] Also, the recent studies of mice with non-functional tPA or uPA genes point in the same direction. With the double knockouts, the animal suffered from generalized deposition of fibrin.[52] The tPA gene knockouts did not get any measurable thrombotic problems, but regulation of fibrinolysis might be different in mice as compared to humans, uPA being relatively more important in the mice.

V. IMPAIRED FIBRINOLYSIS IN POSTOPERATIVE DVT

Venous thromboembolism remains a significant problem in patients who undergo major surgical procedures, and fibrinolytic function has been extensively studied in a variety of surgical settings. In particular, these studies have documented a transient postoperative "fibrinolytic shutdown" caused by a temporary increase in plasma PAI-1 activity as part of an acute phase reaction.[6] The value of measuring preoperative plasma PAI-1 or tPA levels for assessing the risk of postoperative DVT is still unclear. In two studies of patients subjected to total hip replacement, preoperative PAI-1 levels in plasma correlated significantly with the risk of developing postoperative DVT.[53,54] Furthermore, the magnitude of the increase in plasma PAI-1 concentration observed on the first postoperative day predicted a later DVT. Studies of fibrinolytic function in connection with major abdominal surgery failed to confirm such a relationship.[55] In early studies of women undergoing gynecological surgery, in which specific measurements of the fibrinolytic components were not available, the preoperative euglobulin clot lysis time was found to be one of the most important predictors of postoperative DVT.[56] Thus, more studies are needed before we can finally evaluate the importance of impaired fibrinolytic function in the process of postoperative DVT.

VI. IMPAIRED FIBRINOLYSIS IN PATIENTS WITH CORONARY HEART DISEASE

The early epidemiological and clinical studies of fibrinolytic function in CHD were performed with "global" assays measuring the overall fibrinolytic function, such as euglobulin clot lysis time or fibrin plate lysis. The early phases of the Northwick Park Heart Study, the one large prospective epidemiological study of middle-aged men that included measurement of fibrinolytic function, failed to demonstrate a clear relation between impaired fibrinolysis and increased risk of future cardiovascular events.[57] A non-specific assay was used, and samples were taken only at rest. Men who later developed clinical CHD had a lower fibrinolytic activity, although statistical independence was not found for this association when multivariate models were applied. However, with the accumulation of further CHD episodes in the Northwick Park Heart study, a strong, independent relation subsequently emerged between low fibrinolytic activity, as measured by dilute clot lysis time, and increased risk of future CHD in men aged 40-54 at entry in the study, suggesting that low fibrinolytic activity is a strong determinant of CHD in younger men.[58]

Prospective studies of initially healthy individuals that included specific determinations of the individual components of the fibrinolytic enzyme system are unfortunately not yet available, whereas a few longitudinal cohort studies of patients with manifest CHD or atherosclerosis have been reported. Although a reduced fibrinolytic capacity cannot yet be considered as an established risk factor in the conventional epidemiological sense, the data produced so far strongly suggest that the fibrinolytic enzyme system must be taken into consideration in forthcoming prospective studies.

A. CASE-CONTROL STUDIES

The introduction of sensitive and specific methods to determine the individual components of the fibrinolytic enzyme system rapidly resulted in an abundance of cross-sectional studies of patients with angina pectoris or previous myocardial infarction (for a review see ref. no. 6). These studies have consistently shown a decreased fibrinolytic activity in patients as compared to controls. Data from our group and others have indicated that reduced fibrinolytic capacity, mainly due to elevated plasma levels of PAI-l, may be of importance for myocardial infarction, especially in young patients with hypertriglyceridemia.[26] A few studies, which have focused on patients without metabolic risk factors, have provided discrepant results in failing to show any associations between activities of PAI-1 or tissue plasminogen activator (t-PA) and CHD.[59,60] Considering the general pattern that emerges from all case-control studies, it appears that elevated PAI-1 activity in plasma is more strongly related to myocardial infarction than to angina pectoris or to angiographically ascertained coronary artery disease.[61]

A minor proportion of young postinfarction patients with normal plasma PAI-1 activity show impaired fibrinolytic capacity caused by a decreased release of tPA. In what appears to be a contradiction, basal tPA antigen levels are also generally elevated among patients with coronary atherosclerosis. However, as mentioned above, there is no correlation between tPA activity and tPA antigen in plasma samples taken at rest. On the contrary, many studies have shown a fairly strong positive correlation between basal tPA antigen and PAI-1 activity. The reason for this is that the major portion of tPA antigen in plasma taken at rest is contained in an inactive complex between tPA and PAI-1.

There is no general indication that the firm relation between elevated plasma PAI-1 activity or reduced tPA activity and CHD depends on a relation between fibrinolytic components and severity of coronary atherosclerosis. However, a recent angiographic study of middle-aged men, evaluated because of chest pain and/or abnormal exercise stress tests, revealed a positive association between plasma PAI-1 activity and severity of coronary artery disease.[62]

B. LONGITUDINAL COHORT STUDIES

Support for a causal relationship between impaired fibrinolytic function and myocardial infarction was first obtained from a follow-up study of men who had survived a myocardial infarction before the age of 45 years.[63] The study suggested that a high plasma concentration of PAI-1 activity is independently related to reinfarction within 3 years of a primary event, along with dyslipoproteinemia involving VLDL and HDL, poor left ventricular performance, and multiple vessel coronary artery disease. Two additional small-scale longitudinal studies of unselected postinfarction patients and patients with unstable angina pectoris have provided confirmatory information on the role of impaired fibrinolysis as a marker for a high-risk state.[64,65] An elevated basal tPA antigen level was also found to be associated with increased risk of cardiovascular events during a 4-year follow-up period in a larger cohort of patients with severe angina pectoris and angiographically documented coronary artery disease.[66] However, multivariate analysis indicated that only a diagnosis of hypertension and left ventricular performance each made an independent contribution to the prediction of cardiovascular events. A predictive value of tPA antigen concentration on long-term mortality was subsequently found in this cohort.[67] Furthermore, Ridker et al recently reported higher tPA antigen concentrations among participants who later suffered myocardial infarction in the prospective Physicians Health Study.[68] Adjustment for CHD risk factors abolished the statistical significance of the association between tPA antigen and long-term mortality. No support for a causal relationship was therefore obtained. Indeed, it was suggested that increased plasma tPA antigen concentration was a consequence of silent atherosclerosis. However, it seems more plausible that the increased plasma tPA antigen merely reflects increased plasma PAI-1 concentrations.

Recently, Cortellaro et al studied hemostatic function in a case-control study of 953 patients with atherosclerotic disease.[69] During a one year follow up, 60 patients suffered a thrombotic event, in most cases a myocardial infarction, but in some instances transient ischemic attacks and occasionally peripheral arterial thrombosis. The patients with events were compared with 94 patients without any event during the same time period. A highly statistically significant difference in plasma PAI-1 activity was observed between the two groups, those with events having higher levels. In addition, elevated levels of the fibrin degradation product D-dimer were associated with thrombotic events.

From the available clinical and epidemiological evidence, it seems reasonable to assume that the predictive value of fibrinolytic activators and inhibitors is likely to vary depending on the age, sex, risk factor burden, and primary clinical manifestation of coronary atherosclerosis of the individual. Because of the marked inter- and intra-personal variability of plasma PAI-1 activity and the multiple interrelations with other risk factor mechanisms, future clinical and epidemiological studies would certainly be expected to give somewhat deviating results regarding the predictive power of PAI-1. Nevertheless, the present data strongly suggest that determinations of fibrinolytic function, especially PAI-1 activity and tPA antigen concentrations, should be included in future prospective studies evaluating the role of hemostatic function in arterial thrombosis. Further support for this statement comes from genotyping for the 4G/5G polymorphism in the PAI-1 promoter region in young postinfarction patients and population-based controls. The frequency of the 4G-allele, which is associated with higher plasma PAI-1 concentration, was significantly higher among the patients, and the genotype distribution differed significantly between the two groups.[36] In addition, a group of patients subjected to coronary bypass surgery contained a significantly larger proportion of individuals homozygous for the 4G-allele than age-matched controls (unpublished data by Nordenhem, Moor, Blombäck, Rydén, Hamsten and Wiman). Taken together these data strongly suggest that PAI-1 has an independent etiological role in CHD.

VII. CONCLUSIONS

Impaired fibrinolytic function is a quite common finding in patients with thrombotic disease, mainly due to an elevation of the plasma PAI-1 concentration. In patients with idiopathic DVT no reliable prospective or genetic studies have been published. Therefore, in this instance, it is difficult to draw firm conclusions about cause or consequence. Regarding postoperative DVT, a preoperative increase in PAI-1 seems to predict a postoperative DVT in patients subjected to hip surgery. Furthermore, the immediate postoperative elevation of PAI-1, as part of the acute phase response, seems to be predictive for the development of a later DVT.

Several longitudinal cohort studies of patients with manifest CHD have linked elevated plasma PAI-1 or tPA antigen concentrations to future cardiovascular events, particularly myocardial infarction. The tPA antigen level in basal plasma is quite strongly correlated with the PAI-1 concentration and not with tPA activity, and therefore most likely reflects the PAI-1 concentration. Before PAI-1 can be regarded as a risk factor in the conventional epidemiological sense, its relationship to myocardial infarction must be demonstrated in prospective studies of healthy populations.

Regulation of the plasma concentration of PAI-1 is at present not well understood. Multiple interactions with disturbances of both carbohydrate and lipoprotein metabolism are evident. Recently, knowledge of the importance of genetic factors in regulating plasma PAI-1 concentration has become available and will certainly shed new light on the importance of impaired fibrinolytic function in the etiology of CHD in the near future.

ACKNOWLEDGEMENTS

This study was financially supported in part by the Swedish Medical Research Council (projects nos 5193 and 8691), "Konung Gustaf V:s och Drottning Victorias Stiftelse", Swedish Heart-Lung Foundation and Karolinska Institute.

REFERENCES

1. **Virchow, R.**, Ein vortrag über die Thrombose vom Jahre 1845, in *Gesammelte Abhandlungenzur wissenschaftligen Medizin,* Frankfurt, Germany, Meidinger, 478, 1856.
2. **Bertina, R. M., Koeleman, B. P. C., Koster, T., Rosendaal F. R., Dirven, R. J., de Ronde H., van der Velden, P. A. and Reitsma P. H.**, Mutation in blood coagulation factor V associated with resistance to activated protein C, *Nature,* 369, 64, 1994.
3. **Chmielewska, J., Rånby, M. and Wiman, B.**, Evidence for a rapid inhibitor to tissue plasminogen activator in plasma, *Thromb. Res.,* 31, 427, 1983.
4. **Kruithof, E. K. O., Tran-Thang, C., Ransijn, A. and Bachmann, F.**, Demonstration of a fast-acting inhibitor of plasminogen activators in human plasma, *Blood,* 64, 907, 1984.
5. **Wiman, B. and Hamsten, A.**, The fibrinolytic enzyme system and its role in the etiology of thromboembolic disease, *Semin. Thromb. Hemostas.,*16, 207, 1990.
6. **Wiman, B. and Hamsten, A.**, Impaired fibrinolysis and risk of thromboembolism, *Progr. Cardiovasc. Dis.,* 34, 179, 1991.
7. **Juhan-Vague, I. and Alessi, M. C.**, Plasminogen activator inhibitor 1 and atherothrombosis, *Thrombos. Haemost.,* 70 (1), 138, 1993.
8. **Andreotti, F., Davies, G. J., Hackett, D. R., Khan, M. I., de Bart, A. C., Aber, V. R., Maseri, A. and Kluft, C.**, Major circadian fluctuations in fibrinolysis factors and possible relevance to time of onset of myocardial infarction, sudden cardiac death and stroke, *Am. J. Cardiol.,* 62, 635, 1988.
9. **Grimaudo, V., Hauert, J., Bachmann, F. and Kruithof, E.K.O.**, Diurnal variation of the fibrinolytic system, *Thromb. Haemostas,.* 59, 495, 1988.
10. **Angelton, P., Chandler, W. L. and Schmer, G.**, Diurnal variation of tissue-type plasminogen activator and its rapid inhibition. *Circulation,* 79, 101, 1989.
11. **Colucci, M., Paramo, J. A. and Collen, D.**, Generation in plasma of a fast acting inhibitor of plasminogen activator in response to endotoxin stimulation, *J. Clin. Invest.,* 75, 818, 1985.
12. **Emeis, J.J. and Kooistra, T.**, Interleukin-1 and lipopolysaccharide induce a fast-acting inhibitor of tissue-type plasminogen activator in vivo and in cultured endothelial cells, *J. Experimental Med.,* 163, 1260, 1986.
13. **Alessi, M. C., Juhan-Vague, I., Kooistra, T., Declerck, P. J. and Collen, D.**, Insulin stimulates the synthesis of plasminogen activator inhibitor 1 by hepatocellular cell line HepG2. *Thromb. Haemostas.,* 60, 491, 1988.
14. **Schneider, D. J. and Sobel, B. E.**, Augmentation of synthesis of plasminogen activator inhibitor type-1 by insulin and insulin-like growth factor type-1: Implications for vascular disease by hyperinsulinemic states, *Proc. Natl. Acad. Sci.,* USA, 88, 9959, 1991.
15. **Schneider, D. J., Nordt, T. K. and Sobel, B. E.**, Stimulation by proinsulin of expression of plasminogen activator inhibitor type-1 in endothelial cells. *Diabetes,* 41, 890, 1992.
16. **Nordt, T. K., Schneider, D. J. and Sobel, B. E.**, Augmentation of the synthesis of plasminogen activiator inhibitor type-1 by precursors of insulin. A potential risk factor for vascular disease, *Circulation,* 89, 321, 1994.
17. **Anfosso, F., Chomiki, N., Alessi, M. C., Vague, P. and Juhan-Vague, I.**, Plasminogen activator inhibitor-1 synthesis in the human hepatoma cell line HepG2. Metformin inhibits the stimulating effects of insulin. *J. Clin. Invest.,* 91, 2185, 1993.
18. **Stiko-Rahm, A., Wiman, B., Hamsten, A. and Nilsson, J.**, Secretion of plasminogen activator inhibitor-1 from cultured human umbilical vein endothelial cells is induced by very low density lipoprotein. *Arteriosclerosis,* 10, 1067, 1990.
19. **Latron, Y., Chautan, M., Anfosso, F., Alessi, M. C., Nalbone, G., Lafont, H. and Juhan Vague, I.**, Stimulating effect of oxidized low density lipoproteins on plasminogen activator inhibitor-1 synthesis by endothelial cells, *Arterioscler. Thromb.,* 11, 1821, 1991.
20. **Mussoni, L., Mannucci, L., Sirtori, M., Camera, M., Maderna, P., Sironi, L. and Tremoli, E.**, Hypertriglyceridemia and regulation of fibrinolytic activity, *Arterioscler. Thromb.,* 12, 19, 1992.
21. **Tremoli, E, Camera, M., Maderna P., Sironi, L., Prati, L., Colli, S., Piovella, F., Bernini, F., Corsini, A. and Mussoni, L.**, Increased synthesis of plasminogen activator inhibitor-1 by cultured human endothelial cells exposed to native and modified LDLs. An LDL receptor-independent phenomenon. *Arterioscler. Thromb.,* 13, 338, 1993.
22. **Hamsten, A. and Wiman, B.**, Fibrinolysis and Atherosclerotic cardiovascular disease, in *Atherosclerotic Cardiovascular Disease, Hemostasis, and Endothelial Function,* Francis, R.B., Jr., Ed., 107, 1993.
23. **Phillips, G. B.**, Relationship between sex hormones and the glucose-insulin-lipid defect in men with obesity, *Metabolism* 42, 116, 1993.
24. **Caron, P., Bennet, A., Camare, R., Louvet, J. P., Boneu, S. and Pie, P.**, Plasminogen activator inhibitor in plasma in related to testosterone in men, *Metabolism* 38, 1010, 1989.

25. **Yang, X. C., Jing, T. Y., Resnick, L. M. and Phillips, G. B.**, Relation of hemostatic risk factors to other risk factors for coronary heart disease and to sex hormones in men, *Arterioscler. Thromb.*, 13, 167, 1993.

26. **Hamsten, A., Wiman, B., de Faire, U. and Blombäck, M.**, Increased plasma levels of a rapid inhibitor of tissue plasminogen activator in young survivors of myocardial infarction, *N. Engl. J. Med.*, 313, 1557, 1985.

27. **Mehta, J., Mehta, P., Lawson, D. and Saldeen, T.**, Plasma tissue plasminogen activator inhibitor levels in coronary artery disease: correlation with age and serum triglyceride concentrations, *J. Am. Coll. Cardiol.*, 9, 263, 1987.

28. **Juhan-Vague, I., Vague, P., Alessi, M., Badier, C., Valadier, J., Aillaud, M. and Atlan, C.**, Relationships between plasma insulin triglyceride, body mass index, and plasminogen activator inhibitor 1, *Diabetes Metab.*, 13, 331,1987.

29. **Sundell, I. B., Dahlgren, S., Rånby, M., Lundin, E., Stenling, R. and Nilsson, T. K.**, Reduction of elevated plasminogen activator inhibitor levels during modest weight loss, *Fibrinolysis* 3, 51, 1989.

30. **Andersen, P., Smith, P., Seljeflot, I., Brataker, S. and Arnesen, H.**, Effects of gemfibrozil on lipids and haemostasis after myocardial infarction, *Thromb. Haemostas.*, 63, 174, 1990.

31. **Mehrabian, M., Peter, J. B., Barnard, R. J. and Lusis, A. J.**, Dietary regulation of fibrinolytic factors, *Atherosclerosis* 84, 25, 1990.

32. **Juhan-Vague, I., Alessi, M. C. and Vague, P.**, Increased plasma plasminogen activator inhibitor-1 levels. A possible link between insulin resistance and atherothrombosis. *Diabetologia* 34, 457, 1991.

33. **Juhan-Vague, I., Thompson, S. G. and Jespersen, J.**, on behaft of the ECAT Angina Pectoris Study Group, Involvement of the hemostatic system in the insulin resistance syndrome, a study of 15000 patients with angina pectoris, *Arterioscler. Thromb.*, 13, 1865, 1993.

34. **Folsom, A. R., Qamhieh, H. T., Wing, R. R., Jeffery, R. W., Stinson, V. L., Kuller, L. H. and Wu, K. K.**, Impact of weight loss on plasminogen activator inhibitor (PAI-1), factor VII and other hemostatic factors in moderately overweight adults, *Arterioscler. Thromb.*, 13, 162, 1993.

35. **Potter van Loon, B. J., Kluft, C., Radder, J. K., Blankenstein, M. A. and Meinders, A. E.**, The cardiovascular risk factor plasminogen activator inhibitor type 1 is related to insulin resistance, *Metabolism,* 42, 945, 1993.

36. **Hamsten, A. and Eriksson, P.**, Fibrinolysis and atherosclerosis: an update. *Fibrinolysis.* 8, Suppl. 1, 253-262,1994.

37. **Dawson, S., Hamsten, A., Wiman, B., Henney, A. and Humphries, S.**, Genetic variation at the plasminogen activator inhibitor-1 locus is associated with altered levels of plasma plasminogen activator inhibitor-1 activity, *Arterioscler. Thromb.*,11, 183, 1991.

38. **Dawson, S. J., Wiman, B., Hamsten, A., Green, F., Humphries, S. and Henney, A. M.**, The two allele sequences of a common polymorphism in the promoter of the plasminogen activator inhibitor-1 (PAI-1) gene respond differently to interleukin-1 in HepG2 cells, *J. Biol. Chem.*, 268, 10739, 1993.

39. **Mansfield, M. W., Stickland, M. H., Carter, A. M. and Grant P. J.**, Polymorphisms of the plasminogen activator inhibitor-1 gene in type 1 and type 2 diabetes, and in patients with diabetic retinopathy, *Thromb. Haemost.*, 71, 731, 1994.

40. **McLean, J.W., Tomlinson, J. E., Kuang, W. J., Eaton, D. L., Chen, E. Y., Fless, G.M., Scanu, A. M. and Lawn, R. M.**, cDNA sequence of human apolipoprotein(a) is homologous to plasminogen, *Nature* 330, 132, 1987.

41. **Loscalzo, J., Weinfeld, M., Fless, G. M. and Scanu, A. M.**, Lipoprotein (a), fibrin binding and plasminogen activation, *Arteriosclerosis* 10, 240, 1990.

42. **Harpel, P. C., Gordon, B. R. and Parker, T.S.**, Plasmin catalyzes binding of lipoprotein(a) to immobilized fibrinogen and fibrin, *Proc. Natl. Acad. Sci.*, USA 86, 3847, 1989.

43. **Miles, L.A., Fless, G.M., Levin, E.G., Scanu, A.M. and Plow, E. F.**, A potential basis for the thrombotic risks associated with lipoprotein(a), *Nature* 339, 301, 1989.

44. **Hajjar, K.A., Gavish, D., Breslow, J. L. and Nachman, R.L.**, Lipoprotein (a) modulation of endothelial cell surface fibrinolysis and its potential role in atherosclerosis, *Nature* 339, 303, 1989.

45. **Gonzales-Gronow, M., Edelberg, J. M. and Pizzo, S.V.**, Further characterization of the cellular plasminogen binding site: evidence that plasminogen and lipoprotein(s) compete for the same site, *Biochemistry,* 28, 2374, 1989.

46. **Edelberg, J.M., Gonzales-Gronow, M. and Pizzo, S.V.**, Lipoprotein(a) inhibits streptokinase-mediated activation of human plasminogen, *Biochemistry,* 28, 2370, 1989.

47. **Kluft, C. and Verheijen, J. H.**, The Leiden Fibrinolysis Working Party, Blood collection and handling procedures for assessment of tissue-type plasminogen activator (t-PA) and plasminogen activator inhibitor-1 (PAI-1), *Fibrinolysis,* 4, 155, 1990.

48. **Isaksson, S. and Nilsson, I. M.**, Defective fibrinolysis in blood and vein walls in recurrent idiopathic venous thrombosis, *Acta Chir. Scand.*, 138, 313, 1972.

49. **Korninger, C., Lechner, K., Niessner, H., Gossinger, H. and Kundi, M.**, Impaired fibrinolytic capacity predisposes for recurrence of venous thrombosis. *Thromb. Haemost.*, 52, 127, 1984.

50. **Ridker, P. M., Vaughan, D.E., Stampfer, M.J., Manson, J. E., Shen, C., Newcomer, L.M., Goldhaber, S.Z. and Hennekens, C.H.**, Baseline fibrinolytic state and the risk of future venous thrombosis. A prospective study of endogenous tissue-type plasminogen activator and plasminogen activator inhibitor, *Circulation,* 85, 1822, 1992.

51. **Erickson, L. A., Fici, G. J., Lund, J. E., Boyle, T.P., Polites, H.G. and Marotti, K.R.**, Development of venous occlusions in mice transgenic for the plasminogen activator inhibitor-1 gene, *Nature,* 346, 74, 1990.

52. **Carmeliet, P., Schoonjans, L., Kieckens, L., Ream, B., Degen, J., Bronson, R., De-Vos, R., van-den-Oord, J. J., Collen, D., Mulligan, R. C.**, Physiological consequences of loss of plasminogen activator gene function in mice, *Nature,* 368, 419, 1994.

53. **Paramo, J. A., Alfaro, M. J. and Rocha, E.**, Postoperative changes in the plasmatic levels of tissue-type plasminogen activator and its fast-acting inhibitor - Relationship to deep vein thrombosis and influence of prophylaxis, *Thromb. Haemost.*, 54, 713, 1985.

54. **Eriksson, B., Eriksson, E., Gyzander, E., Teger-Nilsson, A-C., Thorsen, S. and Risberg B.**, Thrombosis after hip replacement, relationship to the fibrinolytic system, *Acta Orthop. Scand.*, 60, 159, 1989.

55. **Mellbring, G., Dahlgren, S., Reiz, S. and Wiman, B.**, Fibrinolytic activity in plasma and deep vein thrombosis after major abdominal surgery, *Thromb. Res.*, 32, 575, 1983.

56. **Rakoczi, I., Chamone, D., Verstraete, M. and Collen, D.**, The relevance of clinical and haemostasis parameters for the prediction of postoperative thrombosis of the deep veins of the lower extremity in gynecologic patients. *Surg. Gynecol. Obstet.*, 151, 225, 1980.

57. **Meade, T. W., North, W. R., Chakrabarti. R., Stirling, Y., Haines, A.P., Thompson, S. G., Brozovie, M.**, Haemostatic function and cardiovascular death: early results of a prospective study., *Lancet,* 1, 1050, 1980.

58. **Meade, T. W., Ruddock, V., Stirling, Y., Chakrabarti, R. and Miller, G. J.**, Fibrinolytic activity, clotting factors, and long-term incidence of ischaemic heart disease in the Northwick Park Heart Study, *Lancet,* 342, 1076, 1993.

59.   **Oseroff, A., Krishnamurti. C., Hassett, A., Tang, D. and Alving, B.,** Plasminogen activator and plasminogen activator inhibitor activities in men with coronary artery disease, *J. Lab. Clin. Med.,* 113, 88, 1989.

60.   **Vandekerckhove, Y., Baele, G., de Puydt, H., Weyne, A and Clement, D.,** Plasma tissue plasminogen activator levels in patients with coronary heart disease, *Thromb. Res.,* 50, 449, 1988.

61.   **Aznar, J., Estelles, A., Tormo, G., Sapena, P., Tormo, V., Blanch, S. and Espana, F.,** Plasminogen activator inhibitor activity and other fibrinolytic variables in patients with coronary artery disease, *Br. Heart. J.,* 59, 535, 1988.

62.   **Phillips, G. B., Pinkernell, B. H. and Jing, T-Y.,** The association of hypotestosteronemia with coronary artery disease in men, *Arterioscler. Thromb.,* 14, 701, 1994.

63.   **Hamsten, A., de Faire, U., Walldius, G., Dahlén, G., Szamosi, A., Landou, C., Blombäck, M. and Wiman, B.,** Plasminogen activator inhibitor in plasma: risk factor for recurrent myocardial infarction, *Lancet,* 2, 3, 1987.

64.   **Gram, J., Jespersen, J., Kluft, C. and Rijken D.C.,** On the usefulness of fibrinolysis variables in the characterization of a risk group for myocardial reinfarction, *Acta Med. Stand.,* 221, 149, 1987.

65.   **Munkvad, S., Gram, J. and Jespersen, J.,** A depression of active tissue plasminogen activator in plasma characterizes patients with unstable angina pectoris who develop myocardial infarction, *Eur. Heart J.,* 11, 525, 1990.

66.   **Jansson, J. H., Nilsson, T.K. and Olofsson, B.O.,** Tissue plasminogen activator and other risk factors as predictors of cardiovascular events in patients with severe angina pectoris, *Eur. Heart J.,* 12, 157, 1991.

67.   **Jansson, J-H., Olofsson, B-O. and Nilsson, T-K.,** Predictive value of tissue plasminogen activator mass concentration on long-term mortality in patients with coronary artery disease. A 7-year follow-up, *Circulation,* 88, 2030, 1993.

68.   **Ridker, P. M., Vaughan, P. E., Stampfer, M. J., Manson, J. E. and Hennehens, C. H.,** Endogenous tissue-type plasminogen activator and risk of myocardial infarction. *Lancet,* 341, 1165, 1993.

69.   **Cortellaro, M., Cofrancesco, E., Boscheti, C., Mussoni, L., Donati, M.B., Cardillo, M., Catalano, M., Gabrielli, L., Lombardi, B., Specchia, G.,Specchia, G., Tavazzi, L., Tremoli, E., Pozzoli, E. and Turri, M.,** for the PLAT Group, Increased fibrin turnover and high PAI-1 activity as predictors of ischemic events in artherosclerotic patients - a case-control study, *Arterioscler. Thromb.,* 13, 1412, 1993.

Fundamental Aspects and Laboratory Approaches

C. Drug and Blood Products Induced Hypercoagulability

DRUG INDUCED HYPERCOAGULABILITY

M. Greaves and F. E. Preston
Department of Haematology, Royal Hallamshire Hospital, Sheffield

Iatrogenic thrombosis resulting from drug therapy has been recognised for several decades: it is now a quarter century since Vessey and Doll presented their case - control data which supported the suspected link between oestrogen-containing oral contraceptive use and a predisposition to "spontaneous" venous thromboembolic disease.[1] As well as the epidemiological importance, early recognition of the possible link between a medication and a thrombotic complication may be lifesaving - as in the frequently extensive arteriovenous thrombosis which develops in the syndrome of "heparin-induced thrombocytopenia". Furthermore, the study of mechanisms whereby drug therapy can lead to a prothrombotic state may provide insights into physiological and pathological aspects of haemostasis. (Table I).

Table I : Drug Related Thrombosis

Estrogens and thrombosis	
Chemotherapy-related thrombosis	
Thrombosis due to anticoagulant drugs -	Heparin-induced thrombocytopenia Warfarin-induced skin necrosis
Drug-induced lupus inhibitors and thrombosis	
Thrombosis complicating haemostatic therapy -	Coagulation factor concentrates DDAVP
Radiographic contrast media and thrombosis	

I. ESTROGEN THERAPY AND THROMBOSIS

The evidence for a causal relationship between therapy with estrogen-containing drugs, including the oral contraceptive, and thrombosis is strong. Jordan, in 1961, reported pulmonary embolism in a woman taking a combined oral contraceptive preparation[2] and since then numerous cases and series have been recorded. Thrombosis in visceral and intracerebral veins and arterial thrombosis have been reported, as well as limb vein thrombosis. Epidemiological data, supporting a relationship, have also accumulated. Case-control studies have suggested an increase in the risk of "spontaneous" venous thromboembolism of 4 to 11 fold in estrogen-containing oral contraceptive users, with a similar or possibly lower relative increase in the risk of post-operative thrombosis.[1,3-7] Prospective (cohort) studies have suggested a similar increased risk.[4,8-10] In the study carried out by the Royal College of General Practitioners[9] death in oral contraceptive users was associated with a wide range of vascular diseases. However, it is unfortunate that bias has not been confidently excluded in these studies of estrogen use and thrombosis. It remains possible that more diagnoses of thrombosis were made due to knowledge of estrogen usage. In the only reported controlled clinical trial[11] an 8 year follow up of a large population of women randomised to oral or other contraceptive methods was presented. Unfortunately objective methods were not used for diagnosis of venous thrombosis and although there was no apparent difference in incidence between the two groups the validity of this observation is open

0-8493-5804-3/96/$0.00+$.50

to doubt. Despite these reservations regarding the possibility of bias, on balance, current evidence supports an association between estrogen-containing oral contraceptive use and venous thromboembolism.

There is also evidence for an increased incidence of venous thromboembolism where estrogens have been used for suppression of lactation[12] the highest risk being in those women who undergo operative delivery.[13] Somewhat surprisingly the Veterans Administration Co-operative Urological Research Group[14] found no evidence of increased mortality from thromboembolism in subjects with prostate cancer treated with estrogens. Estrogen usage as part of a secondary prevention strategy against myocardial infarction in males was however associated with an increased risk of pulmonary embolism.[15]

In view of the recent major increase in usage of Hormone Replacement Therapy (HRT) it is important to know whether this exposure to lower estrogen doses is associated with an increased thrombotic risk. There is no evidence to date that this is the case. The few available studies have given negative results although all had methodological flaws and confidence limits have been wide.[6,8,16] Therefore consideration should be given to any possible risks, and assessed against the benefits, where use of HRT is considered in a woman with a history of venous thromboembolism or known thrombophilia.

Mechanism of Increased Thrombotic Risk:

Several essentially prothrombotic changes in the haemostatic system have been noted in association with use of estrogen-containing oral contraceptives, but most attention has been directed toward the undoubted reduction in plasma antithrombin concentration, first noticed by von Kaulla.[17] This occurs in the first cycle of treatment and is dose-dependent[18,19] and consistent.[20-24] The reduction involves functional activity, levels of antithrombin antigen remaining unaffected.[23,24] Progestogens do not have such an effect.[25,26]

Whilst this reduction in antithrombin activity is likely to be a major contributor to the increased thrombotic risk, estrogen usage is also associated with increases in prothrombin, factor VII and factor X, and probably in fibrinogen[21,27] some or all of which could contribute.

The recent discovery of activated protein C resistance as a frequent finding in subjects with venous thromboembolism raises the possibility that interaction between this, usually genetically determined, prothrombotic state and estrogen use may at least in part underly the increased thrombotic risk associated with oral contraception. Vandenbroucke et al.[28] have calculated a greater than 30 fold risk of venous thrombosis in women with the factor V Leiden mutation (which most commonly produces activated protein C resistance) and estrogen therapy compared with women with neither risk factor.

II. THROMBOSIS AND CANCER CHEMOTHERAPY

Cancer is associated with thrombotic complications. In some malignancies the association is particularly striking, for example that between acute promyelocytic leukaemia and disseminated intravascular coagulation (DIC) or mucin-secreting adenocarcinoma and DIC. Numerous reports have suggested that drugs used in the treatment of malignancies may further increase the incidence of thrombotic events. In some instances the evidence is strong and insights are available into possible mechanisms: there are many reports of venous thrombosis due to asparaginase therapy for ALL and this drug appears to cause a marked reduction in the plasma concentration of antithrombin in some subjects. In other situations the association is more tenuous and little is known of the pathogenesis; combination chemotherapy for breast cancer may increase thrombotic risk, but precisely which drugs are responsible and how they act remain unanswered questions.

A. CANCER AND THROMBOSIS

Over 100 years ago Trousseau described the association between venous thrombosis and gastric cancer. The risk of thrombosis in cancer sufferers is difficult to quantitate, but a prevalence of up to 15% has been reported[30] with much higher rates in postmortem studies.[30] The increased risk may be, in part, due to immobilisation associated with the disease state, the need for surgery or direct involvement of blood vessels by the tumour, for example in renal carcinoma. However, a variety of mechanisms relating to activation of coagulation have also been postulated, in some cases with supporting laboratory evidence.

Thrombocytosis of a reactive type is not uncommon in malignancy and may contribute to the prethrombotic state. Increased plasma concentrations of fibrinogen and factor VIII also occur, but whether these represent thrombotic risk factors in this context is open to doubt. Some types of tumour cell seem able to directly or indirectly activate the coagulation system.[31] Tumour cell-mediated platelet activation is one possible mechanism. Several tumours appear to elaborate a protease capable of the direct activation of factor X.[32] Tumour cells may also be associated with tissue factor, allowing abnormal coagulation activation through the extrinsic pathway.[33] Indirect coagulation activation through release of procoagulants by monocytes and macrophages stimulated by the presence of tumour cells may also occur. A multifactorial pathogenesis of thrombosis in malignancy seems likely, but, whatever the mechanisms, it seems possible that the risk can be compounded by the exposure to chemotherapeutic agents.

B. CANCER THERAPY AND THROMBOSIS
1. Breast Cancer

Combination chemotherapy and adjuvant therapy in breast cancer have been associated with venous and arterial thrombotic complications.[34-37] Levine and colleagues[36] found 14 episodes of thrombosis (13 venous) in 205 patients with stage II disease during 979 patient-months of multiagent chemotherapy or chemohumoral therapy whilst no event occurred during 2413 patient-months off treatment. This finding led the authors to conclude that the relationship between chemotherapy and thrombosis in breast cancer patients is causal. In 159 patients with stage IV breast cancer who were receiving combination chemotherapy Goodnough et. al.[35] reported a 17.6% thrombosis incidence and events were more common whilst on active treatment and were apparently unrelated to other risk factors such as ambulatory status or presence of thrombocytosis. Again, venous events predominated, although DIC and myocardial infarction were also reported. The reasons for the perceived increased thrombotic risk have not been identified - shortening of clotting times during the treatment phase was described by Canobbio et. al.,[38] and minor adverse changes in haemorheological variables by another group.[39] More interestingly there are reports of a reduction in the plasma concentration of the natural anticoagulant protein C, as well as protein S.[40,41] Protein C levels fell to 32-70% of mean normal in the 9 subjects treated with cyclophosphamide, methotrexate and 5-fluorouracil reported by Feffer et al.[41] Although factor X also fell, the effect was less marked; there was no significant change in antithrombin. Whether there is a direct effect of chemotherapeutic agents on vitamin K metabolism, or whether the reduced plasma concentrations are due to a broader effect on protein synthesis is open to question.

Tamoxifen treatment has been implicated as a risk factor for thrombosis in breast cancer patients in several studies.[42-48] In contrast, Mouridsen et. al.,[49] reported only 11 cases of thrombophlebitis in 1122 evaluable patients on Tamoxifen and concluded that "in view of the widespread use of Tamoxifen it is difficult to ascertain the denominator in relation to venous or arterial thromboembolism". However in a recent randomised, placebo controlled trial on the efficacy of Tamoxifen in patients with localised disease 12 of 1318 subjects receiving the drug suffered thrombosis, in contrast to 2 of the 1326 receiving placebo.[50]

There are experimental data which would support a prothrombotic effect of the drug.[51,52] Enck and Rios[52] reported low functional antithrombin levels in 10 of 24 women with metastatic breast cancer treated with Tamoxifen for a median of 36 weeks, whereas only 1 of 11 untreated women with comparable disease had a subnormal plasma concentration of antithrombin. Although Auger and

Mackie[53] reported no change in antithrombin on Tamoxifen, their data suggest that 3 of 16 women treated with the drug for localised breast cancer had a subnormal level (below 70%) but none of the 15 untreated women was affected. No difference was found in protein C, fibrinopeptide A or in vitro monocyte procoagulant activity. Interpretation of such studies is confounded by the observation that a reduction in plasma antithrombin concentration may be a feature of advanced breast cancer, even in the absence of drug exposure.[54]

Although the efficacy of Tamoxifen is believed to be due to a blocking of the growth-enhancing effects of oestrogen on the breast tumour tissue, Tamoxifen itself has weak oestrogenic activity and has been reported to have oestrogen-like effects on the concentration of proteins in plasma, a possible link to the increased thrombotic risk.[55]

The perceived risk of thrombotic complications in women receiving chemotherapy for metastatic breast cancer has led to investigation of low dose warfarin (INR 1.3 to 1.9) as prophylaxis. A relative risk reduction of 85% for venous thromboembolism was achieved.[56]

2. Other Cancers

Chemotherapy for other solid tumours has been considered to be associated with a thrombotic risk.[57-59] Ruiz et al.[60] found a reduction in tPA (functional activity) and increase in fibrinopeptide A after chemotherapy with regimes containing cisplatin, mitomycin C and vindesine or adriamycin, cyclophosphamide and methotrexate, in subjects with stage III-IV lung cancer. After 3 cycles of therapy, plasminogen activator inhibitor levels also rose, a prothrombotic change. Cisplatin has been implicated in cases of myocardial infarction and stroke.[61,62] An increase in plasma von Willebrand factor on treatment with this drug is consistent with damage to the vascular endothelium due to chemotherapy.[62] Bleomycin also produces endothelial injury in animal studies[63] and has been implicated in the development of Raynaud's phenomenon and coronary artery occlusion in man, often when given combined with cisplatin.[64,65] Bleomycin and mitomycin occasionally cause a pulmonary veno-occlusive syndrome, possibly due to direct vascular toxicity principally affecting the pulmonary vessels.[61] A thrombotic mircoangiopathy has also been reported in subjects treated with cisplatin and bleomycin[66,67] but is more common with mitomycin; with this drug microangiopathic haemolysis, often with renal failure, may occur in 5% or more of those exposed[61] with an even higher incidence of renal failure alone. The complication occurs most commonly after several months of therapy and has been described even after discontinuation of the drug. It seems likely that the compound induces nephrotoxicity by directly damaging the renal vascular endothelium with, in some cases, systemic coagulation activation, fibrin deposition and microangiopathic haemolysis. Cyclosporin, used to prevent graft rejection for example after bone marrow transplantation, also produces a microangiopathic syndrome with renal impairment as well as being implicated in venous thromboembolism[68] although others have found no increased incidence of large vessel thrombosis with this drug.[69,70]

L-asparaginase is a serine protease derived from E.coli and both bleeding and thrombotic complications of its use have been described, usually in acute lymphoblastic leukaemia.[71] The authors have seen both fatal cerebral haemorrhage secondary to sagittal sinus thrombosis and axillary vein thrombosis with plasma antithrombin <20% of mean normal, resulting from asparaginase therapy. Asparaginase use frequently results in a reduction in plasma fibrinogen, factor V, factor VIII, von Willebrand factor, plasminogen, α_2-plasmin inhibitor and protein C as well as antithrombin.[72-74] A regimen for antithrombin replacement has been devised in an attempt to reduce the thrombotic risk associated with asparaginase therapy in ALL.[75]

C. HEPATIC VENO-OCCLUSIVE DISEASE

As indicated above, several chemotherapeutic agents have been suspected of causing vascular endothelial damage. Veno-occlusive disease of the liver is a common complication of allogeneic bone marrow transplantation and appears to be induced by the preparatory chemotherapeutic regimens used, and possibly by radiotherapy also.[76] Alkylating agents in particular have been implicated but many drugs have been associated with the development of this complication. Histologically, intimal thickening is seen in the intrahepatic tributaries of the hepatic vein.

In one series 21% of subjects undergoing bone marrow transplantation for malignant disease suffered this complication[77] and it has been described in autologous as well as allogeneic marrow transplantation.[77,78] Hepatomegaly is often accompanied by abdominal discomfort and distension due to ascites. A fatal outcome is not uncommon, although apparently full recovery may also ensue.

Less commonly a similar clinical picture is caused by major hepatic vein thrombosis - Budd-Chiari syndrome - following cancer chemotherapy.[79]

III. THROMBOSIS DUE TO ANTICOAGULANT DRUGS

A. HEPARINS AND THROMBOSIS

A small proportion of subjects treated with heparin develop life-threatening thromboembolic complications. Because the thrombosis occurs at a time of falling platelet counts the rather deceptive term "heparin-induced thrombocytopenia (HIT)" incompletely describes this important iatrogenic condition. Although rare, the prompt recognition of HIT may be lifesaving.

Heparin therapy has long been known to result in thrombocytopenia, but this is most commonly trivial (platelets >100 x 10^9/l), transient despite continuation of heparin therapy, and clinically unimportant. The term HIT Type 1 has been used to describe this common situation, which is distinct from HIT with thrombosis, designated HIT Type 2.[80,81] Type 1 HIT may be due to a degree of in vivo platelet aggregate formation and clearance, as heparin is well known to have a minor pro-aggregatory effect on platelets ex vivo[82] and also enhances the effect of other agonists such as ADP and immune complexes. This type of thrombocytopenia requires no therapeutic intervention, although differentiation from early Type 2 HIT may be problematic.

Type 2 HIT occurs later in relation to the initiation of heparin therapy, often after 7 days or more, and never before 4 days in the absence of prior exposure to heparin. This time course is entirely consistent with the immune pathogenesis which is now widely accepted.[80,83,84] Evidence for this includes increased bone marrow megakaryocytes and reduced platelet survival,[85] and the presence in serum of a platelet activating IgG.[86] It may be that the thrombocytopenia results, at least in part, from phagocytosis of antibody coated platelets by reticuloendothelial cells, but the associated thrombosis indicates platelet consumption due to activation within the circulation. Studies in vitro, which have demonstrated platelet aggregation and release ex vivo in the presence of patient IgG and therapeutic concentrations of heparin, strongly support this concept.[86]

The precise mechanisms of heparin antibody interaction with platelets are becoming more clear. An immune complex mechanism is currently favoured, and involvement of platelet factor 4 (PF4) suggested. Thus IgG binding to PF4-heparin coated microtitre plates is noted when plasma from a subject with HIT Type 2 is added. This is not seen with normal plasma, and the binding does not occur when β-thromboglobulin or antithrombin III are substituted for PF4.[87] Also, HIT sera failed to cause release in platelets from a subject with grey platelet syndrome - these lack the alpha granules which are the cellular repository for PF4.[88] Interestingly, the antibody may be PF4 specific rather than heparin specific as HIT serum activates platelets when heparin is replaced by other negatively charged compounds, including dextran sulphate and pentosan polyphosphate, in the experimental system.[89,90] Binding of the immune complex (heparin + PF4 + antibody) to platelets probably occurs via Fcγ receptors.[91]

1. Clinical Features:

Thrombosis usually accompanies the onset of thrombocytopenia but may occur whilst the falling platelet count remains within the normal range. New events may occur for several days after withdrawal of heparin once the syndrome is established. Arterial events - limb ischaemia and gangrene, stroke, myocardial infarction and renal impairment are described. Major deep venous thrombosis and pulmonary embolism may occur and arterial and venous thrombosis may coexist. Further arterial events are more common in those subjects given heparin for an initial arterial thrombus and, similarly, new venous thrombosis or embolism tends to occur in those treated for venous thromboembolism. Skin necrosis and disseminated intravascular coagulation may occur.[92-98]

Mortality is high, particularly if diagnosis is delayed. Possibly 30% of subjects with HIT Type 2 fail to survive.[99]

A recent well-conducted investigation by Warkentin et al.[100] has demonstrated a lower incidence of development of heparin-induced antibody and HIT type 2 in subjects undergoing lower limb orthopaedic surgery when the low molecular weight heparin enoxaparin is used as prophylaxis, compared with that with use of unfractionated heparin.

2. Diagnosis and Management:

Diagnosis is primarily clinical and a high index of suspicion is required. In the UK the Committee on Safety of Medicines now recommends monitoring of the platelet count whenever heparin is given for more than 4 days. Differentiation from other causes of thrombocytopenia such as disseminated intravascular coagulation or sepsis, in a sick patient, or from HIT Type 1 in the early stages, may be difficult. For these reasons confirmatory laboratory tests have been developed. These include complement fixation, passive haemagglutination, platelet aggregation and platelet release assays. The measurement, in an aggregometer, of platelet aggregation induced by HIT serum in the presence of a therapeutic concentration of heparin can be carried out in most laboratories. One drawback is marked variability in the sensitivity of donor platelets to the HIT antibody/immune complex. However, when conditions are optimised a sensitivity of around 90% and specificity of 80% or more may be achievable.[101] Slightly better results may be obtained by measurement of 14C-serotonin release, rather than aggregation,[102] but the test is technically more demanding and time-consuming. The efficacy and applicability of other tests which measure heparin-dependent IgG binding to normal platelets by ELISA[103] or flow cytometry remain to be determined. The progress in our understanding of the pathogenesis of HIT has led to the development of possibly more specific assays using heparin-PF4 as the antigen.

In the presence of strong clinical suspicion of the diagnosis of HIT2, even without a confirmatory test result, it is prudent to discontinue heparin if the perceived balance of risks supports this. In the presence of active thrombosis warfarin should be used. If warfarin has already been introduced no other anticoagulant therapy may be required, but other drugs have been used as an alternative or until adequate warfarin effect can be achieved. These include aspirin, dipyridamole, dextran, ancrod, prostacyclin analogue, hirudin and argatroban.[104-108] Only anecdotal data on efficacy are available, and as resolution of the syndrome occurs in the majority of cases after withdrawal of heparin only, the choice of therapy remains problematic.

An alternative approach is the substitution of a heparinoid[109,110] or low molecular weight (LMW) heparin.[111-115] LMW heparins frequently show cross-reactivity with unfractionated heparin in platelet aggregation or release assays for HIT Type 2 - possibly with a frequency in excess of 80%.[109] Although favourable outcome has been reported it is unwise to substitute LMW heparin for the unfractionated material in HIT where in vitro testing suggests cross-reactivity. In contrast the heparinoid (designated Orgaran) has a low cross-reaction rate (around 10%)[109] and clinical data to date are encouraging.[109,110,116,117]

Further clinical experience may clarify the optimal therapeutic strategy for this potentially catastrophic complication of heparin therapy.

B. VITAMIN K ANTAGONISTS AND THROMBOSIS

Warfarin and other oral anticoagulant drugs - coumarins and indanediones - cause a reduction in the plasma concentration of the fully carboxylated forms of all vitamin K dependent proteins. This includes the anticoagulant protein C and its cofactor protein S as well as coagulation factors II, VII, IX and X.

In inherited thrombophilia due to deficiency of protein C or S institution of warfarin therapy may induce a transient prothrombotic state due to the further reduction of protein C/S before an effective anticoagulant effect is achieved. This may result in a progression of thrombosis in a deficient subject when oral anticoagulation is introduced without adequate heparin cover. Many cases of "warfarin-induced skin necrosis" - a purpura fulminans-like area of skin infarction, usually affecting an area of adiposity such as buttock or thigh - result from this mechanism, although it can occur in non-deficient individuals.[118-120] Introduction of warfarin therapy in subjects deficient in protein C or S should be cautious and in combination with heparin therapy.

IV. DRUG INDUCED LUPUS INHIBITORS AND THROMBOSIS

An association between the presence in serum or plasma of antiphospholipid antibody (APA) and arteriovenous thromboembolic disease has been recognised. APA are usually detected by solid-phase assays for anticardiolipin (ACA) or by coagulation-based assays for lupus anticoagulant (LA). The dilute Russell's viper venom time and the kaolin clotting time have been found to be especially sensitive. Diagnosis of LA requires confirmation of lipid specificity, most commonly determined by quenching of the in vitro anticoagulant effect using washed platelets disrupted by freezing and thawing. Guidelines for the procedures for detection of APA have been published.[121]

APA are commonly detectable in subjects with systemic lupus erythematosus (SLE) and in other collagen vascular disorders, as well as in association with a range of infections and malignant conditions. APA can also be induced by medications. Occasionally they are detected in otherwise healthy subjects. Where persistent APA positivity occurs against a background of thrombosis, without the presence of a more broad-based autoimmune disorder such as SLE, the term "Primary Antiphospholipid Syndrome" (PAPS) has been applied. Some females with PAPS also give a history of poor pregnancy outcome, especially recurrent miscarriage, and those subjects with persistently positive tests and two or more consecutive miscarriages are also considered to have the syndrome. Thrombocytopenia is an additional association.

Thrombotic complications in PAPS may be arterial, venous or both. Deep venous thrombosis affecting the limbs is most common, but thrombosis in unusual sites is also a feature, and, importantly, stroke occurring at a young age and with a high risk of recurrence has been reported frequently.[122-124]

The pathogenesis of thrombosis and miscarriage in PAPS remains unclear. Causality for the anticardiolipin or lupus anticoagulant has not been demonstrated. APA containing IgG interferes in the proteins C/S anticoagulant system in various ways.[125] A prothrombotic influence on fibrinolysis and on platelet activation have also been considered important. It remains possible, however, that APA are surrogate markers for other antibodies which are pathogenic in thrombotic disease. APA-containing sera also frequently demonstrate anti-vascular endothelial cell activity.[126]

It has recently been demonstrated that the antigens for APA are not, or not solely, negatively-charged phospholipids as previously thought but, rather, highly lipid-bound proteins. β_2-glycoprotein I (β_2-GPI) is one such protein and prothrombin a second. Galli and colleagues[127] have classified APA into three categories, two of which have an in vitro anticoagulant effect. Two types of ACA can be identified. Type A prolongs phospholipid-dependent coagulation assays, the inhibitory effect being β_2-GPI-dependent and due to the potentiation of the inhibitory effect of β_2-GPI on the conversion of prothrombin by the complex of factors Xa and Va and negatively charged phospholipid. Type B are devoid of anticoagulant effect. The third category is LA, which may coexist in plasma with ACA Types A or B. LA also prolong phospholipid dependent coagulation times, and are detected in this way. This effect is species specific and independent of β_2-GPI. Current evidence suggests that antibodies recognise an epitope which becomes exposed when human prothrombin binds to anionic phospholipids.[128]

A range of medications has been linked to the development of APA (Table II). Chlorpromazine and related drugs are by far the most important group. It has been found that up to 75% of patients treated with chlorpromazine for more than 2.5 years develop LA.[129] ACA may also be detected,[130,131] and antinuclear antibodies.[132] The isotype is, unusually, almost always IgM. With some other drugs, such as procainamide, IgG autoantibodies may develop. It has been suggested that an increased incidence of thrombosis is not a feature of drug-induced APA. For example, in the analysis of 219 subjects with LA reported by Gastineau et. al.[133] thrombosis was not noted in any of the 14 with drug-induced LA, whereas 26% of the 205 with apparently "spontaneous" LA or LA in SLE, gave a history or arterial and/or venous thrombotic events. Canoso and Sise[130] reported a similar experience. Others have, however, reported thrombotic events in subjects with chlorpromazine-induced APA.[134,135]

Table II : Drugs Linked to the Development of APA

Frequently Reported:
  Phenothiazines (especially Chlorpromazine)
  Quinidine
  *Procainamide
  Phenytoin
  *Hydralazine
Occasionally Reported (possibly fortuitous):
  Amoxycillin
  Valproic acid
  Streptomycin
  Propranolol
  Acebutalol

*Procainamide and Hydralazine may produce a lupus-like clinical syndrome.

APA which occur against a background of systemic infection appear not to be associated with an increased risk of thromboembolism. It may be that drug-induced APA are similar in this respect, but sufficient data have not yet accumulated for a firm conclusion to be reached on this. It would therefore perhaps be prudent to assume that drug-induced LA or ACA could be important in the thrombotic risk factor assessment in an individual subject.

V. THROMBOSIS DUE TO MATERIALS USED IN TREATMENT OF BLEEDING DISORDERS AND TO ERYTHROPOIETIN THERAPY

There is little doubt that the administration of prothrombin complex concentrates, used primarily for the management and prophylaxis of bleeding in haemophilia B, has been associated with the development of a prothrombotic state and clinical thrombosis. Concerns have also been raised in relation to DDAVP and fibrinolytic inhibitors tranexamic acid and Epsilon-amino caproic acid, and to intravenous immunoglobulin therapy for immune thrombocytopenia (ITP).

A . PROTHROMBIN COMPLEX CONCENTRATES (PCC) AND THROMBOSIS

PCC contain approximately equal amounts of coagulation factors II, IX and X and sometimes factor VII. Thromboembolic complications of their use have been reported not infrequently, and these include arterial and venous thromboembolism, as well as DIC.[136,137] Complications are especially likely to occur when PCC is administered to subjects with severe liver disease[136] and their use is generally contra-indicated in these circumstances.

Using assays for markers of coagulation activation, such as those for fibrinopeptide A, prothrombin activation peptide (F_{1+2}) and thrombin-antithrombin complexes, it has been demonstrated that in vivo coagulation activation is a feature of PCC administration in haemophilia B.[138,139]

The prothrombotic effect of PCC has been variously ascribed to the zymogen content, with generation of high plasma concentrations,[140] to the presence of activated clotting factors[141] and to coagulation-active phospholipid as a contaminant.[142] The use of "purified" factor IX concentrates in haemophilia B may well reduce the risk of thrombosis; there is already strong evidence of reduced thrombogenicity with these products, compared with PCC.[138,139] Factor XI concentrates have also recently given cause for concern with regard to possible thrombogenicity.

B. DDAVP AND THROMBOSIS

This vasopressin analogue is widely used in the treatment of subjects with von Willebrand's disease and mild haemophilia A as well as those with some qualitative platelet disorders. Given intravenously or intranasally it results in a rise in the plasma concentrations of von Willebrand factor and factor VIII. Although generally and justifiably regarded as safe, its use has occasionally been linked to the development of myocardial infarction and stroke.[143-146]

Venous thrombosis has also been reported.[147] Although pooled data from the use of DDAVP in what could be considered the high-risk situation of cardiac surgery suggest a low risk of thrombosis,[148] the drug is probably best avoided in subjects with symptomatic arterial occlusive disease.

C. INHIBITORS OF FIBRINOLYSIS AND THROMBOSIS

Fibrinolytic inhibitors have been widely used as adjuncts to haemostatic therapy in bleeding disorders, as well as in the treatment of menorrhagia, for many years. Reports of intracranial and other thrombotic events have appeared.[149-151] However these drugs are widely used and risk of thrombosis must be low, but may perhaps be compounded by other factors, such as the post-operative state. This observation is supported by the finding of only 11 reported episodes of thrombosis in 238,000 women treated with tranexamic acid for menorrhagia, a thrombotic incidence which is probably no different from that expected to occur "spontaneously".[152] There is a risk of increased tissue ischaemia if these drugs are administered in DIC.

D. INTRAVENOUS IMMUNOGLOBULIN FOR ITP

Woodruff et. al.[153] briefly reported on two episodes of stroke and two of myocardial infarction in elderly patients treated with intravenous immunoglobulin for ITP. All had pre-existing vascular disease or hypertension. Frame and Crawford[154] reviewed the data on 34 subjects older than 60 years treated with the Scottish Blood Transfusion Service intravenous immunoglobulin preparation. Only one of three deaths within 14 days of treatment could be attributed to thrombosis-myocardial infarction in a man with hypertension.

It seems likely that the rising platelet count may be the contributory factor if there is indeed a thrombotic risk associated with the use of these products in ITP.

E. ERYTHROPOIETIN

Exacerbation of hypertension and development of shunt thrombosis have been widely reported with the use of erythropoietin in the anaemia of chronic renal failure. There are also anecdotal reports of other thrombotic episodes.[155] Erythropoietin has also been widely used as a "performance enhancer" in endurance sports, especially cycling. The report of sudden death among cyclists, often shortly after competition, has been linked to this use of erythropoietin.[156] Hyperviscosity due to raised haematocrit, compounded by dehydration, may explain this suggested association.

VI. INTRAVASCULAR CONTRAST MEDIA AND THROMBOSIS

Although invasive radiological techniques involving vascular catheterisation carry an inherent thrombotic risk, especially as they are carried out in high risk patients, an additional possibility of thrombosis has been attributed to the use of contrast media, including the more sophisticated nonionic agents now in common usage. These contrast media have a lower osmolality than their "ionic" predecessors. Although thrombosis has been reported[157] this is an uncommon complication of these procedures: Gabriel et al.,[158] noted only 12 instances of unexplained coronary thrombosis or adherent clot at the catheter tip in 10,000 patients undergoing cardiac catheterisation.

Despite this concern in vitro studies suggest that radiographic contrast media exert an anticoagulant and possibly antiplatelet effect.[158,159] The major effect of nonionic contrast media may be on fibrin assembly.[158] It seems likely that the thrombotic risk of catheterisation procedures relates more strongly to technique, patient selection and other factors such as catheter design than to an inherent prothrombotic influence of contrast media, but more experimental data are required to fully resolve this question.

VII. CONCLUSIONS

Iatrogenic thrombosis due to medications is a clinically significant problem. Further studies are required to define the risks more precisely and to further delineate the pathogenic mechanisms underlying thrombotic complications of therapy.

ACKNOWLEDGEMENT
The authors are grateful to Mrs. L. Wattam for her expertise in the preparation of the manuscript.

REFERENCES

1.   **Vessey M. P., Doll R.,** Investigation of relation between use of oral contraceptives and thromboembolic disease, *Brit. Med. J.,* 2, 199, 1968.
2.   **Jordan W. M.,** Pulmonary embolism, *Lancet,* ii, 1146, 1961.
3.   **Sartwell P. E., Masi A. T., Arthes F. G. et. al.,** Thromboembolism and oral contraceptives: an epidemiologic case-control study, *Am. J. Epidemiol.,* 90,365, 1969.
4.   **Vessey M. P., Doll R., Fairbairn A. S., Glober G.,** Post-operative thromboembolism and the use of oral contraceptives, *Brit. Med. J.,* 3, 123, 1970.
5.   **Greene G. R., Sartwell P. E.,** Oral contraceptive use in patients with thromboembolism following surgery, trauma or infection, *Am. J. Pub. Health,* 62, 680, 1972.
6.   **Boston Collaborative Drug Surveillance Programme:** Oral contraceptives and venous thromboembolic disease, surgically confirmed gallbladder disease, and breast tumours, *Lancet,* I, 1399, 1973.
7.   **Stolley P. D., Tonascia J. A., Tockman M. S., et. al.,** Thrombosis with low-estrogen oral contraceptives, *Am. J. Epidemiol.,* 102, 197, 1975.
8.   **Petitti D. B., Wingerd J., Pellegrin F., Ramcharan S.,** Oral contraceptives, smoking, and other factors in relation to risk of venous thromboembolic disease, *Am. J. Epidemiol.,* 108, 480, 1978.
9.   **Royal College of General Practitioners' Oral Contraception Study,** Oral contraceptives, venous thrombosis, and varicose veins, *J. Roy. Coll. Gen. Practitioners,* 28, 393, 1978.
10. **Royal College of General Practitioners' Oral Contraception Study,** Further analysis of mortality in oral contraceptive users, *Lancet,* I, 541, 1981.
11. **Fuertas-de la Haba A., Curet J. O., Pelegrina I., Bangdiwala I.,** Thrombophlebitis among oral and non-oral contraceptive users, *Obstet. Gynecol.,* 38, 259, 1971.
12. **Daniel D. G., Campbell H., Turnbull A. C.,** Puerperal thromboembolism and suppression of lactation, *Lancet,* ii, 287, 1967.
13. **Jeffcoate T. N. A., Miller J., Roos R. F., Tindall V. R.,** Puerperal thromboembolism in relation to the inhibition of lactation by oestrogen therapy, *Brit. Med. J.,* 4, 19, 1968.
14. **Veterans Administration Co-operative Urological Research Group,** Treatment and survival of patients with cancer of the prostate, *Surg., Gynecol., Obstet.,* 124, 1011, 1967.
15. **Coronary Drug Project Research Group,** Initial findings leading to modifications of its research protocol, *JAMA,* 214, 1303, 1970.
16. **Gow S., MacGillivray I.,** Metabolic, hormonal and vascular changes after synthetic oestrogen therapy in oophorectomized women, *Brit. Med. J.,* 2, 73, 1971.
17. **von Kaulla E., Droegemuller W., Aoki N., von Kaulla K. N.,** Antithrombin III depression and thrombin generation acceleration in women taking oral contraceptives, *Am. J. Obstet. Gynecol.,* 109, 868, 1971.
18. **Conard J., Samama M., Salomon Y.,** Antithrombin III and the oestrogen content of combined oestro-progestogen contraceptives, *Lancet,* ii, 1148, 1972.
19. **Bell A. P., McKee P. A.,** Fibrin formation and dissolution in women receiving oral contraceptive drugs, *J. Lab. Clin. Med.,* 80, 751, 1977.
20. **Zuck T. F., Bergin J. J., Raymond J. M., Dwyre W. R.,** Implications of depressed antithrombin III activity associated with oral contraceptives, *Surg., Gynecol., Obstet.,* 133, 608, 1971.
21. **Meade T. W., Brozovic M., Chakrabarti R., et. al.,** An epidemiological study of the haemostatic and other effects of oral contraceptives, *Brit. J. Haematol.,* 34, 353, 1976.
22. **Sagar S., Stamatakis J. D., Thomas D. P., Kakkar V. V.,** Oral contraceptives, antithrombin III activity, and post-operative deep vein thrombosis, *Lancet,* I, 509, 1976.
23. **Wessler S., Gitel S. N., Wan L. S., Pasternack B. S.,** Estrogen-containing oral contraceptive agents: a basis for their thrombogenicity, *J. Am. Med. Assoc.,* 236, 2179, 1976.

24. **Petersen C., Kelly R., Minard B., Cawley L. P.,** Antithrombin III: comparison of functional and immunologic assays, *Am. J. Clin. Pathol.,* 69, 500, 1978.

25. **Howie P. W., Mallinson A. C., Prentice C. R. M. et. al.,** Effect of combined oestrogen-progestogen oral contraceptives, oestrogen, and progestogen on antiplasmin and antithrombin activity, *Lancet,* II, 1329, 1970.

26. **Larsson-Cohn U., Fagerhol M. K., Abilgaard U.,** Concentration of Antithrombin III during combined and progestogen-only oral contraceptive treatment, *Acta. Obstet. et Gynecol. Scand.,* 51, 315, 1972.

27. **Ogston D.,** *The Physiology of Hemostasis,* Croom Helm, London, 1983.

28. **Vandenbroucke J.P., Koster T., Briet E., et. al.,** Increased risk of venous thrombosis in oral-contraceptive users who are carriers of factor V Leiden mutation, *Lancet,* 344, 1453, 1994.

29. **Luzzatto G., Schafer A. I.,** The prethrombotic state in cancer, *Sem. Oncol.,* 17, 147, 1990.

30. **Ambrus J. L., Ambrus C. M., Pickren J. W.,** Causes of death in cancer patients, *J. Med.,* 6, 61, 1975.

31. **Rickles F. R., Hancock W. W., Edwards R. L., et. al.,** Antimetastatic agents, *Semin. Thrombos. Haemostas.,* 14, 88, 1988.

32. **Falanga A., Gordon S. G.,** Isolation and characterization of cancer procoagulant: A cysteine proteinase from malignant tissue, *Biochem.,* 24, 558, 1985.

33. **Rickles F. R., Edwards R. L.,** Activation of blood coagulation in cancer: Trousseau's syndrome revisited, *Blood,* 62, 14, 1983.

34. **Weiss R. B., Tormey D. C., Holland J. F., et. al.,** Venous thrombosis during multinodal treatment of primary breast carcinoma, *Cancer Treat Rep.,* 65, 677, 1981.

35. **Goodnough L. T., Saito H., Manni A., et. al.,** Increased incidence of thromboembolism in stage IV breast cancer patients treated with a five-drug chemotherapy regimen: A study of 159 patients, *Cancer,* 54, 1264, 1984.

36. **Levine M. N., Gent M., Hirsh J., et. al.,** The thrombogenic effect of anticancer drug therapy in women with stage II breast cancer, *New Eng. J. Med.,* 318, 404, 1988.

37. **Saphner T., Tormey D. C., Gray R.,** Venous and arterial thrombosis in patients who received adjuvant therapy for breast cancer, *J. Clin. Oncol.,* 9, 286, 1991.

38. **Canobbio L., Fassio T., Ardizzoni A., et. al.,** Hypercoagulable state induced by cytostatic drugs in stage II breast cancer patients, *Cancer,* 58, 1032, 1986.

39. **Miller B., Heilmann L.,** Hemorheologic variables in breast cancer patients at the time of diagnosis and during treatment, *Cancer,* 62, 350, 1988.

40. **Rogers J. S., Murgo A. J., Fontana J. A., Raich P. C.,** Chemotherapy for breast cancer decreases plasma protein C and protein S, *J. Clin. Oncol.,* 2, 276, 1988.

41. **Feffer S. E., Carmosino L. S., Fox R. L.,** Acquired protein C deficiency in patients with breast cancer receiving cyclophosphamide, methotrexate, and 5-fluorouracil, *Cancer,* 63, 1303, 1989.

42. **Nevasaari K., Heikkinen M., Taskinen P. J.,** Tamoxifen and thrombosis, *Lancet,* 2, 946, 1978.

43. **Fisher B., Redmond C., Brown A., et. al.,** Treatment of primary breast cancer with chemotherapy and tamoxifen, *New Eng. J. Med.,* 305, 1, 1981.

44. **Jacquot C., Craterol R., Bariety J., et. al.,** DES versus Tamoxifen in advanced breast cancer, *New Eng. J. Med.,* 304, 1042, 1981.

45. **Ribeiro G., Palmer M. K.,** Adjuvant tamoxifen for operable carcinoma of the breast: report of a clinical trial by the Christie Hospital and Holt Radium Institute, *Brit. Med. J.,* 286, 827, 1983.

46. **Lipton A., Harvey H. A., Hamilton R. W.,** Venous thrombosis as a side-effect of tamoxifen treatment, *Cancer Treat. Rep.,* 68, 887, 1984.

47. **Dahan R., Espie M., Mignot L., et. al.,** Tamoxifen and arterial thrombosis, *Lancet,* I, 638, 1985.

48. **Healey B., Tormey D. C., Gray R., et. al.,** Arterial and venous thrombotic events in ECOG adjuvant breast cancer trials, *Proc. Am. Soc. Clin. Oncol.,* 6, 54, 1987.

49. **Mouridsen H., Palshof T., Patterson J., Battersby L.,** Tamoxifen in advanced breast cancer, *Cancer Treat. Rep.,* 5, 131, 1978.

50. **Fisher B., Costantino J., Redmond C., et. al.,** Clinical Trial evaluating tamoxifen in treatment of patients with node-negative breast cancer who have estrogen receptor-positive tumors, *New Eng. J. Med.,* 320, 479, 1989.

51. **Enck R. E., Rios C. N.,** Tamoxifen treatment of metastatic breast cancer and antithrombin III levels, *Cancer,* 53, 2607, 1984.

52. **Jordan U. C., Fritz N. F., Tormey D. C.,** Long-term adjuvant treatment with tamoxifen: effects on sex hormone binding globulin and antithrombin III, *Cancer Res.,* 47, 4517, 1987.

53. **Auger M. J., Mackie M. J.,** Effect of tamoxifen on blood coagulation, *Cancer,* 61, 1316, 1988.

54. **Kies M. S., Posch J. J., Giolma J. P., Rubin R. N.,** Haemostatic function in cancer patients, *Cancer,* 46, 831, 1980.

55. **Fex G., Adielsson G., Mattson W.,** Oestrogen-like effects of tamoxifen on the concentration of proteins in plasma, *Acta Endocrin.,* 97, 109, 1981.

56. **Levine M., Hirsh J., Gent M., et. al.,** Double-blind randomised trial of very low dose warfarin for prevention of thromboembolism in stage IV breast cancer, *Lancet,* 343, 886, 1994.

57. **Kaismis B. S., Spiers A. D.,** Thrombotic complications in patients with advanced prostatic carcinoma treated with chemotherapy, *Lancet,* I, 1194.

58. **Krauss S., Sonoda T., Solomon A.,** Treatment with advanced gastrointestinal cancer with 5-fluorouracil and mitomycin C., *Cancer,* 48, 1598, 1979.

59. **Seifter E. J., Young R. C., Longo D. L.,** Deep venous thrombosis during therapy for Hodgkin's Disease, *Cancer Treat. Rep.,* 69, 1011, 1985.

60. **Ruiz M. A., Marugan I., Estelles E., et. al.,** The influence of chemotherapy on plasma coagulation and fibrinolytic systems in lung cancer patients, *Cancer,* 63, 643, 1989.

61. **Doll D. C., Ringenberg Q. S., Yarbro J. W.,** Vascular toxicity associated with antineoplastic drugs, *J. Clin. Oncol.,* 4, 405, 1986.

62. **Licciardello J. T. W., Moake J., Rudy C. K., et. al.,** Elevated plasma von Willebrand Factor levels and arterial occlusive complications associated with cisplatin-based chemotherapy, *Oncology,* 42, 296, 1985.

63. **Orr F. W., Adamson I. Y. R., Young L.,** Promotion of pulmonary metastasis by bleomycin-induced endothelial injury, *Cancer Res.,* 46, 891, 1983.

64. **Bodensteiner D. C.,** Fatal coronary artery fibrosis after treatment with bleomycin, vinblastine and cisplatin, *South. Med. J.,* 74, 898, 1981.

65. **Ricci J. A., Goldstein L.,** Coronary artery disease in the presence of bleomycin therapy, *Cancer Treat. Rep.,* 66, 440, 1982.

66. **Harrell R. M., Sibley R., Vogelzang N.,** Renal vascular lesions after chemotherapy with vinblastine, bleomycin and cisplatin, *Am. J. Med.,* 73, 429, 1982.
67. **Jackson A. M., Rose B. D., Graff L. G. et. al.,** Thrombotic microangiopathy and renal failure associated with antineoplastic chemotherapy, *Ann. Int. Med.,* 104, 41, 1984.
68. **Vanrenterghem Y., Roels L., Lerut T., et. al.,** Thromboembolic complications and haemostatic changes in cyclosporin-treated cadaveric renal allograft recipients, *Lancet,* I, 999, 1985.
69. **Bergentz S-E., Bergquist D., Bornmyr S., et. al.,** Venous thrombosis and cyclosporin, *Lancet,* ii, 101, 1985.
70. **Choudhury N., Neild G. H., Brown Z., Cameron J. S.,** Thromboembolic complications in cyclosporin-treated kidney allograft recipients, *Lancet,* ii, 606, 1985.
71. **Priest J. R., Ramsay N. K. C., Steinherz P. G., et. al.,** A syndrome of thrombosis and hemorrhage complicating L-asparaginase therapy for childhood acute lymphoblastic leukemia, *J. Pediatr.,* 100, 984, 1982.
72. **Pui H. C., Jackson C. W., Chesney C. M., et. al.,** Involvement of von Willebrand factor in thrombosis following asparaginase-prednisone-vincristine therapy for leukemia, *Am. J. Hematol.,* 25, 291, 1987.
73. **Saito M., Asakura H., Jokaji H., et. al.,** Changes in haemostatic and fibrinolytic proteins in patients receiving L-asparaginase therapy, *Am. J. Hematol.,* 32, 20, 1989.
74. **Gugliotta L., D'Angelo A., Mattioli B. M., et. al.,** Hypercoagulability during L-asparaginase treatment: the effect of antithrombin III supplementation in vivo, *Brit. J. Haematol.,* 74, 465, 1990.
75. **Mattioli-Belmonte M., Gugliotta L., Delvos U., et. al.,** A regimen for antithrombin III substitution in patients with acute lymphoblastic leukaemia under treatment with L-asparaginase, *Haematologica,* 76, 209, 1991.
76. **Reed G. B., Cox A. J.,** The human liver after radiation injury: A form of veno-occlusive disease, *Am. J. Pathol.,* 48, 597, 1966.
77. **McDonald G. B., Sharma P., Mattews D. E., et. al.,** Veno-occlusive disease of the liver after bone marrow transplantation: possible association with graft-versus-host disease, *Hepatology,* 4, 116, 1984.
78. **Woods W. G., Dehner L. P., Nesbit M. E., et. al.,** Fatal veno-occlusive disease of the liver following high dose chemotherapy, irradiation and bone marrow transplantation, *Am. J. Med.,* 68, 285, 1980.
79. **Zafrani S., Pinaudeau V., Dhumeaux D.,** Drug-induced vascular lesions of the liver, *Arch. Intern. Med.,* 143, 495, 1987.
80. **Green D.,** Heparin-induced thrombocytopenia, *Med. J. Australia,* 144, 7, 1986.
81. **Chong B. H.,** Heparin-induced thrombocytopenia, *Aust. & N. Z. J. Med.,* 22, 145, 1992.
82. **Salzman E. W., Rozenberg R. D., Smith M. H., et. al.,** Effect of heparin and heparin fractions on platelet aggregation, *J. Clin. Invest.,* 65, 64, 1980.
83. **Ansell J., Deykin D.,** Heparin-induced thrombocytopenia and recurrent thromboembolism, *Am. J. Hematol.,* 8, 325, 1980.
84. **Warkentin T. E., Kelton J. G.,** Heparin-induced thrombocytopenia, *Ann. Rev. Med.,* 40, 31, 1989.
85. **Wahl T. O., Lipschitz D. A., Stechschute D. J.,** Thrombocytopenia associated with antiheparin antibody, *J. Am. Med. Assoc.,* 240, 2560, 1978.
86. **Chong B. H., Pitney W. R., Castaldi P. A.,** Heparin-induced thrombocytopenia: association of thrombotic complications with heparin-dependent IgG antibody that induces thromboxane synthesis and platelet aggregation, *Lancet,* ii, 1246, 1982.
87. **Amiral J., Bridey F., Dreyfus M., et. al.,** Platelet factor 4 complexed to heparin is the target for antibodies generated in heparin-induced thrombocytopenia, *Thrombos. Haemostas.,* 68, 95, 1992.
88. **Gruel Y., Boizard-Boval B., Wautier J. L.,** Further evidence that alpha-granule components such as platelet factor 4 are involved in platelet - IgG - heparin interactions during heparin-associated thrombocytopenia, *Thrombos. Haemostas.,* 70, 374, 1993.
89. **Anderson G. P.,** Insights into heparin-induced thrombocytopenia, *Brit. J. Haematol.,* 80, 504, 1992.
90. **Greinacher A., Michels I., Mueller-Eckhardt C.,** Heparin-associated thrombocytopenia: the antibody is not heparin specific, *Thrombos. Haemostas.,* 67, 545, 1992.
91. **Chong B. H., Fawaz I., Chesterman C. N., Berndt M. C.,** Heparin-induced thrombocytopenia: mechanism of interaction of the heparin-dependent antibody with platelets, *Brit. J. Haematol.,* 73, 235, 1989.
92. **Bell W. R., Tomasulo P. A., Alving B. M., Duffy T. P.,** Thrombocytopenia occurring during the administration of heparin: a prospective study in 52 patients, *Ann. Intern. Med.,* 85, 155, 1976.
93. **Leroy J., Leclerc M. H., Delahousse B., et. al.,** Treatment of heparin-associated thrombocytopenia with low molecular weight heparin (CY216), *Sem. Thrombos. Haemostas.,* 11, 326, 1985.
94. **Buge A., Poisson M., Vidhaillet M., et. al.,** Thrombopenia and disseminated intravascular coagulation during treatment with heparin: 2 cases with neurological complications, *Rev. Neurolog.,* 144, 289, 1988.
95. **Hartman A. R., Hood R. M., Anagnostopoulos C. E.,** Phenomenon of heparin-induced thrombocytopenia associated with skin necrosis, *J. Vasc. Surg.,* 7, 781, 1988.
96. **Chong B. H., Ismail F., Cade J., et. al.,** Heparin-induced thrombocytopenia: studies with a new low molecular weight heparinoid, Org 10172, *Blood,* 73, 1592, 1989.
97. **Feng W. C., Singh A. K., Bert A. A., et. al.,** Perioperative paraplegia and multiorgan failure from heparin-induced thrombocytopenia, *Ann. Thor. Surg.,* 55, 1555, 1993.
98. **Singer R. L., Mannion J. D., Bauer T. L., et. al.,** Complications from heparin-induced thrombocytopenia in patients undergoing cardiopulmonary bypass, *Chest,* 104, 1436, 1993.
99. **King D. J., Kelton J. G.,** Heparin-induced thrombocytopenia, *Ann. Intern. Med.,* 100, 536, 1984.
100. **Warkentin T.E., Levine M.N., Hirsh J., et. al.,** Heparin-induced thrombocytopenia in patients treated with low-molecular-weight heparin or unfractionated heparin, *New Eng. J. Med.,* 332, 1330, 1995.
101. **Chong B. H., Burgess J., Ismail F.,** The clinical usefulness of the platelet aggregation test for the diagnosis of heparin-induced thrombocytopenia, *Thrombos. Haemostas.,* 69, 344, 1993.
102. **Sheridan D., Carter C., Kelton J. G.,** A diagnostic test for heparin-induced thrombocytopenia, *Blood,* 67, 27, 1986.
103. **Gruel Y., Rupin A., Darnige L., et. al.,** Specific quantification of heparin-dependent antibodies for the diagnosis of heparin-associated thrombocytopenia using an enzyme-linked immunosorbent assay, *Thrombos. Res.,* 62, 377, 1991.
104. **Rhodes G. R., Dixon R. H., Silver D.,** Heparin-induced thrombocytopenia. Eight cases with thrombotic-haemorrhagic complications, *Ann. Surg.,* 186, 752, 1977.
105. **Sobel M., Adelman B., Szentpetery S., et. al.,** Surgical management of heparin-associated thrombocytopenia. Strategies in the treatment of venous and arterial thromboembolism, *J. Vasc. Surg.,* 8, 395, 1988.

106. **Demers C., Ginsberg J. S., Brill-Edwards P., et. al.,** Rapid anticoagulation using ancrod for heparin-induced thrombocytopenia, *Blood,* 78, 2194, 1991.
107. **Matsuo T., Kario K., Chikahira Y., et. al.,** Treatment of heparin-induced thrombocytopenia by use of argatoroban, a synthetic thrombin inhibitor, *Brit. J. Haematol.,* 82, 627, 1992.
108. **Nand S., Robinson J. A.,** Plasmapheresis in the management of heparin-associated thrombocytopenia with thrombosis, *Am. J. Hematol,* 28, 204, 1988.
109. **Chong B. H., Magnani H. N.,** Lomoparan in heparin-induced thrombocytopenia, *Haemostasis,* 22, 85, 1992.
110. **Magnani H. N.,** Heparin-induced thrombocytopenia (HIT): an overview of 230 cases treated with Orgaran (Org 10172), *Thrombos. Haemostas.,* 70, 554, 1993.
111. **Vitoux J. F., Mathieu J. F., Roncato M., et. al.,** Heparin-associated thrombocytopenia: treatment with low molecular weight heparin, *Thrombos. Haemostas.* 55, 37, 1990.
112. **Benhamou A. C., Gruel Y., Barsotti J., et. al.,** The white clot syndrome of heparin-associated thrombocytopenia and thrombosis (WCS or HATT): 26 cases, *Int. Angiol.,* 4, 303, 1985.
113. **Faivre R., Kieffer Y., Bassand J. P., Maurat J. P.,** Severe thrombopenia from heparin: value of the use of low molecular weight heparin. A propos of 6 cases, *Arch. des Maladie due Coeur et des Vaisseaux,* 78, 27, 1985.
114. **Goualt-Heilmann M., Huet Y., Adnot S., et. al.,** Low molecular weight heparin fractions as an alternative therapy in heparin-induced thrombocytopenia, *Haemostas.,* 17, 134, 1987.
115. **Glock Y., Szmil E., Boudjeria B., et. al.,** Cardiovascular surgery and heparin-induced thrombocytopenia, *Int. Angiol.,* 7, 238, 1988.
116. **Ortel T. L., Gockerman J. P., Califf R. M., et. al.,** Parenteral anticoagulation with the heparinoid Lomoparan (Org 10172) in patients with heparin-induced thrombocytopenia and thrombosis, *Thrombos. Haemostas.,* 67, 292, 1992.
117. **Greinacher A., Drost W., Michels I., et. al.,** Heparin-associated thrombocytopenia: successful therapy with the heparinoid Org 10172 in patients showing cross-reaction to LMW heparins, *Ann. Haematol.,* 64, 40,1992.
118. **Verhagen H.,** Local haemorrhage and necrosis of the skin and underlying tissues at starting therapy with dicumarol or dicumacyl, *Acta. Med. Scand.,* 148, 455, 1954.
119. **Broekmans A. W., Bertina R. M., Loeliger E. A., et. al.,** Protein C and the development of skin necrosis during anticoagulant therapy, *Thrombos. Haemostas.,* 49, 244, 1983.
120. **Samama M., Horellou M. H., Soria J., et. al.,** Successful progressive anticoagulation in a severe protein C deficiency and previous skin necrosis at the initiation of oral anticoagulant treatment, *Thrombos. Haemostas.,* 51, 132, 1984.
121. **Machin S. J., Giddings J., Greaves M., et. al.,** Detection of the lupus like anticoagulant: current laboratory practice in the United Kingdom, *J. Clin. Pathol.,* 43, 73, 1990.
122. **APASS,** Recurrent thromboembolic and stroke risk in patients with neurological events and antiphospholipid antibodies, *Ann. Neurol.,* 78, 226, 1990.
123. **Greaves M.,** Clinical associations and prognostic significance of antiphospholipid antibodies, *Thrombos. Haemostas.,* 69, 244, 1993.
124. **Greaves M.,** Coagulation abnormalities and cerebral infarction, *J. Neruol., Neurosurg. & Psychiatr.,* 56, 433, 1993.
125. **Malia R. G., Kitchen S., Greaves M., Preston F. E.,** Inhibition of activated protein C and its cofactor protein S by antiphospholipid antibodies, *Brit. J. Haematol.,* 76, 101, 1990.
126. **Linsey N. J., Henderson F. I., Malia R. G., et. al.,** Inhibition of prostacyclin release by endothelial binding anticardiolipin antibodies in thrombosis-prone patients with SLE and APS, *Brit. J. Rheumatol.,* 33, 20, 1994.
127. **Galli M.,** Involvement of protein cofactors in the expression of antiphospholipid antibodies, *Haematologica,* In press, 1994.
128. **Bevers E. M., Galli M., Barbui T., et. al.,** Lupus anticoagulant IgG's (LA) are not directed to phospholipids only, but to a complex of lipid-bound human prothrombin, *Thrombos. Haemostas.,* 66, 629, 1991.
129. **Zarrabi M., Zucker S., Miller F., et. al.,** Immunologic and coagulation disorders in chlorpromazine-treated patients, *Ann. Intern. Med.,* 91, 194, 1979.
130. **Canoso R. T., Sise H. S.,** Chlorpromazine-induced lupus anticoagulant and associated immunologic abnormalities, *Am. J. Hematol.,* 13, 121, 1982.
131. **Canoso R. T., deOliveira R. M.,** Characterisation and antigenic specificity of chlorpromazine-induced antinuclear antibodies, *J. Lab. Clin. Med.,* 108, 213, 1986.
132. **Canoso R. T., deOliveira R. M.,** Chlorpromazine-induced anticardiolipin antibodies and lupus anticoagulant: Absence of thrombosis, *Am. J. Hematol.,* 27, 272, 1988.
133. **Gastineau D. A., Kazmier F. J., Nichols W. C., Bowie E.J.W.,** Lupus anticoagulant: An analysis of the clinical and laboratory features of 219 cases, *Am. J. Hematol.,* 19, 265, 1985.
134. **Mueh J. R., Herbst K. D., Rapaport S. I.,** Thrombosis in patients with the lupus anticoagulant, *Ann. Intern. Med.,* 92, 156, 1980.
135. **Triplett D. A., Brandt J. T., Musgrave K. A., Orr C. A.,** The relationship between lupus anticoagulants and antibodies to phospholipid, *JAMA,* 259, 550, 1988.
136. **Kasper C. K.,** Thromboembolic complications, *Thrombos. Diath. Haemorrhagica,* 33, 640, 1975.
137. **Lusher J. M.,** Thrombogenicity associated with factor IX complex concentrates, *Sem. Hematol.,* 28, 3, 1991.
138. **Hampton K. K., Preston F. E., Lowe G. D. O., et. al.,** Reduced coagulation activation following infusion of a highly purified factor IX concentrate compared to a prothrombin complex concentrate, *Brit. J. Haematol.,* 84, 279, 1993.
139. **Thomas D. P., Hampton K. K., Dasari H., et. al.,** A crossoveer pharmacokinetic and thrombogenicity study of a prothrombin complex concentrate and a purified factor IX concentrate, *Brit. J. Haematol.,* 87, 782, 1994.
140. **White G. C., Roberts H. R., Kingdon H. S., Lundblad R. L.,** Prothrombin complex concentrates: potentially thrombogenic material and clues to the mechanisms of thrombosis in vivo, *Blood,* 49, 159, 1977.
141. **Seligsohn U., Kasper C. K., Osterud B., Rapaport S. I.,** Activated factor VII: presence in factor IX concentrates and persistence in the circulation after infusion, *Blood,* 53, 827, 1979.
142. **Giles A. R., Nesheim M. E., Hoogendorn H., et. al.,** The coagulant active phospholipid content is a major determinent of in vitro thrombogenicity of prothrombin complex (factor IX concentrates) in rabbits, *Blood,* 59, 401, 1982.
143. **Bond L., Bevan D.,** Myocardial infarction in a patient with haemophilia treated with DDAVP, *New Eng. J. Med.,* 318, 121, 1988.
144. **Byrnes J. J., Larcada A., Moake J. L.,** Thrombosis following desmopressin for uremic bleeding, *Am. J. Hematol,* 2, 63, 1988.
145. **O'Brien J. R., Green P.J., Salmon G., et. al.,** Desmopressin and myocardial infarction, *Lancet,* i, 664, 1989.

146.   **van Dantzig J. M., Durec D. R., Witen C. J. W.,** Desmopressin and myocardial infarction, *Lancet,* i, 664, 1989.
147.   **Albert S. G., Salvato-Lechner V., Joist J. H.,** Venous thromboembolism and transient thrombocytopenia in a patient with diabetes insipidus treated with DDAVP, *Thrombos. Res.,* 50, 695, 1988.
148.   **Mannucci P. M. and Lusher J. M.,** Desmopressin and thrombosis, *Lancet,* ii, 675, 1989.
149.   **Naeye L.,** Thrombotic state after hemorrhagic diathesis, a possible complication of therapy with epsilon-aminocaproic acid, *Blood,* 19, 694, 1962.
150.   **Sharp A. A.,** Pathological fibrinolysis, *Brit. Med. Bull.,* 20, 240, 1964.
151.   **Hoffman E. P., and Koo A. H.,** Cerebral thrombosis associated with Amicar, *Radiol.,* 131, 687, 1979.
152.   **Astedt B., Bekarsy Z.,** Treatment with the fibrinolytic inhibitor tranexamic acid - risk for thrombosis? *Acta. Obstet. et Gynecol. Scand.,* 69, 353, 1990.
153.   **Woodruff R. K., Grigg A. P., Firkin F. C., Smith I. L.,** Fatal thrombotic events during treatment of autoimmune thrombocytopenia with intravenous immunoglobulin in elderly patients, *Lancet,* ii, 217, 1986.
154.   **Frame W. D., Crawford R. J.,** Thrombotic events after intravenous immunoglobulin, *Lancet,* ii, 468, 1986.
155.   **Raine A. E.,** Hypertension, blood viscosity and cardiovascular morbidity in renal failure: Implications of erythropoietin therapy, *Lancet,* I, 97, 1988.
156.   **Eichner E. R.,** Better dead than second, *J. Lab. Clin. Med.,* 120 359, 1992.
157.   **Grollman J. H., Liu C. K., Astone R. A., Lurie M. D.,** Thromboembolic complications in coronary angiography associated with the use of nonionic contrast medium, *Cath. & Cardiovasc. Diag.,* 14, 159, 1988.
158.   **Gabriel D. A., Jones M. R., Reece N. S., et. al.,** Platelet and fibrin modification by contrast media, *Circ. Res.,* 68, 881, 1991.
159.   **Parvez Z., Vik H.,** Intravascular contrast media and thrombin generation, *Acta Radiologica,* 35, 172, 1994.

DRUG - DEPENDENT PLATELET ACTIVATING IgG: HEPARIN AND STREPTOKINASE

T. Lecompte
Laboratoire d'hématologie: exploration de l'hémostase et de la thrombose
CHU de Nancy - France

Since the seventies much attention has been paid to thrombocytopenia occurring during heparin therapy. One reason is probably that, by contrast to other drug associated thrombocytopenias, its main risk is not haemorrhage, but thrombosis. Many authors believe that this peculiarity is related to the platelet activating ability of the heparin-dependent immunoglobulins G (IgGs) found in the blood of these patients. It is intriguing that IgGs directed against streptokinase are also able to activate platelets in vitro, and they have been invoked as a potential cause of limited efficacy of streptokinase for coronary artery recanalization. This kind of human IgG is reminiscent of some murine monoclonal antibodies directed to platelets that were reported to activate them[1].

I. HEPARIN

A. MAIN FEATURES OF IMMUNE HEPARIN-ASSOCIATED THROMBOCYTOPENIA (HAT)[2,3]

Typically thrombocytopenia has a delayed onset. The high risk interval extends from day 5 to day 15. The platelet count is not very low, and haemorrhage seldom occurs. By contrast, a substantial number of these patients were reported to have thrombotic complications, some of them (mainly with arterial thrombosis) with devastating consequences, especially if heparin is not discontinued. When the drug is stopped, platelet count usually returns to baseline promptly. HAT has not only been reported with unfractionated heparins (in the following, "heparin" will mean unfractionated heparin), but also in patients receiving low molecular weight heparins[4]. The existence of two distinct types of thrombocytopenia (immune and non immune) related to heparin therapy remains a matter of debate [3,5].

For several reported patients a heparin-dependent platelet activating factor (HD-PAF) was evidenced; moreover purified IgGs retain this activating property. A platelet releasable cationic protein, platelet factor 4 (PF4) which binds heparin and other polysulfated polysaccharides, is most probably involved in IgG binding to the platelet[6-8]. The reason why an immunologic response to PF4/heparin complexes appears in some patients remains to be elucidated[5]. Platelet activation is the result of a two-point interaction of IgG with platelets: specific binding, F(ab) portion, to a complex formed of a protein (such as PF4) and heparin and deposited onto the platelet surface; interaction of the Fc portion of platelet-associated IgG with its platelet receptor, CD32[1,5,9,10].

Thrombocytopenia is generally thought to result from consumption into ongoing, platelet rich thromboses and/or removal of activated but re-circulating platelets. The process could be self-limited as suggested by the inter-platelet model of Fc/CD32 dependent activation[1], explaining that thrombocytopenia is rarely severe; in most series the mean nadir platelet count lies around 40-60 x 10^9/L.

Thus HAT differs from common drug associated thrombocytopenia - i.e. quinine - where the Fc portion of platelet bound IgG interacts with resident tissue phagocytic cells, leading to platelet removal and destruction. The interaction of the Fc portion with the platelet Fc receptor CD32 was thought to be unique for heparin (explaining the peculiar clinical features of HAT), but, as discussed below, it is also responsible for platelet activation by anti-SK antibodies. A two-point interaction of IgG with platelets resulting in platelet activation in vitro might also hold true in vivo. Other factors could contribute to the thrombotic risk such as: IgG binding to the endothelial cells covered with endogenous heparan sulfate; neutralization by released PF4 of the anticoagulant, beneficial effect of heparin; predisposing, and now unopposed factors, since these patients were administered heparin for having thrombosis, or a risk for it.

B. CLINICAL USEFULNESS OF A BIOLOGIC TEST

Difficulties for diagnosis of HAT on clinical grounds alone are common. For instance, cases of suggestive thromboses have been reported with only a mild decline in platelet count, or with transient thrombocytopenia despite continuing heparin; in some patients previously treated with heparin (a fact that cannot always be reliably ruled out), an early drop in platelet count may occur, attributable to an anamnestic response. As mentioned above, it has been repeatedly suggested that two types of HAT would exist: type I, due to a direct effect of heparin on platelets, that would be benign and transient; or type II, immune mediated, with a high risk of thrombosis if treatment is continued. Even if one agrees with such a hypothesis, the features of the two types do overlap to such an extent that a priori distinction in a given patient while on heparin is very difficult[5]. Above all, many patients, especially critically ill ones, are receiving other drugs, or have comorbid conditions which can cause thrombocytopenia.

Thus, during the acute phase, even if the clinician facing a potential case has already suspended heparin, and despite the unavoidable delay required for the laboratory to provide a biologic result, a reliable test would be of some help in clinical decision-making. In a patient requiring continuing antithrombotic treatment, a positive result would support a switch to other therapies with their own potential adverse effects, or less convenient, or with limited evaluation. A negative result would reinitiate a search for other causes of the thrombocytopenia. Here, the result of the biologic test is aimed at replacing the a posteriori crucial piece of information obtained from follow up of the platelet count after discontinuing heparin. Additionally, if another drug was also considered to be the likely cause and stopped, even this clinical criterion will remain ambiguous.

Furthermore even if diagnosis based on simple discontinuation of therapy was thought to be feasible and proved to be successful, these patients are at risk of requiring later anticoagulant treatments (for instance for cardiopulmonary bypass or for hemodialysis). At that time the careful biologic follow-up of the HD-PAF, if present during the first episode, may help to manage these settings.

Finally, laboratory studies can be useful to compare unfractionated and low molecular weight heparins, and to test new heparinoïd anticoagulants such as Orgaran in order to select new preparations with lesser risk for this adverse effect than heparins[11] , and eventually to try to solve the debate about the actual existence of a non immune (type I) HAT.

C. PROPOSED TESTS AND VALIDATION PROCESS

The biologic, diagnostic tests for HAT may be classified into two main groups[12]. Thus the assays of group I indirectly measure heparin dependent Ig by detecting nonspecific platelet-dependent functional endpoints such as aggregation or serotonin release. The assays of group II document the interaction of immunoglobulins with platelets. The functional response is influenced by more parameters than the binding. There are however general methodologic difficulties in platelet immunology techniques.

Recently, Amiral and colleagues described an ELISA for "heparin-induced antibodies" based on their reaction with immobilized complexes of heparin and PF4[6]; it seems to be very promising but remains to be extensively studied[8]. Other molecules than PF4 might be involved in some patients[13]. Conversely, the ELISA is able to detect immunoglobulins M, which are not able to activate platelets, at least by the mechanism described above.

As for every diagnostic test, there may be false negative and false positive results, determining sensibility and specificity. It has proven difficult to evaluate the performances of the various laboratory procedures that have been used, despite a methodology greatly improved by the pioneering works of the Hamilton group[14,15]. There is neither a gold standard (although the serotonin release assay seems to be a good candidate) nor accepted and unequivocal criteria for defining an authentic, immune type, HAT. This reflects the frequent difficulties in the diagnosis in clinical practice since: (i) another cause should be excluded; (ii) type I HAT, if it exists, is itself a diagnosis by excluding type II; (iii) idiopathic thrombocytopenic purpura due to auto-antibodies, despite the improvements in assay technology, also remains a diagnosis by exclusion.

The group I platelet function tests will now be presented with more details since several attempts have been made to assess their value. Platelet aggregation was used in the very first in vitro assays for HAT. It remains widely used, for practical reasons, and despite the fact that for several years attention has been called to its low sensitivity[14,15]. For instance, a survey performed in 1993 in France[16] including 54 laboratories showed that all of them used the platelet aggregation in a conventional apparatus.

Donor's platelets are separated from other blood cells and kept in donor's citrated plasma: usually referred to as platelet-rich plasma, or PRP [17]. The proportion of patient's sample (plasma or serum, see below) to PRP is quite variable between laboratories: from 1 volume to 1 volume, to 1 to 3 [10,16]. Most often the reaction takes place in an aggregometer, under stirring at 37°C, and aggregation is continuously monitored as an increase in light transmission (LT). There is at least one heparin concentration between 0.1 to 1.0 unit / mL. In typical cases of HAT there is a rapid aggregation with formation of large aggregates occurring after a lag or, occasionally, after a period of slow aggregation. It must be kept in mind that an apparatus monitoring changes in LT is not sensitive to small aggregates. Conversely an increase in LT may also be due to platelet lysis. The observation time varies: up to 20 minutes. Of note in the often quoted study pointing to a low sensitivity it was only 10 minutes [14]. Fifteen minutes has been used in the extensive recent study by Chong and colleagues [18]. The following controls with normal donor's platelets should be performed: heparin without patient's sample, and patient's sample without heparin. The test is regarded as positive if the increase in LT is of more than 20 % of the controls'.

The so called HIPA test [19] is also a platelet aggregation test, but it is performed in the wells of a microtiter tray, and donor's platelets are separated from plasma by one washing step. Platelets are prepared from four donors. The test volume is low: 100 μL. Two concentrations of heparin are used: 0.2 and 100 units / mL. Aggregation is detected by visual inspection of the wells. The reaction is positive when the suspension becomes transparent with the low, but not the high concentration of heparin. The overall result is said positive when aggregation is detected with at least two donors, and questionable when it occurs with the platelets of one donor only.

In order to carry out the serotonin release assay [15], platelets must first be loaded with labeled serotonin; they are then washed once. The incubation is carried out in a similar manner as for the HIPA test. The radioactivity released in the supernatant is counted after centrifugation, and the result is expressed as the percentage of platelet associated radioactivity. Here also two concentrations of heparin are used (0.1 and 100 units / mL), and a positive result was set at 20 % of release with the therapeutic concentration but not with the high concentration. The serotonin release assay was demontrated to be highly specific. Moreover such an assay was used with samples from 387 patients treated with unfractionated heparin or enoxaparin (a LMWH) for about 10 days as a prophylaxis of thrombosis after elective hip surgery; the frequencies of HD-PAF were 7.8 % and 2.2 % respectively [20].

The assays with washed platelets (HIPA and serotonin release) are reported to be more sensitive than the aggregation test with platelets kept in donor's citrated plasma [13,19]. However, in the extensive work of Chong and associates [18], the difference in sensitivity between aggregation (normal platelets in plasma) and serotonin release (washed normal platelets) tends to be small.

D. SOME QUESTIONS AND ANSWERS REGARDING THE TEST

The questions concern the three test components: patient's sample, normal platelets, heparin.

1. Patient.

Since the presence of heparin in patient's sample may cloud the results of the biological test [21,22], it has been widely recommended to draw blood after heparin discontinuation. The advisable delay depends on the route of administration and the kind of heparin used.

Although there are many obvious differences between plasma and serum which could affect the result of the test, to our knowledge, no systematic comparison has been reported. When serum is used, heat inactivation in order to destroy thrombin is mandatory (this will also destroy complement). However aggregation of IgGs might also ensue, and aggregated IgGs do stimulate normal platelets through binding to CD32.

2. Platelets

First care must be taken that the final (after dilution with patient's sample) concentration of platelets in the assay is sufficiently high (preferably at least.250 x 10^9 / L)

Second the considerable variability among donors of the platelet response to the HD-PAF [23-25] seems to be mainly related to the CD32-dependent pathway [10,26]. The use of platelets with a prompt response to a carefully selected murine monoclonal antibody which activates platelets in a Fc/CD32-dependent manner[27] might help.

3. Heparin

The unimodal relationship between the concentration of heparin and the platelet functional response in the presence of a HAT patient's sample is now well known. The two-point assay (positive result with a "therapeutic" concentration, negative with 100 U / mL) has been proposed[15] to improve the specificity and to overcome the problem generated by the residual amounts of heparin that may be present in patient's sample (under such a circumstance, a positive result might be obtained without further addition of heparin in vitro). The removals from the sample of heparin by using commercial reagent is another possibility.

The use of the heparin the patient has received (even same lot) has been recommended, but it appeared that the reaction can occur with a variety of polysulfated polysaccharides[28], and even non-saccharadic but negatively charged macromolecules[9]. Nevertheless it remains possible that heterogeneity among heparin preparations for therapeutic use leads to different outcomes[3], both in vivo and in vitro, especially if poorly responsive normal platelets are used to detect a low titer HD-PAF.

E. PRACTICAL RECOMMENDATIONS REGARDING HAT

1/ The platelet count must be checked in order to rule out pseudo-thrombocytopenia due to anticoagulant- or temperature- dependent agglutinins[29].

2/ A biologic test is useful for every patient with thrombocytopenia and/or thrombosis during heparin therapy, mainly in order to manage them on a long term basis (at risk for requiring future parenteral anticoagulation). Despite the apparent simplicity of the platelet aggregation test (using donor platelets not isolated from plasma), there are several pitfalls, and it seems wise to restrict its performance to laboratories used to carrying out platelet function tests. Moreover one should be aware of the potential difficulties of testing a sample still containing heparin. The use of non-washed platelets from normal donors seems acceptable, but the experimental conditions mentioned above should be rigidly followed. Healthy donors for platelets must be carefully selected, in order to improve the sensitivity of the test; in particular, platelets must be reactive to CD32-dependent stimuli.

3/ When a seemingly questionable result is obtained (on technical grounds or considering the patient's clinical data), (i) a sample should be referred to a laboratory that performs a test with washed platelets; (ii) the test can be repeated with another patient's blood sample collected a few days later. In the latter case, its is worthwhile to concomitantly run the two samples with the same donor's platelets.

4/ It has been suggested that in vitro testing is required before using a low molecular weight heparin (LMWH), or to the compound Orgaran, in a patient thrombocytopenic while receiving unfractionated heparin and requiring further anticoagulation. Such a recommendation is difficult to be formally validated. Furthermore a high rate of "cross-reaction" is expected when a sensitive assay is used[5,10]. Orgaran is often preferred to LMWH[5]; heparins and heparinoïds can be ranked according to their interactions with platelets in vitro, and presumably in vivo: unfractionated > low molecular weight > Orgaran[5,10]. The use of rapidly acting antithrombotic drugs not chemically related to heparin, such as ancrod or hirudin or argatroban, seem to be the best choice, but unfortunately these drugs are not yet readily available to most clinical centres in the world.

5/ When facing complex settings (threatening thombosis, re-exposure) it is advisable to refer the patient to centres used to managing such cases, where the different needed skills are gathered.

II. ANTI-STREPTOKINASE ANTIBODIES AND PLATELET FUNCTION

Streptokinase is a foreign protein, produced by ß-hemolytic streptococci, clinically used as a thrombolytic agent. Antibodies to SK may appear in the blood either as the result of streptococcal infection, or of treatment with SK[30,31]. In the latter case, an increase up to 100-fold in antibody titers has been reported[32,33].

These antibodies have been known for a long time since they may neutralize the ability of SK to activate plasminogen into plasmin[34], being responsible for the so called resistance to SK: hence they are called SK-neutralizing antibodies. Furthermore SK is cleared rapidly from the circulation when complexed with specific immunoglobulins[30].

Platelet activation is another functional property of anti-SK antibodies, suspected after one anecdotal report of thrombus propagation within coronary arteries of a patient with acute myocardial infarction and receiving SK[35]. The prevalence of such anti-SK antibodies might be quite high, since the addition of 5,000 units / mL of SK to platelet-rich plasma caused aggregation for 14 out of 100 normal subjects[36]. When SK is added to platelet-rich plasma in vitro, the effect is generally inhibition of platelet aggregation by classical agonists such as ADP; this inhibition is mainly related to fibrinogenolysis[37,38]. With the PRP of some subjects however, a suitable (rather high) concentration of SK may trigger aggregation[39]. A lower concentration of SK (1,000 units / mL) was reported to potentiate the aggregating effect of ADP on platelets of some, but not all, subjects[40]. Platelet aggregation occurs much more frequently in whole blood than in PRP, presumably because there are additional pro-aggregatory factors in the former milieu[41].

The antibodies able to activate and aggregate platelets could be different from those inhibiting the lytic effect of SK. The immune complexes (in fact, ternary complexes of plasminogen • SK • anti-SK) would bind to platelets since SK binds to plasminogen and plasminogen has binding sites on platelets[36].

We have shown, by using purified (by means of affinity chromatography) anti-SK IgGs and washed human platelets, that activation requires plasminogen, is complement independent, and involves the interaction of the Fc portion of the IgG with the CD32 molecule[39]. The role of CD32 has been also suggested by Heptinstall et al.[42]

Previous treatment with SK is a contra-indication to its re-use, because of the high titers in SK-neutralizing antibodies[33]; one should also now consider the potential deleterious effects of platelet activation by the above-mentioned ternary complex. It remains to be studied whether the presence, as a result of infection, of the subset of anti-SK antibodies which can activate platelets, might influence the clinical outcome after SK administration. In a study involving 333 patients treated with SK or anistreplase (anisoylated lys-plasminogen SK activator complex) for acute myocardial infarction, no influence of pretreatment anti-SK antibody levels on angiographic or clinical end-points was evidenced; anti-SK antibody levels were measured however by means of a radioimmunoassay[43]. Aspirin is currently widely used in association with SK in acute myocardial infarction, but might not be always sufficient to block the immune mediated platelet activation[40]. Finally it should be noticed that thrombocytopenia is not recorded as an adverse reaction to SK infusion, and thus the platelet activating immunoglobulins G related to SK and to heparin might not be totally similar; it is intriguing however that in a patient summary given as an example of nonimmune HAT by Warkentin and Kelton[3], thrombocytopenia occurred early after SK administration.

REFERENCES

1. **Rubinstein E., Boucheix C., Worthington R. E., Caroll R. C.**, Anti-platelet antibody interactions with Fc gamma receptor, *Sem. Thromb. Hemost.*, 21, 10, 1995.
2. **Chong B. H., Berndt M. C.**, Heparin-induced thrombocytopenia, *Blut*, 58, 53, 1989.
3. **Warkentin T. E., Kelton J. G.**, Interaction of heparin with platelets, including heparin-induced thrombocytopenia, in *Low-molecular weight heparins in prophylaxis and therapy of thromboembolic diseases*, Bounameaux H., Ed., Marcel Dekker, Inc, New York, Basel, Hong Kong, 1994, 75.
4. **Lecompte T., Luo S. K., Stieltjes N., Lecrubier C., Samama M. M.**, Thrombocytopenia associated with low molecular weight heparin, *Lancet*, 338, 1217, 1991.
5. **Greinacher A.**, Antigen generation in heparin-associated thrombocytopenia: the nonimmunologic type and the immunologic type are closely linked in their pathogenesis, *Semin. Thromb. Hemost.*, 21, 106, 1995.
6. **Amiral J., Bridey F., Dreyfus M., et al**, Platelet factor 4 complexed to heparin is the target for antibodies generated in heparin-induced thrombocytopenia, *Thromb. Haemost.*, 68, 95, 1992.
7. **Greinacher A., Pötzsch B., Amiral J., et al**, Heparin-associated thrombocytopenia: isolation of the antibody and characterization of a multimolecular PF4-heparin complex as the major antigen, *Thromb. Haemostas.*, 71, 247, 1994.
8. **Visentin G. P., Ford S. E., Scott J. P., Aster R. H.**, Antibodies from patients with heparin-induced thrombocytopenia / thrombosis are specific for platelet factor 4 complexed with heparin or bound to endothelial cells. *J. Clin. Invest.*, 93, 81, 1994.
9. **Anderson G. P.**, Insights into heparin-induced thrombocytopenia, *Br. J. Haematol.*, 80, 504, 1992.
10. **Lecompte T., Stieljes N., Luo S. K., et al**, Heparin- and streptokinase-dependent platelet-activating immunoglobulin G: mechanism and diagnosis, *Semin. Thromb. Hemost.*, 21, 95, 1995.
11. **Chong B. H., Ismail F., Cade J., et al**, Heparin-induced thrombocytopenia: studies with a new low molecular weight heparinoid, Org 10172, *Blood*, 73, 1592, 1989.
12. **Warkentin T. E., Kelton J. G.**, Heparin-induced thrombocytopenia, in *Progress in Hemostasis and Thrombosis*, Coller B., Ed., 1991, 1.

13.   **Greinacher A., Amiral J., Dummel V., et al.**, Laboratory diagnosis of heparin-associated thrombocytopenia and comparison of platelet aggregation test, heparin-induced platelet activation test, and platelet factor 4 / heparin enzyme-linked immunosorbent assay, *Transfusion*, 34, 381, 1994.

14.   **Kelton J. G., Sheridan D., Brain H., et al.**, Clinical usefulness of testing for a heparin-dependent platelet-aggregating factor in patients with suspected heparin-associated thrombocytopenia, *J. Lab. Clin. Med.*, 103, 606, 1984.

15.   **Sheridan D., Carter C., Kelton J. G.**, A diagnostic test for heparin-induced thrombocytopenia, *Blood*, 67, 27, 1986.

16.   **Nguyen P., Lecompte T., et le Groupe d'Etude sur l'Hémostase et la Thrombose (GEHT) de la Société Française d'Hématologie**, Heparin-induced thrombocytopenia: a survey of tests employed and attitudes in haematology laboratories, *Nouv. Rev. Fr. Hematol.* 36, 353, 1994.

17.   **Lecrubier C, Lecompte T., Potevin F., et al.**, Heparin-induced thrombocytopenia: methodological and diagnostic problems and therapeutics aspects (a study of 26 cases), *J. Mal. Vasc.*, 12, 128, 1987.

18.   **Chong B. H., Burgess J., Ismail F.**, The clinical usefulness of the platelet aggregation test for the diagnosis of heparin-induced thrombocytopenia, *Thromb. Haemost.*, 69, 344, 1993.

19.   **Greinacher A., Michels I., Kiefel V., Mueller-Eckhardt C.**, A rapid and sensitive test for diagnosing heparin-associated thrombocytopenia, *Thromb. Haemostas.*, 66, 734, 1991.

20.   **Warkentin T. E., Levine M. N., Hirsh J., et al.**, Heparin-induced thrombocytopenia in patients treated with low-molecular-weight heparin or unfractionated heparin, *N. Engl. J. Med.*, 332, 1330, 1995.

21.   **Gibson J., Uhr E., P Motum P., Rickard K. A., Kronenberg H.**, Platelet aggregometry for the diagnosis of heparin induced thrombocytopenia-thrombosis syndrome, *Pathology*, 19, 105, 1987.

22.   **Mc Cabe White M., Siders L., Jennings L. K., White F. L.**, The effect of residual heparin on the interpretation of heparin-induced platelet aggregation in the diagnosis of heparin-associated thrombocytopenia, *Thromb. Haemost.*, 68, 88, 1992.

23.   **Salem H. H., van de Weyden M. B.**, Heparin-induced thrombocytopenia: variable platelet rich plasma reactivity to heparin dependent platelet aggregating factor, *Pathology*, 15, 297, 1983.

24.   **Pfueller S.L., David R.**, Different platelet specificities of heparin-dependent platelet aggregating factors in heparin-associated immune thrombocytopenia, *Br. J. Haematol.*, 64, 149, 1986.

25.   **Isenhart C. G., Brandt J. T.**, Platelet aggregation studies for the diagnosis of heparin-induced thrombocytopenia, *Am. J. Clin. Pathol.*, 1993, 324, 1993.

26.   **Warkentin T. E., Hayward C. P. M., Smith C. A., Kelly P. M., Kelton J. G.**, Determinants of donor platelet variability when testing for heparin-induced thrombocytopenia, *J. Lab. Clin. Med.*, 120, 371, 1992.

27.   **Morel M. C., Lecompte T., Champeix P., et al**, A monoclonal murine antibody, PL2-49, which is a platelet activator, *Br. J. Haematol.*, 71, 57, 1989.

28.   **Greinacher A., Michels I., Mueller-Eckhardt C.**, Heparin-associated thrombocytopenia: the antibody is not heparin specific, *Thromb. Haemost.*, 67, 545, 1992.

29.   **Farkas J. C., Brossel C., Boyer J. M., Brisset D., Laurian C.**, Cold-reactive platelet agglutinins, *Thromb. Haemost.*, 70, 879, 1993.

30.   **Fletcher A. P., Alkjaersig N., Sherry S.**, The clearance of heterologous protein from the circulation of normal and immunized man, *J. Clin. Invest.*, 37, 1306, 1958.

31.   **Spöttl F., Kaiser R.**, Rapid detection and quantitation of precipitating streptokinase-antibodies, *Thrombos. Diathes. Haemorrh.*, 32, 608, 1974.

32.   **Lynch M., Littler W. A., Pentecost B. L., Stockley R. A.**, Immunoglobulin response to intravenous streptokinase in acute myocardial infarction, *Br. Heart J.*, 66, 139, 1991.

33.   **Declerck P. J., Vanderschueren S., Billiet J., Moreau H., Collen D.**, Prevalence and induction of circulating antibodies against recombinant staphylokinase, *Thromb. Haemost.* 71, 129, 1994.

34.   **Tillet W., Edwards L., Garner R.**, Fibrinolytic activity of hemolytic streptocci. The development of resistance to fibrinolysis following acute streptococcus infection, *J. Clin. Invest.*, 13, 47, 1934.

35.   **Vaughan D. E., Kirshenbaum J. M., Loscalzo J.**, Streptokinase-induced, antibody-mediated platelet aggregation: A potential cause of clot propagation in vivo, *J. Am. Coll. Cardiol.*, 11, 1343, 1988.

36.   **Vaughan D. E., van Houtte E., Declerck P. J., Collen D.**, Streptokinase-induced platelet aggregation. Prevalence and mechanism, *Circulation*, 84, 84, 1991.

37.   **Gouin I., Lecompte T., Morel M. C., et al**, In vitro effect of plasmin on human platelet function in plasma. Inhibition of aggregation caused by fibrinogenolysis, *Circulation*, 85, 935, 1992.

38.   **Lebrazi J., Abdelouahed M., Mirshahi M., Samama M.M., Lecompte T.**, Streptokinase and APSAC inhibit platelet aggregation in vitro by fibrinogenolysis: Effect of plasma fibrinogen degradation products X and E, *Fibrinolysis*, 9, 113, 1995.

39.   **Lebrazi J., Helft G., Mirshahi M., Samama M. M., Lecompte T.**, L'agrégation plaquettaire induite par les IgGs anti-streptokinase nécessite l'interaction du domaine Fc avec le récepteur plaquettaire FcfiRII/CD32, *Nouv. Rev. Fr. Hematol.*, 36, 29, 1994.

40.   **Terres W., Krüger K., Bleifeld W.**, Prevalence and mechanism of streptokinase-induced platelet stimulation. Effect of acetylsalicylic acid, *Eur. Heart J.*, 13, 1514, 1992.

41.   **Heptinstall S., Berridge D. C., Judge H.**, Effects of streptokinase and recombinant tissue plasminogen activator on platelet aggregation in whole blood, *Platelets*, 1, 177, 1990.

42.   **Heptinstall S., Sanderson H. M., Fox S., et al.**, Factors that potentiate or inhibit platelet activation by streptokinase, *Thromb. Haemost.*, 69, 1074, 1993.

43.   **Fears R., Hearn J., Standring R., JL Anderson J. L., Marder V. J.**, Lack of influence of pretreatment antistreptokinase antibody on efficacy in a multicenter patency comparison of intravenous streptokinase and anistreplase in acute myocardial infarction, *Am. Heart. J.*, 124, 305, 1992.

WARFARIN INDUCED HYPERCOAGULABILITY: STANDARDISATION OF LABORATORY ASPECTS AND MANAGEMENT OF SKIN NECROSIS

M.J. Seghatchian* and M.M. Samama **
* NBS, Colindale, London ; ** Hôtel-Dieu, University Hospital, Paris

I. INTRODUCTION

Oral anticoagulant therapy with vitamin K antagonists is widely used as the method of choice in the prevention/treatment of thrombotic disease[1-3]. There are at least two distinct groups of vitamin K antagonists: the coumarin derivatives (e.g. Warfarin) and Indanedione derivative (e.g. phenindione). Warfarin is the anticoagulant of choice in North America and in many other countries. Its biological half life is about 35h [1]. It is now well established that Warfarin intake rapidly decreases circulating protein C activity (with a half life of about 6-7h), in relation to factors IX, X, II and protein S. This leads to an imbalance in the natural anticoagulant capability of blood, with occasional consequence of thrombosis, in particular during the initial phase of oral anticoagulation[1-3].

Pharmacology of orally ingested Warfarin has also been the focus of much intensive study[1,4]. According to Kelly et al[4] Warfarin is completely absorbed, with peak plasma concentration within 30 minutes to 9 hours after ingestion of drug. It appears that 99% of Warfarin binds to albumin in the plasma, hence the volume of distribution of Warfarin is identical to that of the albumin space[4]. Only the free Warfarin is therapeutically active, therefore concurrent administration of drugs or therapeutic products which compete with Warfarin for binding to albumin, or compounds which inhibit Warfarin metabolism, may markedly influence its anticoagulant effect[1-4]. Warfarin undergoes metabolic transformation in the liver. Drugs which interact with Warfarin may also influence the stereoselective inhibition of Warfarin metabolism, affecting the outcome of therapy (see refs 2,4 for review).

The clinical importance of certain laboratory observations of Warfarin is still incompletely understood. A rapid depression of the components of the protein C system is thought to contribute to the pathogenesis of Warfarin induced - hypercoagulability and skin necrosis. These are rare but devastating side effects of Warfarin[5,6]. The optimal anticoaglation effect of Warfarin is delayed until the normal vitamin K proteins are cleared from the circulation (between 36 to 72 hours after drug administration)[7]. The induced hypercoagulability commonly occurs in the early phase due to a differential rate of clearance of the functionally active vitamin K dependent protein C and/or alteration in its activation states[8]. Factors V and VIII are also activated during this period, supporting the view that thrombin is produced during the early phase of anticoagulation[8]. Care also should be taken during the withdrawal period as imbalance between procoagulant and anticoagulant vitamin K dependent proteins, induced by differential rate of synthesis/clearance, can also lead to thrombotic complications[9,10]. Care also should be taken during the institution of Warfarin therapy to prevent skin necrosis.

This chapter highlights some unresolved aspects of laboratory monitoring of the therapeutic range, focusing on the standardisation of prothrombin time (PT). The recent use of recombinant tissue factor (RTF) compared to human placenta-derived conventional tissue factor (HPD-CTF) is summarised. The issue of induced hypercoagulability and skin necrosis is briefly discussed, including its prevention and treatment.

II. STANDARDISATION ASPECTS OF THERAPEUTIC RANGE

Since Warfarin inhibits the vitamin K-dependent synthesis of factors II, VII, IX and X the best laboratory test used to monitor Warfarin therapy is the prothrombin time. It is sometimes forgotten that the main attribute of a laboratory investigation is primarily to be reproducible while the accuracy or closeness to the "true" value is secondary. Thus it is important to obtain reproducible results with consistency, wherever the test is performed, manually or by automated methodology.

A. Reproducibility and uniformity in Standard :

There are may ways to achieve reproducibility: i) develop reference methods. This often goes against habit, making the implementation of the modifications rather difficult. ii) identify the shortcoming through collaborative studies. Although Inter-laboratory studies are important for achieving laboratory comparability, from a standardisation point of view the apparently simple global tests such as PT are actually the hardest to standardise. The measurements have two major sources of variability. These are the reagents (different thromboplastins) and the methods (instruments) which may lead to different absolute results even if the ratio of control to test is the same.

The basic problem which remains to be resolved is how to convert a clotting time to an internationally agreed scale, when different reagents and instruments are used in different areas of the world. The establishment of an International Reference Thromboplastin and reporting the data in terms of International Normalised Ratio (INR) is one step in the right direction[2,6]. In practice however, there are a multiplicity of different reference thromboplastins having different sensitivity. The International Sensitivity Index (ISI) is used so that separate thromboplastins may be cross calibrated[11,12] and the prothrombin time is then expressed in terms of ISI for the reagent used. This may add complexity and confusion rather than resolving it. Some manufacturers of thromboplastin reagents have been changing the sensitivity of their thromboplastins from more intense to less intense ISI. Therefore, a typical thromboplastin reagent does not truly exist [13]. The INR system is supposed to overcome such a heterogeneity.

Moreover, with recent technological advances using capillary blood samples, the self monitoring of Warfarin therapy by the patient at home becomes feasible[14,15]. In one randomised trial, patients doing home monitoring achieved superior anticoagulant control in the range of 2.0. - 3.0 INR compared with those receiving standard clinical care. This difference was related to subtherapy in home monitoring[14] as the accuracy of the portable prothrombin time monitor was found to be best at an INR of 3.0[16]. While the accuracy and precision of the portable prothrombin time monitor justify its usage, a randomised clinical trial is needed to ascertain the clinical effectiveness and safety of this instrument in the outpatient clinic. Another important issue is to establish whether low dose Warfarin is in effect safe in certain subclinical/clinical settings. Low dose could eliminate dose adjustment, which would also eliminate the inconvenience for both patient and laboratory and the cost of laboratory monitoring. As far as the reagents are concerned, it is fair to say that the availability of non-standardised commercial reagents with different sensitivity contributed to an increased frequency of bleeding complications and discrepancies between the USA and European laboratories[2,6]. Hence the way forward is thought to be to simplify the calibration process by developing reference plasmas which can be used instead of the patient samples. This approach is under active consideration by international bodies.

B. Recombinant Versus Conventional Thromboplastin:

With the availability of recombinant tissue factor (RTF) a highly defined, sensitive and reproducible reagent, with enormous potential as the standard thromboplastin reagent for monitoring oral anticoagulation, attention was focused on comparative analysis.

In a French multicenter collaborative study[17], we have evaluated the effect of recombiplastin. This is a clear water soluble human tissue factor solution, without any particulate matter, (produced by Ortho Diagnostics from Baculevirus and relipidated with a highly purified phospholid) in different clinical settings. The prothrombin time in seconds and in INR was assessed for reliability by intra and inter laboratory evaluation. Several participating laboratories determined on each of 10 days on KC10 (Baxter Instrument) PT of the usual normal plasma pool calibration curve, 3 identical calibration plasmas, and plasmas from 20 normal and 50 patients on oral anticoagulant therapy. Comparison was made with two other commercial extraction thromboplastins (so called ISI #1 & ISI #2). In each conflicting data factors VII, X and V were also measured. In normals, PT values were comparable for the 3 reagents but in plasma from anticoagulated patients the longest time (64.2 sec) was observed with RTF as compared to neoplastin (32.8 sec) and thromborell (54.4 sec). Furthermore, RTF was found to be the most sensitive reagent for factors VII and X deficiency. The correlation coefficient between RTF:INR and the INR from other reagents was good (0.85 <R <0.95). However the slope produced break point in the regression curve when INR was above 3.0. This emphasises the need for a new set of norms to be established for RTF to help clinicians in their decision making, if such a preparation has developed wide spread usage. The RTF was found to be stable and there was no difference in sensitivity after the 24h incubation, at 37°C. Thus the use of such a product would be helpful in a standardisation and harmonisation program.

Finazzi et al[18] carried out a prospective randomised double blind clinical trial in a single centre to compare the clinical and laboratory quality of oral anticoagulant therapy using RTF and a human placenta-derived conventional thromboplastin (HPD-CTF). On 757 consecutive patients receiving OA for various indications the therapeutic INR was found to be in the same proportion (70.2% vs 68.8%). The incidence of bleeding was 18.5 versus 16.5% for RTF and HPD-CTF patients respectively.

Brien et al[19] evaluated a new synthetic reagent (innovin[TM], Baxter Diagnostics Inc.) and found that at higher INR values, some discrepant results were observed with innovin[TM] compared to HPD-CTF. This supports the earlier finding of Bader et al[20], based on a multicenter evaluation of a new reagent based on RTF and synthetic phospholipids. These variations were attributed to instruments used and the calculation of sensitivity to depletion of vitamin K dependent factors, especially factor VII, in the upper therapeutic range of some anticoagulant patients[20].

These trials indicate that RTF is as effective and as highly sensitive as conventional reagent in monitoring oral anticoagulation, however the source of thromboplastin (recombinant vs extractive) may have some relevant clinical impact for the therapeutic regimen, adding another complexity to the INR equation[17].

III. CLINICAL ASPECTS

Skin necrosis is a complication which occurs during the early phase of oral anticoagulant intake, when the rapid decrease in protein C, due to its short half-life (6 to 7h) leads to thrombosis in the microvasculature. Other factors such as the levels of thrombomodulin/thrombin complex, the potent activator of protein C and protein S may play a role in induced hypercoagulability. The half life of protein S is relatively longer (24h), than the protein C half life. Skin necrosis has been observed in rare patients with congenital protein C deficiency especially in homozygous individuals and exceptional cases of heterozygous patients with protein S deficiency [21-24].

Acquired deficiency of protein C/S often reflects either some pathological states (e.g. liver disease, DIC, respiratory distress syndrome, acute leukaemia, post-operative period, lupus-like anticoagulant) or drug-induced abnormalities such as from L-Asparaginase and Vitamin K-antagonists[25]. The most likely explanation for this, for example, in DIC phenomena is that protein C becomes activated, possibly by thrombin forming complexes with its inhibitors, and rapidly cleaned from the circulation[25]. The decrease in circulating protein C, due to oral anticoagulant, is different, as during the early phase protein C is cleared relatively fast[26] while other vitamin K dependent factors (except factor VII) remain relatively unchanged in the short term. This can lead to a poor antithrombotic effect during the early phase of anticoagulant therapy and/or the occurrence of skin necrosis in particular in protein C deficiency[21]. The fall in protein C level may be associated with formation of a certain intermediate complex between components of a protein C modulatory system. The risk of Warfarin induced skin necrosis in protein S deficiency is minimal as protein S has a relatively longer half life (24h).

To prevent skin necrosis in patients with severe congenital protein C deficiency, a low initial dose of oral anticoagulant is recommended. Administer heparin concomitantly for 7 to 10 days while progressively increasing the oral anticoagulant dose as needed[22]. Protein C concentrates have been used in anecdotal cases of protein C deficiency at the initiation of oral anticoagulant treatment to prevent skin necrosis[27].

In newborns with purpura fulminans, fresh frozen plasma (10ml/Kg, twice a day) for at least 4 to 10 weeks is indicated until all the necrotic lesions disappear. Warfarin is then used for long term treatment, with the PT maintained at an INR of 2.5-4.0. The infusion of FFP should be maintained without overloading until satisfactory prolongation of PT is achieved [26]. An alternative strategy is 100U/Kg protein C concentrate every 48h over a period of 9 months, allowing the complete resolution of the thrombotic conditions[28,29]. In adults with homozygous protein C deficiency, Conard et al [30] found a normalization of coagulation activation with a purified protein C concentrate

IV. CONCLUSION

Warfarin in the early phase of anticoagulation therapy has a dramatic effect on protein C synthesis (by introducing abnormal molecules) and on its activation states. The latter influences its overall regulatory mechanism. Any acquired deficiency in protein C, including Warfarin induced abnormality, is likely to contribute to thrombotic tendencies, identifiable by increased levels of markers of hypercoagulability associated with thrombin generation, including the release of prothrombin fragment 1+2 and protein C activation peptide. While PT measurement remains as the essential assay for monitoring the therapeutic dose of Warfarin, standardisation of this assay remains unresolved, despite the use of recombinant tissue factor. Skin necrosis is a rare but dramatic side effect of oral anticoagulant treatment, the mechanism of which is now becoming understood. At the initiation of an oral anticoagulant, a transient hypercoagulable state can occur specially in patients with protein C deficiency. Protein C concentrates may prove useful for the prevention and treatment of this particular complication of warfarin therapy.

ACKNOWLEDGEMENT

The authors wish to express their sincere thanks to Usha Mistry for typing and rearranging this manuscript.

REFERENCES

1.   **Freedman, M.D.** Oral anticoagulants: pharmacodynamics, clinical indications and adverse effects, *J. Clin. Pharmacol.*, 32, 196, 1992.
2.   **Hirsh, J., Dalen, J.E., Deykin, D., et al.** Oral anticoagulants. Mechanism of action, clinical effectiveness and optimal therapeutic range. *Chest.* 120, 312S, 1992.
3.   **Cook, D.J., Guyatt, G.H., Laupacis, A., et al.** Rules of evidence and clinical recommendation on the use of antithrombtic agents, *Chest*, 102, 305S, 1992.
4.   **Kelly, J.G., and O'Malley, K.** Clinical pharmacokinetics of oral anticoagulants, *J. Clin. Pharmacokinetics*, 4, 1, 1979.
5.   **Clouse, L.H. and Comp, P.C.** The regulation of haemostasis: The protein C system, *N. Engl. J. Med.*, 314, 1298, 1986.
6.   **Loellger, E.A.** The optimal therapeutic range in oral anticoagulation. History and proposal, *Thromb. haemostasis,* 42, 1141, 1979.
7.   **D'Angelo, S.V., Comp. P.C., Esmon, C.T., et al.** Relationship between protein C antigen and anticoagulant activity during oral anticoagulation and in selected disease states, *J. Clin. Invest.*, 77, 416, 1986.
8.   **Stirling, Y., and Seghatchian, M.J.** Further studies in the heterogeneity of protein C in normal and Warfarinised plasmas, evaluated by crossed immunoelectropheresis, *Br. J. Haematol.*, 71 (Suppl. 1), 34, 1989.
9.   **Conard, J., Horellou, M.H., van Dreden, P., et al.** Homozygous protein C deficiency with late onset and recurrent coumarin-induced skin necrosis, *Lancet*, 339, 743, 1992.
10.   **Conway, E.M., Bauer, K.A., Barzegar, S., et al.** Suppression of hemostatic system activation by oral anticoagulants in the blood of patients with thrombotic diatheses, *J. Clin. Invest.*, 80, 1535, 1987.
11.   **Wright, I., Marple, C.D., and Bech, D.F.** Report of the Committee for the Evaluation of Anticoagulants in the Treatment of Coronary Thrombosis with Myocardial Infraction. *Am. Heart J.*, 36, 801, 1948.
12.   **Hirsh, J.** Is the dose of Warfarin prescribed by American physicians unnecessarily high? *Arch. Intern. Med.*, 147, 769, 1987.
13.   **Bussey, H.I., Force, R.W., Bianco, T.M., and Leonard, A.D.** Reliance on prothrombin time ratios causes significant errors in anticoagulation therapy. *Arch. intern. Med.*, 152, 278, 1992.
14.   **Ansell, J., Holden, A. And Knapk, N.** Patient self-management or oral anticoagulation guided by capillary (fingerstick) whole blood prothrombin times. *Arch. Intern. Med.*, 149, 2509, 1989.
15.   **White, R.H., McCurdy, S.A., von Marensdorff, H., et al.** Home prothrombin time monitoring after the initiation of Warfarin therapy. A randomised, prospective study. *Ann. Intern. Med.*, 111, 730, 1989.
16.   **McCurdy, S.A., White, R.H.** Accuracy and precision of a portable anticoagulation monitor in a clinical setting. *Arch. Intern. Med.*, 152, 589, 1992.
17.   **Roussi, J., Drouet, L., Samama M., Sié, P.,** French multicentric evaluation of recombinant tissue factor (recombiplastin) for determination of prothrombin time. *Thromb. Haemostas.*, 72, 698-704, 1994.
18.   **Finazzia, A., Falanga, A., Galli, M. et al.** Recombinant versus high-sensitivity conventional thromboplastin: A randomised clinical study in patients on oral anticoagulant. *Thromb. Haemost.* 72, 804, 1994.
19.   **Brien, W.F., Crawford, L., Wood, D.E.** Discrepant results in INR testing. *Thromb. Haemost.* 76, 985, 1994.
20.   **Bader, R., Mannucci, P.M., Tripodi, A., et al.** Multicentric evaluation of a new PT reagent based on recombinant human tissue factor. *Thromb. Haemost.* 71, 292, 1994.
21.   **Broekmans, A.W., Bertian, A.M., Loeliger, E.A., et al.** Protein C and the development of skin necrosis during anticoagulant therapy. *Thromb. Haemost.* 49, 251, 1983.
22.   **Samama, M., Horellou, M.H., Soria, J., et al.** Successful progressive anticoagulation in a severe protein C deficiency and previous skin necrosis at the initiation of oral anticoagulant treatment. *Thromb. Haemost.* 51, 132, 1984.

23. **Conard, J., Horellou, M.H., Van Dreden, P., et al.** Homozygous protein C deficiency with late onset and reccurent coumarin-induced skin-necrosis. *Lancet,* 339, 743-744, 1992.

24. **Grimaudo, V., Gueissaz, F., Hauert, J., et al .** Necrosis of skin induced by coumarin in a patient deficient in protein S. *Br Med J,* 298,233,1989.

25. **Mannucci, P.M., and Viagano, S.** Deficiencies of protein C, an inhibitor of blood coagulation. *Lancet.* ii, 463, 1982.

26. **Mimuro, J., Sakata, Y., Wakabayashi, K., et al.** Level of protein C determined by combined assays during disseminated intravascular coagulation and oral anticoagulation. *Blood.* 69,1704, 1987.

27. **Dreyfus M, Magny JF, Bridey F, Schwarz HP, Panche C, Dehan M, Tchernia G.** Treatment of homozygous protein C deficiency and neonatal purpura fulminans with a purified protein C concentrate. *N Engl J Med,* 325, 1565, 1991.

28. **Marlar, R.A., Montgomery, R.R., Broekmans, A.W.** and the Working Party. Diagnosis and treatment of homozygous protein C deficiency. *J. Pediatr.* 114, 528, 1989.

29. **Vukovich, T., Auberger, K., Weil, J., et al.** Replacement therapy for a homozygous protein C deficiency-state using a concentrate of human protein C and S. *Br. j. Haematol.* 70, 435, 1988.

30. **Conard, J., Bauer, K.A., Gruber, A., et al.** Normalization of markers of coagulation activation with a purified protein C concentrate in adults with homozygous protein C deficiency. *Blood,* 82, 1159-1164, 1993.

PARADOXICAL HYPERCOAGULABILITY INDUCED BY THROMBOLYTIC DRUGS

G. Helft*, MM. Samama**
*Clinique Cardiologique Hôpital Necker, Paris
**Service d'Hématologie biologique, Hôtel-Dieu, Paris

Coronary artery disease leading to myocardial infarction is a major cause of death and disability.The triggering event is thrombotic obstruction of a coronary artery. One approach to the restoration of vascular continuity is pharmacologic dissolution of the blood clot. Currently, six thrombolytic agents are either approved for clinical use or under clinical investigation in patients with acute myocardial infarction. These are: streptokinase, anisoylated plasminogen streptokinase activator complex (APSAC), recombinant tissue plasminogen activator (rt-PA), urokinase, recombinant single chain u-PA (pro-urokinase) and staphylokinase. Reduction of infarct size, preservation of ventricular function and significant reduction in mortality have been obtained from the earlier thrombolytic agents used,[1,2] and are highly probable for the newer ones. Consequently, thrombolytic therapy has become a standard component of the treatment of acute myocardial infarction.

The benefits of coronary thrombolysis depend on achieving and maintaining coronary artery patency. But failure of coronary thrombolysis or recurrent occlusion occurs in up to 40% of patients treated with thrombolytics. In the Gusto angiographic study, flow through the infarct-related artery 90 minutes after the initiation of thrombolytic therapy was normal in only 54% of the group given t-PA and heparin. Reocclusion between the 90th minute and the fifth day occurred in about 6%.[3] This secondary occlusion could be related to the fact that despite their powerful activity, thrombolytic agents may paradoxically activate the coagulation system.

Rapid and complete restoration of flow through the infarct-related coronary artery results in improved ventricular performance and lower mortality among patients with acute myocardial infarction. Reocclusion of the infarct artery negates the potential benefits associated with early reperfusion. The pathophysiological basis for reocclusion is therefore important to understand and combat. The mechanisms are probably the same as for initial thrombotic occlusion: severe stenosis, disruption of the intimal surface, increased shear forces, and exposed surface thrombin promoting platelet activation and coagulation.

The importance of inhibition of procoagulant activity following successful coronary thrombolysis has recently been documented. Additional reduction of mortality in patients treated with various thrombolytics for myocardial infarction requires inhibition of platelet activation with aspirin and it may be further reduced by adjunctive anticoagulation with intravenous heparin. According to the Gusto study comparing four thrombolytic strategies for acute myocardial infarction, the lowest mortality was obtained from accelerated t-PA and intravenous heparin.[4] Previous studies[5] have shown that heparin enhanced the likelihood of persistent patency of the infarct artery optimizing the benefit of thrombolysis. Early and maintained patency of the infarct-related artery clearly improved survival after myocardial infarction.

Presumably, the benefits conferred by adjunctive antithrombotic regimens are attributable to prevention of recurrent coronary thrombosis. The mechanisms responsible for recurrent thrombosis after coronary thrombolysis are complex and numerous. They are not fully known but include increased procoagulant activity induced by pharmacological activation of plasminogen, local expression of procoagulant activity when the vessel is reperfused, presence of high shear forces that promote platelet deposition, and attenuation of physiologic fibrinolytic activity after pharmacologic thrombolysis.[6] Thus, recurrent thrombosis after coronary thrombolysis depends on a complex interaction between procoagulant factors associated with the atherosclerotic plaque, procoagulant activity induced by the residual thrombus, and paradoxical procoagulant activity which pharmacological thrombolysis promotes.[7]

I. MECHANISMS OF PROTHROMBIN ACTIVATION
ACCOMPANYING THROMBOLYSIS

Elevated plasma levels of fibrinopeptide A[8,9] and of thrombin-antithrombin III complexes (TAT) [10-12] are found in patients in the first hours after the beginning of thrombolytic therapy. Patients with acute myocardial infarction treated with heparin only did not have these elevated plasma levels. These authors suggested that this paradoxical increase in thrombin activity after administration of thrombolytics may be responsible for reocclusion in some patients. Some investigators suggested that TAT levels occurring during thrombolytic therapy may serve as predictors of reocclusion.[9] For patients with thrombin-antithrombin III complex levels greater than 6 ng/ml 120 minutes into thrombolysis with urokinase or rt-PA, an unfavorable clinical course was predicted with 96.2% sensitivity and 93.1% specificity. This result was not confirmed by others[13] who found no significant difference in these coagulation parameters between patients with and without reinfarction. TAT complex concentration was not a useful indicator of reinfarction in the 543 patients studied and neither was the concentration of prothrombin activation fragments 1+2. This latter finding concerns the multicentre trial comparing saruplase (recombinant single-chain, non-glycosylated human pro-urokinase) and urokinase. Actually, evidence for continued thrombosis despite intense fibrinolysis is described for various thrombolytics. Increase in platelet support of thrombin generation after thrombolytic therapy by rt-PA is also reported.[14]

There is a strong relationship between the extent of clot lysis and the intensity of clot-associated procoagulant activity. Factors causing increase in procoagulant activity following thrombolysis include plasmin-mediated activation of coagulation factors, exposure of procoagulant factors bound to residual thrombus and platelet activation. The most important determinant of recurrent thrombosis seems to be the extent to which thrombin activity is increased. Indeed, generation of thrombin is the ultimate consequence of activation of coagulation, inducing the formation of fibrin, activation of platelets and increased activity of factors IXa and Xa by thrombin-mediated activation of cofactors V and VIII.

In vitro experiments indicated a possible mechanism. Increased fibrinopeptide A and TAT levels were found in normal plasma or uncoagulated blood after incubation with thrombolytics.[15] Eisenberg et al.[16] found that recalcified plasma incubated with various thrombolytic agents (streptokinase, urokinase, rt-PA) shortened the clotting time of a second plasma.[16] Clotting times of this second-stage plasma were more markedly accelerated by addition of first-stage plasma incubated with streptokinase and urokinase than by addition of plasma incubated with t-PA and was accelerated more with higher than with lower concentrations of each agent. These results confirm a causative relationship between the extent of plasminogen activation and the intensity of procoagulant activity induced. Other results suggested that in a purified system plasmin may induce a weak activation of factor X and a more pronounced direct activation of prothombin. Activation of prothrombin associated with stimulation of fibrinolysis has been demonstrated.[17]

Plasmin-dependent activation of factor X and subsequent activation of prothrombin is not the sole mechanism. Brommer[18] proposed that streptokinase, and to a lesser extent other thrombolytic agents, activates the prothrombinase complex directly or indirectly through a calcium-dependent mechanism, independent of the presence of plasminogen, with a resulting acceleration of thrombin generation.[18] Thrombin generation induced by the addition of thromboplastin together with calcium was greatly accelerated in the presence of thrombolytics (mainly with streptokinase). Similar effects were seen after activating the intrinsic pathway. Aprotinin did not affect the results. The effect of streptokinase was also observed in plasminogen-depleted plasma. The findings proved that thrombin generation induced by the intrinsic or extrinsic pathway is accelerated by streptokinase independent of the presence of plasminogen.

II. OTHER MECHANISMS

Plasminogen activators may attenuate the effects of heparin by depleting the heparin cofactor, antithrombin III.[19] An additional interaction that can contribute to an unfavorable imbalance between thrombosis and fibrinolysis is platelet release of plasminogen activator inhibitor type-1 (PAI-1) which can attenuate activity of endogenous plasminogen activators well after an administered pharmacologic fibrinolytic agent has been cleared from the circulation.[20] Another study provides some support for the idea that an increased synthesis of fibrinogen in circulation may result in a procoagulant tendency. If this is so, the high molecular weight fraction and phosphorylated fibrinopeptide A content may serve as a risk index for thrombosis.[21]

III. PROCOAGULANT ACTIVITY INDUCED BY THE RESIDUAL THROMBUS

This procoagulant activity is explained in part by the fact that thrombin binds to fibrin and remains bound to cross-linked fibrin within the thrombus. This bound thrombin is protected from inactivation by antithrombin III and may induce recurrent thrombosis.[22,23] Furthermore, proteolysis of fibrin caused by plasmin releases bound thrombin which can be secondarily active.[24] This can enhance the procoagulant state but the local procoagulant activity may be modulated by circulating factors. In addition to thrombin bound to fibrin, factor Xa contributes to procoagulant activity. Factor Xa is also protected from antithrombin III in presence of fibrin and when bound to phospholipid membranes in the complex with Va.[25]

Heparin, the most used antithrombotic, is not an ideal antithrombotic agent: it requires antithrombin III as a cofactor, does not have affinity for clot-bound thrombin, and is bound or inactivated by plasma proteins and platelet factor 4. Because of these deficiencies of heparin, direct thrombin inhibitors, which bind to the catalytic site of thrombin, bind to thrombin in the clot and are resistant to agents that degrade heparin, have been sought and studied in patients with acute coronary syndromes. The prototypic direct thrombin inhibitor is hirudin, a 65-amino-acid peptide derived from the medicinal leech, now available in clinically useful quantities through recombinant technology.[26]

IV. PLATELET ACTIVATION RESULTING FROM THROMBOLYSIS

The relationship of thrombolysis and platelet activation is complex and still debated. Multiple and counterbalancing effects come into play. These include: platelet secretion of both fibrinolytic and antifibrinolytic components, assembly of fibrinolytic components on the platelet surface causing enhanced plasmin generation which may be pro- or antifibrinolytic and the influence of plasmin on platelet function. However, although plasmin has been shown to directly induce platelet activation in some systems,[27] the concentrations of plasmin used are higher than those present during pharmacological thrombolysis. Nonetheless, there is a marked platelet activation after pharmacologic coronary thrombolysis.[28,29] One potential mechanism for platelet activation is the formation of thrombin (see above) which is the most potent platelet agonist. For streptokinase, there is still perhaps another mechanism of platelet activation involving antistreptokinase antibody. A plasminogen-streptokinase-antistreptokinase antibody ternary complex seems to induce platelet aggregation.[30]

V. CLINICAL IMPLICATIONS

Effective coronary thrombolysis depends on prompt production of a favorable balance between fibrinolysis and ongoing thrombosis. Without adjunctive anticoagulation, the clinical benefit seems partly compromised. Anticoagulation with intravenous agents is particularly important with clot-selective fibrinolytic agents such as t-PA. Three big trials have tested the benefits of effective adjunctive anticoagulation.[31-33] Unfortunately, for different reasons, these reports show unexpectedly high rates of intracranial bleeding associated with administration of two plasminogen activators (streptokinase and t-PA) and two intravenously administered anticoagulants (heparin and hirudin). It appeared absolutely necessary to reduce the anticoagulant regimen for the future. The trials are going on with lower regimens.

VI. CONCLUSION

Paradoxically, pharmacological thrombolysis is associated with increases in procoagulant activity. The numerous mechanisms of this observation are still imperfectly elucidated, but procoagulant activity may explain some of the failures of coronary thrombolysis, in particular the phenomenon of reocclusion. The mechanisms include increase in procoagulant activity induced by pharmacological activation of plasminogen, local expression of procoagulant activity when the vessel is reperfused, presence of high shear forces that promote platelet deposition, and attenuation of physiologic fibrinolytic activity. Procoagulant activity can be reduced by adjunctive anticoagulation with heparin or hirudin. The preliminary encouraging results of both antithrombotics correctly used are certainly in part explained by inhibition of procoagulant activity.

REFERENCES

1.   **ISIS-2 Collaborative Group**. Randomized trial of intravenous streptokinase, oral aspirin, both or neither among 17187 cases of suspected acute myocardial infarction , ISIS-2, *Lancet* 2, 349, 1988.
2.   **Yusuf, S., Sleight, P., Held, P., MacMahon, S.**, Routine medical management of acute myocardial infarction. Lessons from overviews of recent randomized controlled trials. *Circulation* 82 , suppl II, II-117, 1990.
3.   **The GUSTO Angiographic Investigators,** The effects of tissue plasminogen activator, streptokinase, or both on coronary-artery patency, ventricular function, and survival after acute myocardial infarction. *N. Engl. J. Med.* 329, 1615, 1993.
4.   **The GUSTO Investigators,** An international randomized trial comparing four thrombolytic strategies for acute myocardial infarction. *N. Engl. J. Med.* 329, 673, 1993.
5.   **Hsia, J., Kleiman, N., Aguirre, F., Chaitman, R., Roberts, R.**, Heparin-induced prolongation of partial thromboplastin time after thrombolysis: relation to coronary artery patency. *J. Am. Coll. Cardiol* 20, 31, 1992.
6.   **Coller, B.S.**, Platelets and thrombolytic therapy. *N. Engl. J. Med.* 322, 33, 1990.
7.   **Eisenberg, P.R.**, Procoagulant effects of fibrinolytic agents in : *Coronary thrombolysis in perspective* edited by Marcel Dekker, Inc. New York Basel Hong Kong 1993: 77-99.
8.   **Eisenberg, P.R., Sherman, L.A., Jaffe, A.S.**, Paradox elevation of fibrinopeptide A after streptokinase : evidence for continued thrombosis despite intense fibrinolysis. *J. Am. Coll. Cardiol.* 10, 527, 1987.
9.   **Owen. J., Friedman, K.D., Grossman, B.A., Wilkins, C., Berke, A.D., Powers, E.R.**, Thrombolytic therapy with tissue plasminogen activator or streptokinase induces transient thrombin activity. *Blood* 72, 616, 1988.
10.   **Gulba, D.C., Barthels, M., Reil, G.H., Lichtlen, P.R.**, Thrombin/antithrombin complex level as early predictor of reocclusion after successful thrombolysis. *Lancet* 2, 97,1988.
11.   **Tripodi, A., Botasso, B., Mannucci, P.M.**, Elevation of thrombin-antithrombin complexes during thrombolytic therapy in patients with myocardial infarction. *Res. Clin. Lab.* 20, 197, 1990.
12.   **Gulba, C.G., Barthels, M., Westhoff-Bleck, M., Jost, S., Rafflenbeul, W., Daniel, W.G., Hecker, H., Lichtlen, P.R.**, Increased thrombin levels during thrombolytic therapy in acute myocardial infarction. *Circulation* 83, 937, 1991.
13.   **Hoffmann, J.J., Michels, H.R., Windeler, J., Gunzler, W.A.**, Plasma markers of thrombin activity during coronary thrombolytic therapy with saruplase or urokinase: no prediction of reinfarction. *Fibrinolysis* 7, 330, 1993.
14.   **Chang, P., Aronson, D.L., Scott. J., Kessler, C.M.**, Increase in platelet support of thrombin generation after thrombolytic therapy. *Am. J. Cardiol.* 70, 406, 1992.
15.   **Eisenberg, P.R., Miletich, J.P.**, Induction of marked thrombin activity by pharmacological concentrations of plasminogen activators in nonanticoagulated whole blood. *Thromb. Res.* 55, 635, 1989.
16.   **Eisenberg, P.R, Miletich, J.P., Sobel, B.E.**, Factors responsible for the differential procoagulant effects of diverse plasminogen activators in plasma. *Fibrinolysis* 5, 217, 1991.
17.   **Seitz, R., Pelzer, H., Immel, A., Egbring, R.**, Prothrombin activation by thrombolytic agents. *Fibrinolysis* 7, 109, 1993.
18   **Brommer, E.J.P, Meijer, P.**, Thrombin generation induced by the intrinsic or extrinsic coagulation pathway is accelerated by streptokinase, independently of plasminogen. *Thromb. Haemost.* 70, 995, 1993.
19.   **Kornowski, R., Battler, A.**, Activated protein C and antithrombin-III activity during arterial thrombolysis with recombinant tissue-type plasminogen activator in rabbits. *Coron. Art. Dis.* 4, 1115, 1993.
20.   **Torr-Brown, S.R., Sobel, B.E.**, Attenuation of thrombolysis by release of plasminogen activator inhibitor type-1 from platelets. *Thromb. Res.* 72, 413, 1993.
21.   **Reganon, E.,Vila, V., Aznar, J., Lacueva, V., Martinez, V., Ruano, M.**, Studies on the functionality of newly synthesized fibrinogen after treatment of acute myocardial infarction with streptokinase, increase in the rate of fibrinopeptide release. *Thromb. Haemostas.* 70, 978, 1993.
22.   **Mirshahi M, Soria J, Soria F, Faivre F, Lu H, Courtney M, Roitsch C, Tripuier C, Caen JP.** Evaluation of the inhibition by heparin and hirudin of coagulation activation during rt-PA-induced thrombolysis. *Blood* 74, 1026, 1989.
23.   **Weitz, J.I, Hudoba, M., Massel. D., Maraganore, J., Hirsh, J.**, Clot-bound thrombin is protected from inhibition by heparin-antithrombin III but is susceptible to inactivation by antithrombin III-independent inhibitors. *J. Clin. Invest.* 86, 385, 1990.
24.   **Bloom, A.L.**, The release of thrombin from fibrin by fibrinolysin. *Brit. J. Haemat.* 8, 129, 1962.
25.   **Eisenberg, R., Siegel, J.E., Abenschein, D.R., Miletich, J.P.**, Importance of factor Xa in determining the procoagulant activity of whole-blood clots. *J. Clin. Invest.* 91, 1877, 1993.
26.   **Marki, W.E., Wallis, R.B.,** The anticoagulant and antithrombotic properties of hirudins. *Thromb. Haemost.* 64, 344, 1990.
27.   **Guccione, M.A., Kinlough-Rathbone, R.L, Packham, M.A. et al,** Effects of plasmin on rabbit platelets. *Thromb. Haemost.* 53, 8, 1985.

28. **Griguer, P., Brochier, M., Leroy, J., Leclerc, M.H., Antoine, G., Bertrand, H., Chalons, F.,** Platelets aggregation after thrombolytic therapy. *Angiology,* 31,91,1980.

29. **Fitzgerald, D.J., Catella, F., Roy, L., FitzGerald, G.A.,** Marked platelet activation in vivo after intravenous streptokinase in patients with acute myocardial infarction. *Circulation* 77, 142, 1988.

30. **Lebrazi, J., Helft, G., Vacheron, A., Samama, M.M, Mirshahi, M., Lecompte, T.,** Human anti-streptokinase antibodies induce platelet aggregation in a Fc/CD32 dependent manner. *Fibrinolysis* 8, suppl 1, 40, 1994.

31. **Antman, E.M. for the TIMI 9A** Investigators, Hirudin in acute myocardial infarction. Safety report from the thrombolysis and thrombin inhibition in myocardial infarction (TIMI) 9A trial. *Circulation* 90, 1624, 1994.

32. **The Global Use of Strategies to Open Occluded Coronary Arteries (GUSTO) IIa Investigators,** Randomized trial of intravenous heparin versus recombinant hirudin for acute coronary syndromes. *Circulation* 90, 1631, 1994.

33. **Neuhaus, K.L., Essen, R., Tebbe, U., Jessel, A., Heinrichs, H., Mäurer, W., Döring, W., Harmjanz, D., Kötter, V., Kalhammer, E., Simon, H., Horacek, T.,** Safety observations from the pilot phase of the randomized r-hirudin for improvement of thrombolysis (HIT-III) study. *Circulation* 90, 1638, 1994.

UPDATE ON THROMBOGENICITY OF FIX AND FXI CONCENTRATES: LABORATORY AND CLINICAL ASPECTS OF THE INDUCED HYPERCOAGULABILITY

J. Goudemand* and M.J. Seghatchian**

* Centre Hospitalier Régional Universitaire, Hématologie, Lille

** NBS, Colindale, London

I. INTRODUCTION

Human plasma is a unique source of many of the haemostatic components of blood and still remains the essential starting material for the extraction of several blood products concentrates. Modern transfusion practice nevertheless requires that the safest and most efficacious products are consistently produced and used without overloading the patient with unwanted sub-components that may contribute to untoward effects. The goal of any haemostatic replacement therapy is to achieve an optimal level of haemostasis by adjusting the dose and frequency of administration with the most appropriate blood product concentrate of the highest purity. Replacement therapy should always be accompanied by adequate laboratory monitoring, as often the response of an individual patient varies. The induced imbalance between procoagulant and anticoagulant activities can lead in some cases to transient hypercoagulability, occasionally with serious thrombotic complications. This is of particular relevance to Factor IX (FIX) concentrate preparations (activated or non-activated) that are effectively used to "bypass" the high titre FVIII inhibitor, particularly during active bleeding. However, some serious thrombogenic complications may occur when frequent and/or large quantities of FIX are administered or in the presence of liver dysfunction compromising the clearance of activated coagulation factors.

This report deals with some properties of FIX concentrate preparations with particular reference to the quality monitoring of untoward thrombogenicity. A brief resumé of clinical experience with high purity FIX concentrates is presented. There need be no cause for clinical concern when "state of the art" preparations are used. Reference is also made to the *in vivo* thrombogenicity of FXI concentrates.

A. HISTORICAL BACKGROUND

Prothrombin Complex Concentrates (PCCs) are plasma products that contain vitamin K-dependent factors including FIX. PCCs have been available in Europe since 1958 and in the United States since the late 1960s. Numerous preparations (probably more than twenty) are available around the world. For several years PCCs remained the sole treatment of haemophilia B patients.

Relatively soon after the introduction of PCCs, thrombotic complications associated with their use were reported.[1] This situation was not changed after the recommendation of the ISTH in 1974 to add heparin to the concentrate. [2] The complications included superficial or deep vein thrombosis, pulmonary embolism, cerebral embolism, arterial thrombosis (especially acute myocardial infarction) and disseminated intra-vascular coagulation (DIC). Most complications occurred in patients treated with large and repeated doses of PCCs (as needed in surgery) or in those with advanced liver disease.[3]

However, it seems necessary to distinguish two groups of patients:

- those with haemophilia A (or B) with an inhibitor treated with high daily dosages of activated or non-activated PCCs for severe bleeding.[4-11]

- those with haemophilia B without inhibitor who developed thrombosis after receiving doses of PCCs that often did not appear to be excessive (see examples in Table I).

The latter cases only really illustrate the thrombogenic risk associated with the use of PCCs.

Table I

Thrombotic manifestations occurring in haemophilia B patients under treatment with PCCs

N°	FIX level (%)	Age (yr)	Operation	PCC	Daily Dosage		Day of ocurrence	Outcome	Ref.
1	<1	27	knee replacement	D.E.FIX (Edinburgh)	D1 165 U/kg D2 130 U/kg D3 130 U/kg	DIC Thrombophlebitis of the arm	D3	resolved	Small et al 1982 (12)
2	<1	45	inguinal hernia	Bebulin (Immuno)	D1 100 U/kg D2 - D4 80 U/kg	DIC MI	D4	death on D8	Chistolini et al 1990 (13)
3	<1	28	osteotomy	PPSB (Biotransfusion)	D1 6 200 U D2 - D14 6 000 U Total: 92 000 U	Thrombosis of the sylvian artery	D14	resolved	Bardin & Sultan 1990 (14)
4	4	2	circumcision	PPSB (Biotransfusion)	D1 600 U D2 900 U D3 1 000 U Total: 2 500 U	DIC	D4	resolved	Bardin & Sultan 1990 (14)
5	13	40	excision of thigh pseudotumor	Konyne (Cutter)	D1 100 U/kg D2 ev 24 hrs	DIC	D3	resolved	Conlan et al 1990 (15)
6	<1	32	bilateral knee replacement	Konyne (Cutter)	D1 100 U/kg D2 ev 14 hrs	DIC	D5	resolved	Conlan et al 1990 (15)
7	<1	21	bronchoscopy lumbar puncture intubation	Konyne (Cutter)	D1-D3 30 U/kg Total: 6 000 U D4 3 000 U	DIC MI	D4	death on D9	Green et al 1990 (16)
8	5	41	ventriculostomy	Profilnine (Alpha) Konyne (Cutter)	D1 12 970 U D2 7 960 U D3 9 500 U D4 9 500 U	DIC	D4	resolved	Hadly et al 1991 (17)
9	<1	22	polytraumatism	Christmassin (Green cross)	D1 - D3 65 U/kg	DIC	D3	resolved	Ohga et al 1993 (18)

B. THROMBOTIC INCIDENCE ASSOCIATED WITH PCCs

The incidence of thrombosis in haemophilia B patients undergoing surgery treated with PCCs is 38% (8/24) as reported by Kasper *et al.*[19] and 9% (3/34) in a French study.[20] In the absence of high-risk situations the incidence of thrombosis is probably much lower.[21]

These thrombotic manifestations have led to the preparation of more purified FIX concentrates [22,23] and to the use of thrombogenicity tests in order to try to select non-thrombogenic batches of each product.

II. COMPOSITION OF FIX CONCENTRATES

A. PCCs AND THEIR POTENTIAL THROMBOGENIC COMPONENTS

PCCs are prepared from Cohn fraction I supernatant, Cohn fraction IV or cryosupernatant and adsorbed on DEAE Sephadex, DEAE cellulose or tricalcium phosphate. The adsorbed vitamin K dependent factors are eluted and concentrated using ultrafiltration, polyethylene glycol or lyophilisation. The specific activity of PCCs is around 1 to 5 units of FIX per mg of protein which corresponds to a 10 to 50 fold purification from plasma. PCCs contain equivalent amounts of FIX, FII, FX but variable amounts of FVII depending on the nature of the adsorption material (adsorption on DEAE cellulose or tricalcium phosphate results in a higher concentration in FVII than DEAE Sephadex). The other proteins present in PCCs are FVIII:Ag (mainly with tricalcium phosphate), high molecular weight kininogens, C1 inhibitor, inter alpha trypsin inhibitor (ITI) (mainly in DEAE preparations), Hageman factor, antithrombin III, alpha 2 macroglobulin (tricalcium phosphate), ceruloplasmin, fibronectin and immunoglobulins.[24] PCCs also contain variable levels of anticoagulant vitamin K-dependent proteins such as Protein C and S.

Classical explanations for the thrombogenicity of PCCs include the presence of small amounts of activated FVIIa, IXa, Xa[25] or coagulant-active phospholipids[26,27] or zymogen excess due to the difference in the respective half life of FIX and the other vitamin K-dependent factors FII, VII, X.[28] Proteins C and S as well as fibrinolysis cofactors proteins such as Plasminogen Activator Inhibitor Type I (PAI-1) content of PCCs could also modulate their thrombogenic effect.[29]

B. HIGH PURITY (HP) FIX CONCENTRATES

Several HP FIX concentrates have been prepared through conventional or immunoaffinity chromatography (Table II). Compared to PCCs the main characteristics of HP FIX concentrates are their high specific activity (generally higher than 150 units of FIX per mg of protein) and their variable levels of other factors, *ie* vitamin K-dependent factors, fibrinogen, fibronectin and immunoglobulins which are either absent or present in small amounts;[38] C4 and ITI are detected in some products.[39] Heparin is added in low quantities in some concentrates.

III. CURRENT TESTS FOR THROMBOGENICITY

A. *IN VITRO* THROMBOGENICITY TESTS
1. NAPTT

The non activated partial thromboplastin time is one of the most used thrombogenicity tests.[40] It measures the clotting time of a recalcified mixture of 1/10 or 1/100 diluted test samples, phospholipids and normal plasma. According to the rules of the European Pharmacopoeia the clotting time of a 1/10 dilution must be > 150 sec (for a buffer blank time of 230-250 sec). NAPTT is well correlated with IXa and IIa, partly sensitive to ATIII and not influenced by coagulant-active phospholipids.[25,41] It emphasizes the key role of IXa. It has been shown that as little as 200-400 ng of IXa are thrombogenic in the rabbit.[25]

2. TFCT

The thrombin fibrinogen clotting time is performed by observing, over 24 hours, the clot formation of a mixture of pure or 1/10 diluted test sample and fibrinogen.[42] The minimum clotting time must be 24 hours at 20° or 6 hours at 37° after neutralisation of heparin (European Pharmacopoeia). This test provides a sensitive measure of the thrombin activity.[43]

Table II
Characteristics of some purified FIX concentrates

Product	Method of purification	Viral inacti-vation	Heparin	SA U/mg	FIXa U/ml (45)	TAT mg/ml (45)	F1+2 nM (45)	Ref.	Effect of a single infusion (ref.)	Experience in surgery (ref.)
ARC/ Baxter	DEAE Sephadex Dextran Sulphate	SD	0	9 (37) 28(37)	<20ng/ml (39)			Menache et al (39)		
Alphanine (Alpha)	DEAE Cellulose Barium citrate precipitation Polysaccharide affinity chro.	heat/ heptane	<2U/ 50UFIX	69 (42) 124(45)	<0,0005	16	>40	Herring et al (31)	PCC vs FIX (30)	13 cases (60)
Alphanine SD (Alpha)	DEAE Cellulose Barium citrate precipitation Polysaccharide affinity chro.	SD	<2U/ 50UFIX	184				Herring et al (32)	PCC vs FIX (54)	
FIX HP SD (LFB)	DEAE Sephadex DEAE Sepharose Heparin Sepharose	SD	5U/ml	119	<0,0005	56	5	Burnouf et al (33)	PCC vs FIX (55)	18 cases (14,61)
Mononine (Armour)	DEAE Sephadex Immunoaffinity chro.	Na thiocya-nate	0	188	<0,0005	4	1	Hrinda et al (34)	FIX (59)	59 cases (62)
Immunine (Immuno)	DEAE Fraktogel Hydrophobic chro. interaction	steam	5U/ 100UFIX	196 (45)	<0,0005	22	5	Wöber et al (35)	FIX (38)	20 cases (64,63)
Nanotiv (Novo)	DEAE Sepharose Heparin sepharose Cation exchange chro.	SD	0	200	<0,0005	7	3	Östlin et al (36)	FIX (38)	3 cases (38)
9MC (BPL)	DEAE Sepharose Metal chelate affinity chro.	SD	0	166				Feldman et al (48)	PCC vs FIX (56)	14 cases (65)

3. TGT

The thrombin generation test is performed in two stages. First, the test sample is mixed with buffer and $CaCl_2$. Fibrinogen is then added to a sample of the mixture and the clotting time is recorded. Results are expressed in TGt50 which is the time required to clot the fibrinogen in 50 sec.[42] To be considered as safe, the tested materials must have a TGt50 higher than 10 min.[44] The test can be done before or after heparin neutralisation. TGT measures the tendency of a concentrate to form thrombin during incubation with calcium. It is usually associated with a short TFCT and well correlated with IIa and Xa.[41]

4. FIXa Chromogenic test

Gray *et al.*[45] have proposed the inclusion of the measurement of FIXa using FXa chromogenic substrate in a battery of thrombogenic tests. In this assay the test sample (or IXa standard) is incubated for 30 minutes with a reagent mixture containing FX (160nM), recombinant FVIII (1nM), phospholipid (10microg/mL), Ca Cl_2 (5mM) and hirudin (15nM). FXa generation is measured with the chromogenic substrate, S2765 and its concentration calculated by comparison with the standard curve.

B. *IN VIVO* TESTS: ANIMAL MODELS
1. Stasis rabbit model

In this model loose ligatures are applied to the jugular veins of a rabbit. The product is infused over 15 sec in the marginal ear vein. Ligatures are tied off 15 sec exactly after the end of the infusion. Formation of thrombi in the jugular veins is expressed in score (from 0 = no thrombi to 4 = total obstruction)[46] or in ED50 which is the dose producing thombi (regardless of their size) in half of all examined veins.[47]

2. Non-stasis animal models

These models have been developed in the rabbit,[44] the dog[48] and the rat[49] by the Scottish group. They consist of the infusion of the product over 15 or 30 min in a peripheral vein and in the measurement of various haemostasis markers: coagulation factors, platelets, including the release of some activated peptides such as fibrinopeptide A (FpA), from blood samples taken from a collateral vein or artery at various intervals before, during and after the infusion.

C. COMPARATIVE ANALYSES
1. Comparison between Conventional Tests and Animal Models

When infused (100U/kg) in a non-stasis model PCCs characterised by a short NAPTT and TGt50 behave similar to thrombin (50 NIH U/kg) and induce a rapid and transient drop in fibrinogen, FVIII and platelets. Maximum score of thrombi is also recorded in the Wessler model (30 U/kg). In contrast, the administration of PCCs with long NAPTT and TGt50 has no significant effect in either model. PCCs with short NAPTT and long TGt50 induce an immediate drop in fibrinogen and platelets with a gradual return to normal and maximum thrombosis in the Wessler model. PCCs with long NAPTT and short TGt50 have a delayed and less limited effect in the both stasis and non-stasis models.[44] These experiments reveal that PCCs active in NAPTT have the most immediate and extensive effects in the stasis model, probably as a result of the direct infusion of partially activated coagulation factors, vasoactive peptides, or high molecular weight kininogens. Certain PCCs with long NAPTT produced slow *in vivo* activation of coagulation via an intermediate step. This mechanism is best explored by non-stasis models that yield more information than the stasis models.

2. The use of activation markers of hypercoagulability

The essential difference between PCCs and HP FIX concentrates can be demonstrated by measuring sensitive coagulation activation peptide markers in canine non-stasis models. PCCs induce a characteristic elevation of FpA which reaches a peak 30 minutes after the infusion whereas HP FIX concentrates do not.[48] This time interval contrasts with the rapid response in the Wessler model showing that the thrombogenic effect is due to thrombin generated *in vivo* via activation of coagulation. As there is no difference between the thrombogenicity of PCCs in FVII deficient versus normal dogs, the FVII/tissue pathway probably plays a small role in the thrombogenicity of PCCs as compared to the intrinsic clotting system.[50] PCCs contain significant amounts of coagulant-active phospholipids[26] that may potentiate the activity of any Xa (and IXa) present in the product when infused in a stasis[27] or non-stasis model.[48] In this respect the added advantage of the solvent/detergent (SD) process would be its ability to remove these phospholipid contaminants (however Mononine which is not SD treated is also devoid of these components). All the products listed in Table II fulfil the criteria of non-thrombogenicity in *in vitro* tests and stasis[30,33,35,36,51] or non-stasis[48,49,51] animal models.

On the other hand, it has been shown that HP FIX concentrates with short NAPTT or FCT generated FpA levels similar to those observed after albumin when infused (200 U/kg) in a non-stasis dog model.[48] The same results were observed in a non-stasis rat model.[49] So a short NAPTT would not be predictive of the thrombogenicity of HP FIX concentrates in a non-stasis model. This lack of correlation between *in vitro* and *in vivo* thrombogenicity tests has been also demonstrated in stasis models.[30,33] Furthermore, some batches with short NAPTT and FCT did cause thrombus formation in the Wessler model but not in a non-stasis model. This suggests that traces of activated clotting factors may be rapidly inhibited or cleared before causing further activation.[52] Most of the *in vitro* thrombogenicity tests currently used appear to be inappropriate for HP FIX products.

IV. CLINICAL EXPERIENCE

In humans, infusion of a single dose (50 U/kg) of PCCs can result in heightened FX activation, prothrombin activation and thrombin activity expressed by a significant elevation of FX activation peptide, prothrombin fragment 1+2 (F1+2) and FpA. As a consequence of thrombin generation, thrombin-antithrombin (TAT) complexes are formed. This sequence has been observed with different products by several authors.[38,53-56] The rise in F1+2 and TAT is immediate and sustained whereas the peak FpA is relatively delayed (60 min). Although PCCs contain significant amount of F1+2[53-55] it is unlikely that the rise in F1+2 is the result of administration of exogenous F1+2 since the half-life of F1+2 is only 90 min.[57] This could not explain sustained increases in F1+2 for up to 6 hours. The half-life of FpA is even shorter (3-5 min)[58] and the presence of FpA in PCCs could not explain the FpA peak that occurs 60 min post-infusion. *In vivo* prothrombin activation and thrombin generation is the only explanation for these findings and is highly suggestive of a pre-thrombotic state. However, the augmentation in thrombin activity is not sufficient to elevate levels of fibrin monomer or to cause enhanced fibrinolytic activity.[53]

In contrast to earlier PCCs, HP FIX concentrates infused in combined cross-over studies at the same or even higher dosage (100 U/kg) in the same patients did not cause an increase of these markers.[53-56] Furthermore, no significant modifications of F1+2, TAT, FpA were observed in patients receiving a single infusion of the other products.[38,59] These findings show that infusion of HP FIX concentrates results in less activation of coagulation than other less pure PCCs.

However, as most of the thrombotic complications associated with the use of PCCs occurred after repeated infusions, the effects of multiple doses of HP FIX concentrates on activation of the haemostatic effect had also to be established. There is now a growing clinical experience with HP FIX concentrates in patients undergoing surgery.[14,38,60-62,64,65] No thrombotic events have been reported in any of these patients. Moreover, repeated measurement of markers of hypercoagulability in patients treated for several days with HP FIX concentrate did not give evidence of abnormal activation of coagulation. This was regardless of the type of surgery and the fact that orthopaedic procedures are usually considered as high-risk thrombotic situations.[61,66]

V. THROMBOGENIC POTENTIAL OF FXI CONCENTRATES

Severe or partial congenital deficiency of FXI occurs primary in Ashkenazi Jews and with a lesser frequency in other ethnic groups.[67,68] Approximately 200 cases of FXI deficiency have been reported in the United States, mostly in New York and Los Angeles. In most patients there is no correlation between bleeding episodes and the level of FXI.[69] Individuals who are homozygotes or compound heterozygotes for FXI gene mutations have levels below 15U/dL and may show excessive bleeding after dental extraction, surgery, and injuries to certain sites, in particular in areas with a high fibrinolytic activity (e.g. oral cavity, nose, bladder and uterus).[70] Circumcision has been performed on many severely deficient patients without causing excessive bleeding. Patients with partial deficiency (FXI between 15 to 70 U/dL) are also at risk of excessive bleeding, but FXI level is not a good predictor of the bleeding tendency in such patients.

Bleeding episodes are treated with frozen plasma. Since 1985 plasma derived FXI concentrates have become available (in UK and in France) for patients with congenital FXI deficiency.[71,72] Some batches of the British product elicited significant thrombogenic responses in animal models, so heparin (10 U/mL) was added by the manufacturer to reduce activation of coagulation.[73] Care should be taken if such a product is given to patients who are sensitive to heparin induced thrombocytopenia. While it is justifiable to use FXI concentrates to cover major surgery (e.g. heart surgery), or in a site particularly prone to fibrinolysis (e.g. tonsillectomy, prostatectomy), the dose used should raise the FXI level to above 70 U/dL and not exceed 100 U/dL. The use of an antifibrinolytic agent should be considered first.[70] It is also important to note that although patients with severe FXI deficiency with a history of vascular disease have received FXI concentrate to cover for surgery without adverse events, thrombotic events after administration of FXI concentrates have been reported in four patients with cardiovascular disease treated with the product from BPL.[74] Activation of coagulation has been also reported in two patients treated with the French product from LFB.[75] All the reported patients were elderly or had other risk factors (cancer). In view of the possibility that FXI concentrate may have contributed to the events, the potential risks and benefits should be carefully considered before treatment and care should be taken to avoid peaks of greater than 100 U/dL FXI. The current recommendations are : i) the total dose given should not exceed 30 U/kg; this is calculated from the rise required, multiplied by Wt in Kg (except in children and in pregnancy) and divided by 2. ii) treatment should be carried out in special centres by the specialist with regular monitoring of FXI clotting activity. iii) early screening for evidence of hypercoagulability and thrombosis is indicated.[76]

VI SUMMARY

With the advent of a purification system the conventional tests for the thrombogenicity of FIX concentrates become redundant. Attention is focused on the monitoring of the patient's response to a prescribed effective dose. Accumulated clinical experiences with the new HP FIX concentrates indicate that these products are safe and effective. Patients can be treated safely even in situations that need large and repeated administration of FIX. The risk/benefit ratio of FXI concentrates should be carefully considered before treatment. Peaks greater than 100 U/dL of FXI *in vivo* should be avoided.

A highly promising approach of viral filtration (a process called nano-filtration, which consists of passing protein solution onto small pore membranes of 15 to 35 nm) is applied to certain preparations, allowing steric removal of any known viruses.[77] This limits the potential risk of viral contaminants. In the near future, the conventional thrombogenicity testing may become obsolete.

Note: Part of this manuscript was presented at the BBTS Component SIG Meeting.[78]

REFERENCES

1. **Lusher, J.M.,** Thrombogenicity associated with factor IX complex concentrates, *Semin. Hematol.,* 28, 3,1991.
2. **Ménaché, D. and Roberts, H.R.,** Report and recommendations of task force members and consultants, *Thromb . Haemostas .,* 33, 645, 1975.
3. **Cederbaum, A.I., Blatt, P.M. and Roberts, H.R.,** Intravascular coagulation with uses of human prothrombin complex concentrates, *Ann. Intern. Med.,* 84, 683, 1976.
4. **Gruppo, R.A., Bove, K.E. and Donaldson, V.H.,** Fatal myocardial necrosis associated with prothrombin complex concentrate therapy in hemophilia B., *N. Engl. J. Med.,* 309, 242, 1983.
5. **Agrawall, B.L., Zelkowitz, L. and Hletko, P.,** Acute myocardial infarction in a young hemophilic patient during therapy with factor IX concentrate and epsilon amino caproic acid, *J. Pediatrics.,* 98, 931, 1981.
6. **Fuerth, J.H. and Mahrer, P.,** Myocardial infarction after factor IX therapy, *JAMA,* 245, 1455, 1981.
7. **Sullivan, D.W., Purdy, L.J., Billingham, M. and Gladner, B.E.,** Fatal myocardial infarction following therapy with prothrombin complex concentrates in a young man with hemophilia A, *Pediatrics,* 74, 279, 1984.
8. **Fukui, H., Fujimura, Y., Takahashi, Y., Mikami, S. and Yoshioka, A.,** Laboratory evidence of DIC under Feiba treatment of a hemophilic patient with intracranial bleeding and high titre factor VIII inhibitor, *Thromb. Res.,* 22, 177, 1981.
9. **Rodeghiero, F., Castronovo, S. and Dini, E.,** Disseminated intravascular coagulation after infusion of Feiba (Factor VIII inhibitor by passing activity) in a patient with acquired haemophilia, *Thromb. Haemostas.,* 48, 339, 1982.
10. **Chavin, S.I., Siegel, D.M., Rocco, T.A. and Olson, J.P.,** Acute myocardial infarction during treatment with an activated prothrombin complex concentrate in a patient with a factor VIII deficiency and a factor VIII inhibitor, *Am. J. Med.,* 85, 245, 1988.
11. **Mizon, P., Goudemand, J., Jude, B. and Marey, A.,** Myocardial infarction after Feiba therapy in a hemophilia B patient with a factor IX inhibitor, *Ann. Hemat.,* 64, 309, 1992.
12. **Small, M., Love, G.D.O., Douglas, J.T., Forbes, C.D. and Prentice, C.R.M.,** Factor IX thrombogenicity: in vivo effects on coagulation activation and a case report of disseminated intravascular coagulation, *Thromb. Haemostas.,* 48, 76, 1982.

13.   Chistolini, A., Mazzucconi, M.G., Tirindelli, M.C., La Verde, G., Ferrari, A. and Mandelli, F., Disseminated intravascular coagulation and myocardial infarction in a haemophilia B patient during therapy with prothrombin complex concentrates, *Acta Haematol.*, 83, 163, 1990.

14.   Bardin, J.M. and Sultan, Y., Factor IX concentrate versus prothrombin complex concentrate for the treatment of hemophilia B during surgery, *Transfusion*, 30, 441, 1990.

15.   Conlan, M. and Hoots, W.K., Disseminated intravascular coagulation and hemorrhage in hemophilia B following elective surgery, *Am. J. Hemat.*, 35, 203, 1990.

16.   Green, D., Snapper, H., Abu-Jawdeh, G. and Reddy, J., Acute myocardial infarction, non bacterial thrombotic endocarditis and disseminated intravascular coagulation in a severe hemophiliac, *Am. J. Hemat.*, 35, 210, 1990.

17.   Hadley, T. and Djulbegovic, B., Disseminated intravascular coagulation after factor IX complex resolved using purified factor IX concentrate, *Ann. Intern. Med.*, 115, 621, 1991.

18.   Ohga, S., Saito, M., Matsuki, A., Kai, T. and Ueda, K., Disseminated intravascular coagulation in a patient with haemophilia B during factor IX replacement therapy, *Br. J. Haematol.*, 84, 343, 1993.

19.   Kasper, C.K., Rickard, K. and Aledort, L., Report of factor VIII and IX subcommittee meeting, paper presented at 13th Cong. ISTH, Amsterdam, the Netherlands, July 1-6, 1989.

20.   Verroust, F., Ferrer-Le Coeur, F., Laurian, Y., Fressinaud, E., Sultan, Y., Gazengel, C., Bosser, C., Goudemand, J., Parquet, A., Saint Paul, E., Durin, A., Derlon, A., Négrier, C., Vicariot, M., Benion, L., Berthier, A.M., Roche, M., Surgery in hemophiliacs B with french FIX concentrates: a multicomparative review, paper presented at 14th Cong. ISTH, New York, USA, July 4-9,1993.

21.   Bray, G.L. and Aledort, L.M., Consideration governing factor IX product choice in hemophilia B, *Transfusion*, 34, 554, 1994.

22.   Smith, K.J., Factor IX concentrates: the new products and their properties, *Transf. Med. Rev.*, 6, 124, 1992.

23.   Thompson, A.R., Factor IX concentrates for clinical use, *Sem. Thromb. Hemostas.*, 19, 25, 1993.

24.   Pejaudier, L., Kichenin-Martin, V., Boffa, M.C. and Steinbuch, M., Appraisal of the protein composition of prothombin complex concentrates of different origins, *Vox Sang.*, 52, 1, 1987.

25.   Hultin, M.B., Activated clotting factors in factor IX concentrates, *Blood*, 54, 1028, 1979.

26.   Giles, A.R., Nesheim, M.E., Hoogendoorn, H., Tracy, P.B. and Mann, K.G., The coagulant-active phospholipid content is a major determinant of in vivo thrombogenicity of prothrombin complex (factor IX) concentrates in rabbits, *Blood*, 59, 401, 1982.

27.   Giles, A.R., Nesheim, M.E., Hoogendoorn, H., Tracy, P.B. and Mann, K.G., Stroma free human platelet lysates potentiate the in vivo thrombogenicity of factor Xa by the provision of coagulant-active phospholipid, *Br. J. Haematol.* 51, 457, 1982.

28.   Aronson, D.L. and Ménaché, D., Thrombogenicity of factor IX complex: in vivo investigation, *Dev. Biol. Stand.*, 67, 149, 1987.

29.   Mikaelsson, M. and Oswaldsson, U., Factor IX complex concentrates contain plasminogen activator inhibitor type 1 (PAI-1), paper presented at 14th Cong. ISTH, New York, USA, July 4-9,1993.

30.   Ménaché, D., Behre, H.E., Orthner, C.L., Nunez, H., Anderson, H.D., Triantaphyllopoulos, D.C. and Kosow, D.P., Coagulation factor IX concentrate: method of preparation and assessment of potential in vivo thrombogenicity in animal models, *Blood*, 64, 1220, 1984.

31.   Herring, S.W. and Hildebrant, C.M., Heat-treated pure factor IX, paper presented at 5th Intern. Symp. on Hemophilia Treatment, Tokyo, Japan, 1986.

32.   Herring, S.W., Shitanishi, K.T., Peddala, L., Goei, S. and Vemura, Y., Characteristics and safety of a coagulation factor IX product, paper presented at 21th Intern. Cong. of the WFH, Mexico City, Mexico, April 24-29, 1994.

33.   Burnouf, T., Michalski, C., Goudemand, M. and Huart, J.J., Properties of a highly purified human plasma factor IX:c therapeutic concentrate prepared by conventional chromatography, *Vox Sang.*, 57, 225, 1989.

34.   Hrinda, M.E., Huang, C., Tarr, G.C., Weeks, R., Feldman, F. and Schreiber, A.B., Preclinical studies of a monoclonal antibody-purified factor IX, Mononine TM, *Semin. Hematol.*, 28, 6, 1991.

35.   Wöber, G., Szgary, M. and Linnau, Y., Partitioning by chromatography of HIV-1 and H-1 parvovirus during the manufacture of a highly purified FIX concentrate (Immunine), paper presented at 35th Ann. Meet. of the GTH, Göttingen, FRG, Feb. 20-23, 1991.

36.   Östlin, A., Löf, A.L., Eriksson, B., Mattson, C. and Moberg, U., Characterisation of Nanotiv, a highly purified factor IX concentrate, paper presented at 14th Cong. ISTH, New York, USA, July 4-9, 1993.

37.   Feldman, P.A., Harris, L., Evans, D.R. and Evans, H.E., Preparation of a high-purity factor IX concentrate using metal chelate affinity chromatography, in *Biotechnology of Blood proteins*, Rivat, C. and Stoltz, J.F., Eds., INSERM John Libbey Eurotext, Paris, London, 1993, pp 63-68.

38.   Berntorp, E., Björkman, S., Carlsson, M., Lethagen, S. and Nilsson, I.M., Biochemical and in vivo properties of highly purified factor IX concentrates, *Thromb. Haemostas.* , 70, 768, 1993.

39.   Moberg, V.U., Ekblad, M., Löf, A.L., Novak, V. and Oswaldsson, U., Biochemical characterization of various factor IX concentrates, paper presented at 21th Intern. Cong. of the WFH, Mexico City, Mexico, April 24-29, 1994.

40.   Kingdon, H.S., Lundblad, R.L., Veltkamp, J.J. and Aronson, D.L., Potentially thrombogenic materials in human FIX concentrates, *Thromb. Diath. Haemorrh.*, 33, 617, 1975.

41.   Prowse, C.V., Chiruside, A. and Elton, R.A., In vitro thrombogenicity tests of factor IX concentrates. I A survey of available assays, *Thromb. Haemostas.*, 42, 1355, 1979.

42.   Sas, G., Owens, R.E., Smith, J.K., Middleton, S. and Cash, J.D., In vitro spontaneous thrombin generation in human factor IX concentrates, *Br. J. Haematol.*, 31, 25, 1975.

43.   Feldman, P.A., Mc Grath, S. and Evans, H., Sensitivity of the fibrinogen clotting time: an in vitro test of potential thrombogenicity, *Vox Sang.*, 66, 1, 1994.

44.   Prowse, C.V. and Williams, A.E., A comparison of the in vitro and in vivo thrombogenic activity of factor IX concentrates using stasis (Wessler) and non stasis rabbit models, *Thromb. Haemostas.*, 4, 81, 1980.

45.   Gray, E., Tubbs, J., Cesmeli, S. and Barrowcliffe, T.W., Thrombogenicity of FIX concentrates: in vitro and in vivo results, *Thromb. Haemostas.*, 69, 1285, 1993.

46.   Wessler, S., Reimer, S.M., Sheps, M.C., Biologic assay of a thrombosis-inducing activity in human serum., *J. Appl. Physiol.*, 14, 943, 1959.

47.   Vinazzer, H., Comparison between two concentrates with factor VIII inhibitor bypassing activity, *Thomb. Res.*, 26, 21, 1982.

48.   Mc Gregor, I.R., Ferguson, J.M., Mc Laughlin, L.F., Burnouf, T. and Prowse, C.V., Comparison of high purity factor IX concentrates and a prothrombin complex concentrate in a canine model of thrombogenicity, *Thromb.*

Haemostas., 66, 609, 1991.

49. **Mc Laughlin, L.F., Drummond, O. and Mc Gregor, I.R.,** A novel rat model of thrombogenicity: its use in evaluation of prothrombin complex concentrates and high purity factor IX concentrates, *Thromb. Haemostas.*, 68, 511, 1992.

50. **Ferguson, J.M., Mc Gregor, I.R., Mc Laughlin, L.F. and Prowse, C.V.,** Use of factor VII deficient beagles bred by artificial insemination to evaluate mechanism of thrombosis associated with prothrombin complex concentrates, *Blood Coag. Fibrinol.*, 2, 731, 1991.

51. **Feldman, P.A., Mc Gregor, I.R., Ferguson, J.M., Mc Laughlin, L.F. and Sims, G.E.,** Pre-clinical evaluation of thrombogenicity of a high purity factor IX concentrate, *Thromb. Haemostas.*, 69, 1281, 1993.

52. **Mc Gregor, I.R., Mc Laughlin, L.F., Drummond, O., Ferguson, J.M., and Prowse, C.V.,** Limitation of in vitro thrombogenicity tests applied to high purity factor IX concentrates, in *Biotechnology of Blood proteins*, Rivat, C. and Stoltz, J.F., Eds., INSERM John Libbey Eurotext, Paris, London, 1993, pp 87.

53. **Mannucci, P.M., Bauer, K.A., Gringeri, A., Barzegar, B., Simoni, L. and Rosenberg, D.,** Thrombin generation is not increased in the blood of hemophilia B patients after the infusion of a purified factor IX concentrate, *Blood*, 76, 2540, 1990.

54. **Hampton, K.K., Preston, F.E., Lowe, G.D.O., Walker, I.D. and Sampson, B.,** Reduced coagulation activation following infusion of a highly purified factor IX concentrate compared to a prothrombin complex concentrate, *Br. J. Haematol.*, 84, 279, 1993.

55. **Mannucci, P.M., Bauer, K.A., Gringeri, A., Barzegar, S., Santagostino, E., Tradati, F.C. and Rosenberg, R.D.,** No activation of the common pathway of the coagulation cascade after a highly purified factor IX concentrate, *Br. J. Haematol.*, 79, 606, 1991.

56. **Thomas, D.P., Hampton, K.K., Dasani, H., Lee, C.A., Giangrande, P.L.F., Harman, C., Lee, M.L. and Preston, F.E.,** A cross-over pharmacokinetic and thrombogenicity study of a prothrombin complex concentrate and a purified factor IX concentrate, *Br. J. Haematol.*, 87, 782, 1994.

57. **Bauer, K.A., Broekmans, A.W., Bertina, R.M., Conard, J., Horellou, M.H., Samama, M.M. and Rosenberg, R.D.,** Hemostatic enzyme generation in the blood of patients with hereditary protein C deficiency, *Blood*, 71, 1418, 1988.

58. **Nossel, H.L., Yudelman, T., Canfield, R.E., Butler, V.P., Spanondis, K., Wildner, G.D. and Qureshi, G.D.,** Measurement of fibrinopeptide A in human Blood, *J. Clin. Invest.*, 54, 43, 1974.

59. **Kim, H.C., Mc Millan, C.W., White, G.C., Bergman, G.E., Horton, M.W. and Saidi, P.,** Purified factor IX using monoclonal immunoaffinity technique: clinical trials in hemophilia B and comparison to prothrombin complex concentrate, *Blood*, 79, 568, 1992.

60. **Goldsmith, J.C., Kasper, C.K., Blatt, P.M., Gomperts, E.D., Kessler, C.M., Thompson, A.R., Herring, S.W. and Novak, P.L.,** Coagulation factor IX: successful surgical experience with a purified factor IX concentrate, *Am. J. Hemat.*, 40, 210, 1992.

61. **Goudemand, J., Marey, A., Caron, C., Wibaut, B. and Mizon, P.,** Clinical efficacy of a highly purified SD-treated factor IX concentrate prepared by conventional chromatography, *Transf. Med.*, 3, 299, 1993.

62. **White, G.C., Shapiro, A., Pitel, P., Bergman, G.E. and the Mononine study group,** Safety and efficacy of a monoclonal antibody purified factor IX concentrate in hemophilia B patients undergoing surgical procedures, paper presented at 21th Intern. Cong. of the WFH, Mexico City, Mexico, April 24-29, 1994.

63. **Berntorp, E., Anderle, K., Elyster, E., Kunschak, M., Rivard, G.,** Clinical efficacy of a new factor IX concentrate: Immunine, paper presented at 21th Intern. Cong. of the WFH, Mexico City, Mexico, April 24-29, 1994.

64. **Tengborn, L., Stigendal, L., Gustafsson, G., Strömberg, C. and Hultmark, P.,** Treatment with a pure factor IX concentrate in a patient with moderate hemophilia B undergoing bilateral hip replacement, *Transfusion*, 33, 936, 1993.

65. **Thomas, D.P., Lee, C.A., Colvin, B.T., Dasani, H., Dolan, G., Giangrande, P.L.F., Jones, P., Lucas, G., Cantwell, O. and Harman, C.T.,** Clinical experience with a highly purified factor IX concentrate in patients undergoing surgical operation, *Haemophilia*, 1, 17, 1995.

66. **Santagostino, E., Mannucci, P.M., Gringeri, A., Tagariello, G., Baudo, F., Bauer, K.A. and Rosenberg, G.R.D.,** Markers of hypercoagulability in patients with hemophilia B given repeated, large doses of factor IX concentrates during and after surgery, *Thromb. Haemostas.*, 71, 737, 1994.

67. **Seligsohn, U.,** Factor XI deficiency, *Thromb. Haemostas.*, 70, 68, 1993.

68. **Asakai, R., Chung, D.W., Davie E.W. and Seligsohn, U.,** Factor XI deficiency in Ashkenazi Jews in Israel, *N. Engl J. Med.*, 325, 153, 1991.

69. **Bolton-Maggs, P.H.B., Patterson, D.A., Wensley, R.T. and Tuddenham, E.G.D.,** Definition of the bleeding tendency in Factor XI-deficient kindreds. A clinical and laboratory study, *Thromb. Haemostas.*, 73, 194, 1995.

70. **Berliner, S., Horowitz, I., Martinowitz, U., Brenner, B. and Seligsohn, U.,** Dental surgery in patients with severe factor XI deficiency without plasma replacement, *Blood Coag. Fibrinol.*, 3, 465, 1992.

71. **Bolton-Maggs, P.H.B., Wensley, R.T., Kernoff, P.B.A., Kasper, C.K., Winkelman, L., Lane, R.S. and Smith, J.K.,** Production and therapeutic use of a factor XI concentrate from plasma, *Thromb. Haemostas.*, 67, 314, 1992.

72. **Burnouf-Radosevich, M. and Burnouf, T.,** A therapeutic, highly purified factor XI concentrate from human plasma, *Transfusion*, 32, 861, 1992.

73. **Winkelman, L., Mc Laughlin, L.F., Gray, E. and Thomas,S.,** Heat-treated factor XI concentrate: evaluation of *in vivo* thrombogenicity in two animal models, *Thromb. Haemostas.*, 69, 1286, 1993 (Abst.).

74. **Bolton-Maggs, P.H.B., Colvin B.T., Satchi, G., Lee, C.A. and Lucas, G.S.,** Thrombogenic potential of Factor XI concentrate, *Lancet*, 344, 748, 1994.

75. **Mannucci, P.M., Bauer, K.A., Santagostino, E., Faioni, E., Barzegar, S., Cappola, R. and Rosenberg, R.D.,** Activation of the coagulation cascade after infusion of a factor XI concentrate in congenitally deficient patients, *Blood*, 84, 1314, 1994.

76. **Lee, C.A. and Bolton-Maggs, P.H.B.,** Guidelines for the use of FXI concentrate on behalf of the United Kingdom Haemophilia Centre Director Organisation, personal communication, 1994.

77. **Burnouf-Radosevich, M., Appourchaux, P., Huart, J.J. and Burnouf, T.,** Nanofiltration, a new specific virus elimination method applied to high-purity factor IX and factor XI concentrates, *Vox Sang.*, 67, 132, 1994.

78. **Goudemand J. and Seghatchian M.J.,** Thrombogenicity of Factor IX concentrates : current state of the art, *Clin. Lab. Haemat.*, 16, 400, 1994.

ARTIFICIAL SURFACES AND HYPERCOAGULABILITY

M.J. Seghatchian
NBS, Colindale, London

I. INTRODUCTION

Major technological advances in the past three decades have led to widespread use of prosthetic devices for the replacement or support of various organs and tissues[1]. Today, the use of various long-term implants (eg mechanical and bioprosthetic devices, total artificial hearts, bioprosthetic heart valves, total joint replacements, ventricular assist devices, vascular grafts, dental implants and contact lenses and devices involving for example catheters and equipment for cardiopulmonary bypass and hemodialysis) are widespread in modern clinical medicine. More recently stents are used frequently in peripheral arterial intervention. The use of such an implant obviously, at the initial phase and some weeks after, until endothelialisation is completed, is associated with hemostatic activation requiring antithrombotic therapy. Many attempts have been made to develop protein resistance artificial surfaces. However, there is still no such thing as a completely inert artificial surface, and thromboembolic complications remain a major managment problem in this area. Fibrinogen adsorption and surface hydrophilicity are strongly related. The hydrophilicity is distinctly increased after photochemical rather than thermal grafting. Biomaterial can induce platelet, leucocyte and complement activation. Newer techniques such as the measurement of platelet microparticules, by flowcytometry, leukocyte activation (shedding of L-selectin) and complement activation measured by ELISA are currently providing useful information in laboratory flow models. It appears that mechanisms of biomaterial's failure are different and the main hemostatic complications more related to complement, leukocytes and platelet activation and microvesiculation rather than thrombin generation. This brief review highlights some of the unresolved technical and clinical aspects of artificial surfaces including "stents" which are becoming a popular angioplasty implant.

II. DEVELOPMENT OF ARTIFICIAL SURFACES

A. HISTORICAL PERSPECTIVE

As early as 1935 Carrel and Lindberg[2] developed a perfusion pump (artificial heart), with the long term aim of supporting patients' defective organs, and in 1957 Akutsus and Kolff[3] reported the initial success with an experimental animal implant of an air-driven total artificial heart. In 1963 a high priority was given to the development of mechanical circulatory support devices[4].

The early devices produced significant hemolysis and coagulation disturbance (thrombosis and embolism due to abnormal blood flow patterns in areas of stasis) and it soon became clear that a smooth surface, washed more effectively by blood flowing at physiological velocity, prevented the accumulation of critical concentrations of activated factors responsible for thrombosis[5,6]. Despite many advances in the past 30 years problems related to thrombogenicity of biomaterial and problems associated with artificial-implant such as bleeding; emboli; implant calcification; component dysfunction and failure of biomaterial due to infection[7,8] still remain unresolved.

0-8493-5804-3/96/$0.00+$.50

B. BIOCOMPATIBILITY AND THROMBOEMBOLIC COMPLICATIONS OF ARTIFICIAL DEVICES

The "biocompatibility" of a device refers to not only its resistance to thrombosis but also to several other processes including cellular proliferation, complement activation, hemolysis, infection, calcification, biomaterial degradation and release of toxic products[9]. In practice, no devices made from artificial or natural biological materials fulfill all of these criteria.

Thrombosis within or around indwelling catheters or devices may occur by two principal mechanisms:

1. The effect of artificial surfaces on the blood.

This depends upon the physical and chemical characteristic properties of the materials employed (eg roughness of the inner surface; irregularities induced in flow particularly in high shear-stress regions and/or relatively slow flow or complete stasis). These may result in contact phase and complement activation and increased platelet adhesion or the release of substances that stimulate platelet aggregation and thrombin generation.

2. The effect of artificial devices on the vessel wall itself.

Endothelial cells can be easily detached from vessel walls exposing the highly thrombogenic subcomponents (eg collagen, Von Willebrand factor, fibronectin and other matrix components) through the denudation of vessel walls[9].

Despite improvements in hemodynamic design and the use of more thromboresistant materials, thrombosis associated with artificial devices remains to be resolved.

Insufficient anticoagulation during hemodialysis may also result in clot formation within the dialysis tubing and membrane, while excessive anticoagulation may cause haemorrhage, complement activation, activation of contact system/fibrinolysis, platelet degranulation and consumption of coagulation factors. These abnormalities nevertheless are not of major clinical importance. However, anticoagulant related haemorrhage, platelet-related dysfunction and thromboembolism are among the major clinical complications reported with the use of long-term prosthetic devices[1,9]. In addition, non-bacterial vasculitis results from chronic irritation of the vascular lumen by the artificial surfaces; for example, catheter and bacterial arteritis/phlebitis reportedly may ensue owing to introduction of bacteria with the catheter, or to inadequate aseptic technique following catheter insertion[1,9].

III. ARTIFICIAL SURFACES AND
ENDOTHELIAL/ HEMATOLOGICAL MODIFICATIONS

Certain pathophysiologic conditions contributing to stasis, hypercoagulability or hyperviscosity, due to injury to blood cells can play a major role in thromboembolism. However, according to Didisheim and Watson[9] the thrombogenicity of biomaterials is caused not so much by the biophysical/biochemical properties of the materials as by their lack of power to stimulate the active processes of thrombus prevention and dissolution. It is well known that endothelial derived molecules such as prostacyclin (PGI_2), endothelial-derived relaxing factor (EDRF), ADPase, heparin and related glycosaminoglycans, surface bound antithrombin, thrombomodulin and tissue plasminogen activator (TPA) play an important role in maintaining endothelial surfaces non-thrombogenic[10-11]. For example:

i. Prostacyclin is a vasodilator and potent inhibitor of platelet aggregation and adhesion.
ii. EDRF is also a vasodilator, contributing to platelet antiaggregatory properties.
iii. ADPase metabolises ADP released from circulating cells or vessel wall components, transforming it to AMP which inhibits platelet aggregation.

iv. Antithrombins in the presence of heparin on endothelial surface prevent thrombin generation and the conversion of fibrinogen to fibrin.

v. Thrombin upon binding to thrombomodulin on the endothelial cell membrane activates protein C, and surface bound activated protein C converts several plasma coagulation factors such as activated factors V and VIII to their inactive forms. Free protein S which is released from endothelium acts as cofactor for protein C activation.

vi. TPA digests fibrin, which is formed locally if all the above antithrombotic mechanisms are overwhelmed by the magnitude of the thrombogenic stimulus.

Apart from the above mentioned antithrombotic mechanisms which work in concert, the physiological flow itself prevents the local accumulation of products of cellular release in situ thus maintaining the activated factors to non-critical concentrations. Nevertheless, with the implanted device thromboembolism is common and usually arises in regions of non-physiological flow[9].

Different types of artificial surface are currently used in patients requiring cardiac valve replacement and other artificial devices. The main problems with such surfaces are the potential for thromboembolism and the need for life-long anticoagulation[1,9]. The problems can be related to three distinct areas involving the mechanical part; the biomaterial part and/or the individual pathophysiological variations.

The pathogenesis of clotting by artificial surfaces is thought to involve the following:

a. Activation, surface adhesion and aggregation of platelets, followed by release reactions in response to the numerous triggering factors (eg collagen, thrombin, ADP)[12]. Those mediated by prostaglandins and the products of their metabolism can be inhibited by acetyl salicylic acid (ASA)[13].

b. Stimulation of intrinsic coagulation systems on foreign surfaces, leading to thrombin generation, irreversible platelet aggregation and shortening of platelet survival[14].

The megathrombocytic index (percentage of platelets which are higher than or equal to 0.29 μm in diameter)[15] or release platelet activation markers are useful diagnostic strategies[16,17].

IV. CLINICAL FEATURES

The major types of thrombosis in relation to artificial surfaces are:

1. **Obstructive**, in which the fibrinous sediment settles at the bottom of the implantation base. This occurs with relatively high frequency.

2. **Acute or chronic**, acute types are usually massive and destructive whereas chronic thromboses are more often fibrinous and organised.

3. **Precocious or delayed**, these appear during the first month of the postoperative period as acute, massive thrombus depending upon hemodynamic conditions, favoured by the low flow.

The two major types of thromboembolic events are:

1. **Systemic events**, the majority are localised in cerebral arteries (82%) with 14% fatal cases. The risk is higher in the first year. The recurrence incidence is high in the first 18 months for wherever the prosthesis was located, though the probability for the first event to occur is higher in the case of a mitral prosthesis[18].
2. **Valve Thrombosis**. Thrombosis of bioprostheses is rare and its incidence is influenced by the site and type of the prosthesis. It can be acute or chronic. The sudden deaths are probably related to this complication[19].

V. ANTITHROMBOTIC MANAGEMENT

The therapeutic modalities for preventing thrombotic complications associated with the use of artificial devices depend on the particular device as well as the clinical status of the individual.

This is exemplified here for stents implant. Platelet activation is observed immediately following the implantation of stent, whatever its composition. In fact, negatively charged stents (Strecker, Wiktor) despite the similarity with the platelet membrane behave exactly like metallic stents (Palmaz-Schatze, Medinvent). To avoid the occlusion from the start, every angioplasty patient should be given aspirin (250 mg) and heparin (10,000 to 15,000 units). Long term anticoagulation is said to be essential for the acute phase of implant[20].

In the first clinical trial with wall stent two types of antithrombotic treatment dipyridamole (300 mg/day) and aspirin (100 mg/day) and the combined regimen of dipyridamole/aspirin plus oral anticoagulant with an INR>2-3 were compared[20]. Thrombotic occlusion within 15 days for the former mode of therapy were 39% versus 24% for the combined mode of therapy. Different results are nevertheless obtained with different types of stent implant. Of course, aggressive antithrombotic therapy is always associated with higher risk of hemorrhage.

Several modes of antithrombotic therapy are currently proposed for the management of patients during the critical period of up to 2 to 4 weeks, aiming at an INR close to 2.5 for patient/control as the standard. In principal a therapeutic dose of heparin is given before warfarin is initiated and after implant and this therapy is followed during 3 months.

Because of early high incidence of thromboembolism the use of oral anticoagulants is recommended, as the preventative measure, though the incidence of haemorrhages is a matter of concern. Combined therapy; Warfarin in combination with aspirin (ASA) or dipyridamole has been tried without significant difference but the rate of gastrointestinal haemorrhage increases heavily in ASA as compared to dipyridamole group[21]. Antiplatelet drugs are not as effective as Warfarin therapy. Therefore the antivitamin K therapy remains the basic treatment in patients with mechanical heart valve prostheses[22].

In the therapy of valve thrombosis the fibrinolytic agents alone or combined with heparin have a good success rate[23]. However, such therapy can generate transient peripheral or cerebral emboli. In selecting the treatment of choice clinicians should take into account the usual contraindications of fibrinolytic therapy, particularly after recent surgery (less than 15d) or recent and non-transient cerebral embolism.

During hemodialysis, sufficient heparin is given to prolong the APTT to 1.5 to 2.5 times the basal level. In contrast, cardiopulmonary bypass requires a much larger doses of heparin resulting in very long APTT, which is then of no value in monitoring coagulability[22]. Nevertheless, the prothrombotic state of the patients should be determined prior to the procedure, because it might influence therapy.

Patients with mechanical heart valves require lifetime oral anticoagulation. Infection remains the most frustrating complication of the long-term use of artificial devices, deserving attention to maintaining absolutely sterile technique during the implant procedure as well as in all aspects of postoperative care.

VI. FUTURE TRENDS

There is an urgent need for small diameter vascular grafts which can survive for longer than 10 years. Major progress has been made in several areas, such as in the development of materials that inhibit coagulation fibrinolysis and platelet aggregation. The use of resorbed and replaced materials and "test tube vessels", where the cell culture is used to create a new blood vessel, has been advanced. Stents are now frequently used in arterial intervention. In a recent French study[24] on 272 stented patients, treated with 250 mg/day ticlopidine, 100 mg/day aspirin, a bolus of 10,000 IU of standard heparin was injected before coronary angioplasty, and then 5000 IU at the end of stent implantation. The stents were deployed with 2.5 - 5.0 mm balloon at 11.8 ATM (mean), subacute occlusion within the first month occurred in 2.2% of patients, with no death or surgery in 97.8% of patients. This new therapeutic protocol using ticlopidine at a moderate dose may not be sufficient in all patients. The low dose of aspirin without heparin use after sheath removal appears to be highly effective and safe in coronary stent-implant patients. The protocol using the combination ticlopidine-aspirin on the theoretical basis is more appropriate as these drugs are active in different pathways of platelet activation. This therapeutic strategy nevertheless should be proven by large controlled trials. Nevertheless thromboembolism and infection remain the two principal current limitations of long-term usage of artificial surfaces. Special attention is also needed regarding optimal therapeutic anticoagulant and antibiotic therapy in this area of clinical medicine.

While undoubtedly the biomaterials of the future will offer exciting progress, thoughtful clinical management will always be required for the control and prevention of thrombotic complications of artificial surfaces in certain types of patients.

Contact of blood with artificial surfaces involves participation of cellular components of blood such as erythrocytes and leucocytes in complex cell-protein and cell-cell interactions[25]. Platelet adhesion is promoted by absorption of fibrinogen and vWF fibronectin on surfaces. The timing of the fibrinogen absorption and removal from the artificial surface may have important clinical consequences. Gammaglobulin absorption also promotes platelet reactivity and may induce leucocyte adhesion. On the other hand absorbed albumin reduces platelet and leucocyte adhesion thus inhibiting thrombus formation. The hydrodynamic behaviour of erythrocytes, and deposition of erythrocytes on surfaces can influence platelet adhesion and thrombus formation on artificial surfaces.

Thrombus formation on an artificial surface involves FXIIa-induced release of ADP from platelets, which brings about the participation of the complement system and the modulation of immunological and inflammatory reactions. Activation of the contact system can also increase fibrinolytic activity, as identified by increased levels of FDP.

Leucocyte adhesion is also influenced by the nature of the absorbed protein layer. Leucocyte adhesion may be followed by activation and stimulation of cell functions such as protein synthesis, promoting the production and release of substances such as superoxide and other free radicals, leukotrienes, interleukins, tumour necrosis factor, plasminogen activator, prostaglandin, histamine and platelet activated factors. Adhered granulocytes have reduced ability to combat infection.

Activation of the complement system and release of the anaphylactotoxins C3a and C5a can result from blood contact with an artificial surface[26]. C5a release is important because of it role as a potent mediator of granulocyte response, including, aggregation, degranulation, chemotaxis, and toxic oxygen radical production. C5a normally contributes to host defence by promoting leucocyte accumulation and activation at local sites of inflammation. In contrast, systemic or intravascular complement activation and C5a formation are believed to induce diffuse granulocyte activation and damage to multiple organ systems[27].

Heparin in combination with an anti-platelet agent are useful in combating thrombosis. However it is to be expected that the implant will be in place within the circulation for many years. Accordingly, one is dealing with rather different long term problems. In such a condition anticoagulation may not always be justifiable.

A comprehensive review of thrombosis on foreign surfaces; the issue of biocompatibility and monitoring of blood response reviewed by Courtney and Forbes[27-30] has recently become available.

ACKNOWLEDGEMENT

I am grateful to Dr David Cummins for his fruitful comments and guidance in the preparation of this manuscript and to Mrs. Gillian Lucas for the typing and amendments.

REFERENCES

1.   **Acar, J., Michel P.L., Berdah J.,** Thromboembolic events in prosthetic valves. In Clinical Thrombosis (Eds) Kwaan H.C.K. and Samama M:M., *CRC Press Florida.*, 225, 1989.
2.   **Carrel, A. and Lindbergh, C.A.,** Culture of whole organs, *Science,* 81, 621, 1935.
3.   **Akutsu, T. and Kolff, W.J.,** Permanent substitutes for valves and hearts, *Trans. Am. Soc. Artif. Intern Organs,* 4, 230, 1958.
4.   **Working Group on Mechanical Circulatory Support of the NHLBI, Artificial Heart and Assist Devices**: Directions, Needs, Costs, Societal and Ethical Issues, NIH Publ. NO. 85-2723, National Institutes of Health, Bethesda, MD, 1985.
5.   **Kolff, W.J.,** The artifical heart; research, development or invention?, *Dis. Chest,* 56, 314, 1969.
6.   **Bernhard, W.F., Husain, M., and Robinson, T.C.,** An appraisal of blood trauma and the blood-material interface following prolonged assisted circulation. *J. Thorac. Cardiovasc. Surg.,* 58, 801, 1969.
7.   **Colman, R.W., Hirsh, J., Marder, V.J., and Salzman, E.W., Eds.,** *Hemostasis and Thrombosis: Basic Principles and Clinical Practice,* Lippincott, New York, 1994.
8.   **Gristina, A.G.,** Biomaterial-centered infection; microbial adhesion versus tissue integration, *Science,* 237, 1588, 1987.
9.   **Didisheim, P. and Watson.** Thromboembolic complications of cardiovascular devices and artificial surfaces. In Clinical Thrombosis (Eds) Kwaan, H.C.K. and Samama, M.M., *CRC Press,* Florida, 275, 1989.
10. **Farah. E.,** Complications thromboemboliques chez les porteurs de prothèses valvulaires, in *Cardiopathies Valvulaires Acquises,* Acar J., Ed., Flammarion, Paris, 1985, 637.
11. **Gimbrone, M.A., Jr., Ed.,** *Vascular Endothelium in Hemostasis and Thrombosis,* Churchill Livingstone, New York, 1986.
12. **Cella, G., Schivazappa, L., Casonato, A., et al.,** In vivo platelet release reaction in patients with heart valve prosthesis, *Haemostasis,* 9, 263, 1980.
13. **Dale, J., Myhre, E., Storstein, O., Stormorken, H.,** Prevention of arterial thromboembolism with acetyl-salicyclic acid. *Am. Heart J.,* 94, 101, 1977.
14. **Harker, L.A., and Schlichter, S.I.,** Studies of platelet and fibrinogen kinetics in patients with prosthetic heart valves. *N. Engl. J. Med.,* 283, 1302, 1970.
15. **Dumoulin-Lagrange, M., Tirmarche, M., Horellou, M.H., et al.,** Modification des plaquettes dans les cardiopathies valvulaires acquises, *Coeur,* 11, 335, 1980.
16. **Conard, J., Horellou, M.H., Baille, T.M., et al.,** Plasma beta thromboglobulin in patients with valvular heart disease with or without valve replacement; relationship with thromboembolic accidents, *Eur. Heart J.,* 5 (Suppl. D), 13, 1984.
17. **Dudczak, R., Niessner H., Thaler, E., et al.,** Plasma concentration of platelet specific proteins and fibrinopeptide A in patients with artificial heart valves, *Haemostasis,* 10, 186, 1981.
18. **Acar, J., Enriquez-Sarano, M., Farah, E., et al.,** Recurrent systemic embolic events with valve prosthesis, *Eur. Heart J.,* 5 (Suppl. D), 33, 1984.
19. **Beeunsaert, R., Denef, B., and De Geest, H.,** Diagnosis and treatment of obstruction of a tricuspid Björk-Sheiley prosthesis, *Acta Cardiol.,* 1, 13, 1983.
20. **Serruys, P.W., Strauss, B.H., et al,** Angiographic follow-up after replacement of a self-expanding coronary-artery stent *N Engl J Med* 324,13,1991.
21. **Starkman, G., Estampes, B., Vernant, P., and Acar, J.,** Prévention des accidents thromboemboliques systémiques chez les patients porteurs de prothèses valvulaires artificielles, *Arch. Mal. Coeur,* 75, 85, 1982.
22. **Loeliger, E.A. and Lewis, S.M.,** Progress in laboratory control of oral anticoagulants, *Lancet,* 2, 318, 1982.
23. **Witchitz, S., Veyrat, C., Moisson, P., et al.,** Fibrinolytic treatment of thrombosis in prosthetic heart valves, *Br. Heart J.,* 44, 545, 1980.
24. **Faivre, R., Petiteau, P.Y., Aubry, P. et al,** Coronary stenting without coumadin : Phase V without heparin. *Thromb haemostas* 73,1700 (abstr.), 1995.
25. **Forbes, C.D., Courtnery, J.M.,** Thrombosis and artificial surfaces. In: Bloom AL, Forbes CD, Thomas DP, Tuddenham EGD (eds). Hemostasis and thrombosis. Edinburgh: Churchil Livingstone, 1301, 1994.
26. **Kazatchkine, M.D., Carreno, M.P.,** Activation of the complement system at the interface between blood and artificial surfaces. *Biomaterials* 9, 30,1987.
27. **Courtney, J.M., Sundaram, S., Forbes, C.D., et al.,** Extracorporeal circulation: biocompatibility of biomaterials. In: Forbes C.D., Cushieri A (eds). *Management of bleeding disorders in surgical practice.* Oxford: Blackwell Scientific, 236, 1993.
28. **Sundaram, S., Courtney, J.M., Taggart, D.P., et al.,** Biocompatibility of cardiopulmonary bypass: influence on blood compatibility of device type, mode of blood flow and duration of application. *Int J. Artif Orans* 17:118,1994.
29. **Courtney, J.M., Sundaram, S., Lamba, N.M.K., Forbes, C.D.,** Monitoring of the blood response in blood purification. *Artif Organs* 17:260, 1993.
30. **Courtney, J.M., Forbes, C.D.,** Thrombosis on foreign surfaces. *British Medical Bulletin* 50, 966, 1994.

Acquired Disorders and Congenital Thrombophilia

A. Acquired Disorders: Epidemiology, Pathophysiological Conditions

HAEMOSTATIC VARIABLES AND ARTERIAL THROMBOTIC DISEASE: EPIDEMIOLOGICAL EVIDENCE

P.Y. Scarabin

Unité INSERM 258, Hôpital Broussais, Paris

INTRODUCTION

After more than a century of debate, the relative contribution of atherogenesis and thrombosis to the development of ischemic heart disease (IHD) remains controversial. Over the past decades, the lipid hypothesis has dominated the epidemiological study of IHD and the role played by lipoproteins in the pathogenesis of the arterial disease has been extensively emphasized. However, there is now evidence that thrombosis may contribute to the onset of clinically manifest IHD (e.g. myocardial infarction, unstable angina, sudden death) not only as an acute complication of atheroma and plaque rupture, but also as a cause of the chronic process of atherogenesis[1].

The relation between haemostatic variables and the IHD risk has not so far been a mainstream topic for investigation. Cross-sectional studies provided little relevant information on haemostatic function in relation to IHD. Longitudinal studies of recurrence in survivors of myocardial infarction are also subject to important drawbacks. Epidemiological surveys in apparently healthy subjects are more adequate but few prospective studies included measures of haemostatic function. This lack of data may be partly due to the difficulties in assessing blood coagulation and fibrinolytic system on a large scale. Most coagulation factors are subject to a large within-subject variability and a single measurement of a haemostatic variable does not necessarily provide a reliable estimation of the actual value in a subject [2-4]. This source of variation may result in a strong underestimation of a relation to IHD. Another problem is the difficulty to detect a prethrombotic state in apparently healthy subjects. Whether high levels of clotting factors as well as a decrease in fibrinolytic activity may be relevant to arterial thrombosis remains questionnable and the usefulness of activation peptides of blood coagulation as markers of IHD risk has still to be assessed.

Early results of cohort studies in healthy subjects are now available. They suggest that plasma fibrinogen, factor VII coagulant activity and other haemostatic variables may be involved in the development of IHD. These data as well as some other epidemiological evidences that support this hypothesis are reviewed here.

I. PROSPECTIVE STUDIES

A. NORTHWICK PARK HEART STUDY

This study was the first one to investigate the relation between a set of haemostatic variables and the IHD risk[5]. Study population consisted of men recruited in occupational groups in North-West London. Baseline examination included platelet count, platelet adhesiveness to glass beads, fibrinolytic activity (dilute clot lysis time), fibrinogen concentration (gravimetric method) and factor V, factor VII, factor VIII, antithrombin III activity. The principal results were based upon 1511 white men aged 40-64 years. After a mean follow-up period of 10 years, 109 subjects had experienced first major events of IHD. Raised factor VII activity and high fibrinogen levels were associated with an increased IHD risk. Multivariate analysis showed independent associations between each of these clotting factors and IHD risk but not for serum cholesterol level (Table I). However, the independent contribution of factor VII to the prediction of IHD was significant only for events occurring within 5 years after initial examination, especially for IHD deaths[6].

A further analysis recently showed a significant interaction between age and dilute clot lysis time in relation to IHD risk. A fall of one standard deviation in fibrinolytic activity was associated with an

0-8493-8481-8/96/$0.00+$.50

increase in IHD risk of about 40% in men aged 40-54 years at the initial examination. In contrast, low fibrinolytic activity was not a significant predictor of IHD in older men[7].

No significant association between other haemostatic variables and IHD incidence was found. Surprisingly, both low and high levels of antithrombin III were associated with increased IHD deaths[8].

Table I : Independent associations with IHD for events occurring within 5 years and in total follow-up period in the Northwick Park Heart Study (After Meade et al , 1985).

IHD < 5 years				All IHD		
Variable	**SRE**	**p**		**Variable**	**SRE**	**p**
Fibrinogen	1.57	0.003		Age	1.65	<0.0001
Age	1.54	0.006		Fibrinogen	1.41	0.0002
Factor VII	1.37	0.03		Systolic BP	1.32	0.008
Systolic BP	1.27	0.09		Cholesterol	1.18	NS
Cholesterol	1.17	NS		Factor VII	1.14	NS
Smoking	-	NS		Smoking	-	NS

SRE : standardised regression effect (increased risk of an event for a one standard deviation rise in each variable).

B. GÖTEBORG STUDY

The relation between haemostatic variables and the incidence of arterial diease was investigated in a random sample of 792 men aged 54 years. During 13.5 years of follow-up, myocardial infarction occurred in 92 subjects and 37 had experienced a stroke. Conventional IHD risk factors as well as factor II-VII-X (Owren method), factor VIII activity, plasminogen concentration and fibinolytic capacity were measured at the baseline examination. Plasma fibrinogen concentration was positively related to the incidence of both myocardial infarction and stroke. After adjustment for smoking, blood pressure and serum cholesterol, the association between fibrinogen level and stroke remained significant but the impact of fibrinogen on IHD risk was of borderline significance. There was a positive interaction between blood pressure and fibrinogen concentration with respect to the risk of stroke[9].

C. THE LEIGH STUDY

Plasma fibrinogen was measured in a sample of 297 men aged 40-69 years. During a mean follow-up interval of 7 years, myocardial infarction occurred in 40 men. There was a strong and independent association between fibrinogen level and IHD incidence[10].

D. FRAMINGHAM STUDY

Fibrinogen levels were measured at the tenth biennial examination of the Framingham Study in 1315 participants. During a follow-up period of 12 years, arterial disease occurred in 165 men and 147 women. Fibrinogen levels were positively associated with the incidence of cardiovascular disease in both sexes. After allowance for the main IHD risk factors, fibrinogen level made significant contribution to the prediction of IHD risk in both sexes. The relationship between fibrinogen value and the incidence of stroke was significant only in men[11].

E. CAERPHILLY AND SPEEDWELL COLLABORATIVE HEART DISEASE STUDIES

The results of these two studies are based upon a combined cohort of 4,860 middle-aged men recruited from the general population. Two hundred fifty one major IHD events had occurred within a mean follow-up period of about 4 years. Both fibrinogen concentration and plasma viscosity made independent contributions to the prediction of IHD risk[12].

F. PROCAM STUDY

This study recently provided information on the association of plasma fibrinogen and factor VII coagulant activity to the subsequent risk of IHD. The clotting factors were measured in 2116 healthy subjects aged 40-65 years. After 6 years of follow-up, 82 major IHD events (9 sudden deaths, 14 fatal and 59 nonfatal myocardial infarctions) were recorded. Multivariate analysis showed that a high level of fibrinogen was an important risk factor for IHD. In addition, there was a positive interaction between fibrinogen and LDL cholesterol levels with respect to IHD risk. Interestingly, the incidence of IHD was similar at any level of LDL cholesterol in men with low fibrinogen concentration. There was no clear association between factor VII and IHD risk. However, there was a borderline significant higher factor VII activity in subjects who experienced fatal events than in the non-event group[13].

G. PHYSICIANS' HEALTH STUDY

The association between endogenous tissue-type plasminogen activator (tPA) and cardiovascular risk has been tested in two nested case-control studies using the Physicians' Health Study cohort. The concentration of tPA antigen was measured in 231 healthy subjects who later developed myocardial infarction and in an equal number of subjects matched for age and smoking who remained free of cardiovascular disease within a follow-up period of 5 years. High levels of tPA antigen were associated with an increased risk of myocardial infarction. Multiple regression analysis showed that HDL-cholesterol, total cholesterol, tPA antigen, and systolic blood pressure were the most powerful predictors of IHD risk[14]. Using a similar study design, level of tPA antigen was found to be positively associated with the risk of stroke, even after adjustment for blood pressure and other confounders[15].

II. INFLUENCE OF CARDIOVASCULAR RISK FACTORS

Associations between haemostatic variables and the risk of subsequent IHD do not necessarily imply cause-effect relationships. However, general epidemiological characteristics of fibrinogen and factor VII are consistent with the hypothesis that these clotting factors may play a role in the pathogenesis of IHD (Table II). It is quite conceivable that adverse effects of some cardiovascular risk factors on the development of IHD may be partly due to changes in the coagulation system.

A. AGE

Advancing age is probably the most powerful predictor of IHD risk. Both fibrinogen concentration and factor VII activity are positively correlated with age in both sexes[16-19]. Fibrinogen level increases about 2 mg/dl and 1 mg/dl per year in men and women, respectively[20]. The rise in factor VII with age is steeper in women than in men (about 1% and 0.5% per year, respectively) within the range 20-64 years[21]. A positive correlation between age and the ratio of factor VII activity to factor VII antigen has been reported[18]. This association is consistent with an increased level of activated factor VII form in the elderly. Using a more direct approach to estimate activated factor VII, similar results have been recently found[22].

B. SMOKING

A number of cross-sectional studies have consistently shown higher levels of plasma fibrinogen in current smokers than in non-smokers and ex-smokers[16,17,19,20]. Cigarette consumption is likely the strongest environmental determinant of plasma fibrinogen level. In several cohort studies, an important part of the relationship between smoking and IHD risk is mediated through fibrinogen concentration[6,11,12]. There is some evidence for a positive dose-response effect of smoking on fibrinogen[19]. A positive association between the lifetime duration of smoking and plasma fibrinogen has been reported[23]. After stopping cigarette consumption, fibrinogen concentration falls to a level found in life-long non-smokers in 5 to 10 years[19,23]. Longitudinal data showed that smoking cessation and resumption of the habit was associated with a decrease or an increase in fibrinogen level of about 15 mg/dl[23].

C. PLASMA LIPIDS AND DIETARY FAT

There is clear evidence for a strong and positive association of both serum cholesterol and triglyceride levels with factor VII activity[5,24-26]. In the Northwick Park Heart Study, the relation between factor VII and the incidence of IHD was significant after adjustment for cholesterol level while the impact of cholesterol on IHD risk was not substantial in multivariate analysis[6]. Further studies have suggested that the relation between plasma lipids and factor VII activity was explained in part by factor VII activation and not only in terms of total factor VII concentration[24,25].

Experimental studies have shown a positive association between the day-to-day variation in total fat intake and factor VII activity[27]. There is some evidence that triglyceride-rich lipoproteins generated in response to fat intake may result in increased activity state of factor VII perhaps through the production of free fatty acids during alimentary lipemia [28-30]. A long-term study of a diet lower in fat and cholesterol (American Heart Association phase 2 diet) has recently shown a decrease in both serum cholesterol and factor VII activity (about 6 % and 11%, respectively) without any change in total factor VII concentration and plasma fibrinogen concentration[31].

D. ORAL CONTRACEPTIVES AND MENOPAUSAL STATUS

Raised factor VII coagulant activity and, to a lesser extent, high level of plasma fibrinogen concentration have been found in women taking oral contraceptives[17,32-34]. A dose-response effect of ethinyloestradiol on factor VII has been reported in pill users[33]. Whether the rise in factor VII activity is due to a higher proportion of activated factor VII rather than to an increase in the concentration of native factor VII protein is not yet well documented. Two recent cross-sectional studies failed, however, to show an increased factor VII activation in oral contraceptive users[22,34].

Population-based studies reported higher levels of both factor VII activity and fibrinogen concentration in postmenopausal than in premenopausal women of the same age[17,19,20,35-37]. A further rise in factor VII activity was observed in women having undergone bilateral oophorectomy[36]. This finding may be relevant to the two-fold increase in IHD risk which follows castration in women[38]. Observational studies suggested that the putative beneficial effect of hormone replacement therapy on the development of IHD could be partly mediated through a decrease in both factor VII activity and fibrinogen concentration[39,40].

Table II : Determinants of fibrinogen levels and factor VII activity

Factor VII		Fibrinogen
	Increased	
Age		Age
Obesity		Obesity
Oral contraceptive		Oral contraceptive
Hyperlipidemia		Smoking
Saturated fat intake		Low employment grade
Menopause		Menopause
Diabetes		Diabetes
	Decreased	
Low fat diet		Moderate alcohol intake

E. OTHER CHARACTERISTICS

Fibrinogen level has been shown to be negatively correlated with alcohol consumption[16,19,20] and positively associated with body mass index [16,17,19,20]. Both factor VII activity and fibrinogen level are higher in diabetic patients than in control subjects[20]. A negative association between fibrinogen concentration and employment grade has been reported[37]. This finding may be relevant to the higher rate of IHD in lower employment grades. Familial history of myocardial infarction has been related to high levels of fibrinogen in young people[41]. Seasonal variations in fibrinogen levels are well documented [42-45]. Higher concentrations of fibrinogen in cold months may partly account for the increased risk of IHD in winter.

III. GENETIC CONTRIBUTION

The relative contribution of genetic and environmental factors to plasma concentrations of haemostatic proteins related to IHD risk is not yet well documented. Most studies were performed in small population samples and confidence intervals of estimates were large.

A . FIBRINOGEN

Heritability has been shown to account for about 50% of the total phenotypic variance of plasma fibrinogen levels in Swedish nuclear families[46]. In Norwegian monozygotic twins, the intraclass correlation coefficient was only 0.27[47]. Several restriction fragment length polymorphisms (RFLPs) at the A- and B-fibrinogen loci have been used to investigate the genetic variations in plasma fibrinogen levels. In a British study of three RFLPs, the strongest association was found with the *Bcl*I polymorphism at the B-fibrinogen locus. Genetic variation at this locus accounted for 9% of the variance of fibrinogen[48]. By contrast, a Norwegian study and a Scottish study failed to detect any association between *Bcl*I polymorphism and the plasma fibrinogen concentrations[47,49]. In a subsequent British study, a *Hae*III RFLP located in the promoter region of the B-fibrinogen gene was significantly associated with fibrinogen levels and this genetic variation explained about 3% of the total phenotypic variance[50]. In a large French case-control study of myocardial infarction (ECTIM study), the *Hae*III RFLP at the B-fibrinogen locus was also significantly related to plasma fibrinogen concentrations, but it explained only 1% of the total phenotypic variation[51]. There was some evidence for a positive interaction of smoking and *Hae*III RFLP in determining plasma fibrinogen levels[51,52].

Whether fibrinogen genotype is related to cardiovascular risk has to be further investigated. A Scottish case-control study has recently reported an association between genetic variation at the B-fibrinogen locus and increased risk of peripheral atherosclerosis[53]. The ECTIM study fails to detect any association between the *Hae*III genotype of fibrinogen and the risk of myocardial infarction[51]. However, the case-control approach tends to select survivors of myocardial infarction and it is quite conceivable that the association between *Hae*III genotype and the MI risk might differ in patients who experienced a fatal event. Prospective data are clearly needed to explore this possibility.

B . FACTOR VII

A common genetic polymorphism of factor VII has been identified in healthy sujects from the United Kingdom[54]. This RFLP of factor VII gene changes arginine (Arg) at residue 353 to glutamine (Gln). The frequency of the allele for Gln_{353} (absence of the *Msp*I cutting site) was 10%. There was a strong association between *Msp*I RFLP at the factor VII locus and the factor VII coagulant activity Heterozygotes had factor VII activity 22% lower than the sample mean. The *Msp*I genotype accounted for about 20% of the total phenotypic variation.

A further study of healthy men from the United Kingdom showed a significant interaction between plasma triglycerides and factor VII *Msp*I genotype in determining factor VII activity[55]. There was a strong and positive correlation between factor VII activity and triglyceride levels in subjects who carry the allele for Arg_{353} whereas no association was found in those carrying the allele for Gln_{353}.

The ECTIM study failed to provide evidence for a significant association between factor VII *Msp*I genotype and the risk of myocardial infarction[56].

CONCLUSIONS AND FUTURE DEVELOPMENTS

The measurement of plasma fibrinogen concentration substantially improves the prediction of arterial disease and high levels of this clotting factor should be added to major cardiovascular risk factors. Whether the association between plasma fibrinogen and CHD risk is one of cause and effect remains to be clarified. Increased plasma fibrinogen concentration may result from the presence of the inflammatory process associated with both chronic and acute phases of atherosclerosis. However, even if high fibrinogen levels may be the consequence of vessel wall damage, they can also be relevant to the pathogenesis of IHD through effects on blood viscosity, platelet aggregation, fibrin formation, and atheroma itself[57].

The association between factor VII activity and IHD risk has to be clearly confirmed. Availability of a novel clot-based assay that directly measures activated factor VII[22] should make it possible to clarify the relevance of raised factor VII activity to thrombogenesis. There is increasing evidence that hypofibrinolysis mainly due to a rise in plasminogen activator inhibitor activity may be involved in the development of atherothrombosis[58,59]. No prospective data are available in healthy subjects. The value of activation peptides of blood coagulation in the assessment of arterial thrombosis risk needs to be investigated. Large cohort studies including haemostatic measurements at the baseline examination are in progress in USA and Europe[60-62] and they should address these issues.

Plasma fibrinogen concentration and factor VII activity can be modified through changes in lifestyle. Smoking and saturated fat intake are major determinants of fibrinogen and factor VII levels, respectively. Therefore, central policies affecting dietary habits or tobacco advertising appear to be further justified to reduce the IHD incidence. However, environmental factors may have limited effects on the haemostatic system. Pharmacological approaches such as low-dose warfarin[63] or fibrinogen-lowering drugs[57] should be considered in the primary prevention of IHD.

REFERENCES

1.   **Fuster, V., Badimon, L., Badimon, J.J., and Chesebro, J.H.,** The pathogenesis of coronary artery disease and the acute coronary syndromes, *N Engl J Med.*, 326, 242, 1992.
2.   **Meade, T.W., North, W.R.S., Chakrabarti, R., Haines, A.P., and Stirling, Y,**Population-based distribution of haemostatic variables, *Br Med Bull*, 33, 283, 1977.
3.   **Thompson, S.G., Martin, J.C., and Meade, T.W,**Sources of variability in coagulation factor assays, *Thomb Haemos*, 58, 1073, 1987.
4.   **Scarabin, P.Y, , Strain, L., Ludlam, C.A., Jones, J., and Kohner, E.M.,** Reliability of a single B-thromboglobulin measurement in a diabetic population: importance of PGE1 in anticoagulant mixture, *Thromb Haemost*, 57, 201, 1987.
5.   **Meade, T.W., Chakrabarti, R., Haines, A.P., North, W.R.S., Stirling, Y., and Thompson, S.G,** Haemostatic function and cardiovascular death : early results of a prospective study, *Lancet*, 1050, 1980.
6.   **Meade, T.W., Mellows, S., Brozovic, M., Miller, G.J., Chakrabarti, R.R., North, R.R., Haines, A.P., Stirling, Y., Imeson, J.D., and Thompson. S.G,** Haemostatic function and ischaemic heart disease: principal results of the Northwick Park Heart Study, *Lancet*, ii,, 533, 1986.
7.   **Meade, T.W., Ruddock, V., Stirling, Y., Chakrabarti, R., and Miller, G.J.,** Fibrinolytic activity, clotting factors, and long-term incidence of ischaemic heart disease in the Northwick Park Heart Study, *Lancet*, 342, 1076, 1993.
8.   **Meade, T.W., Cooper, J., Miller G.J., Howarth, D.J.,and Stirling, Y.,** Antithrombin III and arterial disease, *Lancet*, 337, 850, 1991.
9.   **Wilhelmsen, L., Svardsudd, K., Korsan-Bengsten, K., Larsson, B., Welin, L., and Tibblin, G.,** Fibrinogen as a risk factor for stroke and myocardial infarction, *N Engl J Med*, 311, 501, 1983.
10.   **Stone, M.C., and Thorp, J.M.,** Plasma fibrinogen: a major coronary risk factor., *J R Coll Gen Pract* , 35, 565, 1985.
11.   **Kannel, W.B., Wolf, P.A., Castelli, W.P., and D'Agostino, R.B.,** Fibrinogen and risk of cardiovascular disease: the Framingham Study, *JAMA*, 258, 1183, 1987.
12.   **Yarnell, J.W.G., Baker, I.A., Sweetnam, P.M., Bainton, D., O'Brien, J.R., Whitehead, P.J., and Elwood, P.C.,** Fibrinogen, viscosity, and white blood cell count are major risk factors for ischemic heart disease. The Caerphilly and Speedwell Collaborative Heart Disease Studies, *Circulation*, 83, 836, 1991.
13.   **Heinrich, J., Balleisen, L., Schulte, H., Assmann, G., and Van de Loo, J.,** Fibrinogen and factor VII in the prediction of coronary risk : results from the PROCAM Study in healthy men, *Arterioscler Thromb*, 14, 54, 1994.
14.   **Ridker, P. M., Vaughan, D. E., Stampfer, M. J., Manson, J. M., and Hennekens, C. H.,**Endogenous tissue - type plasminogen activator and risk of myocardial infarction, *Lancet,* 341, 1165, 1993.
15.   **Ridker, P. M., Hennekens, C.H., Stampfer, M. J., Manson, J. R., and Vaughan, D. E.,** Prospective study of endogenous tissue plasminogen activator and risk of stroke, *Lancet*, 343, 940, 1994.
16.   **Meade, T.W., Chakrabarti, R., Haines, A.P., North, W.R.S., and Stirling, Y.,** Characteristics affecting fibrinolytic activity and plasma fibrinogen concentrations, *British Med J*, 1, 153, 1979.
17.   **Balleisen, L., Bailey, J., Epping, P.H., Schulte, H., and Van de Loo, J.,** Epidemiological study on factor VII, factor VIII and fibrinogen in an industrial population-I. Baseline data on the relation to age, gender, body weight, smoking, alcohol, pill using and menopause, *Thromb Haemos*, 54, 475,1985.
18.   **Scarabin, P.Y., Van Dreden, P., Bonithon-Kopp, C., Orssaud, G., Bara, L., Conard, J., and Samama, M.,** Age-related changes in factor VII activation in healthy women, *Clin Sci*, 75, 341, 1988.
19.   **Lee, A.J., Smith, W.C.S., Lowe, G.D.O., and Tunstall-Pedoe, H.,** Plasma fibrinogen and coronary risk factors: the Scottish Heart Health Study, *J Clin Epidemiol* , 43, 913, 1990.
20.   **Folsom, A.R., Wu, K.K., Davis, C.E., Conlan, M.G., Sorlie, P.D., and Szklo, M.,** Population correlates of plasma fibrinogen and factor VII, putative cardiovascular risk factors, *Atherosclerosis*, 91, 191,1991.
21.   **Brozovic, M., Stirling, Y., Harricks, C., North, W.R.S., and Meade, T.W.,** Factor VII in an industrial population, *Brit J Haematol*, 28, 381, 1974.
22.   **Morissey, J.H., Macik, B.G., Neuenschwander, P.F., and Comp, P.C.,** Quantitation of activated factor VII levels in plasma using a tissue factor mutant selectively deficient in promoting factor VII activation, *Blood*, 81, 734, 1993.
23.   **Meade, T.W., Imeson, J., and Stirling, Y.,** Effects of changes in smoking and other characteristics on clotting factors and the risk of ischaemic heart disease, *Lancet*, 31, 986, 1987.
24.   **Miller G.J, Walter S.J, Stirling Y, Thompson S.G, Esnouf M.P, and Meade T.W,** Assay of factor VII activity by two techniques: evidence for an increased conversion of VII to A-VIIa in hyperlipidemia, with possible implications for ischaemic heart disease. *Br J Haematol*, 59, 249, 1985.
25.   **Scarabin, P.Y., Bara, L., Samama, M., and Orssaud, G.,** Further evidence that activated factor VII is related to plasma lipids, *Brit J Haematol*, 59, 186, 1985.
26.   **Bruckert, E., Carvalho de Souza, J., Giral, P., Soria, C., Chapman, M.J., Caen, J., and De Gennes, J.L.,** Interrelationship of plasma triglyceride and coagulant factor VII levels in normotriglyceridemic hypercholesterolemia, *Atherosclerosis*, 75, 129,1989.

27. **Miller, G.J, Martin, J.C., Webster, J., Wilkes, H., Miller, N.E., Wilkinson, W.H., and Meade,T.W.,** Association between dietary fat intake and plasma factor VII coagulant activity - A predictor of cardiovascular mortality, *Atherosclerosis*, 60, 269, 1986.

28. **Miller, G.J., Martin, J.C., Mitropoulos K.A., Reeves, B.E.A., Thompson, S.G., Meade, T.W., Cooper, J.A., and Cruickshank, JK,** Plasma factor VII is activated by postprandial triglyceridaemia, irrespective of dietary fat composition, *Atherosclerosis*, 86,163,1991.

29. **Mitropoulos, K.A., Miller, G.J., Martin, J.C., Reeves, B.E.A., and Cooper, J.,** Dietary fat induces changes in factor VII coagulant activity through effects on plasma free stearic acid concentration, *Arterioscler Thromb*, 14, 214, 1994.

30. **Silveira, A., Karpe, F., Blomback, M., Stelner, G., Walldius, G., and Hamstcn, A.,** Activation of coagulation factor VII during alimentary lipemia, *Arterioscler Thromb*, 14, 60, 1994.

31. **Brace, L.D., Gittler-Buffa, C., Miller, G.J., Cole, T.G., Schmeisser, D., Prewitt, T.E., and Bowen, P.E.,** Factor VII coagulant activity and cholesterol changes in premenopausal women consuming a long-term cholesterol-lowering diet, *Arterioscler Thromb*, 14, 1284, 1994.

32. **Poller, L., and Thompson, J.M.,** Clotting factors during oral contraception. Further report. *Brit MedJ*, 2, 23, 1992.

33. **Meade, T.W., Haines, A.P., North, W.R.S., Chakrabarti, R.R., Howarth, D.J., and Stirling, Y.,** Haemostatic, lipid and blood pressure profiles of women on oral contraceptives containing 50 ug and 30 ug oestrogen, *Lancet*, 2, 948, 1977.

34. **Plu-Bureau, G., Scarabin, P.Y., Bara, L.., Malmejac, A., Guize, L., and Samama, M.,** Factor VII activation and oral contraceptives, *Thromb Res* , 70, 275, 1993.

35. **Meade, T.W., Imeson, J.D., Haines, A.P., Stirling, Y., and Thompson, S.G.,** Menopausal status and haemostatic variables. *Lancet* ; i:22, 1986.

36. **Scarabin, P.Y., Bonithon-Kopp, C., Bara, L., Malmejac, A., Guize, L., and Samama, M.,** Factor VII activation and menopausal status. *Thromb Res* ; 57:227, 1990.

37. **Brunner, E.J., Marmot, M.G., White, I.R., O'Brien, J.R., Etherington, M.D, Slavin, B.M, Kearnet, E.M., and Smith, G.D.,** Gender and employment grade differences in blood cholesterol apoliproteins and haemostatic factors in the Whitehall II Study, *Atherosclerosis*, 102, 195, 1993.

38. **Colditz, G.A., Willett, W.C., Stampter, M.J., Rosnerc, B., Speizer, F.E. and Hennekens C.H.,** Menopause and the risk of coronary heart disease in women. *N Engl J Med.*, 316, 1105, 1987.

39. **Nabulsi, A.A., Folsom, A.R., White, A., Patsh, W., Heiss, G., Kenneth, K.W., and Szklo, M.,** Association of hormone-replacement therapy with various cardiovascular risk of factors in postmenopausal women, *N Engl J Med*, 328, 1069, 1993.

40. **Scarabin, P.Y., Plu-Bureau, G., Bara, L., Bonithon-Kopp, C., Guize, L, and Samama M.M.,** Haemostatic variables and menopausal status : influence of hormone replacement therapy, *Thromb Haemost*, 70, 584, 1993.

41. **Bara, L., Nicaud, V., Tiret, L., Cambien, F., and Samama, M.M.,** On behalf of the EARS Group., Expression of a paternal history of premature myocardial infarction on fibrinogen, factor VIIc and PAI-1 in European offspring - The EARS Study, Thromb Haemos, 71,144, 1994.

42. **Stout, R.W., and Crawford, V.,** Seasonal variations in fibrinogen concentrations among elderly people, *Lancet*, 338, 9, 1991.

43. **Woodhouse, P.R., Khaw, T.K., Foley, A., and Meade, T.W.,** Seasonal variations of plasma fibrinogen and factor VII activity in the elderly : winter infections and death from cardiovascular disease, *Lancet*, 343, 435, 1994.

44. **Elwood, P.C., Beswick, A. Obrien, J.R., Renaud, S., Fifield, R., Limb, E.S., and Bainton, D.,** Temperature and risk factors for ischaemic heart disease in the Caerphilly prospective study, *Brit Heart J*, 70, 6, 520, 1993.

45. **Scarabin, P.Y., Bara, L, Nicaud, V., Cambou, J.P., Arveiler, D., Luc, G., Evans, A.E., and Cambien F.,** Seasonal variations of plasma fibrinogen in elderly people, *Lancet*, 343, 975, 1994.

46. **Hamsten A, Iselius D, De Faire U, and Blomback M.,** Genetic and cultural inheritance of plasma fibrinogen concentration, *Lancet*, ii, 988,1987.

47. **Berg K, and Kierulf P.,** DNA polymorphisms at fibrinogen loci and plasma fibrinogen concentration, *Clin Genet* , 36, 229, 1989.

48. **Humphries, S.E., Cook, M., Dubowitz M, Stirling, Y., and Meade, T.W.,** Role of genetic variation at the fibrinogen locus in determination of plasma fibrinogen concentration, *Lancet*, i, 1452, 1987.

49. **Connor, J.M., Fowkes, F.G.R., Wood, J., Smith, F.B., Donnan, P.T., and Lowe, G.D.O.,** Genetic variation at fibrinogen loci and plasma fibrinogen levels, *J Med Genet*, 29, 480, 1992.

50. **Thomas, A.E., Green, F.R., Kelleher, C.H., Wilkes, H.C., Brennan, P.J., Meade, T.W., and Humphries, S.E.,** Variation in the promoter region of the B-fibrinogen gene is associated with plasma fibrinogen levels in smokers and non-smokers, *Thromb Haemost*, 65, 487, 1991.

51. **Scarabin, P.Y., Bara, L., Ricard, S., Poirier, O., Cambou, J.P., Arveiller, D., Luc, G., Evans, A.E., Samama, M., and Cambien, F.,** Genetic variation at the B-fibrinogen locus in relation to plasma fibrinogen concentrations and risk of myocardial infartion, *Arterioscl Thromb*, 886, 1993.

52. **Green, F., Hamsten, A., Blomback, M., and Humphries, S.,** The role of β-fibrinogen genotype in determining plasma fibrinogen levels in young survivors of myocardial infarction and healthy controls from sweden, *Thromb Haemost*, 70, 915, 1993.

53. **Fowkes, F.G.R., Connor, J.M., Smith, F.B., Wood, J., Donnan, P.T., and Lowe G.D.O.,** Fibrinogen genotype and risk of peripheral atherosclerosis, *Lancet*, 339, 693, 1992.

54. **Green, F., Kelleher, C., Wilkes, H., Temple, A., Meade, T.W., and Humphries, S.E.,** A common genetic polymorphism associated with lower coagulant factor VII levels in healthy individuals. *Arterioscl Thromb*, 11, 540,1991.

55. **Humphries, S., Lane, A., Green, A., Green, F., Cooper, J., and Miller, G.J,** Factor VII coagulant activity and antigen levels in healthy men are determined by interaction between factor VII genotype and plasma triglyceride concentration. *Arterioscler Thromb*, 14,193, 1994.

56. **Lane, A., Green, F., Scarabin, P.Y., Nicaud, V., Bara, L., Humphries, S., Evans, A., Luc, G., Cambou, J.P., Arveiler, D., and Cambien, F.,** The factor VII Arg/Gln$_{353}$ polymorphism determines factor VII coagulant activity in patients with myocardial infarction (MI) and control subjects in Belfast and in France but is not a strong indicator of the MI risk in the ECTIM Study. *Atherosclerosis* (in press).

57. **Ernst, E,** The role of fibrinogen as a cardiovascular risk factor, *Atherosclerosis*, 100, 1, 1993.

58. **Juhan-Vague, I., and Alessi, MC.,** Plasminogen activator inhibitor 1 and atherothrombosis, *Thromb Haemostas*, 70, 138, 1993.

59.   **Hamsten, A,** The haemostatic system and coronary heart disease, *Thromb Res,* 70, 1, 1993.
60.   **The ARIC Investigators.,** The atherosclerosis risk in communities (ARIC) study : design and objectives, *Am J Epidemiol,* 129, 4, 687, 1989.
61.   **Miller, G.J.,** Hemostasis and cardiovascular risk, the British and European experience, *Arch Pathol Lab Med,* 116, 1318,1992.
62.   **Scarabin, P.Y., Juhan-Vague, I., and Cambien F.,** The PRIME Study, personal communication, 1994.
63.   **Meade,T.W., Wilkes, H.C., Stirling, Y., Brennan, P.J., Kelleher, C., and Browne, W.,** Randomised controlled trial of low-dose warfarin in the primary prevention of ischaemic heart disease : design and pilot study, *Eur Heart J,* 9, 836, 1988.

HYPERLIPIDEMIA AND BLOOD COAGULATION

M.P. Esnouf
Nuffield Dept of Clinical Biochemistry, Radcliffe Infirmary, University of Oxford.

I. INTRODUCTION

Epidemiological studies suggest that the predominant effect of hyperlipidemia is to increase the thrombogenic potential of the plasma giving rise to an increased risk of ischaemic heart disease. The emphasis of this review will be on the interactions of the proteins of the contact phase of coagulation with the surface of lipoprotein particles. However, it is still a matter of debate as to what extent the activation of the contact-phase proteins by these surfaces contributes to the hypercoagulable state.

Hyperlipidemia is a state that everybody achieves, albeit temporarily, at least once or twice a day and is induced simply by eating. Two hours or so after ingestion, lipoprotein particles can be detected in the plasma and their concentration is proportional to the lipid content of the meal. During this phase, the triglycerides in the chylomicron particles are hydrolysed by lipoprotein lipase and the free fatty acids are transported across the vascular endothelium. The fatty acid carboxyl groups confer a negative charge onto the surface of the lipid particles and these negatively charged particles become a potent surface for activating factor XII. It is the physical nature of the surface created by these fatty acids which determines their reactivity with the contact phase proteins. In the normal course of events this effect is minimised by the neutralisation of the negative charge by the positively charged lipid binding proteins such as β_2-glycoprotein I and annexin V. It could also be argued that the fibrinolytic pathway is also stimulated through the increased rate of activation of the contact phase. However, the physiological significance of this route remains to be proved.

II. HUMAN HYPERLIPIDEMIAS

The feeding of a high fat diet to human volunteers shows a strong association between VIIc and the amount of fat consumed two hours earlier[1] . The rise in the coagulant activity of factor VII (VIIc) is most closely related to the increase in the triglyceride rich VLDL and chylomicron fractions of the plasma lipoproteins[2] and is not associated with an increase in the concentration of factor VII[3,4]. There is, in the general population, a positive association between the habitual consumption of fat and VIIc[5]. Women during late pregnancy are also hyperlipidaemic and this is associated with an increased concentration of large lipoprotein particles[6], an increased concentration of free fatty acids[7] and a raised VIIc[8]. In these cases and in those individuals who have sustained hyperlipidemia, the rise in VIIc is also associated with an increase in the factor VII concentration[1,8]. In contrast, patients with a deficiency of functional lipoprotein lipase have a massive hyperlipidemia, do not have a high VIIc nor elevated levels of factorVII[9] ,which suggests that the lipolysis of the lipoprotein particles is a prerequisite for factor VII activation. It is likely that sustained factor VII activation leads to the increased rate of production of prothrombin F1.2, which in turn stimulates the hepatic synthesis of the vitamin K-dependent clotting factors, including factor VII[10] (see later).

III. THE INTERACTION OF
THE CONTACT-PHASE PROTEINS WITH FACTOR VII

The four proteins of the contact-phase, factor XII, prekallikrein, high molecular-weight kininogen and factor XI all interact on a negatively charged surface to produce a number of activated products some of which remain associated with the surface (α-factor XIIa and factor XIa) while kallikrein and bradykinin, having lost their binding domains, leave the surface[11]. It has been known for many years that the cold-activation of factor VII in citrated plasma is caused by β-factor XIIa[12]. At 37°C the activation of factor VII by β-factor XIIa is normally inhibited by C $\overline{1}$ esterase inhibitor but at 0°C the activity of the inhibitor is reduced fifteen fold[13]. If factor VII is activated by the contact phase *in* vivo, at 37°C and in the presence of Ca++, there most be an endogenous activator of factor XII, which is not blocked by C $\overline{1}$ esterase inhibitor, but is able to activate factor VII.

The first stage in this process to consider is contact activation. This occurs when factor XII is exposed to an electronegative surface such as ellagic acid, dextran sulphate or cerebroside sulphatides[14-18]. In purified systems the presence of the surface promotes "autoactivation" of factor XII first to two-chain α-XIIa and subsequently to a degradation product, β-XIIa, which has no direct coagulant activity[19]. The autoactivation is catalysed by traces (0.7-0.3%) of factor αXIIa[20] contaminating the preparations of factor XII by traces. In plasma, the contact phase involves three other proteins, namely, prekallikrein, high molecular weight kininogen and factor XI [21,22] and the co-operative effect of these other proteins amplifies the initial activation of factor XII. The structural and functional relationship of the interactions of the proteins involved in the contact phase have been reviewed comprehensively[23]. Nuijens et al [24] describe a monoclonal antibody directed against an N-terminal fragment (Mr 40,000) of factor XII which activates the contact phase in the absence of a surface. The authors conclude that factor XII can exist in two forms, one active and the other inactive and that their antibody or an electronegative surface can stabilise the single chain form in an "active" conformation. Thus factor XII in the active conformation would convert some prekallikrein to kallikrein which in turn would stabilise the active conformation of factor XII by proteolytic cleavage. The α-XIIa generated by exposure to a suitable surface activates factor XI [25] which in turn activates factor IX[26]. Activated factor XII, kallikrein, and factor IXa all activate factor VII[12], thus providing a link between the contact phase and the first step of the extrinsic system.

The presence of an endogenous surface capable of activating factor XII in plasma can be demonstrated by the storage of citrated plasma, taken from women in late pregnancy, overnight in plastic tubes at 4°C[15]. In contrast, plasma taken from non-pregnant controls and stored under the same conditions, shows little or no increase in XIIa or VIIc. The extent of " cold-activation " of factor VII in samples of plasma taken during late pregnancy was reduced by 67% in the presence of a Mab directed against factor IX as compared with 22% by an anti-factor XI Mab[27]. This suggests that under these conditions factor VII appears to be activated directly by factor IXa and since the anti-XI Mab was less effective than the anti-factor IX, it is possible that the factor IX was activated directly by kallikrein. In the presence of EDTA (2mM) the rate of factor VII activation was depressed, whereas there was no effect on the rate of factor XII activation. The activation of factor VII seen in the presence of EDTA may reflect its direct activation by XIIa (α or β).

We have suggested[13] that large lipoprotein particles with negatively charged long-chain saturated fatty acids at their interface with plasma, provide the physiological activating surface. The negative charge arises in all probability from the action of lipoprotein lipase. Patients with a deficiency of the enzyme[10], whose plasma has a very high triglyceride content, have normal values of XIIa and VIIc, and show a rapid activation of factor XII following the addition of lipoprotein lipase.

Recently, the role of factor XII in coagulation has been questioned because patients with factor XII deficiency show no haemostatic complications and also by the demonstration that factor XI bound to an electronegative surface is rapidly activated by thrombin[28,29]. However, the interpretation of these experiments has been challenged[30,31] because they were carried out with purified reagents. When the experiments were repeated in plasma or in the presence of fibrinogen, the preferred substrate for thrombin, little or no factor XI activation could be detected.

IV. THE ACTIVATION OF FACTOR XII BY FATTY ACIDS

The incubation of purified factor XII (0.15 - 1.4 µM) with long chain saturated fatty acids such as stearate (C-18) or behenate (C-22) emulsified with albumin (15.6 : 1), results in the activation of the zymogen with kinetics similar to those obtained from the incubation of factor XII with sulphatide vesicles or dextran sulphate[32]. It was concluded that the factor XII was activated by the crystalline non-bound stearate or behenate, while the fatty-acids bound at the high or low affinity sites were ineffective. In contrast, an emulsion prepared with an unsaturated fatty acid (oleic) did not activate the factor XII. It was suggested that factor XII was activated on a surface which had immobile negatively charged groups with an optimal charge density. More recently we[20] have extended this study using factor XII (0.025 - 0.25 µM) containing < 0.05% XIIa. The XIIa generated was measured by an ELISA rather than by amidolytic activity. This enabled us to measure XIIa formation within 5 sec of exposure to the surface. The reaction was stopped by dilution in buffer containing Tween-20 (0.05%). Under these conditions the optimal XII concentration was 0.15 µM and the optimal ratio of fatty acid to albumin was 3.9:1. We also investigated the effect of emulsions made with the *cis*- and *trans*-isomers of C 18-1 and C18-2 fatty acids. Factor XII activation only occurred when the reaction was studied below the melting point of the particular isomer.

V. ACTIVATION OF FACTOR VII

Factor VII is converted *in vitro* to α-factor VIIa in the presence of tissue factor and calcium ions by all the activated coagulation factors except by the enzymes from the contact-phase[12] . The activation by Xa which is the most potent activator of factor VII, is inhibited by Tissue Factor Pathway Inhibitor[33] secreted from the endothelium. Unlike the other activated coagulation factors VIIa is only poorly inhibited by the plasma protease inhibitors[34] thus increasing its half-life in plasma. Therefore the coagulant activity of factor VII (VIIc) is an indicator of the flux of the coagulation system.

Factor VII also binds to triglyceride rich plasma lipoprotein fractions coated on wells of a microtitre plate[35] associating most strongly with the chylomicron and VLDL fractions; this interaction is not calcium dependent and does not take place in the presence of the detergent Tween-20. This suggests that the association of factor VII with the lipoproteins is hydrophobic, in contrast to the interaction with tissue factor. It is, therefore, possible that factors XII and VII may associate on a lipoprotein surface and the factor VII is activated directly by the XIIa generated on the same surface. Experiments in which rabbits were fed a diet supplemented with 1% cholesterol resulted in a considerable increase in large lipoprotein particles and a three-fold rise in VIIc[36], which could be attributed to an increase in the rise in the specific activity of the factor VII. Since native factor VII has no coagulant activity[37,38,39] it means that an increase in VIIc is due to a rise in the proportion of activated factor VII (αVIIa). It should be emphasised that the response of the single-stage assay to VIIa depends very much on the reagents used for the assay[40]. The increase in VIIc in the hypercholesterolaemic rabbit is also associated with a 150 - 200% rise in the plasma concentration of prothrombin, factor X[41] and factor XII[42] There was also an increase in the mean absolute catabolic rates for prothrombin and factor X being 1.8 times that of the control group. It has already been shown[43] that the rate of synthesis of the vitamin K dependent coagulation factors by hepatocyte cultures could be doubled following the addition of fragments which contained the first forty-five residues of prothrombin to the culture medium. This stimulation in the rate of transcription of these proteins was dependent on the presence of γ-carboxyglutamic acid in the fragment. We proposed[9] that the increase in the rate of synthesis of prothrombin and factor X in the hypercholesterolaemic rabbits was caused by an increase in the steady state concentration of the prothrombin activation peptide fragment 1.2 arising from the increase in the catabolic rate. To test this hypothesis normal rabbits were injected with 10 mg of bovine fragment 1. It was found that there was a transient increase in the plasma concentration of the two clotting factors reaching a maximum after 32 hours (factor X) and 55 hours (prothrombin). We were surprised to find in a second series of experiments[42] in rabbits that there was a similar increase in the absolute catabolic rate of factor XII in response to the high cholesterol diet. In pregnant women and in those taking oral contraceptives, conditions associated with an increase in the flux of the coagulation system, there is also a rise in the concentration of factor XII antigen[42,44,45].

VI. ACTIVATED FACTOR XII IN PLASMA

The sequence of events described above would be credible if it could be shown that plasma contained activated factor XII. Until recently the only available methods were based on the measurement of the amidolytic activity of diluted plasma samples in the presence of protease inhibitors to inhibit kallikrein and other proteases. In an attempt to overcome the uncertainties inherent in this technique we have developed an ELISA based on a monoclonal antibody which is specific for XIIa and has no detectable recognition for factor XII[46]. The mean XIIa concentration in the plasma of 360 middle aged men was 4.2 ± 2.9 ng/ml in a skewed distribution in a range from 2.5 - 27 ng/ml. Plasma contains between 12 - 47 µg/ml factor XII[47], so the amount of XIIa in plasma is about 1/10,000 that of the zymogen. It would seem unlikely that such a wide distribution of XIIa could be accounted for by variations in the plasma factor XII concentration. A more reasonable interpretation is that the difference in the steady state concentration of XIIa arises from varying amounts of large lipoprotein particles (activating surface) in the plasma. This is supported by the finding that there is an association between plasma triglyceride and the amount of XIIa. Western blots of plasma samples, with a high XIIa content, initially separated by SDS-PAGE showed that the majority of the XIIa was free and not associated with C $\overline{1}$ esterase inhibitor. It is likely that the XIIa was originally associated with an activating surface which shields it from interacting with C $\overline{1}$ esterase inhibitor[48].

VII. THE PHOSPHOLIPID BINDING PROTEINS

The negative charge created on the surface of the lipoprotein particles by the action of lipoprotein lipase may be partially neutralised by the lipid binding protein β_2-Glycoprotein 1 which thereby inhibits the activation of factor XII[49]. We[20] have recently isolated from the plasma of a number of subjects a complex of α-factor XIIa asociated with a number of proteins including β_2-Glycoprotein 1. In preliminary experiments, the amount of β_2-Glycoprotein I associated with the factor XII appears to be inversely proportional to the amount of α-factor XIIa. Presumably both the proteins are in competition for the same positively charged sites. It is not yet established whether the calcium mediated phospholipid-binding proteins such as Annexin V have a role in the inhibition of the contact phase.

VIII. SUMMARY

This brief review suggests a pathway for the activation of factor VII by factor XII, activated on the surface of lipoprotein particles in the plasma, thus "priming" the coagulation system. The only difficulty with this simplistic idea is that factor XII deficient patients do not show any tendency to bleed. It may be that in these patients there is an alternative pathway, such as the activation of factor XI by thrombin on a suitable surface.

The generation of activated factor VII via the contact-phase in healthy individuals is probably of little significance, in contrast to older subjects, who have developed atheroma over several years. If in these subjects a plaque sheers from the endothelial wall in a coronary artery exposing tissue factor, then coagulation will procede rapidly and possibly obstruct the coronary circulation.

In model experiments it has been shown that emulsions of *cis*-unsaturated free fatty-acids do not cause factor XII activation, whereas *trans*- unsaturated fatty acids, which invariably have a melting point well above that of the *cis*- isomer and saturated fatty acids form a potent factor XII activating surface, always provided that the melting point of the fatty acid is above that at which the experiment is being carried out. However, it is not clear how the proportion of low melting point fatty acids in the diet affect the thrombogenic potential of the lipoprotein particles.

REFERENCES

1. **Miller GJ, Martin JC, Webster J, et al.** Association between dietary fat intake plasma factor VII coagulant activity - a predictor of cardiovascular mortality. *Atherosclerosis*, 60, 269, 1986.
2. **Mitropoulos K A, Miller G J, Reeves B E A, Wilkes H C, Cruickshank J K.** Factor VII coagulant activity is strongly associated with the plasma concentration of large lipoprotein particles in middle-aged men. *Atherosclerosis*, 76, 203, 1989.
3. **Carvalho de Sousa J, Bruckett E,Giral P, et al.** Plasma factor VII triglyceride concentration and fibrin degradation products in primary hyperlipidemia: a clinical and laboratory study. *Haemostasis*, 19, 83, 1989.
4. **Scarabin P Y, Bara L, Samama M, Orssaud G.** Further evidence that activated factor VII is related to plasma lipids. *Brit J Haematol*, 61, 186, 1985.
5. **Miller GJ, Cruickshank JK, Ellis LJ, et al.** Fat consumption and factor VII coagulant activity in middle-aged men. An association between a dietary and thrombogenic coronary risk factor. *Atherosclerosis*; 78, 19,1989.
6. **Warth M R, Arky R A, Knopp R H.** Lipid metabolism in pregnancy. III altered lipid composition in intermediate, very low, low and high-density lipoprotein fractions. *J Clin Endocrinol Metab*; 41, 649, 1975.
7. **McDonald-Gibson R G, Young M, Hytten F E.** Changes in plasma non esterified fatty acids and serum glycerol in pregnancy. *Br J Obstet Gynaecol*, 82, 473, 1975.
8. **Stirling Y, Woolf L, North W R S, Segatchian M J, Meade T W.** Haemostasis in normal pregnancy. *Thromb Haemost*, 52: 176, 1984.
9. **Mitropoulos KA, Miller GJ, Watts GF, Durrington PN,** Lipolysis of triglyceride-rich lipoproteins activates coagulant Factor XII: A study in familial lipoproteinnnnnn-lipase deficiency. *Athersclerosis*,94, 119, 1992.
10. **Mitropoulos K A, Esnouf M P.** The prothrombin activation peptide regulates synthesis of the vitamin K-dependent proteins in the rabbit. *Thrombosis Res*, 57: 541, 1990.
11. **Cochrane CC, Griffin JH**: Molecular assembly in the contact phase of the Hageman factor system. *Amer.J.Med*, 67, 657, 1979.
12. **Seligsohn U, Osterud B, Brown S F, Griffin J H, Rapaport S I.** Activation of human factor VII in plasma and in purified system. Role of activated factor IX, kallikrein and activated factor XII. *J Clin Invest*, 64, 1049, 1979.
13. **Mitropoulos K A, Martin J C, Reeves B E A, Esnouf M P.** The activation of the contact phase of coagulation by physiological surfaces in plasma: the effect of large negatively charged liposomal vesicles. *Blood*, 73, 1525, 1989.
14. **Margolis J.** The interrelationship of coagulation of plasma and release of peptides. *Ann NY Acad Sci*, 104, 133, 1963.
15. **Kluft C.** Determination of prekallikrein in human plasma: optimal conditions for activating prekallikrein. *J Lab Clin Med*, 91, 83, 1978.
16. **Bock P E, Srinivasan K R, Shore J D.** Activation of intrinsic blood coagulation by ellagic acid: insoluble ellagic acid-metal ion complexes are the activating species. *Biochemistry*, 20, 7258,1981.
17. **Fujikawa K, Heimark R L, Kurachi K, Davie E W.** Activation of bovine factor XII (hageman factor) by plasma kallikrein. *Biochemistry*, 19, 1322, 1980.
18. **Revak S D, Cochrane C G, Bouma B N, Griffin J H.** Surface and fluid phase activities of two forms of activated hageman factor produced during contact activation of plasma. *J Exp Med*, 147, 719, 1978.
19. **Mandle R Jr, Kaplan A P.** Hageman factor substrates. Human plasma prekallikrein: mechanism of activation by Hageman factor and participation in Hageman factor-dependent fibrinolysis. *J Biol Chem*, 252, 6097, 1977.
20. **Esnouf M P, Sarphie A F, Burgess A I.** (unpublished observations).
21. **Kaplan A P, Silverberg M.** The coagulation-kinin pathway of human plasma. *Blood*, 70, 1, 1987.
22. **Berrettini M, L‰mmle B, Griffin JH.** Initiation of coagulation and relationships between intrinsic and extrinsic coagulation pathways.In: Verstraete M, Vermylen J., Lijnen R, Arnout J (eds) : Thrombosis XIth Congress Haemostasis, Leuven, *The Netherlands Leuven University Press* 1987, p473.
23. **Meijers J C, McMullen B A, Bouma B N.** The contact activation proteins: a structure/function overview. *Agents Actions* Suppl, 38, 219, 1992.
24. **Nuije**ns J H, Huijbregts C C M, Eerenberg-Belmer A J M, Meijers J C M, Bouma B N, Hack C E. Activation of the contact system by a monoclonal antibody directed against a neodeterminant in the heavy chain region of human coagulation factor XII (Hageman factor). *J Biol Chem*, 264, 12941, 1989.
25. **Ratnoff O D, Davie E W, Mallett D L.** Studies on the action of Hageman factor : evidence that activated hageman factor in turn activates plasma thromboplastic antecedent. *J Clin Invest*, 40, 803, 1961.
26. **Rosenthal R L, Dreskin O H, Rosenthal N.** New Hemophilia-like disease caused by deficiency of a third plasma thromboplastic factor. *Proc Soc Exp Biol Med*, 82, 171, 1953.
27. **Mitropoulos K A, Reeves B E A, OíBrien D P, Cooper J A, Martin J C.** The relationship between factor VII coagulant activity and factor XII activation induced in plasma by endogenous or exogenously added contact surface. *Blood Coag & Fibrinolysis*, 4, 223, 1993.

28.   **Naito K, Fujikawa K.** Activation of blood coagulation factor XI independent of factor XII. *J Biol Chem*, 266, 7353, 1991.

29.   **Gailani D, Broze G J Jr.** Factor XI activation in a revised model of blood coagulation. Science, 253, 909, 1991.

30.   **Scott C F, Colman R W.** Fibrinogen blocks the autoactivation and thrombin-mediated activation of factor XI on dextran sulfate. *Proc Soc Natl Acad Sci USA*, 89, 11189, 1992.

31.   **Brunnee T, La Porta C, Reddigari S R, Salerno V M, Kaplan A P, Silverberg M.** Activation of factor XI in plasma is dependent on factor XII. *Blood*, 81, 580, 1993.

32.   **Mitropoulos K A, Esnouf M P.** The autoactivation of factor XII in the presence of long-chain saturated fatty acid - a comparison with the potency of sulphatides and dextran sulphate. Thromb Haemostas, 66, 446, 1991.

33.   **Novotny W F, Girard T J, Miletich J P, Broze G J.** Purification and characterizetion of a lipoprotein associated coagulation inhibitor from human. *J Biol Chem*, 264, 18832, 1989.

34.   **Broze G J , Majerus P W.** Purification and properties of human coagulation factor VII. *J Biol Chem*, 225,1242, 1980.

35.   **Carvalho de Sousa J,Soria C, Ayrault-Jarrier M, et al.** Association between coagulation factors VII and X with triglyceride rich lipoproteins. *J Clin Path,* 41, 940, 1988.

36.   **Mitropoulos K A, Esnouf M P, Meade T W.** Increased factor VII coagulant activity in the rabbit following diet-induced hypercholesterolaemia. Evidence for increased conversion of VII to aVIIa and higher flux within the coagulation pathway. *Atherosclerosis*, 63, 43,1987.

37.   **Rao L V M, Rapaport S I.** Activation of VII bound to tissue factor: a key early step in the tissue factor pathway of blood coagulation. *Proc Soc Natl Acad Sci USA*, 85, 6687, 1988.

38.   **Wildgoose P, Berkner K L, Kisiel W.** Synthesis, purification and characterization of an Arg[152] --->Glu site-directed mutant of recombinant human blood clotting factor VII. *Biochemistry*, 29, 3413, 1990.

39.   **Williams E B, Krishnaswamy S, Mann K G.** Zymogen/enzyme discrimination using peptide chloromethyl ketones. *J Biol Chem*, 264, 7536, 1989.

40.   **Miller G J, Stirling Y, Esnouf M P, Heinrich J, van der Loo J, Kienast J, Wu K K, Morrisey J H, Meade T W, Martin J C, Imeson J D, Cooper J A, Finch A.** Factor VII-deficient substrate plasmas depleted of protein C raise the sensitivity of the factor VII bio-assay to activated-factor VII: an international study. *Thrombosis and Haemostasis*, 71, 38, 1994.

41.   **Mitropoulos K A, Esnouf M P.** Turnover of factor X and prothrombin in rabbits fed on a standard or cholesterol-supplemented diet. *Biochem J*, 244, 263, 1987.

42.   **Esnouf M P , Mitropoulos K A, Burgess A I.** The relation of G F, Abbate R, Prisco D. Eds. Thrombosis: An Update. *Scientific Press*. Florence. 1992 : p 715.

43.   **Graves C B, Munns T W, Carlisle T L, Grant G A, Strauss A W.** Induction of prothrombin synthesis by prothrombin fragments. *Proc Soc Acad Sci USA*, 78, 4772, 1981.

44.   **Gordon E M, Ratnoff O D, Jones P K.** The role of augmented Hageman factor (factor XII) titers in the cold-promoted activation of factor VII and spontaneous shortening of the prothrombin time in women using oral contraceptives. *J Lab Cli Med*, 99, 363, 1982.

45.   **Schved J F, Gris J C, Neveu S, Mares P, Sarlat C.** Variations of factor XII level during pregnancy in a woman with hageman factor deficiency. *Thromb Haemost*, 60, 526, 1988.

46.   **Esnouf M P, Sarphie A F, Burgess A I, Ford R P.** (unpublished observations).

47.   **Wuillemin W A, Furlan M, Lammle B.** A quantitative dot immunobinding assay for coagulation factor XII in plasma. *J Immunol Methods*, 130, 133,1990.

48.   **Pixley R A, Schmaier A, Colman R W.** Effect of negatively charged activating compounds on inactivation of factor XIIa by CEMBED Equation inhibitor. *Archives Biochem Biophys*, 256, 490, 1987.

49.   **Henry M L, Everson B, Ratnoff O D.** Inhibition of the activation of Hageman factor (Factor XII) by ß2-Glycoprotein 1. *J Lab Clin Med*, 111, 519.

ANTIPHOSPHOLIPID ANTIBODY SYNDROME

D.A. Triplett

Hematology, Ball Memorial Hospital, Muncie, Indiana

I. ANTIPHOSPHOLIPID ANTIBODIES

Antiphospholipid antibodies (APA) are a family of autoimmune and alloimmune immunoglobulins (IgG, IgM, IgA, or mixtures) which were originally thought to react specifically with negatively charged or neutral phospholipids.[1-4] The detection of these antibodies and subsequent classification has been based on a variety of in vitro laboratory test systems. Among the various laboratory tests utilized are: complement fixation, coagulation assays, radioimmunoassays (RIA), and microtiter plate ELISA tests. Given the diversity of assays employed as well as the heterogeneity of patient populations studied, the reported incidence of these antibodies in the medical literature varies considerably. Recently, there has been much speculation regarding the true "antigenic target" for this family of immunoglobulins. Many investigators now feel the antibodies recognize complexes of proteins and phospholipids.[5,6] Perhaps a more accurate name is antiphospholipid-protein antibodies. The debate regarding the "true" antigen has largely been centered on evaluating patient plasma/sera in various configurations of the anticardiolipin antibody (ACA) ELISA assay system.[7] Whether the carefully controlled conditions of laboratory assay systems in any way reflect in vivo activity of the APA family of immunoglobulins is unknown.

Historically, the first member of the APA family was described by Wassermann and colleagues in 1906.[8] The Wassermann test was designed for the serologic diagnosis of syphilis. This early complement fixation test was subsequently replaced by flocculation procedures. Pangborn was the first to identify an acidic phospholipid as the antigen present in alcohol extracts of bovine heart.[9] This extract was subsequently named cardiolipin. The most popular test system employed in the initial mass screening programs instituted in the United States and other countries was the Venereal Disease Research Laboratory (VDRL) test. The VDRL reagent consists of a mixture of cardiolipin, lecithin, and cholesterol. With the introduction of mass screening programs to control syphilis, early investigators recognized the phenomenon of a biologic false positive serologic test for syphilis (BFP-STS).[10-13] Individuals with a BFP-STS were categorized as either acute or chronic. By definition, patients with an acute BFP-STS had a duration of positive test results of less than six months while individuals with persistence beyond six months were identified as chronic.[14,15] The chronic BFP-STS patients were more frequently seen in women and, in some instances, the serologic test for syphilis was recognized as a harbinger for subsequent development of systemic lupus erythematosus (SLE). Other autoimmune diseases have also been associated with chronic BFP-STS including rheumatoid arthritis and Sjogren's Syndrome. The antibody responsible for a positive STS was named **reagin**.

The second member of the APA family was first reported by Mueller et. al. and Conley and Hartmann in the early 1950's.[16,17] These two groups described a peculiar circulating anticoagulant (synonym: inhibitor) in patients with SLE. The article by Conley and Hartmann suggested that these patients were at increased risk for bleeding; however, subsequent case reports and patient series have stressed the paradoxical lack of clinical bleeding in patients with this anticoagulant. The patient's plasma did not clot appropriately using various phospholipid (PL) dependent coagulation assays (e.g. Activated Partial Thromboplastin Time [APTT], Kaolin Clotting Time [KCT], dilute Russell Viper Venom Time [dRVVT]). Further analysis of patients with this peculiar anticoagulant reported an apparent increased incidence (usually retrospective patient histories) of either venous or arterial thromboembolic events[2,3,18]. The name **lupus anticoagulant (LA)** was given to this circulating anticoagulant by Feinstein and Rapaport in 1972.[19] It was so named because of the frequency with which it was observed in patients with SLE. Clearly, this is a misnomer since the vast majority of patients detected in routine clinical laboratories do not have underlying SLE. Analogous to a BFP-STS, the finding of an isolated LA may be the first laboratory abnormality observed in a patient who ultimately will develop SLE or another autoimmune disease.

The third member of the APA family was described by Harris and co-workers in 1983.[20] Harris and colleagues described a solid phase RIA which utilized cardiolipin as the antigen. This assay system was stated to be 200 to 400 times more sensitive than conventional serologic tests for syphilis. The stimulus to develop this test was the clinical recognition of an association between chronic BFP-STS and positive LA in patients with a variety of clinical complications. These clinical associations included recurrent arterial and venous thromboembolic events, various complications of pregnancy, the most important being recurrent spontaneous abortion (RSA), and unexplained thrombocytopenia.[21-23] Shortly after the description of the RIA test for **anticardiolipin antibody (ACA)**, a microtiter-based ELISA assay system was described.[7] Because of the regulatory problems associated with radioisotopes and the complexity of the RIA systems, most laboratories now use the ELISA assay for ACA testing.

These three test systems (STS, LA, and ACA) have been utilized to detect APAs either individually or in combination. Early reports suggested LA and ACA were the same antibody.[20] It is now recognized that they are, in fact, different immunoglobulins in most cases.[24,25] Their activities can be separated in vitro utilizing various chromatographic systems or liposome adsorption. Positive laboratory results for LA or ACA may be seen in a variety of different clinical situations. In many cases, the presence of these antibodies is transient. Most often, the transient antibodies are associated with a variety of intercurrent infections (e.g. viral, bacterial, protozoal).[26-30] These antibodies usually disappear within three to six months following the illness. Often they are of IgM isotype and relatively low titer when quantitated in the standard ACA test system. These antibodies are best categorized as alloimmune (Table I). It is useful to consider these antibodies in the same context as the classical BFP-STS. In contrast, persistence of APA positive results by ACA testing or LA testing is of significance particularly in the setting of autoimmune disease such as SLE. When the necessary criteria required for the diagnosis of SLE are not present and there are positive laboratory tests for APA and associated clinical findings, these patients are diagnosed as: Primary Antiphospholipid Antibody Syndrome (PAPS).[31] In Table I, the autoimmune APA are divided into three categories, primary, secondary, and a third category which has been arbitrarily identified: drug-induced. A case could be made to categorize the drug-induced APA with the secondary APA. However, from a clinical standpoint, it is more useful to categorize them separately since the presence and persistence of these antibodies does not in most cases have the same clinical correlation with thromboembolic events or RSA that one sees with other autoimmune APA.[32]

Table I : Classification of APA

   I. **Autoimmune**
            a) Primary
                        Do Not Fulfill Criteria for SLE
            b) Secondary
                        SLE
                        Other Connective Tissue Diseases
            c) Drug Induced

   II. **Alloimmune**
            a) Infections
                        Viral
                        Bacterial
                        Protozoal
                        Fungal
            b) Malignancies
                        Hairy Cell Leukemia
                        Lymphoproliferative

II. ANTIPHOSPHOLIPID ANTIBODY SYNDROME:
HISTORY AND DEFINITION

In the early 1980's, three papers appeared describing an association between LA and ACA and the clinical complications of thrombosis, recurrent abortion, and thrombocytopenia.[20-22] Because of the diverse nature of the clinical findings, a wide spectrum of physicians became interested in the importance of these laboratory observations and their relationship to clinical complications. Hughes suggested the term anticardiolipin syndrome to define the association between positive ACA results and one or more of the observed clinical complications.[34] This term was advanced assuming LA and ACA were the same antibody identified in two different laboratory tests. With the realization that LA and ACA are, in fact, different antibodies, Harris and colleagues proposed the term Antiphospholipid Antibody Syndrome (APS) in 1987.[35,36] Further studies expanded the potential antigenic targets to include other negatively charged phospholipids (phosphatidylserine, phosphatidic acid, and phosphatidylinositol).[24] Indeed, there are reports of antibodies directed against zwitterionic phospholipids and thromboembolic complications.[24,37,38] The immunoglobulin isotype may vary in patients with the APS. IgG ACA is most frequently associated with clinical complications. There is also a correlation between the titer of IgG ACA and the expectation of clinical complications.[2,3] Although IgM and IgA ACA results are less frequently correlated with clinical complications, there are reports in which the isolated presence of either IgA or IgM ACA has been associated with clinical complications.

Table II : Criteria for antiphospholipid antibody syndrome

Clinical	Laboratory
Venous thrombosis	IgG anticardiolipin antibody (>10 GPL units)[a]
Arterial thrombosis	Positive lupus anticoagulant test
Recurrent fetal loss	IgM anticardiolipin antibody (>10 MPL units)[a] and positive LA test

[a] GPL and MPL refer to IgG and IgM phospholipid antibodies. The units refer to the standards proposed by Harris et. al. at the Second International Workshop on Phospholipid Antibodies April 4, 1986.[102]

Taken from Harris.[36] Patients with the APA syndrome should have *at least* one clinical and one laboratory finding during their disease. The APA test(s) should be positive on at least two occasions more than 8 weeks apart. The diagnosis of LA should be established using the criteria established by the SSC Subcommittee for Standardization of Lupus Anticoagulants.(see ref. 95)

Nigel Harris in 1987 proposed criteria to establish the diagnosis of the APS (Table II).[35,36] Following Harris' paper, Asherson proposed the concept of a "Primary" Antiphospholipid Antibody Syndrome (PAPS).[31] In these patients, the diagnostic criteria necessary for SLE are not present; however, the patient does fulfill the necessary criteria for the diagnosis of APS. As noted, PAPS patients may progress to SLE.

III. PRIMARY ANTIPHOSPHOLIPID ANTIBODY SYNDROME (PAPS)

By definition, patients with PAPS do not fulfill clinical or laboratory criteria which define other autoimmune diseases. Asherson and colleagues were the first to describe the PAPS in 1989.[39] Subsequent studies have emphasized the remarkable spectrum of vascular occlusive events seen in patients with PAPS. Virtually every vascular bed (arterial, venous, and capillary) may be affected. The most common location involves the veins of the lower extremity. Approximately 70% of thromboembolic events in the setting of PAPS are venous. On the arterial side of the circulation, the cerebral vasculature is most frequently involved.[40] Cerebral infarction may result from either arterial thrombi or emboli originating from cardiac valve abnormalities. A wide variety of CNS disorders have been linked to APA including visual defects, transient ischemic attacks (TIA), central retinal occlusion, epilepsy, major vessel occlusion, and multi-infarct dementia.[11,42-44] Brey et al. reported the presence of APA in 46% of patients under the age of 50 with a history of cerebral ischemic attacks.[45] Patients with cerebral ischemia and APA have a tendency to be younger (average age 43 years) with an equal distribution of males and females. Approximately a third of patients will have a history of repeated cerebral infarction.[45,46]

Sneddon's Syndrome was originally described as an association of cerebrovascular disease and livedo reticularis without any associated findings of disseminated connective tissue disorder.[43,47,48] More recently, it has been recognized that there is a high frequency of APA in these patients.[48] Pathologic evaluations of skin biopsies in these patients have revealed changes in the small and medium sized arteries in the form of intimal hyperplasia often with accompanying thrombosis. Significantly, there is a lack of atheromatous or inflammatory changes in the vessels.

Occasionally, patients are encountered with the "catastrophic" antiphospholipid syndrome.[49] Also, a clinical picture of thrombotic thrombocytopenic purpura (TTP) may be encountered in the setting of PAPS.[50]

The incidence of cardiac valvular lesions does not appear to be directly related to the presence of APA. The incidence of valvular lesions is similar in patients with PAPS as in patients with SLE and no evidence of APA.

IV. SECONDARY APS (SLE OTHER AUTOIMMUNE DISEASES)

Patients with APS secondary to SLE do appear to differ slightly from patients with PAPS.[51,52] In a recent study by Vianna et. al., they found patients with secondary APS had an increased frequency of autoimmune hemolytic anemia, endocardial valve disease, neutropenia, and low levels of complement 4.[53] The remaining clinical and laboratory findings were similar between PAPS and secondary SLE related to APS.

As noted earlier, patients occasionally may present with the necessary criteria to establish the diagnosis of PAPS. Over the course of time, these individuals may ultimately develop SLE.[54] Consequently, it is important to follow PAPS patients with periodic testing for anti-double stranded DNA antibodies and also complement levels. In some report cases, up to 19 years have elapsed between the initial diagnosis of PAPS and the subsequent diagnosis of SLE. Piette and colleagues have correctly noted that the 1982 ARA revised criteria for classification of SLE cannot be relied upon to distinguish between PAPS and APS secondary to SLE.[55] They have reported a proposed set of criteria necessary to differentiate PAPS and APS secondary to SLE.[56]

Drugs which have been associated with the lupus syndrome often result in production of APA. Among the offending drugs are: procainamide, phenothiazine, ethosuximide, chlorothiazide, hydralazine, quinidine, and oral contraceptives.[24] Although the incidence of thromboembolic complications associated with drug-induced APA is lower than spontaneous appearing APA, a number of cases of thrombosis have been described.[24,57] Certain individuals appear more susceptible to drug-induced APA. Among these are patients with slow acetylating capacity, the presence of HLA DR4 and null alleles at C4A and C4B loci.

V. CATASTROPHIC VARIANT OF APS

In some instances, patients with high levels of APA develop rapid progression of multiorgan failure.[49] Often the patient is comatose with clinical and laboratory findings of renal failure. The sudden onset of multiple thrombotic events and rapid clinical deterioration characterizes this group of patients.[49,58] Aggressive therapeutic measures including plasmapheresis, anticoagulation, and pulse steroid therapy are indicated in these patients.

VI. ARE APA PATHOGENIC?

Virtually all of the early series and case reports associating APA and thromboembolic complications are based on retrospective clinical histories. Whether the APA was present at the time of the historical thrombosis or arose following the thrombosis is a matter of pure speculation. The question of whether APA are a cause, consequence, or coincidence with a thrombotic event remains unanswered although the recent reports of cross-sectional and prospective studies support a causative role for APA in the pathogenesis of arterial and venous thrombosis.[2,59-62] In addition, several animal models have been reported which also point to a pathogenic role of APA in thromboembolic events.[63,64] The recently reported Physician Health Study found an association between initial positivity of ACA test results and subsequent deep vein thrombosis/pulmonary emboli.[61] In this prospective study, there was lack of association between positive ACA results and stroke. Morton et. al. in another prospective study found a trend suggesting positive ACA results were associated with graft failure following coronary artery bypass surgery.[59] A recent cross-sectional study evaluating vascular surgery patients who were admitted for treatment of peripheral arterial disease found a high incidence (26%) of APA in this patient group.[62] Patients who were APA positive had a higher incidence of failure of bypass graft procedures, were disproportionately women and experienced an earlier onset of graft occlusion following bypass surgery.[62] Another cross-sectional analysis was performed when Ginsberg et. al. evaluated patients with SLE.[65] Patients who were ACA positive were found to have elevated levels of prothrombin fragment F1.2 and fibrinopeptide A. Both of these are markers of in vivo activation of coagulation. These results suggest SLE patients with ACA are "hypercoagulable" or prothrombotic.

VII. POTENTIAL PATHOGENIC MECHANISMS FOR APA

Patients with APA may present with thrombi in virtually any vascular site. The complications seen with pregnancy are also thought to be related to thrombotic events or altered perfusion in the placenta.[66] This wide spectrum of anatomic sites suggests multiple mechanisms are involved. This is not unexpected given the marked heterogeneity seen in laboratory testing to identify the presence of APA. Although there is evolving evidence strongly supporting the pathogenic role of APA, a concept which is being recognized in clinical conditions associated with hereditary thrombophilia (e.g. deficiencies of protein C, protein S, AT III, and activated protein C resistance) is applicable to APA related thrombosis.[67] The presence of these hereditary abnormalities as well as acquired APA appears to create a "permissive environment". In this case, the "threshold" for thrombosis is lowered. Thus, a "second hit" (e.g. pregnancy, trauma, oral contraceptives, surgery, prolonged immobilization) may result in a thrombotic event. The recent discovery of APC resistance as the most common cause of hereditary thrombophilia underlines the need to be aware of potential APA positivity in patients with APC resistance.[68,69] The common frequency of APC resistance and superimposed appearance of APA would provide "two hits" thus leading to thromboembolic events. The coexistence of APC resistance and APA may account for many of the venous thrombotic events seen in association with APA. However, the arterial thromboembolic events are not easily explained by this hypothesis. Among the various explanations attempting to link APA and thrombosis, the first to be proposed was altered eicosanoid function. Carreras and colleagues suggested APA inhibited the generation of prostacyclin (PGI-2) by endothelial cells.[70] Their studies were based on in vitro culture of endothelial cells. The APAs studied appeared to inhibit mobilization of arachidonic acid from endothelial cell membranes (inhibition of phospholipase A_2). Since PGI-2 is a potent vasodilator and inhibitor of platelet aggregation, the balance between thromboxane A_2 (TxA$_2$) and PGI-2 is altered with a resulting predisposition to thrombosis.[71] A variety of subsequent studies have yielded variable results.[72-74] This lack of consistency is not surprising given the nature of the assay systems (cell cultures, agonists utilized, patient sample heterogeneity, etc). The ability of APA to inhibit PGI-2 production is a plausible potential pathophysiologic explanation for arterial thrombosis.

Other investigators have focused on the role of APA and the platelet response. In some studies, patient APA have increased generation of thromboxane B_2 (TxB$_2$) in platelet- rich plasma.[75,76] Studies by Carreras and colleagues utilizing urinary metabolites of platelet derived TxA$_2$ have found a significant increase in the urinary excretion of platelet metabolites (2, 3 Dinor TxB$_2$ and 11 dehydro-TxB$_2$).[77] These studies suggest persistent in vivo activation of platelets. Administration of aspirin to a subgroup of patients with elevated thromboxane metabolites resulted in decreased secretion of these platelet thromboxane metabolites.

The protein C system is a complex regulatory system which inactivates the two key cofactors of hemostasis: factor Va and factor VIIIa.[78] Both proteins C and S are vitamin K dependent proteins which bind to negatively charged phospholipid surfaces in the presence of calcium ions. Potentially, APA could interfere with the phospholipid localization of both protein C and protein S. A more exciting hypothesis is the ability of APA to inhibit the activity of Activated Protein C (APC).[79,80] Antibodies to protein C and protein S have also been described in APA patients.[81-83]

Other targets for APA include endothelial cells and the plasma protein Beta$_2$ Glycoprotein I.[84] Endothelial cells have a variety of pro- and anti-coagulant functions. Oosting et. al. demonstrated APA acts synergistically with Tumor Necrosis Factor (TNF) to increase endothelial cell procoagulant activity.[83] Also, a recent paper by Shibata et. al. provides a very interesting hypothesis regarding the ability of APA to react with heparin and heparan sulfate.[85] Heparan sulfate which is found on the surface of endothelial cells acts as an endogenous anticoagulant through its interaction with antithrombin III. Shibata et. al. found that IgG fractions from patients with APA react specifically with a disaccharide sequence found in the critical antithrombin III binding region of heparin and heparan sulfate.

Beta$_2$ Glycoprotein I is a physiologic anticoagulant which binds to a variety of negatively charged molecules.[86] Beta$_2$ Glycoprotein I inhibits the contact activation of blood coagulation, binds heparin and also inhibits the prothrombinase reaction. Beta$_2$ Glycoprotein I enhances the ACA assay system.[87] Some investigators believe the antigenic target for ACA is, in fact, Beta$_2$ Glycoprotein I whereas other contend Beta$_2$ Glycoprotein I is merely a cofactor which accentuates ACA activity.[88,89] Because of its physiologic anticoagulant properties, antibodies to Beta$_2$ Glycoprotein I may create a prothrombotic environment. This possibility, however, seems remote since patients with hereditary deficiency of Beta$_2$ Glycoprotein I do not have a prothrombotic condition.

VIII. LABORATORY IDENTIFICATION OF APA

The laboratory evaluation of APA is an essential part of any work-up of patients with unexplained thromboembolic events. This is particularly true of the so-called "thrombophilic patients". As noted earlier, given the relative frequencies of APC resistance (approximately 3-5% of normal population) and APA (2% of population), it is anticipated that these two abnormalities will often be found in the same individual. APA positivity may be found in virtually any patient population. There is a great deal of accumulating literature pointing out the frequent occurrence of APA in the pediatric population.[89-94] The development of laboratory tests for diagnosis of LA and ACA has accelerated in the last five years. Testing for APA has increased dramatically as a result of the multispecialty interest in the identification of these antibodies as well as their recognized association with thromboembolic events. Through the efforts of the Subcommittee on Lupus Anticoagulants and Antiphospholipid Antibodies of the Scientific and Standardization Committee (International Society of Thrombosis and Haemostasis), progress has been made in defining the necessary criteria for the diagnosis of LA.[95] Also, the efforts of Nigel Harris and colleagues have improved performance of ACA testing. [96] However, there still remains considerable controversy in the area of laboratory testing. Most important is the fact that no laboratory test has, as yet, been identified with predictive value for clinical complications. An indepth discussion of APA testing is beyond the scope of this chapter. There are a number of excellent review articles which detail the perils and pitfalls in establishing the laboratory diagnosis of APA.[97-99] A very important dictum is the necessity to evaluate patient samples for both LA and ACA. Since they are different antibodies in many cases, the laboratory must proceed with parallel evaluation for both of these antibodies. In approximately 60% of patients, both antibodies will be present whereas in the remaining 40%, one will be present and the other absent. The failure to appreciate the requirement to test for both antibodies is the most frequent error made in the laboratory diagnosis of APA.

IX. TREATMENT

Both LA and ACA may be found in a wide variety of normal and symptomatic individuals. Often "benign" APA are seen in the convalescent stage following recent infections. These APA are transient and of no clinical significance. No treatment is indicated for asymptomatic patients. Patients with a history of thromboembolic events and positive APA studies should be treated with appropriate heparin anticoagulation followed by oral anticoagulation. In the study reported by Rosove, there was remarkable fidelity of recurrences (i.e. venous-venous, arterial-arterial) following the first event.[100] Standard intensity of oral anticoagulant therapy (INR 2.0 to 3.0) did not seem to suppress venous recurrences. Indefinite anticoagulation is recommended for patients who have had recurrent thrombosis.

Aspirin has been prescribed for patients with APA and stroke. The doses have varied from 80 mg. to 1300 mg. per day.[101] Presently, it is uncertain whether aspirin does reduce the risk of recurrent stroke in these patients.

In some instances, immunosuppressive therapy or corticosteroids have been used in patients with APS Syndrome. In patients with a catastrophic APS Syndrome, heroic measures such as plasmapheresis have also been employed.

REFERENCES

1. **Triplett, D.A., Brandt, J.T.,** Lupus anticoagulants: misnomer, paradox, riddle, epiphenomenon, *Hematol. Pathol.*, 2, 121, 1988.
2. **Triplett, D.A.**, Antiphospholipid antibodies and thrombosis. a consequence, coincidence, or cause?, *Arch. Pathol. Lab. Med.*, 117, 78, 1993.
3. **Love, P.E., Santoro, S.A.,** Antiphospholipid antibodies; Anticardiolipin and the lupus anticoagulant in systematic lupus erythematosus (SLE) and in non-SLE disorders, *Ann. Int. Med.*, 112, 682, 1990.
4. **Harris, E.N.**, Antiphospholipid antibodies, *Br. J. Haematol.*, 74, 1, 1990.
5. **Vermylen, J., Arnout, J.,** Is the antiphospholipid syndrome caused by antibodies directed against physiologically relevant phospholipid-protein complexes?, *J. Lab. Clin. Med.*, 120, 10, 1992.

6.   **Triplett, D.A.**, Antiphospholipid-protein antibodies: laboratory detection and clinical relevance, *Thromb. Res.*, (in press).
7.   **Loizou, S., McCrea, J.D., Rydge, A.C., Reynolds, R., Boyle, C.L., Harris, E.N.**, Measurement of anticardiolipin antibodies by an enzyme linked immunosorbent assay (ELISA): standardization and quantitation of results, *Clin. Exp. Immunol.*, 62, 738, 1985.
8.   **Wassermann, A., Neisser, A., Bruck, C.**, Eine serodiagnostische reaktion bei syphilis, *Dtsch. Med. Wochenschr.*, 32, 745, 1906.
9.   **Pangborn, M.C.**, A new serologically active phospholipid from beef heart, *Proc. Soc. Exp. Biol. Med.*, 48, 484, 1941.
10.   **Davis, B.D.**, Biologic false positive serologic tests for syphilis, *Medicine*, 23, 359, 1944.
11.   **Moore, J.E., Mohr, C.F.**, Biologically false positive serologic tests for syphilis, *JAMA*, 150, 467, 1952.
12.   **Moore, J.E., Lutz, W.B.**, The natural history of systemic lupus erythematosus: an approach to its study through chronic biologic false-positive reactions, *J. Chronic. Dis.*, 1, 297, 1955.
13.   **Arthur, R.D., Hale, J.M.**, Biologic false positive tests for syphilis associated with routine army immunization, *Mil. Surg.*, 92, 53, 1943.
14.   **Catterall, R.D.**, Collagen disease and chronic biologic false positive phenomenon, *Quart. J. Med.*, 30, 41, 1961.
15.   **Fiumara, N.J.**, Biologic false-positive reaction to syphilis, *N. Engl. J. Med.*, 268, 402, 1963.
16.   **Mueller, J.F., Ratnoff, O., Henile, R.W.**, Observations on the characteristics of an unusual circulating anticoagulant, *J. Lab. Clin. Med.*, 38, 254, 1951.
17.   **Conley, C.L., Hartmann, R.C.**, A hemorrhagic disorder caused by circulating anticoagulants in patients with disseminated lupus erythematosus, *J. Lab. Clin. Invest.*, 31, 621, 1952.
18.   **Bowie, E.J.W., Thompson, J.H., Pascuzzi, C.A., Owen, C.A.**, Thrombosis in systemic lupus erythematosus despite circulating anticoagulants, *J. Lab. Clin. Med.* 62, 416, 1963.
19.   **Feinstein, D.I., Rapaport, S.I.**, Acquired inhibitors of blood coagulation, *Prog. Hemost. Thromb.*, 1, 75, 1972.
20.   **Harris, E.N., Gharavi, A.E., Boey, M.L., Patel, B.M., Macworth-Young, C.G., Loizou, S., Hughes, G.R.**, Anticardiolipin antibodies: detection by radioimmunoassay and association with thrombosis in systemic lupus erythematosus, *Lancet*, 2, 1211, 1983.
21.   **Boey, M.D., Colaco, C.B., Gharavi, A.E., Elkon, K.B., Loizou, S., Hughes, G.R.**, Thrombosis in SLE: Striking association with the presence of circulating "lupus anticoagulant", *Br. Med. J.*, 287, 1021, 1983.
22.   **Hughes, G.R.V.**, Thrombosis, abortion, cerebral disease and the lupus anticoagulant, *Br. Med. J.*, 287, 1088, 1983.
23.   **Harris, E.N., Gharavi, A., Asherson, R.A., Khamashta, M.A., Hughes, G.R.V.**, Antiphospholipid antibodies - middle aged but robust, *J. Rheumatol.*, 21, 978- 981, 1994 (editorial).
24.   **Triplett, D.A., Brandt, J.T., Musgrave, K.A., Orr, C.**, Relationship between lupus anticoagulants and antibodies to phospholipids, *JAMA*, 259, 550, 1988.
25.   **Exner, T., Sahman, N., Trudinger, B.**, Separation of anticardiolipin antibodies from lupus anticoagulant on a phospholipid-coated polystyrene column, *Biochem. Biophysic. Res. Commun.*, 155, 1001, 1988.
26.   **Rugman, F.P., Pinn, G., Palmer, M.F., Waite, M., Hay, C.R.**, Anticardiolipin antibodies in leptospirosis, *J. Clin. Pathol.*, 44, 517, 1991.
27.   **Al-Saeed, A., Makris, M., Malia, R.G., Preston, F.E., Greaves, M.**, The development of antiphospholipid antibodies in haemophilia is linked to infection with hepatitis C, *Br. J. Haematol.*, 88, 845, 1994.
28.   **Daroca, J.C., Gutierrez-Cebollader, J., Yazbeck, H., Berges, A., Rubies-Prat, J.**, Anticardiolipin antibodies and acquired immunodeficiency syndrome: prognostic marker or association with HIV infection?, *Infection*, 20, 140, 1992.
29.   **Jaeger, U., Kapiotis, S., Pabinger, I., Puchhammer, E., Kyrle, P.A., Lechner, K.**, Transient lupus anticoagulant associated with hypoprothrombinemia and factor XII deficiency following adenovirus infection, *Ann. Hematol.*, 67, 95, 1993.
30.   **Yamazaki, M., Asakura, H., Kawamura, Y., Ohka, T., Endo, M., Matsuda, T.**, Transient lupus anticoagulant induced by Epstein-Barr virus infection. *Blood Coagul. Fibrinolysis*, 2, 771, 1992.
31.   **Asherson, R.A.**, A "primary" antiphospholipid syndrome?, *J. Rheumatol.*, 15, 1742, 1988.
32.   **Metzer, W.S., Canoso, R.T., Newton, J.E.O.**, Anticardiolipin antibodies in a sample of chronic schizophrenics receiving neuroleptic therapy, *S. Med. J.*, 87, 190, 1994.
33.   **Hughes, G.R.V.**, The antiphospholipid syndrome: ten years on, *Lancet*, 342, 341, 1993.
34.   **Hughes, G.R.V.**, The anticardiolipin syndrome, *Clin. Exp. Rheumatol.*, 3, 285, 1985.
35.   **Harris, E.N., Baguley, E., Asherson, R.A., Hughes, G.R.V.**, Clinical and serological features of the antiphospholipid syndrome (APS), *Br. J. Rheumatol.*, 26, 19, 1987 (abstract).
36.   **Harris, E.N.**, Syndrome of the black swan, *Br. J. Rheumatol.*, 26, 324, 1987.
37.   **Staub, H.L., Harris, E.N., Khamashta, M.A., Savidge, G., Chahade, W.H., Hughes, G.R.V.**, Antibody to phosphatidylethanolamine in a patient with lupus anticoagulant and thrombosis, *Ann. Rheum. Dis.*, 48, 166, 1989.
38.   **Karmochkine, M., Caloub, P., Piette, J.C., Goldeau, P., Boffa, M.C.**, Antiphosphatidyl-ethanolamine antibody in systemic lupus erythematosus with thrombosis, Clin. Exp. Rheumatol., 10, 603, 1992.
39.   **Asherson, R.A., Khamashta, M.A., Ordi-Ros, J., Derksen, R.H., Machin, S.J., Barquinero, J., Outt, H.H., Harris, E.N., Vilardell-Torres, M., Hughes, G.R.**, The primary antiphospholipid syndrome: major clinical and serological features, *Medicine*, 68, 366, 1989.
40.   **Alarcon-Segovia, D.**, Clinical manifestations of the antiphospholipid syndrome, *J. Rheumatol.*, 19, 1778, 1992.
41.   **Levine, S.R., Deegan, M.J., Futreu, N., Welch, K.M.A.**, Cerebrovascular and neurologic disease associated with antiphospholipid antibodies: 48 cases, *Neurology*, 40, 1181, 1990.
42.   **Coull, B.M., Levine, S.R., Brey, R.L.**, The role of antiphospholipid antibodies in stroke, *Neurol. Clin.*, 10, 125, 1992.
43.   **Piette, J.C.**, The mystery of antiphospholipid antibodies in Sneddon's syndrome, *Arch. Dermatol.*, 130, 519, 1994 (letter to editor).
44.   **Herranz, M.T., Rivier, G., Khamashta, M.A., Blasser, K.U., Hughes, G.R.V.**, Association between antiphospholipid antibodies and epilepsy in patients with systemic lupus erythematosus, *Arthritis Rheum.*, 37, 568, 1994.
45.   **Brey, R.L., Hart, R.G., Sherman, D.G., Tegeler, C.H.**, Antiphospholipid antibodies and cerebral ischemia in young people, *Neurology*, 40, 1190, 1990.
46.   Antiphospholipid Antibodies in **Stroke Study Group Clinical and Laboratory Findings in Patients with Antiphospholipid Antibodies and Cerebral Ischemia**, *Stroke*, 21,1268, 1990.
47.   **Sneddon, I.B.**, Cerebrovascular lesions and livedo reticularis, *Br. J. Dermatol.*, 77, 180, 1965.

48. **Levine, S.R., Welch, K.M.A.,** The spectrum of neurologic disease associated with antiphospholipid antibodies, lupus anticoagulants and anticardiolipin antibodies, *Arch. Neurol.,* 44, 876, 1987.
49. **Asherson, R.A.,** The catastrophic antiphospholipid syndrome, *J. Rheumatol.,* 19, 508, 1992.
50. **Durant, J.M., Lefebre, P., Kaplanski, G., Soubeyrand, J.,** Thrombotic microangiopathy and the antiphospholipid antibody syndrome, *J. Rheumatol.,* 18, 1916, 1991.
51. **Alarcon-Segovia, D.,** Antiphospholipid syndrome within systemic lupus erythematosus, *Lupus,* 3, 289, 1994.
52. **Asherson, R.A., Cervera, R.,** "Primary", "secondary" and other variants of the antiphospholipid syndrome, *Lupus,* 3, 293, 1994.
53. **Vianna, J.L., Khamashta, M.A., Ordi-Ros, J. et. al.** Comparison of the primary and secondary antiphospholipid syndrome: a European multicentre study of 114 patients, *Am. J. Med.,* 96, 3, 1994.
54. **Andrews, P.A., Frampton, G., Cameron, J.S.,** Antiphospholipid syndrome and systemic lupus erythematosus, *Lancet,* 342, 988, 1993.
55. **Piette, J.C., Wechsler, B., Frances, C., Godeau, P.,** Systemic lupus erythematosus and the antiphospholipid syndrome: reflections on the relevance of APA criteria, *J. Rheumatol.,* 19, 1835, 1992.
56. **Piette, J.C., Wechsler, B., Frances, C., Papo, T., Godeau, P.,** Exclusion criteria for primary antiphospholipid syndrome, *J. Rheumatol.,* 20, 1802, 1993.
57. **Asherson, R.A., Zulman, T., Hughes, R.G.V.,** Pulmonary thromboembolism associated with procainamide induced lupus syndrome and anticardiolipin antibodies, *Ann. Rheum. Dis.,* 48, 232, 1989.
58. **Harris, E.N., Bos, K.,** An acute disseminated coagulopathy - vasculopathy associated with the antiphospholipid syndrome, *Arch. Int. Med.,* 151, 231, 1991.
59. **Morton, K.E., Gavahan, T.P., Krilis, S.A., Daggard, G.E., Baron, D.W., Hickie, J.B.,** Coronary artery bypass graft failure - an autoimmune phenomenon?, *Lancet,* 2, 1353, 1986.
60. **Hamsten, A., Norberg, R., Bjorkholm, M., De Firre, U., Holm, G.,** Antibodies to cardiolipin in young survivors of myocardial infarction: an association with recurrent cardiovascular events, *Lancet,* 1, 113, 1986.
61. **Ginsburg, K.S., Liang, M.H., Newcomer, L., Goldhaber, S.Z., Schur, P.H., Hennekens, C.H., Stampfer, M.J.,** Anticardiolipin antibodies and the risk for ischemic stroke and venous thrombosis, *Ann. Intern. Med.* 117, 997, 1992.
62. **Taylor, L.M., Chitwood, R.W., Dalman, R.L., Sexton, G., Goodnight, S.H., Porter, J.M.,** Antiphospholipid antibodies in vascular surgery patients, *Ann. Surg.,* 220, 544, 1994.
63. **Pierangeli, S.S., Barker, J.H., Stikoval, D., Ackerman, D., Anderson, G., Barquinero, J., Acland, R., Harris, E.N.,** Effect of human IgG antiphospholipid antibodies on an in vivo thrombosis model in mice, *Haemostasis,* 71, 670, 1994.
64. **Mizutani, H., Engelman, R.W., Kinjoh, K., Kurato, Y., Ikehara, S., Good, R.A.,** Prevention and induction of occlusive coronary vascular disease in autoimmune (W/B) F1 mice by haploidentical bone marrow transplantation: possible role for anticardiolipin autoantibodies, *Blood,* 82, 3091, 1993.
65. **Ginsberg, J.S., Demers, C., Brill-Edwards, P.,** Johnston, M., Bona, R., Burrows, R.F., Weitz, J., Denburg, J.A., Increased thrombin generation and activity in patients with systemic lupus erythematosus and anticardiolipin antibodies: evidence for a prothrombotic state, *Blood,* 81, 2958, 1993.
66. **Triplett, D.A.,** Antiphospholipid antibodies and recurrent pregnancy loss, *Am. J. Reprod. Immunol.,* 20, 52, 1989.
67. **Miletich, J.P., Prescott, S.M., White, R., Majerus, P.W., Bovill, E.G.,** Inherited predisposition to thrombosis, *Cell,* 72, 477, 1993.
68. **Dahlback, B.,** Inherited resistance to activated protein C, a major cause of venous thrombosis, is due to a mutation in the factor V gene, Haemostasis, 24, 139, 1994.
69. **Koster, T., Rosendaal, F.R., De Ronde, H., Briet, E., Vandenbroucke, J.P., Bertina, R.M.,** Venous thrombosis due to poor anticoagulant response to activated protein C: Leiden Thrombophilia Study, *Lancet,* 342, 1503, 1993.
70. **Carreras, L.O., Defreyn, G., Machin, S.J., Vermylen, J., Deman, R., Spitz, B., Van Assche, A.,** Arterial thrombosis, intrauterine death and "lupus" anticoagulant: detection of immunoglobulin interfering with prostacyclin formation, *Lancet,* 1, 244, 1981.
71. **Carreras, L.O., Maclouf, J.,** The lupus anticoagulant and Eicosanoids, Prostaglandins Leukot. Essent. *Fatty Acids,* 49, 483, 1993.
72. **Watson, K.V., Schorer, A.E.,** Lupus anticoagulant inhibition of in vitro prostacyclin release is associated with thrombosis prone subset of patients, *Am. J. Med.,* 90, 47, 1991.
73. **Schorer, A.E., Wickham, N.W.R., Watson, K.V.,** Lupus anticoagulant induces a selective defect in thrombin mediated endothelial prostacyclin release and platelet aggregation, *Br. J. Haematol.,* 71, 399, 1989.
74. **Walker, T.S., Triplett, D.A., Javed, N., Musgrave, K.,** Evaluation of lupus anticoagulants: antiphospholipid antibodies, endothelium associated immunoglobulin, endothelial prostacyclin secretion, and antigenic protein S levels, Thromb. Res., 51, 267, 1988.
75. **Martinuzzzo, M.E., Maclouf, J., Carreras, L.O., Levy Toledano, S.,** Antiphospholipid antibodies enhance thrombin induced platelet activation and thromboxane formation, Thromb. Haemost., 70, 667, 1993.
76. **Lellouche, F., Martinuzzo, M., Said, P., Maclouf, J., Carreras, L.O.,** Imbalance of thromboxane/prostacyclin biosynthesis in patients with lupus anticoagulant, *Blood,* 78, 2894, 1991.
77. **Carreras, L.O., Maclouf, J.,** Antiphospholipid antibodies and eicosanoids, *Lupus,* 3, 271, 1994.
78. **Esmon, C.T.,** The protein C anticoagulant pathway, *Arterioscler. Thromb.,* 12, 135, 1992.
79. **Marciniak, E., Romond, E.H.,** Impaired catalytic function of activated protein C: a new in vitro manifestation of lupus anticoagulant, *Blood,* 74, 2426, 1989.
80. **Smirnov, M.D., Triplett, D.A., Comp, P.C., Esmon, C.T.,** Role of phosphatidylethanolamine in inhibition of activated protein C by lupus anticoagulants, *Lupus,* 3, 358, 1994 (abstract 184).
81. **Couper, R.T.L., Maxwell, F.C.,** Anticardiolipin and acquired protein S deficiency in early childhood, *J. Paediatr. Child. Health,* 30, 363, 1994.
82. **Sorice, M., Griggi, T., Circella, A., Lenti, L., Arcieri, P., Di Nucci, G.D., Mariani, G.,** Protein S antibodies in acquired protein S deficiencies, *Blood,* 83, 2383, 1994.
83. **Oosting, J.D., Derksen, R.H.W.M., Hackeng, T.M., Van Vliet, M., Preissner, K.T., Bouma, B.N., De Groot, P.G.,** In vitro studies of antiphospholipid antibodies and its cofactor 2 glycoprotein I show negligible effects on endothelial cell mediated protein C activation, *Thromb. Haemost.,* 55, 666, 1991.
84. **Viard, J.P., Amoura, Z., Bach, J.F.,** Anti-B2 Glycoprotein-I antibodies in systemic lupus erythematosus - a marker of thrombosis associated with lupus anticoagulant activity, *C. R. Acad. Sci.* [III], 313, 607, 1991.
85. **Shibata, S., Harpel, P.C., Gharavi, A., Rand, J., Fillit, H.,** Autoantibodies to heparin from patients with antiphospholipid antibody syndrome inhibits formation of antithrombin III-thrombin complexes, Blood, 83, 2537, 1994.
86. **Kandiah, D.A., Krilis, S.A.,** 2 Glycoprotein I, *Lupus,* 3, 207, 1994.

87.   **Galli, M., Comfurius, P., Barbui, T., Zwaal, R.F.A., Bevers, E.M.**, Anticoagulant activity of B2Glycoprotein I is potentiated by a distinct subgroup of anticardiolipin antibodies, *Thromb. Haemost.*, 68, 297, 1992.

88.   **Matsuura, E., Igarashi, Y., Fujimoto, M., Ichikawa, K., Suzuki, T., Sumida, T., Yasuda, T., Koike, T.**, Heterogeneity of anticardiolipin antibodies defined by the anticardiolipin cofactor, *J. Immunol.*, 148, 3885, 1992.

89.   **Matsuda, J., Saitoh, N., Gotchi, K., Gotoh, M., Isukamoto, M.**, Distinguishing 2 glycoprotein I dependent (systemic lupus erythematosus type) and independent (syphilis type) anticardiolipin antibody with tween 20, *Br. J. Haematol.*, 85, 799, 1993.

90.   **Ravelli, A., Martini, A., Burgio, G.R.**, Antiphospholipid antibodies in paediatrics, *Eur. J. Pediatrics*, 153, 472, 1994.

91.   **Ravelli, A., Martini, A., Burgio, R.G., Falcini, F., Taccetti, G.**, Antiphospholipid antibody syndrome as a cause of venous thrombosis in childhood, *J. Pediatrics*, 124, 831, 1994 (letter to editor).

92.   **Carreno, L., Monteagudo, I., Lopez-Longo, F.J., Gonzalez, C., Perez, T., Mahou, M.R., Samson, J., La Pointe, N.**, Anticardiolipin antibodies in pediatric patients with human immunodeficiency virus, *J. Rheumatol.*, 21, 1344, 1994.

93.   **Tucker, L.B.**, Antiphospholipid syndrome in childhood: the great unknown, *Lupus*, 3, 367, 1994 (editorial).

94.   **d'Annunzio, G., Caporali, R., Lorini, R.**, Anticardiolipin antibodies in children and adolescents with insulin-dependent diabetes mellitus, *Diabetes Res. Clin. Pract.*, 23, 63, 1994.

95.   **Exner, T., Triplett, D.A., Taberner, D., Machin, S.J.**, Guidelines for testing and revised criteria for lupus anticoagulants. SSC Subcommittee for Standardization of Lupus Anticoagulants, *Thromb. Haemost.*, 65, 320, 1991.

96.   **Harris, E.N., Pierangeli, S., Birch, D.**, Anticardiolipin wet workshop report, *Am. J. Clin. Pathol.*, 101, 616, 1994.

97.   **Triplett, D.A.**, Screening for the lupus anticoagulant, *Res. Clin. Lab.*, 19, 379, 1989.

98.   **Triplett, D.A.**, New diagnostic strategies for lupus anticoagulants and anti- phospholipid antibodies, *Haemostasis*, 24, 155, 1994.

99.   **Triplett, D.A.**, Assays for detection of antiphospholipid antibodies, *Lupus*, 3,281, 1994.

100. **Rosove, M.H., Brewer, P.M.C.**, Antiphospholipid thrombosis clinical course after the first thrombotic event in 70 patients, *Ann. Intern. Med.*, 117, 303, 1992.

101. **Barbui, T., Finazzi, G.**, Clinical trials on antiphospholipid syndrome: what is being done and what is needed?, *Lupus*, 3, 303, 1994.

102. **Harris, E.N., Gharavi, A.E., Patel, S.P., Hughes, G.R.V.**, Evaluation of the anti- cardiolipin test: report of a standardized workshop held 4 April 1986, *Clin. Exp. Immunol.*, 68, 215, 1987.

PEPTIDE MARKERS IN HYPERCOAGULABILITY ASSOCIATED WITH CORONARY HEART DISEASE

G. J. Miller

Epidemiology and Medical Care Unit, The Medical College of St Bartholomew's Hospital, London

I. INTRODUCTION

Atherothrombotic disease of the coronary arteries evolves silently and unpredictably over many years, eventually presenting in many of those affected as stable or unstable angina pectoris, acute myocardial infarction, cardiac failure or sudden coronary death. The earliest lesion, often present in infancy,[1] is a microscopic focal collection of lipid-laden macrophages within the arterial intima. Progression from this to a more advanced lesion is by no means inevitable, and seems to depend upon continuing injury to the intima in the presence of increased plasma concentrations of atherogenic lipoproteins. With advancement, the collections of macrophages enlarge and coalesce, acquire extracellular deposits of lipid, and gradually become infiltrated with lipid-containing smooth muscle cells.[2] The ultimate lesion is the atheromatous plaque, typically comprised of a basal pool of necrotic debris, cholesterol crystals and calcified material, a middle zone rich in macrophages, smooth muscle cells, connective tissue and lipid, and a dense fibrous cap in which are embedded smooth muscle cells.[3] These plaques encroach upon the vessel's lumen, and some are sufficiently unstable as to fissure or rupture at some point, thereby triggering the coronary thrombosis that precipitates the presenting clinical event.[4]

There is increasing evidence to believe that perturbations in the coagulation and fibrinolytic pathways arise on the endothelial surface in the earliest stages of atherothrombotic disease and that they play an important role in the progression of focal lesions. These disturbances are thought to arise as responses to injury to the arterial wall and to hyperlipidaemia. Thus the possibility arises that markers of these perturbations may afford a measure of the extent and severity of the atheromatous disease and of the risk of a thrombotic complication. In patients who have no primary or hereditable disorder of the haemostatic system, assays which reflect the rates of generation of coagulation factors, the activities of the anticoagulant factors, or the action of thrombin on fibrinogen may be informative in this respect. This chapter reviews what is known so far, and highlights those areas where research is needed.

II. THE ARTERIAL ENDOTHELIUM IN HEALTH

Healthy, resting arterial endothelium is a contiguous monolayer of cells which presents an anticoagulant surface to circulating blood. The cell membranes forming the luminal surface lack both tissue factor (the obligatory cofactor of factor VII required for activation of the extrinsic pathway) and a negative charge sufficient to activate the contact system of coagulation (factor XII, factor XI, prekallikrein and high molecular weight kininogen). Anticoagulant properties are conferred to the surface by heparan sulphate - antithrombin III complexes which inhibit the coagulant proteases factor Xa and thrombin,[5] thrombomodulin-thrombin complexes which activate protein C[6] (a powerful inhibitor of activated factor VIII (VIIIa) and activated factor V (Va)), and secretion of protein S[7] (the cofactor for activated protein C). Fibrinolytic properties are provided by the surface expression of the plasminogen receptor[8] and secretion of both tissue plasminogen activator and plasminogen activator inhibitor type I (PAI-1).[9] In addition, endothelial cells normally produce nitric oxide[10] and prostacyclin[11] which promote vasodilatation and inhibit platelet aggregation. By forming a barrier layer, the intact endothelium prevents blood coming into contact with tissue factor dispersed on cell membranes in the tunica media and adventitia,[12] or with negatively charged contact surfaces on collagen fibres. Thus the fluidity and free flow of blood are protected.

III. ENDOTHELIAL CHANGES IN HYPERCHOLESTEROLAEMIA

Plasma low-density lipoprotein (LDL) particles, the major carriers of circulating cholesterol, are innocuous at physiological concentrations (<3.4 mmol/l)[13] in their native state. At high concentration, however, they provoke changes to endothelial cells in culture akin to activation, facilitating adhesion of monocytes to the cell surface.[14] Those LDL particles exposed to free radicals released by endothelial cells and monocytes become oxidatively modified, and thereby are rendered far more atherogenic.[15,16] Even minimally-modified LDL will stimulate the production of tissue factor mRNA many-fold in human endothelial cells, which express tissue factor at peak levels within about 4 hours of exposure.[17] The same level of exposure to these particles also triggers the endothelial expression of monocyte and granulocyte colony-stimulating factors[18] and monocyte chemotactic factors,[19] thereby promoting the binding of monocytes to endothelial cells. Monocytes release the cytokines interleukin-I and tumour necrosis factor, which both stimulate the expression of tissue factor[20,21] and suppress the expression of thrombomodulin by the endothelial cell in culture.[22] Tumour necrosis factor has also been reported to stimulate the surface-expression of tissue factor by monocytes.[23] Furthermore, oxidatively modified LDL appears to inhibit the activation of protein C on the endothelial cell's surface,[24] presumably by suppressing the expression of thrombomodulin, and Schuff-Werner et al[25] have evidence for its induction of tissue factor-like activity on monocytes. Thus endothelial cell and monocyte activation by oxidatively modified LDL apparently shifts the balance of cell surface properties in favour of procoagulant activity, an alteration reinforced by cytokines liberated at the site of vascular injury.

IV. CYTOKINES AND IN VIVO HAEMOSTATIC ACTIVATION

To test these ideas, Nawroth et al[22] infused recombinant interleukin-I intravenously in rabbits. Scanning electron microscopy of major arteries subsequently revealed strands of fibrin attached to the luminal surface of the endothelial cells, especially at bifurcations, indicating activation of coagulation with thrombin generation. Bauer et al[26] infused recombinant human tumour necrosis factor into patients with active malignancies. Activation of the coagulant pathway was demonstrated by increased concentrations of the peptides that are released from prothrombin and protein C on the conversion to their active enzymes and by raised levels of fibrinopeptide A (FPA) which is released from fibrinogen by thrombin. A similar study was subsequently undertaken in healthy adults given a bolus injection of tumour necrosis factor.[27] The response in plasma factor X activation peptide concentration appeared to be too rapid to have been a consequence of tissue factor synthesis, and may have been due to increased permeability of the endothelium as a response to tumour necrosis factor,[28] thereby allowing access of coagulant zymogens to sub-endothelial structures in the arterial wall. These studies show clearly that exposure of the blood vessel wall to cytokines will raise its capacity to support coagulation.

V. MARKERS OF HYPERCOAGULABILITY

When blood is exposed to a procoagulant surface its coagulation system undergoes a series of linked proteolytic reactions (Figure 1). If exposure is of sufficient magnitude, the intensity of the response will generate a clot or thrombus. Even a sub-thrombotic exposure, however, will nevertheless increase the reaction rates at one or more steps in the coagulation pathway. At each stage, a zymogen such as factor IX, factor X or prothrombin is converted into its respective enzyme responsible for the subsequent proteolytic step in the pathway. Cofactors such as factor VIIIa and factor Va accelerate the reaction rates at the factor IX and factor X steps respectively by enhancing the binding of these zymogens in close proximity to their substrates on the surfaces of endothelial cells, platelets and leucocytes. The substrates for these reactions are all found in large excess in blood, and only small amounts are consumed by the haemostatic mechanism in vivo. Hence, attempts to assess the functional status of the system by measurement of the circulating concentrations of these components are not in general rewarding. Similarly, the enzymes generated at each step of the pathway are difficult to quantify because they exist only transiently before forming complexes with naturally occurring inhibitors. Consequently, another approach is needed to judge the rates of reaction at the several levels of activity within the coagulation pathway.

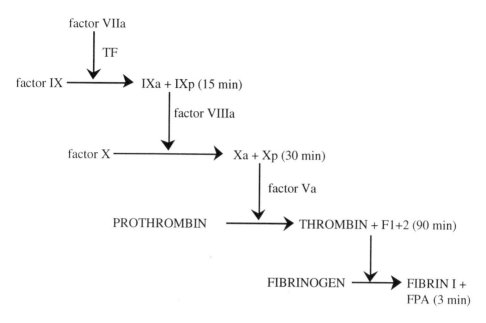

Figure 1. The pathway of fibrin generation. Times in parentheses are the half-lives of the respective peptide fragments. The active form of the factor or cofactor is denoted by 'a', the activation peptide by 'p'. F1+2 is prothrombin's activation peptide fragment 1+2, and FPA is fibrinopeptide A.

In the 1970's, Nossel et al[29-31] developed a radioimmunoassay for the concentration of FPA, which is cleaved from fibrinogen during its proteolytic conversion to fibrin by thrombin. A few years later, Lau et al[32] and Tietel et al[33] extended this approach by establishing a radioimmunoassay for the activation peptide, fragment 1+2 (F_{1+2}), that is cleaved from prothrombin by the prothrombinase complex during the generation of thrombin. These and the activation peptides released during the generation of Factor IXa from factor IX, and factor Xa from factor X, are stable structures with finite half-lives in the circulation. Bauer et al have more recently developed radioimmunoassays for factor IX activation peptide[34] and factor X activation peptide,[35] as well as protein C activation peptide.[36] In the last few years several ELISA systems have been reported for F_{1+2}, and these systems are now available commercially.[37-39] These developments have provided new opportunities to explore the status of the coagulant pathway in the atherothrombotic disorders including coronary heart disease.

VI. HAEMOSTATIC PEPTIDES IN HEALTHY ADULTS

The discovery of basal concentrations of the activation peptides of factor IX, factor X, and prothrombin, as well as FPA, in the plasma of apparently healthy individuals, is indicative of a normal albeit low rate of flux through the coagulation pathway. Average normal values taken from selected studies are presented in Table I, which shows that the great majority of the data currently available are for men of middle age. Published results for men in other age groups suggest that lower values can be expected in younger men and higher values are probably the norm in more elderly males. For example, factor IX activation peptide was found to average 216 pM in 23 men aged 41 to 50 years, rising to 274 pM in 17 aged 71 to 80 years.[34] In 28 men less than 40 years of age, F_{1+2} averaged 1.68nM, while in 25 aged 70 years or more the mean value was 2.78 nM.[42] Plasma FPA levels in these same groups averaged respectively 1.10nM and 1.64nM.[42] Whether these changes reflect an increasing rate of generation or decreasing clearance with increasing age is not certain, but the possibility that they reflect exposure of blood to procoagulant surfaces on an increasingly unhealthy vasculature cannot be excluded. Support for this idea is provided by the raised levels of F_{1+2} and FPA reported in several conditions associated with an increased risk of coronary heart disease and stroke, and in patients with established cardiovascular disorders.

Table I : Normal values for some indices of haemostatic activity in healthy adults

Index[1]	Sex	Age, years Mean	(Range)	Number	Normal values Mean	(SD)	Assay	Reference
IXp, pM								
	Male		(51-60)	14	228	(74)	RIA (non-commercial)	34
	Male	55	(50-61)	443	209	(64)	RIA (non-commercial)	40
Xp, pM								
	Male	<40		23	66	(20)	RIA (non-commercial)	35
	Male	55	(50-61)	445	121	(32)	RIA (non-commercial)	40
F1+2 , nM								
	Male	55	(50-61)	2771	0.70	(0.28)	RIA (non-commercial)	41
	Male		(50-59)	84	1.82	(0.67)	RIA (non-commercial)	42
	Not stated	Not stated		95	0.67	(0.19)	ELISA (Behringwerke)	38
	Male	36	(17-69)	357	0.51		ELISA (Organon-Teknika)	43
FPA, nM								
	Male	55	(50-61)	2771	1.27	(0.87)	RIA (Byk-Sangtec)	41
	Male[2]		(35-54)	137	1.23	(0.70)	RIA (IMCO, Stockholm)	44
	Male		(50-69)	29	1.15	(0.73)	RIA (Mallinckrodt)	42

[1] IXp = factor IX activation peptide; Xp = factor X activation peptide;
F1+2 = prothrombin fragment 1+2; FPA = fibrinopeptide A.

[2] non-smokers only

VII. HAEMOSTATIC PEPTIDES AND CARDIOVASCULAR RISK FACTORS

Lowe et al[44] measured FPA concentration in 412 healthy men aged 35 to 54 years with no history of cardiovascular disease. The mean level was statistically significantly higher in smokers (1.35nM) and ex-smokers (1.50nM) than in non-smokers (1.23nM). Also, individual concentrations increased significantly with systolic blood pressure, body mass index, serum cholesterol concentration and triglyceride concentration (although the correlation coefficients were of low order, ranging from 0.10 to 0.19). Plasma FPA was also found to correlate strongly and positively with fibrinogen concentration, an established marker of risk for atherothrombotic disease.[45,46] Nossel et al[47] studied 130 patients with either a fasting cholesterol concentration above 7.1 mmol/l or a fasting triglyceride higher than 1.81 mmol/l, or both. Although mean FPA levels were slightly raised in his patient groups by between 8% and 38%, as compared with control subjects, none of the differences achieved statistical significance. The conclusion was reached that no steady state elevation in thrombin proteolysis of fibrinogen existed in these hyperlipidaemic patients. In another clinical study of 72 men and 26 women with various presentations of coronary heart disease (none on therapy except nitrates) and an age matched control group of 28 men and 13 women, no significant correlations were observed between FPA concentrations and smoking habit, blood pressure, blood glucose concentration or serum lipid levels.[48]

Scanty though the data are relating FPA concentration to the established coronary risk factors, there is even less information for F_{1+2} concentration in relation to risk status. In a preliminary analysis of baseline data for the second Northwick Park Heart Study, a significant and positive correlation was found between F_{1+2} and factor VII coagulant activity, a strong predictor of fatal coronary heart disease,[49] in 955 healthy middle-aged men.[50] After adjustment for age, Hursting et al[43] found no significant association of F_{1+2} concentration with sex, race (black or white) or smoking habit in their analysis of variance on the data for 357 healthy adults. Donders et al[51] examined 27 men and 27 women with essential hypertension whose ages ranged from 19 years to 70 years. All but 11 were on some form of antihypertensive therapy but nevertheless had raised blood pressure levels at the time of examination. In comparison with a reference group of 50 age- and sex-matched healthy hospital workers, the F_{1+2} concentration in hypertensive patients was raised by about 100% on average, and within the patient group was appreciably higher in those falling in the upper quartile of blood pressure than in those in the lower quartile. Mean levels were reported not to differ significantly between those on therapy and those not taking drugs. There are no published data relating the activation peptides of factor IX or factor X to the established coronary risk factors.

VIII. HAEMOSTATIC PEPTIDES
IN ESTABLISHED CARDIOVASCULAR DISEASE

In contrast to the paucity of data relating indices of haemostatic activation to cardiovascular risk factors, there are a number of reports showing that FPA and F_{1+2} concentrations are frequently elevated in patients with atherothrombotic disease that has presented clinically, the one exception being stable angina pectoris. In 1976, Nossel et al[30] reported increased concentrations of FPA in patients with thrombophlebitis, pulmonary embolism, aortic aneurysm, neoplasia, sepsis and systemic lupus erythematosus. By monitoring the rate of increase in FPA concentration in blood immediately after the venepuncture, it was concluded that the blood of many of these patients had an increased concentration of active thrombin. In the following year, Wajima and Burkett[52] studied 31 patients 2 to 3 days before surgery for obstructive coronary artery disease. Ten of these patients were considered to have an elevated FPA concentration, which decreased to normal levels in the postoperative period. The extent of the coronary artery occlusion was not correlated with the FPA concentration. In view of the absence of any other apparent clinical source, the raised FPA levels were taken to imply locally accelerated haemostatic activity in the diseased coronary arteries. Whether fresh thrombus was observed at the time of surgery was not reported.

Johnsson et al[53] examined 29 patients who had been admitted to coronary care units. In 17 patients a diagnosis of acute myocardial infarction was confirmed by typical signs and symptoms, electrocardiographic changes including the appearance of new pathological Q waves (transmural infarct), and elevated cardiac enzyme concentrations. The remainder were considered to have angina pectoris, myocarditis, or disease of the cervical spine. Blood samples were taken for FPA on the first, second and fourth mornings after admission. No patient had clinical evidence of venous thrombosis, pulmonary embolism or cardiogenic shock. In the patients with myocardial infarction, mean FPA concentrations were two to three times those in the remainder during the first 48 hours, but by the fourth day they had declined toward normal levels. The group of 12 patients without diagnosed myocardial infarction but with central chest pain had lesser increases in FPA concentration which were nevertheless above normal values. Patients with the largest infarctions as judged by peak cardiac enzyme levels appeared to have the highest FPA concentrations in the first 48 hours. A few years earlier, Davies et al[54] had noted occlusive coronary thrombus in 95% of patients who had died of an acute myocardial infarction and had been examined post mortem, and in the following year De Wood et al[55] demonstrated the high frequency of thrombosis in transmural myocardial infarction by performing combined angiography and coronary catheterization shortly after the onset. By this time there was no doubt that the increased FPA concentrations immediately after an acute myocardial infarction reflected the proteolysis of fibrinogen by thrombin at the site of the lesion.

With these discoveries, others have attempted more recently to relate plasma FPA concentrations to the extent of coronary disease and to its clinical manifestations. For example, Serneri et al[48] classified their patients into those with an old myocardial infarction, those with stable or unstable angina pectoris of effort and those with unstable spontaneous angina. All three types of clinical presentation were associated with increased FPA concentrations. They were then classified according to those experiencing daily attacks of chest pain (active) and those free of pain at rest for at least 7 days before examination (quiescent). Mean FPA levels were about sixfold higher in patients with active disease than in those with quiescent disease. There was no apparent relation between the extent of coronary disease on angiography and FPA concentration, supporting the earlier findings of Wajima and Burkett.[52]

Nichols et al[56] studied 82 patients with chest pain, none of whom had had a myocardial infarction within the previous 6 months, and who were clinically free of other cardiac disease, pulmonary embolism and thrombophlebitis. On the basis of coronary arteriography and ventriculography they were categorized into those with normal findings, those with coronary artery disease but no prior myocardial infarction, and those with a previous myocardial infarction. Risk factor status and therapy did not differ significantly between the groups. No differences in mean FPA concentrations were found between the 3 groups. However, their values (0.77, 0.81, and 1.00 nM) were all higher (though not statistically significantly) than the mean reported elsewhere by these investigators for healthy adults (0.64nM).[30] In 3 patients with mural thrombi in the ventricles, FPA concentration was increased.

Differences in FPA levels were sought between patients with a confirmed acute myocardial infarction, others with unstable angina pectoris without infarction, and a third group with non-cardiac acute chest pain examined within 3 days of admission.[57] All three groups had clear elevations in mean FPA concentration, but there were no significant differences between their levels. The non-cardiac sources of chest pain were mostly chest infections, and perhaps accorded with the elevated concentrations reported earlier by Nossel et al in patients with sepsis.[30]

Eisenberg et al[58] have conducted another study which sought to relate FPA concentrations to the extent of myocardial necrosis and the time of blood sampling after the onset of the acute event. Infarction was diagnosed by assay for MB-creatine kinase concentration, and transmural infarction by the evolution of new major Q waves on the electrocardiogram. Mean FPA concentration from the initial blood sample taken on admission from patients with a transmural lesion was found to be significantly greater (42 ng/ml) than that in patients with a non-transmural infarction (5 ng/ml). Plasma FPA levels were most markedly raised when measurement was made within 10 hours of onset of the acute event leading to transmural necrosis. Levels thereafter tended to decline the longer the gap between onset and venepuncture. Unlike the findings of Johnsson et al,[53] no relation was apparent between infarct size and initial or subsequent FPA concentration in patients with a transmural infarction. In one patient with an early recurrent infarction on the third day of admission, a marked increase in FPA concentration was documented soon after the onset of the new episode of chest pain.

Théroux et al[59] conducted a study of 16 consecutive patients with unstable angina and 15 with stable angina pectoris matched for age, sex, coronary risk factors, medication and extent of coronary artery disease. Mean FPA concentration was 5.5 ng/ml in those with unstable angina as compared with a significantly lower and normal value of 2.7 ng/ml in those with stable angina. As did Serneri et al,[48] they concluded that a raised FPA concentration was indicative of active thrombotic disease.

In their study of middle-aged men in Edinburgh, Lowe et al[44] compared FPA concentrations in 117 men who answered positively and 412 answering negatively to a questionnaire for angina pectoris. Although those reporting angina were more frequently smokers and had the higher serum triglyceride concentrations, there was no difference in FPA levels between the two groups. This result contrasted with an earlier finding from the same laboratory, in which men with ischaemic cardiac pain and coronary artery disease demonstrated by arteriography had an increased mean FPA concentration (2.1 nM) in comparison with controls (1.6 nM). No relation was apparent between the extent of disease at arteriography and FPA concentration.[60]

The first reports of an association between F_{1+2} concentration and vascular disease appeared in 1991, when raised levels were noted in patients with deep vein thrombosis confirmed by phlebography and in others with pulmonary embolism demonstrable on lung scan.[38] Whereas the range of concentrations in healthy adults was from 0.32 to 1.2 nM with the particular ELISA used, those in the patients ranged between 1.5 and 9.5 nM. The assay was then applied to patients undergoing coronary arteriography for chest pain, having excluded those with a myocardial infarction within the preceding two months and others with serious non-cardiac disorders. No association was seen between F_{1+2} concentration and the number of stenosed coronary arteries, but patients with any coronary stenosis had a raised mean F_{1+2} concentration about 30% above that of those with no arteriographic changes, a difference of borderline statistical significance.[61]

More recently, Merlini et al[62] measured the plasma of F_{1+2} and FPA on admission to hospital in 80 patients with acute uncomplicated unstable angina, 32 with an acute myocardial infarction, 37 with uncomplicated stable angina and 32 healthy individuals. These measurements were then repeated after 6 months in patients with an uneventful clinical course. All with stable angina pectoris had significant coronary artery disease at arteriography. On admission, those with unstable angina pectoris or myocardial infarction had significant increases in F_{1+2} concentration (1.08 and 1.27nM respectively) as compared with those with stable angina or healthy adults (0.74 and 0.71nM respectively). A similar pattern was seen for FPA concentration, with levels in patients with stable angina not significantly higher than those in healthy controls. Once again, no relations were apparent between the concentrations of either peptide and the extent of coronary artery disease as assessed on the arteriogram.

In those patients who survived 6 months without a new or recurrent myocardial infarction or a need for coronary revascularization, the plasma F_{1+2} concentration at the end of this period remained raised by an amount similar to that found immediately after the acute event, whereas FPA concentrations had returned to normal levels. These results were thought to be indicative of increased thrombin generation at the time of the acute episode sufficient to produce thrombus, followed later by a persistent hypercoagulable state but with insufficient generation of free thrombin to initiate thrombus formation.

There are no published studies to date that have examined factor IX activation peptide or factor X activation peptide at the various stages in the progression of atherothrombotic disorders.

IX. HAEMOSTATIC PEPTIDES AND PREDICTION OF CARDIOVASCULAR DISEASE

The foregoing clinical studies leave little doubt that increased concentrations of FPA are indicative of thrombus formation in vivo. Because the half-life of this 16 amino acid peptide is only about 3 minutes,[29] a high FPA concentration can be taken to reflect ongoing proteolysis of fibrinogen by thrombin. The test is of course neither site nor lesion specific, indicating only free thrombin activity somewhere within the arterial or venous systems. Increased FPA concentrations are found immediately after coronary or cerebral[63] thrombosis, but elevations at later times after the acute event could be due either to recurrences or to complications such as venous thrombosis, pulmonary embolism, mural thrombi in the ventricles, ventricular aneurysm or sepsis. The measurement of FPA is very sensitive to the quality of the venepuncture,[41] and concentrations in blood samples similar to those produced by in vivo thrombosis are easily mimicked by a slightly traumatic insertion of the venepuncture needle. With a good technique for blood sampling, however, repeated measures of FPA concentration may be of some value in monitoring the patient's progress after an acute cardiovascular episode, and in the assessment of the need to initiate or adjust anticoagulant regimens. It does not appear to hold out promise of assessment of risk of clinical coronary heart disease because its concentration can be normal even when there is evidence of a hypercoagulable state in the form of an increased F_{1+2} concentration or a raised factor VII coagulant activity.

The demonstration of a persistent increase in F_{1+2} concentration in patients who have made an uneventful recovery from an episode of unstable angina pectoris or acute myocardial infarction[62] raises the possibility that a similar abnormality may precede the onset of clinical disease. Further evidence in this direction is provided by the positive association between F_{1+2} concentration and factor VII coagulant activity,[50] a known predictor of coronary heart disease.[49] The second Northwick Park Heart Study is a prospective cardiovascular survey designed to assess the relations of the plasma concentrations of the activation peptides of factor IX, factor X and prothrombin with coronary risk factor status and incidence of acute coronary events in healthy middle aged men. The study is now well established and first results are expected about 1996-1997. The survey is based upon the suspicion that in men belonging to a community in which atherosclerosis and clinical coronary heart disease are common, those thrombotic episodes that cause unstable angina, myocardial infarction and sudden cardiac death represent only 'the tip of the iceberg'. The working hypothesis is that with advancing atheromatous disease, subclinical platelet-fibrin deposition becomes more frequent and more extensive, and can be detected by markers of increased rates of turnover at one or more steps 'upstream' or 'midstream' in the haemostatic pathway. On this account, markers of haemostatic activity are being measured annually over five years in all respondents.

X. MONITORING OF ANTICOAGULANT THERAPY IN CORONARY HEART DISEASE

Patients with coronary heart disease are frequently given long-term aspirin, nitrates, beta-blockers or Ca^{++} antagonists according to clinical indication. None of these drugs appears to influence F_{1+2} concentration or FPA concentration significantly.[62,64] In the treatment of acute thrombotic disorders such as venous thromboembolism, heparin reduces the FPA concentration and in sufficient amounts will return it to within the normal range.[29,65] High F_{1+2} levels also decline with heparin treatment, generally returning to normal in about three days.[66] Full dose oral anticoagulant therapy (International Normalised Ratio (INR) of 2.5 or greater) often reduces F_{1+2} to subnormal concentrations,[27] while that sufficient to raise the INR to about 1.5 to 2.5 lowers the concentration to well within the normal range,[64] and even doses which increase the INR only to 1.3 to 1.6 will decrease F_{1+2} concentration by as much as 50% from baseline levels. In one report, although FPA levels declined to normal after recovery from a myocardial infarction, there appeared to be a 'rebound' to raised concentrations within 2 weeks of withdrawal of anticoagulant therapy.[69]

XI. CONCLUSIONS

Studies of peptide markers of the hypercoagulable state are so far in their infancy, especially in coronary heart disease. Injury to the arterial wall in atheromatous disease evidently provokes a loss of the natural anticoagulant properties of the endothelial surface and acquisition of procoagulant characteristics. In theory therefore, the possibility arises that with sufficient advancement of the atheromatous state, sub-thrombotic levels of activation of the coagulation system may give rise to increased circulating concentrations of peptides that are released from certain of the zymogen clotting factors when they are activated. This idea remains to be tested clinically and epidemiologically, but such a mechanism is at least consistent with the increases in the concentrations of the activation peptide of factor IX, F_{1+2}, and fibrinopeptide A between middle age and old age in clinically healthy adults. Studies are required relating the levels of activation peptides to coronary risk factor status, non-invasive measures of atheromatous disease, and the incidence of clinical cardiovascular disease.

An increased FPA concentration appears to be a marker of active thrombus formation somewhere in the vascular system, but is neither site or lesion specific. Blood samples analysed for FPA must be drawn with scrupulous attention to the quality of the venepuncture. There is some preliminary clinical evidence for the persistence of increased F_{1+2} concentrations for at least 6 months after recovery from acute myocardial infarction. This finding, together with the epidemiological association between F_{1+2} and factor VII coagulant activity in healthy men, raises the possibility of increased F_{1+2} concentrations in men at high risk for non-fatal or fatal coronary disease. Studies of the relations of the activation peptides of factor IX, factor X, and protein C to coronary heart disease are in progress but results are awaited.

REFERENCES

1.   **Stary, H. C.,** Macrophages, macrophage foam cells, and eccentric intimal thickening in the coronary arteries of young children, *Atherosclerosis*, 64, 91, 1987.
2   **Stary, H. C., Chandler, A. B., Glagov, S., Guyton, J. R., Insull, W., Rosenfeld, M. E., Schaffer, S. A., Schwartz, C. J., Wagner, W. D., and Wissler, R. W.,** A definition of initial, fatty streak, and intermediate lesions of atherosclerosis. A report from the Committee on Vascular Lesions of the Council on Arteriosclerosis, American Heart Association, *Arterioscler. Thromb.*, 14, 840, 1994.
3.   **Stary, H.,** Evolution and progression of atherosclerotic lesions in coronary arteries of children and young adults, *Arteriosclerosis*, 9 (Suppl I), 1, 1989.
4.   **Davies, M. J., Richardson, P. D., Woolf, N., Katz, D. R., and Mann, J.,** Risk of thrombosis in human atherosclerotic plaques: role of extracellular lipid, macrophage, and smooth muscle cell content, *Br. Heart J.*, 69, 377, 1993.
5.   **Marcum, J. A., McKenney, J. B., and Rosenberg, R. D.,** Acceleration of thrombin-antithrombin complex formation in rat hindquarters via heparinlike molecules bound to endothelium, *J. Clin. Invest.*, 74, 341, 1984.
6.   **Owen, W. G., and Esmon, C. T.,** Functional properties of an endothelial cell cofactor for thrombin-catalyzed activation of protein C, *J. Biol. Chem.*, 256, 5532, 1981.
7.   **Stern, D. M., Brett, J., Harris, K., and Nawroth, P. P.,** Participation of endothelial cells in the protein C - protein S anticoagulant pathway: the synthesis and release of protein S, *J. Cell Biol.*, 102, 1971, 1986.
8.   **Plow, E. F., Freaney, D. E., Plescia, J., and Miles, L. A.,** The plasminogen system and the cell surface: evidence for

plasminogen and urokinase receptors on the same cell type, *J. Cell Biol.*, 103, 2411, 1986.

9. **van Hinsbergh, V. W. M., Binnema, D., Scheffer, M. A., Sprengers, E. D., Kooistra, T., and Rijken, D. C.,** Production of plasminogen activators and inhibitor by serially propagated endothelial cells from human blood vessels, *Arteriosclerosis*, 7, 389, 1987.

10. **Palmer, R. M. J., Ashton, D. S., and Moncada, S.,** Vascular endothelial cells synthesize nitric oxide from L-arginine, *Nature*, 333, 664, 1988.

11. **Moncada, S., Higgs, E. A., and Vane, J. R.,** Human arterial and venous tissues generate prostacyclin (prostaglandin X), a potent inhibitor of platelet aggregation. *Lancet*, 1, 18, 1977.

12. **Wilcox, J. N., Smith, K. M., Schwartz, S. M., and Gordon, D.,** Localization of tissue factor in the normal vessel wall and in the atherosclerotic plaque, *Proc. Natl. Acad. Sci. USA.*, 86, 2839, 1989.

13. **National Cholesterol Education Program.** Report of the Expert Panel on Population Strategies for Blood Cholesterol Reduction: Executive Summary, *Arch. Intern Med.*, 151, 1071, 1991.

14. **Pritchard, K. A., Tota, R. R., Lin, J. H.-C., Danishefsky, K. J., Kurilla, B. A., Holland, J. A., and Stemerman, M. B.,** Native low density lipoprotein. Endothelial cell recruitment of mononuclear cells, *Arterioscler. Thromb.*, 11, 1175, 1991.

15. **Henriksen, T., Mahoney, E. M., and Steinberg, D.,** Enhanced macrophage degradation of low density lipoprotein previously incubated with cultured endothelial cells: recognition by receptor for acetylated low density lipoproteins, *Proc. Natl. Acad. Sci. USA.*, 78, 6499, 1981.

16. **Morel, D. W., Di Corleto, P. E., and Chisholm, G. M.,** Endothelial and smooth muscle cells alter low density lipoprotein in vitro by free radical oxidation, *Arteriosclerosis*, 4, 357, 1984.

17. **Drake, T. A., Hannani, K., Fei, H., Lavi, S., and Berliner, J. A.,** Minimally oxidized low-density lipoprotein induces tissue factor expression in cultured human endothelial cells, *Am. J. Pathol.*, 138, 601, 1991.

18. **Rajavashisth, T. B., Andalibi, A., Territo, M. C., Berliner, J. A., Navab, M., Fogelman, A. M., and Lusis, A. J.,** Induction of endothelial cell expression of granulocyte and macrophage colony-stimulating factors by modified low-density lipoproteins, *Nature*, 344, 254, 1990.

19. **Cushing, S. D., Berliner, J. A., Valente, A. J., Territo, M. C., Navab, M., Parhami, F., Gerrity, R., Schwartz, C. J., and Fogelman, A. M.,** Minimally modified low density lipoprotein induces monocyte chemotactic protein 1 in human endothelial cells and smooth muscle cells, *Proc. Natl. Acad. Sci., USA.*, 87, 5134, 1990.

20. **Bevilacqua, M.P., Pober, J. S., Wheeler, M. E., Cotran, R. S., and Gimbrone, M. A.,** Interleukin 1 (IL-1) activation of vascular endothelium: effects on procoagulant activity and leukocyte adhesion, *Am. J. Pathol.*, 121, 393, 1985.

21. **Nawroth, P. P., and Stern, D. M.,** Modulation of endothelial cell haemostatic properties by tumor necrosis factor, *J. Exp. Med.*, 163, 740, 1986.

22. **Nawroth, P. P., Handley, D. A., Esmon, C. T., and Stern, D. M.,** Interleukin 1 induces endothelial cell procoagulant while suppressing cell-surface anticoagulant activity, *Proc. Natl. Acad. Sci. USA.*, 83, 3460, 1986.

23. **Conkling, P. R., Greenberg, C. S., and Weinberg, J. B.,** Tumor necrosis factor induces tissue factor-like activity in human leukemia cell line U937 and peripheral blood monocytes, *Blood*, 72, 128, 1988.

24. **Weis, J. R., Pitas, R. E., Wilson, B. D., and Rodgers, G. M.,** Oxidised low-density lipoprotein increases cultured human endothelial cell tissue factor activity and reduces protein C activation, *FASEB J.*, 5, 2459, 1991.

25. **Schuff-Werner, P., Claus, G., Armstrong, V. W., Kostering, H., and Seidel, D.,** Enhanced procoagulant activity (PCA) of human monocytes/macrophages after in vitro stimulation with chemically modified LDL, *Atherosclerosis*, 78, 109, 1989.

26. **Bauer, K. A., ten Cate, H., Barzegar, S., Spriggs, D. R., Sherman, M. L., and Rosenberg, R. D.,** Tumor necrosis factor infusions have a procoagulant effect on the hemostatic mechanism of humans, *Blood*, 74, 165, 1989.

27. **van der Poll, T., Buller, H. R., ten Cate, H., Wortel, C. H., Bauer, K. A., van Deventer, S. J. H., Hack, C. E., Sauerwein, H. P., Rosenberg, R. D., and ten Cate, J. W.,** Activation of coagulation after administration of tumor necrosis factor to normal subjects, *N. Engl. J. Med.*, 322, 1622, 1990.

28. **Brett, J., Gerlach, H., Nawroth, P., Steinberg, S., Godman, G., and Stern, D.,** Tumor necrosis factor/cachectin increases permeability of endothelial cell monolayers by a mechanism involving regulatory G proteins. *J. Exp. Med.*, 169, 1977, 1989.

29. **Nossel, H. L., Yudelman, I., Canfield, R. E., Butler, V. P., Spanondis, K., Wilner, G. D., and Qureshi, G. D.,** Measurement of fibrinopeptide A in human blood, *J. Clin. Invest.*, 54, 43, 1974.

30. **Nossel, H. L., Ti, M., Kaplan, K. L., Spanondis, K., Soland, T., and Butler, V. P.,** The generation of fibrinopeptide A in clinical blood samples. Evidence for thrombin activity, *J. Clin. Invest.*, 58, 1136, 1976.

31. **Nossel, H. L., Wasser, J., Kaplan, K L., La Gamma, K. S., Yudelman, I., and Canfield, R. E.,** Sequence of fibrinogen proteolysis and platelet release after intrauterine infusion of hypertonic saline, *J. Clin. Invest.*, 64, 1371, 1979.

32. **Lau, H. K., Rosenberg, J. S., Beeler, D. L., and Rosenberg, R. D.,** The isolation and characterization of a specific antibody population directed against the prothrombin activation fragments F_2 and F_{1+2}, *J. Biol. Chem.*, 254, 8751, 1979.

33. **Tietel, J. M., Bauer, K. A., Lau, H. K., and Rosenberg, R. D.,** Studies of the prothrombin activation pathway utilizing radioimmunoassays for the F_2/F_{1+2} fragment and thrombin-antithrombin complex, *Blood*, 59, 1086, 1982.

34. **Bauer, K. A., Kass, B. L., ten Cate, H., Hawiger, J. J., and Rosenberg, R. D.,** Factor IX is activated in vivo by the tissue factor mechanism, *Blood*, 76, 731, 1990.

35. **Bauer, K. A., Kass, B. L., ten Cate, H., Bednarek, M. A., Hawiger, J. J., and Rosenberg, R. D.,** Detection of factor X activation in humans, *Blood*, 74, 2007, 1989.

36. **Bauer, K. A., Kass, B. L., Beeler, D. L., and Rosenberg, R. D.,** Detection of protein C activation in humans, *J. Clin. Invest.*, 74, 2033, 1984.

37. **Shi, O., Sio, R., Lin, S., Yu, K., Arbuthnutt, K., Ruiz, J., and Gaur, P.,** Performance characteristics of an enzyme-linked immunosorbent assay (ELISA) for prothrombin fragment F1.2., *Thromb. Haemost.*, 65, 1118, 1991.

38. **Pelzer, H., Schwarz, A., and Stuber, W.,** Determination of human prothrombin activation fragment 1+2 in plasma with an antibody against a synthetic peptide, *Thromb. Haemost.*, 65, 153, 1991.

39. **Hursting, M. J., Butman, B. T., Steiner, J. P., Moore, B. M., Plank, M. C., Szewczyk, K. M., Bell, M. L., and Dombrose, F. A.,** Monoclonal antibodies specific for prothrombin fragment 1+2 and their use in a quantitative enzyme-linked immunosorbent assay, *Clin. Chem.*, 39, 583, 1993.

40. **Miller, G. J., Bauer, K. A., Barzegar, S., and Rosenberg, R. D.,** unpublished.

41. **Miller, G. J., Bauer, K. A., Barzegar, S., Foley, A. J., Mitchell, J. P., Cooper, J. A., Rosenberg, R. D.,** The effects

of quality and timing of venepuncture on markers of blood coagulation in healthy middle-aged men, *Thromb Haemost.*, in press.

42.   **Bauer, K. A., Weiss, L. M., Sparrow, D., Vokonas, P. S., and Rosenberg, R. D.**, Aging - associated changes in indices of thrombin generation and protein C activation in humans. Normative Aging Study, *J. Clin. Invest.*, 80, 1527, 1987.

43.   **Hursting, M. J., Stead, A. G., Crout, F. V., Horvath, B. Z., and Moore, B. M.**, Effects of age, race, sex and smoking on prothrombin fragment 1+2 in a healthy population, *Clin. Chem.*, 39, 683, 1993.

44.   **Lowe, G. D. O., Wood, D. A., Douglas, J. T., Riemersma, R. A., MacIntyre, C. C. A., Takase, T., Tuddenham, E. G. D., Forbes, C. D., Elton, R. A., and Oliver, M. F.**, Relationships of plasma viscosity, coagulation and fibrinolysis to coronary risk factors and angina, *Thromb. Haemost.*, 65, 339, 1991.

45.   **Wilhelmsen, L., Svardsudd, K., Korsan-Bengtsen, K., Larsson, B., Welin, L., and Tibblin, G.**, Fibrinogen as a risk factor for stroke and myocardial infarction, *N. Engl. J. Med.*, 311, 501, 1984.

46.   **Meade, T. W., Mellows, S., Brozovic, M., Miller, G. J., Chakrabarti, R. R., North, W. R. S., Haines, A. P., Stirling, Y., Imeson, J. D., and Thompson, S. G.**, Haemostatic function and ischaemic heart disease : principal results of the Northwick Park Heart Study, *Lancet*, 2, 533, 1986.

47.   **Nossel, H. L., Rees Smith, F., Seplowitz, A. H., Dell, R. B., Sciacca, R. R., Merskey, C., and Goodman, D. S.**, Normal levels of fibrinopeptide A in patients with primary hyperlipidemia, *Circ. Res.*, 45, 347, 1979.

48.   **Serneri, G. G. N., Gensini, G. F., Abbate, R., Mugnaini, C., Favilla, S., Brunelli, C., Chierchia, S., and Parodi, O.**, Increased fibrinopeptide A formation and thromboxane A_2 production in patients with ischemic heart disease : relationships to coronary pathoanatomy, risk factors, and clinical manifestations, *Am. Heart. J.*, 101, 185, 1981.

49.   **Meade, T. W., Ruddock, V., Stirling, Y., Chakrabarti, R., and Miller, G. J.**, Fibrinolytic activity, clotting factors, and long-term incidence of ischaemic heart disease in the Northwick Park Heart Study, *Lancet*, 342, 1076, 1993.

50.   **Miller, G. J., Wilkes, H. C., Meade, T. W., Bauer, K. A., Barzegar, S., and Rosenberg, R. D.**, Haemostatic changes that constitute the hypercoagulable state, *Lancet*, 338, 1079, 1991.

51.   **Donders, S. H. J., Lustermans, F. A. T., and van Wersch, J. W. J.**, Prothrombin fragment 1+2 in both treated and untreated hypertensive patients, *Netherlands J. Med.*, 43, 174, 1993.

52.   **Wajima, T., and Burkett, L. L.**, Accelerated hemostasis in coronary artery disease (Abstract), *Thromb. Haemost.*, 38, 269, 1977.

53.   **Johnsson, H., Orinius, E., and Paul, C.**, Fibrinopeptide A (FPA) in patients with acute myocardial infarction, *Thromb. Res.*, 16, 255, 1979.

54.   **Davies, M. J., Woolf, N., and Robertson, W. B.**, Pathology of acute myocardial infarction with particular reference to occlusive coronary thombi, *Br. Heart J.*, 38, 659, 1976.

55.   **De Wood, M. A., Spores, J., Notske, R., Mouser, L. T., Burroughs, R., Golden, M. S., and Lang, H. T.**, Prevalence of total coronary occlusion during the early hours of transmural myocardial infarction, *N. Engl. J. Med.*, 303, 897, 1980.

56.   **Nichols, A. B., Owen, J., Kaplan, K. L., Sciacca, R. R., Cannon, P. J., and Nossel, H. L.**, Fibrinopeptide A, platelet factor 4, and b-thromboglobulin levels in coronary heart disease, *Blood*, 60, 650, 1982.

57.   **Douglas, J. T., Lowe, G. D. O, Forbes, C. D., and Prentice, C. R. M.**, Plasma fibrinopeptide A and beta-thromboglobulin in patients with chest pain, *Thromb. Haemost.*, 50,541, 1983.

58.   **Eisenberg, P. R., Sherman, L. A., Schectman, K., Perez, J., Sobel, B. E., and Jaffe, A. S.**, Fibrinopeptide A : a marker of acute coronary thrombosis, *Circulation*, 71, 912, 1985.

59.   **Théroux, P., Latour, J.-G., Léger-Gauthier, C., and De Lara, J.**, Fibrinopeptide A and platelet factor levels in unstable angina pectoris, *Circulation*, 75, 156, 1987.

60.   **Small, M., Lowe, G. D. O., Douglas, J. T., Hutton, I., Lorimer, A. R., and Forbes, C. D.**, Thrombin and plasmin activity in coronary artery disease, *Br. Heart J.*, 60, 201, 1988.

61.   **Kienast, J., Thompson, S. G., Raskino, C., Pelzer, H., Fechtrup, C., Ostermann, H., and van de Loo, J.**, Prothrombin activation fragment 1+2 and thrombin antithrombin III complexes in patients with angina pectoris; relation to the presence and severity of coronary atherosclerosis, *Thromb. Haemost.*, 70, 550, 1993.

62.   **Merlini, P. A., Bauer, K. A., Oltrona, L., Ardissino, D., Cattaneo, M., Belli, C., Mannucci, P. M., and Rosenberg, R. D.**, Persistent activation of coagulation mechanism in unstable angina and myocardial infarction, *Circulation*, 90, 61, 1994.

63.   **Lane, D. A., Wolff, S., Ireland, H., Gawel, M., and Foadi, M.**, Activation of coagulation and fibrinolytic systems following stroke, *Br. J. Haematol.*, 53, 655, 1983.

64.   **Kistler, J. P., Singer, D. E., Millenson, M. M., Bauer, K. A., Gress, D. R., Barzegar, S., Hughes, R. A., Sheehan, M. A., Maraventano, S. W., Oertel, L. B., Rosner, B., and Rosenberg, R. D.**, Effect of low-intensity warfarin anticoagulation on level of activity of the hemostatic system in patients with atrial fibrillation, *Stroke*, 24, 1360, 1993.

65.   **Peuscher, F. W., van Aken, W. G., Flier, O. T. N., Stoepman-van Dalen, E. A., Cremer-Goote, T. M., and van Mourik, J. A.**, Effect of anticoagulant treatment measured by fibrinopeptide A (fp A) in patients with venous thrombo-embolism, *Thromb. Res.*, 18, 33, 1980.

66.   **Estivals, M., Pelzer, H., Sie, P., Pichon, J., Boccalon, H., and Boneu, B.**, Prothombin fragment 1+2, thrombin-antithrombin III complexes and D-dimers in acute deep vein thrombosis : effects of heparin treatment, *Br. J. Haematol.*, 78, 421, 1991.

67.   **Conway, E. M., Bauer, K. A. Barzegar, S., and Rosenberg, R. D.**, Suppression of haemostatic system activation by oral anticoagulants in the blood of patients with thrombotic diatheses, *J. Clin. Invest.*, 80, 1535, 1987.

68.   **Millenson, M. M., Bauer, K. A., Kistler, J. P., Barzegar, S., Tulin, L., and Rosenberg, R. D.**, Monitoring 'mini-intensity' anticoagulation with warfarin : comparison of the prothrombin time using a sensitive thromboplastin with prothrombin fragment F_{1+2} levels, Blood , 79, 2034, 1992.

69.   **Harenberg, J., Haas, R., Zimmermann, R.**, Plasma hypercoagulability after termination of oral anticoagulants, *Thromb. Res.*, 29, 627, 1983.

HYPERCOAGULABILITY AND CANCER

H.C. Kwaan

Hematology/Oncology Division,Veterans Administration Lakeside Medical Center, Chicago

Gentlemen : Those following my clinical work have surely noticed that there is a frequency of special diseases which attract attention due to the numerous circumstances in which they are observed. *I want to talk about plegmasia alba dolens.* You do remember that we have studied together the white painful edema not only in women with recent parturition but *more often in patients of either sex affected with pulmonary phthisis or internal cancerous tumors.* This is a rare example of generalized intravenous coagulation in the four limbs. What are the conditions where blood acquired this tendency of spontaneous coagulation? You know, gentlemen, *in cachetic states in general, tuberculosis and cancer cachexia in particular, the blood is modified...*

Armand Trousseau (1801-1867)
Lecture at Hôtel-Dieu, Paris 1865

Since Trousseau discussed the changes in blood leading to an increased frequency of "phlegmasia alba dolens" in cancer patients,[1] the association of "hypercoagulability" and cancer has been extensively studied. Today, it is generally recognized that thromboembolism is the second most common cause of death in cancer patients. The incidence cited in 1974 was 1-11%.[2] Since then, increasing survival and new therapies, including the frequent use of venous access catheters, have produced a much higher incidence today. It is likely to be even higher at autopsy. In an individual cancer patient, susceptibility to thrombosis would be enhanced by the concurrence of other risk factors including immobilization, dehydration, advanced age, smoking, diabetes, hypertension, nephrotic syndrome, inflammatory bowel diseases, and a prior history of thromboembolism. Extensive reviews on the general topic of prethrombotic risks are available.[3-5] This chapter will be devoted only to the prethrombotic state in cancer patients.

I. Clinical Manifestations

Not infrequently, thrombosis is the first presentation in a patient without overt clinical cancer. Thromboembolic manifestations may precede the discovery of the cancer by weeks or months.

Table I : Incidence of Cancer Presenting First with Thromboembolism

Author	Thrombo-embolic condition	Method of Diagnosis	Incidence of Cancer	Follow-up Duration	Number of Patients
Gore et al [6]	Pulmonary Embolism	Lung scan		2 yrs	228
		Positive cases	14.5%		
		Negative cases	0%		
Goldberg et al [7]	Deep vein Thrombosis	Impedence Plethysmography		5 yrs	1400
		Positive cases	6.3%		
		Negative cases	2.4%		
	Older subgroup (over age of 50)				490
		Positive cases	4.6%		
		Negative cases	0.3%		
Prandoni et al [8]	DeepVein Thrombosis	Venography		2 yrs	250
	"secondary"group		1,9%		105
	"idiopathic"group		10.5%		145
	recurrence subgroup		17.1%		35

This was recognized by Gore et al.[6] who followed 228 patients for a period of two years after a work-up for pulmonary embolism by lung scan. Those who had a positive lung scan had an incidence of cancer of 14.7%, while no cancer occurred in those with negative lung scans. A similar study by Goldberg et al.[7] was carried out in 1400 patients in whom impedance plethysmography (IPG) was performed for the evaluation of possible deep vein thrombosis. Over a 5-year follow-up period, those with positive tests showed an incidence of cancer of 6.3%, while those with negative tests had 2.4%. The difference was more remarkable among a subgroup of 490 of these patients who were over 50 years of age. The cancer incidence was 4.6% among those with positive IPG and only 0.3% in those with negative tests, an increase of over 15 fold. A more recent study by Prandoni et al. confirmed these observations[8]. They grouped their patients with deep vein thrombosis into those with a well-recognized risk other than cancer as "secondary thrombosis", and the rest as "idiopathic venous thrombosis". During a two year period following the initial presentation of deep vein thrombosis, cancer was diagnosed in 16 of 153 patients (10.5%) with idiopathic venous thrombosis. In 5 of these 16 patients (31%), cancer was discovered at the time of the initial presentation, and in another 9, within the first year (56%). In contrast, only 2 of 107 patients (1.9%) with secondary venous thrombosis were found to have cancer during the two year follow-up period. They also observed that patients with recurrence of their thrombosis had a higher incidence of cancer (17%). Monreal et al. employed more extensive diagnostic searches and observed an even higher incidence of 23% of cancer in those with idiopathic thrombosis.[9] In addition to deep vein thrombosis and pulmonary embolism, occult cancer may first present as ischemic heart disease,[10] or peripheral arterial occlusive disease.[11] These studies point to the necessity that a diligent search for an "occult" malignant disease should be made when a patient who has no obvious thromboembolic risk first presents with deep vein thrombosis or with other forms of thromboembolism. This is especially true when the deep vein thrombosis is refractory to therapy or shows recurrence. This belief is strongly supported by many investigators.[12-15] The thromboembolic presentation is usually that of a deep vein thrombosis, with or without pulmonary embolism. In contrast to the situation in non-cancerous patients, the thrombosis sometimes involves unusual sites, such as the hepatic veins (Budd-Chiari syndrome), of the cerebral sinus or the digital vessels. It is often described as "migratory phlebitis", though in practice, this is not commonly seen as such. The recurrent nature of venous thrombosis, as pointed out by Prandoni et al.[8], should alert the clinician that cancer may be the underlying etiology.

Cancer patients also run a high risk for thromboembolic complications when undergoing surgical operations. The incidence varies from 20% to 60% depending on the type of surgery (Table II). These figures are higher than those encountered in non-cancerous patients undergoing comparable forms of surgical operations.

Table II : Incidence of Thromboembolic Complications
in Cancer Patients Undergoing Different Types of Surgery

TYPE OF SURGERY	RISK :
GENERAL	29%
GYNECOLOGIC	20%
UROLOGIC	41%
ORTHOPEDIC	50-60%
NEUROSURGERY	28%

(Rickles et al) [25]

An uncommon type of thrombosis which sometimes occurs in the cancer patient is non-bacterial thrombotic endocarditis, [16,17] in which an aseptic valvular vegetation becomes the source of arterial emboli to multiple organs such as brain, kidney, spleen, heart and liver. This complication is most often seen in adenocarcinoma of the lung, pancreas and breast.

Generalized coagulopathy is frequently present with cancer and can take several forms. The most common form is disseminated intravascular coagulation (DIC), which is likely to be present in most patients with widespread metastatic disease. This is not surprising since it has long been known that deposition of fibrin[18-22] and of platelets[23,24] occurs in a variety of tumor tissues. Recently, an analysis of blood samples from 719 consecutive patients with advanced cancer of the lung or colon revealed a very high incidence of abnormal coagulation tests,with elevated FDP levels in 27.6% and increased fibrinopeptide A levels in 75.4% of the cases,[25] indicating a state of chronic DIC in these patients. DIC frequently occurs in acute progranulocytic leukemia and is generally acute. Leukemia cells are rich in tissue factors and other procoagulants. At the same time, the bleeding manifestations are more severe because the fibrinolytic activity in these patients is also increased.[26]

Table III : Features of Carcinoma Associated
with Microangiopathic Hemolytic Anemia and of Chemotherapy-Associated HUS/TTP

DISTINGUISHING FEATURES	CARCINOMA ASSOCIATED MICROANGIOPATHIC HEMOLYTIC ANEMIA	CHEMOTHERAPY ASSOCIATED HUS/TTP
Tumor Status	Widely metastatic	Often in remission
Site of Microthrombi	Lung	Kidney
Renal Failure, Hypertension	Rare	Common
Pulmonary Edema	Rare	Common
Intolerance to Transfusion	Rare	Common
Lab. Findings of DIC	Common	Rare
Proposed Etiology	DIC from tumor-associa ted factors	Chemotherapy toxicity + circulating immune complex
Recommended Therapy	Specific antitumor therapy + heparin	Immunoadsorption

(Modified from Murgo[54])

In the acute form found in patients with widespread metastasis, microangiopathic hemolytic anemia may be a notable feature. This picture of microangiopathy should not be confused with the thrombotic microangiopathy (synonyms: thrombotic thrombocytopenic purpura; hemolytic uremic syndrome: TTP/HUS) secondary to chemotherapy. The distinguishing features are shown in Table III. In TTP/HUS, the major site of microthrombi deposition is in the kidneys and thus, renal failure and hypertension are seen. These patients have poor tolerance to blood volume overload, and the high risk of pulmonary edema necessitates great caution with the speed of blood transfusion. Characteristic of this (HUS/TTP) syndrome is the lack of the usual laboratory findings seen in DIC. Instead, the diagnosis is commonly made from the finding of fragmented red blood cells when the peripheral blood is examined during the workup for severe anemia and thrombocytopenia. This complication is associated with a very high mortality rate, estimated to be around 70%, with 50% of the patients dying within the first two months of diagnosis. The most commonly involved chemotherapeutic agent is mitomycin C, but other agents, notably bleomycin, vinblastine and cisplatin are also implicated. How these agents trigger a reaction leading to this complication is unclear. The prominent feature is widespread microthrombi formed from the agglutination of circulating platelets. Although the exact mechanism of the platelet agglutination is unknown, it has been suggested that circulating immune complexes may be responsible.[27] These complexes were recovered from the majority of patients with this complication who underwent immunoadsorptive therapy, and were composed of antibodies against Le^x glypolipid and glycoprotein IIb/IIIa, and are believed to interact with platelets through its surface membrane integrin receptor $\alpha_{IIb}\beta_3$ (IIb/IIIa) leading to agglutination. This forms the hypothetical basis for adsorption therapy in which the patient's blood is extracorporeally passed through a staphylococcal protein A column. In a clinical trial, this form of therapy has been found to yield better survival rates than plasma exchange.[27]

In addition to chemotherapy-related HUS/TTP, other thromboembolic complications may result from therapeutic measures employed in cancer treatment. These are shown in Table IV. The increasing use of venous access devices is associated with an occlusion rate of 10-15%. The thrombus at the catheter tip may also serve as a nidus for infection contributing to an even higher infection rate of one to four infections per 1000 catheter days [28,29] The use of anticoagulants and of a urokinase lock as prophylaxis has shown promising preliminary results.[30-32]

TABLE IV : Thrombosis Complicating Therapeutic Measures

VENOUS ACCESS OCCLUSION

CHEMOTHERAPY ASSOCIATED TTP/HUS

    A. MITOMYCIN ASSOCIATED TTP/HUS

    B. L-ASPARAGINASE ASSOCIATED THROMBOSIS

    C. 5-FU ASSOCIATED CORONARY ARTERIAL OCLUSION

BUDD-CHIARI SYNDROME (Acute Leukemia : Bone Marrow Transplantation)

RAYNAUD'S PHENOMENON

CORONARY ARTERIAL OCCLUSION (5-FU)

HORMONAL THERAPY ASSOCIATED THROMBOSIS:

    A. TAMOXIFEN

    B. ESTROGEN

HEPARIN INDUCED THROMBOCYTOPENIA WITH THROMBOSIS

A unique hypercoagulable state is produced during treatment with L-asparaginase. This agent is a potent inhibitor of hepatic protein synthesis. Following each cycle of therapy, the recovery synthesis of proteins occurs at a varying rate so that the natural inhibitors of thrombosis such as proteins C and S, antithrombin III and plasminogen, may lag behind the coagulation proteins and a period of hypercoagulability may develop[33,34], during which the patient is at risk for thromboembolic complications. Since the plasma plasminogen level is low, thrombolytic therapy with plasminogen activators (tPA, urokinase or streptokinase) during this period will not be effective unless supplemental plasminogen is given.This can be administered in the form of fresh frozen plasma. [33]

Other chemotherapeutic agents have also been implicated in thromboembolic complications including hepatic and pulmonary venous occlusive disease and coronary heart disease [35]. In the case of 5 fluorouracil therapy, an altered protein C with diminished activity may be responsible. [36]

II. PATHOPHYSIOLOGY

The cancer patient is more prone to thromboembolic risk for many reasons. Some of the more significant ones are listed in Table V.

Table V : Pathophysiology of Thromboembolism in Cancer Patients

ABNORMAL BLOOD CONTENTS:

Activation of coagulation
  Tumor-derived tissue factor
  Tumor-derived procoagulant(cysteine protease)
  Tumor-associated leukocyte expression of procoagulants

Activation of platelets
  Tumor cell-derived Le$^\alpha$ and Le^x glycolipid
  Thrombin activation
  Thrombocytosis

Decreased natural anti-thrombotic factors
  Decreased antithrombin III, protein C, free protein S
  Decreased fibrinolytic activity (increased inhibitors)

Lupus Anticoagulant

ABNORMAL BLOOD FLOW

Venous Stasis from:
  Immobilization
  Tumor compression

Hyperviscosity from:
  Leukemic leukostasis
  Paraproteins
  Dehydration
  Erythrocytosis

Tumor cells produce several kinds of procoagulants[37-39], including (a) tissue factor which activates factor VII, forms a complex with factor VIIa and in turn, activates factor X ; (b) cancer procoagulant, a cysteine protease which activates factor X, independent of factor VII[39,40] ; (c) a prothrombinase-like property of tumor-shed vesicles which provides a lipid component of the cell membrane that facilitates the assembly of the prothrombin complex[41], and (d) in addition, the endothelial cells as well as monocytes within a tumor respond to cytokines such as tissue necrosis factor and release their own procoagulants[42].

In addition to thrombin, platelets may be activated by agents derived from tumors. A glycolipid, Le^x antigen, derived from adenocarcinoma, may form an immune complex with platelet membrane glycoprotein IIb/IIIa ($\alpha_{IIb}\beta_3$) and lead to platelet activation.

Tumor cell invasion of the vascular wall may also be a contributing factor to vascular injury and thrombosis.

In certain malignant diseases, hyperviscosity may be a major factor. This is seen in the paraproteinemia associated with plasma cell dyscrasia and in any tumor-associated erythrocytosis. A list of the cancers sassociated with secondary erythrocytosis is shown in Table VI.

TABLE VI : Secondary Polycythemia (Erythrocytosis) In Tumors

	%
RENALCARCINOMA	46
CEREBELLAR HEMANGIOBLASTOMA	21
BENIGN RENAL LESIONS	16
UTERINE FIBROMAS	6
ADRENAL CORTICAL CARCINOMA	3
HEPATOCELLULAR CARCINOMA	3
OVARIAN CARCINOMA	3
PHEOCHROMOCYTOMA	1

III. MANAGEMENT

Prophylactic measures employed in patients at high risk for thrombosis are all applicable to the cancer patient[43,44]. The administration of low dose heparin, singly or in combination with pneumatic leg cuff compression, reduced the incidence of deep vein thrombosis from 24.6% to 11.6% in cancer patients undergoing general surgery[44], from 18.4% to 9.6% in gynecologic surgery[45], and from 41% to 14% in urologic surgery[46]. In neurologic surgery[47-49], where the use of anticoagulants has a potential bleeding risk, the use of pneumatic leg cuff compression alone reduced the incidence from 22-34% to 4-9%.

The management of established venous thrombosis in the cancer patient requires proper anticoagulant therapy. In patients with primary brain tumors or with brain metastasis, the fear of intracranial bleeding has always been a deterrent for the use of anticoagulants, and the insertion of a Greenfield filter is a common practice. However, recent studies indicate that the danger of bleeding may be over-emphasized and that cautious anticoagulation is safe and more effective than Greenfield filters[50]

While there are suggestions of heparin resistance in some cancer patients[51], this has not been shown to be the case on careful analysis of the blood using the heparin assay. The apparent resistance may be due to a more "resistant" aPTT as a result of elevated fibrinogen, factor VIII and other activated clotting factors in the patients' blood. Similarly anecdotal impression of warfarin resistance in cancer patients has also not been proven. Of interest are findings in several clinical trials using low molecular weight heparin in the treatment of deep vein thrombosis and pulmonary embolism, of a lower mortality rate in the cancer patients treated with low molecular weight heparin than in those treated with standard unfractionated heparin[52,53]. At any rate, there does not appear to be any greater risk of bleeding in cancer patients receiving anticoagulant therapy.

In recurrent thrombosis of leg veins, particularly when patients are under anticoagulant therapy, there is a great risk of pulmonary embolism. Thus, interruption of the inferior vena cava is indicated. This is best accomplished by the insertion of a device such as the Greenfield filter.

IV. CONCLUSION

Cancer patients are at increased risk for thromboembolism. Multiple etiologic factors that are unique to the presence of a malignant state are involved and are frequently overlooked during the management of the thromboembolic complications. Though there are variations with each individual cancer patient, it is prudent to consider all of these factors in the overall clinical evaluation.

REFERENCES

1.   **Trousseau, A**, Phlegmasia Alba Dolens. in, Lectures on Clinical Medicine. Delivered at the Hotel-Dieu, Paris. *New Sydenham Society,* London, 1872, 281.
2.   **Goodnight, S.H., Jr.,** Bleeding and intravascular clotting in malignancy, a review. *NY Acad Sci* 230,271, 1974.
3.   **Nachman, R.L., Silverstein, R**, Hypercoagulable states. *Ann Int Med* 1019,819, 1993.
4.   **Schafer A.T,**The hypercoagulable state. *Ann Int Med* 102,814, 1985.
5.   **Kwaan, H.C., Samama, M.M., Lecompte T,** Pathogenesis of thrombosis. in,*Clinical Thrombosis* (eds) HC Kwaan MM Samama. CRC Press, Boca Raton FL,1989,3.
6.   **Gore, J.M., Appelbaum, J.S., Greene, H.L., et al,** Occult Cancer in patients with acute pulmonary embolism. *Arch Int Med* 96 ; 556, 1982.
7.   **Goldberg, R.J., Seneff, M., Gore, J.M., et al,** Occult malignant neoplasm in patients with deep venous thrombosis. *Arch Int Med* 147,251, 1987.
8.   **Prandoni, P., Lensing, S.W.A., Buller, H.R., et al,** Deep vein thrombosis and the incidence of subsequent symptomatic cancer.*N Eng J Med*,1128,1992.
9.   **Monreal, M., Lafoz, E., Cassals, A., et al,** Occult cancer in a patient with venous thrombosis, a systemic a roach. *Cancer* 67,541,1990.
10.   **Naschitz, J.E., Yeshurun, D., Abrahamson, J., et al,** Ischemic heart disease precipitated by occult cancer. *Cancer* 69, 2712, 1992.
11.   **Naschitz, J.E., Schechter, L., Chang J.B,** Intermittent claudication associated with cancer. Case studies. *Angiology* 9,696, 1987.
12.   **Silverstein, R., Nachman, R.L,**Cancer and Clotting-Trousseau's warning. *N Eng J Med* 327,1163, 1992.
13.   **Goldberg, R.J,** Venous thromboembolism and malignancy. *Arch Int Med* 147,1893, 1987.
14.   **Naschitz, J.E., Yeshurun, D., Abramson, J,** Thromboembolism, clues for the presence of occult neoplasia. *Int Angiol* 8, 2001, 1987.
15.   **Naschitz, J.E., Yeshurun, D., Lev, L.M,** Thromboembolism in cancer, Changing trends. *Cancer* 71,1384, 1993.
16.   **Deppish, L.M., Fayuemi, A.O,** Nonbacterial thrombotic endocarditis. Clinicopathologic Correlations. *Am Heart J* 92,723, 1976.
17.   **Guinn, G.A., Ayala, A., Liddicoat, J,** Clinical and therapeutic considerations in nonbacterial thrombotic endocarditis. *Chest* 64,26.1973.
18.   **Billroth, T,** Lectures on Surgical Pathology and Therapeutics. Translated from the 8th ed *New Sydenham Society,* London, 1978.
19.   **Iwasaki T,** Histological and experimental observations on the destruction of tumor cells in the blood vessels. *J Pathol Bacteriol* 20, 85 1915.
20.   **O'Meara, R.A.Q., Jackson, R.D.,**Cytological observations on carcinoma. *Irish J Med Sci* 327, 1958.
21.   **O'Meara, R.A.Q,** Coagulative properties of cancer. *Irish J Med Soc.*474, 1958.
22.   **McCardle, R.J., Harper, P.V., Aspar, I.L, Bake, W.F., Andros, S., Jiminez, F,** Studies with iodine 131-I labelled antibody to human fibrinogen and neohydrin 203-Hg. *Cancer* 20,751, 1967.
23.   **Gasic, G.J., Gasic, T.B., Galanti, N., Johnson, T., Murphy, S,** Platelet tumor cell interaction in mice-the role of platelets in the spread of malignant disease. *Int J Cancer* 11,704, 1973.
24.   **Gaspar, H,** Platelet-tumor cell interaction in metastasis formation. A possible theapeutic a roach to metastasis prophylaxis. *J Med* 8,102, 1977.
25.   **Rickles, F.R., Levine, M., Edwards, R.L., et al,** Abnormalities of blood coagulation in patients with cancer. in, *Thrombosis ; An Update* (eds) GG Neri Serneri, GF Gensini, RA bbate, D Prisco.Scientific Press, Florence, 1992, 241.
26.   **Tallman, M.S., Kwaan, H.C,** Reassessing the hemostatic disorder associated with acute pro-myelocytic leukemia. *Blood* 79,543, 1992.
27.   **Snyder, H.W., Jr., Mittelman, A., Cochran, S. K., Balint, J.P., Jr., Jones, F.R., and the PROSORBA Clinical Trial Group,** Successful treatment of cancer chemotherapy-asoiated thrombotic thrombocytopenic purpura/hemolytic uremic syndrome (TTP/HUS) with protein A immunoadsorption. *Blood* 76,476a (suppl I) 1990.
28.   **Decker, M.D., Edwards, K.M,**Central venous catheter infections. *Ped Clin* 35,579, l988.
29.   **Stillman RM, SolipmanF, GAcia J, Asawyer A,** Etiology of catheter associated sepsis : Correlation with thrombogenicity. *Arch Surg* 112,1497, 1987.
30.   **Fraschini, G., Jadeja, J., Lawson, M., et al,** Local infusion of urokinase for the lysis of thrombosis associated with permanent central venous catheters in cancer patients. *J Clin Oncol* 5, 672, 1987.
31.   **Fraschini, G., Becker, M., Bruso, P., Wang, Z., Raber, M,** Comparative trial of urokinase (UK) vs. heparin (H) as prophylaxis for central venous ports. *Proc A S C O* 10,337, 1991.
32.   **Lawson, M,** Partial occlusion of indwelling central venous catheters. *J Intravenous Nurs* 14,38, 1991.
33.   **Kucuk, O., Kwaan, H.C., Gunnar, W., Vasquez, R.M,** Thromboembolic complications associated with L-Asparaginase therapy. *Cancer* 55, 702, 1985.
34.   **Mitchell, L., Hoogendoorn, H., Giles, A.R., Vegh, P., AndrewM,** Increased endogenous thrombin generation in children with acute lymphoblastic leukemia : Risk of thrombotic complications in L-Asparaginase-induced anti-thrombin III deficiency.*Blood* 83,386, 1994.
35.   **Doll, D.C., Rogenberg, Q.U., Yarbro, J.W,**Vascular toxicity associated with antineoplastic agents. *J Clin Oncol* 4,1405, 1986.
36.   **Kuzel, T.M., Esparaz, B., Green, D., Kies, M.S,** Thrombogenicity of intravenous 5 fluorouracil alone or in combination with cisplatin. *Cancer* 65,885, 1990.
37.   **Gordon, S.C., Franks, J.J., Lewis, B.J,** Comparison of procoagulant activities in extracts of normal and malignant human tissue. *J Natl Cancer Inst* 62,773, 1979.
38.   **Falanga, A., Bolognese-Dalessandro, A.P., Donati, M.B,** Several murine metastasizing tumors possess a cysteine protease with cancer procoagulant characteristics *Intl J Cancer* 39,1774, 1987.
39.   **Gordon, S.G,** Cancer cell procoagulants and their possible role in metastasis.in, *Mechanisms of Cancer and Metastasis* (eds) K CHon, et al, Matinus Nijhoff, Boston, 1984.
40.   **Edwards, R.L., Rickles, F.R,**Macrophage procoagulants. *Prog Hemost Thromb* 7,183, 1984 .
41.   **Van De Water, L., Tracy, P.B., Aronson, D., Mann, KG, Dvorak, H.F,** Tumor cell generation of thrombin via functional prothrombinase assembly. *Cares* 45,5521, 1985.
42.   **Bauer, K.A., tenCate, H., Barzegar, S., et al,** Tumor necrosis factor infusions have a procoagulant effect on the hemostatic mechanism of humans. *Blood* 74,165, 1989.

43. **Salzman, E.W., Hirsh, J**, Prevention of venous thromboembolism. in, *Hemostasis and Thrombosis, Basic Principles and Clinical Practice*.(eds) RWColman, JHirsh, VJMarder, EWSalzman. Lincot, Philadelphia, 1987, 1252.
44. **Clagett, G.P., Reisch, J.S**, Prevention of venous thromboembolism in general surgical patients *Ann Surg*,208,227, 1988.
45. **Clarke-Pearson, D.L., Delong, E., Synan, I.S., et al**, A controlled trial of two low-dose heparin regimens for the prevention of post operative deep vein thrombosis. *Obstet Gynecol*,75,684, 1990 .
46. **Collins, R., Scrimgeour, A., Yusuf, S., et al**, Reduction in fatal pulmonary embolism and venous thrombosis by peri operative administration of subcutaneous heparin, Overview of results of randomized trials in general, orthopedic and urologic surgery. *N Eng J Med*, 318, 1162, 1988.
47. **Turpie, A.G.G., Gallus, A.S., Beattle, W.S, et al,** Prevention o venous thrombosis in patients with intracranial disease by intermittent pneumatic compression of the calf. *Neurology* 27,435, 1977.
48. **Skillman, J.J., Collins, R.E.C., Coe, N.P., et al**, Prevention of deep vein thrombosis in neurosurgical patients, A controlled, randomized, trial of external pneumatic compression boots. *Surgery* 83,354, 1978.
49. **Turpie, A.G.G., Hirsh, J., Gent, M., et al**, Prevention of deep vein thrombosis in potential neurosurgical patients. A randomized trial comparing graduated compression stockings alone or graduated compression stockings plus intermittent pneumatic compression with control. *Arch Int Med* 149,679, 1989.
50. **Schiff, D., DeAngelis, L.M**, Therapy of venous thromboembolism in patients with brain metastases, *Cancer* 73,493, 1993.
51. **Hirsh, J**, Mechanism of action and monitoring of anticoagulants. *Sem Thromb Hemost* 12,1, 1986.
52. **Prandoni, P**, Fixed dose L M W heparin (CY216) as compared with adjusted dose intravenous heparin in the initial treatment of symptomtic proximal venous thrombosis. *Thromb Hemost* 65,872, 1991 (Suppl).
53. **Hull, R.D., Raskob, G.E., Rosenbloom, D., Panju, A.A., et al**, Subcutaneous low molecular weight heparin compared with continuous intravenous heparin in the treatment of proximal vein thrombosis. *N Eng J Med* 326-975, 199.
54. **Murgo AJ**, Thrombotic microangiopathy in the cancer patient including those induced by chemotherapeutic agents. *Sem Haematol* 24, 161, 1987.

HYPERCOAGULABLE STATES AND PREGNANCY

J. Bonnar

Dpt of Obstetrics and Gynaecology, St James Hospital, Dublin

I. INTRODUCTION

A . PHYSIOLOGY OF PREGNANCY AND HYPERCOAGULABLE STATES

Normal pregnancy is associated with major changes in the coagulation and fibrinolytic systems. These appear to relate to the development of the utero-placental circulation and act as a protective mechanism to facilitate haemostasis at delivery. The overall effect of these physiological changes is a state of hypercoagulability and increased thrombotic potential throughout pregnancy and particularly in the immediate post-partum period.[1]

Pregnancy is a well recognised factor for precipitating venous thromboembolism in women with an abnormality of the coagulation or fibrinolytic systems as well as in women where no such abnormality can be identified.The hypercoagulable state of pregnancy presents special problems in women with a familial or acquired predisposition to venous thromboembolism.The identified causes of familial thrombophilia are deficiencies of antithrombin III, and proteins C and S, activated protein C resistance, dysfibrinogenaemias, deficiency of factor VII or factor XII, and factor V abnormalities. Acquired thrombophilia is a feature of the antiphospholipid syndrome which can be associated with recurrent pregnancy loss as well as venous thrombosis. Thrombocythaemia can also increase the risk of thrombosis in pregnancy and may present with recurrent abortion or growth retarded infants due to placental infarction.

Most studies have shown that the level of antithrombin III remains constant during normal pregnancy but is reduced in patients who develop pre-eclampsia.[2] Protein C appears to increase slightly during pregnancy and the increase is maintained into the puerperium.[3] In contrast protein S has been shown to decrease in pregnancy by about 40 % in the second half of pregnancy and returning to normal in the first few days of the puerperium.[3] In women with congenital deficiencies of antithrombin III, protein C and protein S, pregnancy is often the triggering factor for the first thrombotic event. Conard and colleagues[4] have shown the high risk of thrombosis related to pregnancy in women with antithrombin III, protein C and protein S deficiency and the rate was highest with antithrombin III deficiency both during pregnancy and post-partum (Table I).

Table I : Thrombosis related to pregnancy in women with antithrombin III, protein C or S deficiency in absence of prophylactic treatment (Conard et al 1990)

	Antithrombin III	**Protein C**	**Protein S**
No.of pregnancies (no. of women)	63 (n=25)	93 (n=36)	44 (n=17)
Thrombosis related to pregnancy	44 %	24 %	28 %
during pregnancy	18 %	7 %	0 %
in the post-partum	33 %	19 %	17 %

Deficiencies in antithrombin III, protein C and protein S have been estimated at 3 to 8 % or less in patients with a history of venous thrombosis.[5] Among women studied before taking oral contraception the prevalence of antithrombin III deficiency was found to be 1 in 5,000[6] while the prevalence of protein C deficiency was found to be 1 in 300 or 400.[7]

0-8493-5804-3/96/$0.00+$.50

II. ANTITHROMBIN III DEFICIENCY IN PREGNANCY AND PUERPERIUM

In familial antithrombin III deficiency, pregnancy and the puerperium are major precipitating factors for the initial thromboembolic event. Winter and colleagues[8] documented 16 pregnancies in 7 women of 3 families in Scotland. In 15 of the 16 pregnancies thromboembolic complications occurred, 13 during pregnancy and 2 in the puerperium. Thromboembolism can occur very early in the pregnancy and may be the first indication of conception. Antithrombin III deficiency should be suspected where there is a positive family history of thrombosis or a history of recurrent episodes of venous thrombosis before the age of 40 years. Resistance to Heparin treatment also suggests antithrombin III deficiency.

A. MANAGEMENT OF PREGNANCY

The woman with antithrombin III deficiency should understand that both contraceptive pills and pregnancy may precipitate thrombosis. In women with antithrombin III deficiency pregnancy should be carefully planned. Given their very high incidence of thrombosis, prophylaxis with subcutaneous Heparin should be started preferably before conception or as soon as pregnancy is diagnosed. If the patient is receiving long term Warfarin therapy, it should be discontinued before conception or before the sixth week of pregnancy in view of the risk of teratogenesis. Heparin can be given throughout pregnancy by self administered subcutaneous injections in doses similar to those used for the treatment of venous thrombosis,10,000 to 17,500 iu 12-hourly to achieve an APTT ratio of 1.5 - 2.0, 4 to 6 hours after the injection. Lower doses of Heparin do not provide effective prophylaxis. When the anticoagulant effect has been stabilised in early pregnancy regular monitoring should be continued every 2 to 3 weeks during the first 2 trimesters and weekly during the third trimester. Larger doses of Heparin may be required as pregnancy proceeds, especially in the third trimester. With the increasing levels of coagulation factors in late pregnancy the increase of the APTT ratio may not be possible to achieve. If so, an anti-Xa assay can be used to maintain the plasma concentration of Heparin to between 0.20 and 0.40 iu per ml measured as anti-factor Xa activity. Regular monitoring of the platelet count is also advisable. Prolonged Heparin treatment is associated with osteopenia. A recent study estimated the incidence of osteoporotic vertebral fractures to be around 2% in women with long term subcutaneous prophylaxis with Heparin with a mean dose of near 20,000 iu per day and mean duration of 25 weeks.[9]

B. MANAGEMENT OF LABOUR AND DELIVERY

In pregnant women receiving Heparin prophylaxis a detailed protocol for delivery is essential. Delivery by Caesarean section increases the risk of both haemorrhage and thromboembolism. Vaginal delivery is therefore preferable. Patients receiving full therapeutic doses of Heparin should reduce their Heparin dose on the day of delivery either to 10,000 units over 24 hours intravenously or to 5,000 units 12-hourly by subcutaneous injection. Patients taking lower prophylactic doses of Heparin should also reduce the Heparin dosage to 5,000 units 12-hourly for labour and delivery.

In all patients the APTT should be checked to ensure that it has normalised with reduction or discontinuation of Heparin. If the APTT is prolonged induction of labour should be postponed for 24 hours to allow the APTT to return to normal.

During labour antithrombin III concentrate should be infused to maintain the plasma antithrombin level above 80%. An initial dosage of concentrate of 50 to 70 iu per Kg body weight is usually sufficient to normalise the plasma antithrombin III.Normal plasma antithrombin III levels should be maintained post-partum until anti-coagulation with Warfarin has been established. If antithrombin III concentrate is not available fresh frozen plasma should be used.

C. EPIDURAL ANAESTHESIA

If a patient is anticoagulated during labour epidural analgesia should be avoided because of the risk of haematoma formation during insertion and removal of the cannula. If anticoagulant therapy has been discontinued or low dose Heparin is being used and the coagulations screen and platelet count are within normal limits epidural anaesthesia should not be associated with any increased risk of bleeding.

D. MANAGEMENT OF THE PUERPERIUM

Following delivery Heparin should be reintroduced in a dosage of 10,000 to 15,000 iu 12-hourly by subcutaneous injection. Warfarin can be started immediately in a dose of 7 mgs on the first and second day and 5 mgs on the third day. Heparin should be continued until the Warfarin has become fully effective

Following delivery further infusions of antithrombin III should be given every one to two days for the first 5 days post-partum depending on the results of the plasma antithrombin levels. Breast feeding is safe during oral anticoagulant treatment.

E. MANAGEMENT OF THROMBOSIS IN PREGNANCY

If thrombosis occurs during pregnancy in a patient with antithrombin III deficiency, antithrombin III concentrate and Heparin should be given to achieve full anticoagulation for at least 7 to 10 days. Thereafter, twice daily injections of Heparin can be given in a dosage of 10 to 15,000 units 12-hourly to maintain the APTT ratio at 1.5/2.0. If life threatening recurrent thrombosis and emboli occur a vena caval filter should be inserted.

III. DEFICIENCY OF PROTEIN C AND S

Carter and Bellem[10] described the management of protein C deficiency throughout pregnancy. They suggested that the frequency of protein C deficiency in pregnancy could be as high as 1 in 500. Subcutaneous Heparin was used throughout pregnancy. Trauscht-van Horn et al[11] reported on 15 protein C deficient patients and found a good perinatal outcome but the incidence of thromboembolism during pregnancy was 33%. They also found that 5 of 12 protein C deficient women using oral contraception developed thrombosis. Prophylactic Heparin was recommended during pregnancy for protein C deficient women with personal or family histories of thrombosis.

Very few reports are available on the management of pregnancy in women with protein S deficiency. Case reports have described prophylactic oral anticoagulant therapy being used throughout pregnancy. Such therapy will carry a significant hazard of Warfarin embryopathy and perinatal mortality. So far experience is limited in the management of women with a deficiency of either protein C or S. In the meantime management of the pregnancy should be similar to that of the woman with antithrombin III deficiency. Protein C concentrate has been used to prevent peri-partum thrombosis.[12] Fresh frozen plasma 8-hourly has also been used in the management of protein C deficiency.

IV. OTHER CONGENITAL COAGULATION ABNORMALITIES ASSOCIATED WITH THROMBOSIS

A. DYSFIBRINOGENAEMIAS

Ogston[13] reported that about 33% of individuals with dysfibrinogenaemia have a bleeding tendency and less than 10 % have a thrombotic tendency with a few having both a bleeding and thrombotic tendency. The fibrinogen defect may lead to an increase in the half-life of thrombin in the blood or resistance of the fibrin clot to lysis by plasmin. Thrombosis in subjects with dysfibrinogenaemia has been associated with pregnancy and delivery.

B. HEREDITARY DEFICIENCY OF FACTOR VII OR FACTOR XII

In patients with hereditary deficiency of factor VII or factor XII venous thromboembolism has been reported. Whether these deficiencies predispose to or fail to protect against thromboembolism is uncertain.[14]

V. FIBRINOLYTIC SYSTEM ABNORMALITIES

Venous thrombosis has been described in association with congenital abnormalities of a number of components of the fibrinolytic system. Quantitative deficiency of apparently normal fibrinogen was described in a patient who developed thrombosis following delivery.[15] Thrombophilic families with defective release of vascular plasminogen activator in response to venous occlusion have also been reported in association with post-partum thrombosis.[16]

VI. THROMBOCYTHAEMIA AND PREGNANCY

Essential thrombocythaemia has been reported in association with recurrent abortion or fetal growth retardation[17]. Others have reported normal pregnancy in association with thrombocythaemia.[18,19] Randi et al[20] recently reviewed the literature with respect to outcome of pregnancy in patients with essential thrombocythaemia and found that 43 % of published cases had an abnormal outcome. Recurrent abortion was associated with placental infarction. The use of Aspirin and Interferon has been described in patients with essential thrombocythaemia. Normal pregnancy and delivery is also well documented in women with essential thrombocythaemia.[20] Where essential thrombocythaemia is associated with recurrent abortion treatment to reduce the platelet count before conception and low dose Aspirin during pregnancy should be considered.

VII. ANTIPHOSPHOLIPID SYNDROME AND PREGNANCY

The clinical manifestations of the antiphospholipid syndrome include venous and arterial thrombosis and recurrent fetal loss. Late fetal loss and recurrent first trimester abortion may be associated with high levels of lupus anticoagulant or anticardiolipin antibodies.

In pregnancies complicated by antiphospholipid antibodies the vascular supply to the placenta has been the main focus of attention. Fetal loss appears to be secondary to inadequate maternal blood supply through the diseased utero-placental vessels leading to placental infarction. Placental abruption has also been associated with antiphospholipid antibodies. Birdsall et al[21] found that 7 out of 21 women who had a stillbirth due to placental abruption had antiphospholipid antibodies.

Management of pregnancy : the management of patients with antiphospholipid syndrome should be based on the past obstetric history. In women with antiphospholipid antibodies without previous fetal loss or significant medical disease careful monitoring is recommended without any pharmacological intervention. In women with antiphospholipid syndrome and previous fetal loss treatment depends on the level of the antibodies. Where the antibody level is low treatment with low dose aspirin and monitoring of the anticardiolipin or lupus anticoagulant during pregnancy is recommended.

In patients with a high titre of anticardiolipin antibodies and a history of fetal loss or previous thrombotic events, particularly deep vein thrombosis, treatment with Heparin 10,000 units twice daily is recommended and low dose Aspirin 75 mgs daily.

In the presence of lupus anticoagulant with prolongation of the APTT, Prednisone is used to suppress the lupus anticoagulant. The administration of corticosteroids will suppress the lupus anticoagulant but not anticardiolipin. An initial dose of 40-60 mgs daily is recommended with a dose of 10 to 20 mgs of Prednisone daily for maintenance.

Antiphospholipid antibodies are found in 2 to 3 % of the general obstetric population. Because of the low specificity of the tests screening does not seem to be justified. In women with pregnancies complicated by recurrent abortion or fetal death, abruption, growth retardation or severe early on-set pre eclampsia, screening for antiphospholipid antibodies is indicated. Careful obstetric and haematological supervision is required with prophylactic treatment to prevent maternal thrombotic complications and fetal growth retardation.

REFERENCES

1.   **Forbes,C.D. and Greer,I.A.**, Physiology of haemostasis and the effect of pregnancy, *in Haemostasis and Thrombosis Obstetrics and Gynaecology,* Eds., Greer, I.A.,Turpie, A.G.G. and Forbes, C.D, London, Chapman and Hall,1, 1992.
2.   **Weenink,G.H., Treffers,T.E., Vinjn,P .et al**, Antithrombin III levels in preeclampsia correlate with maternal and fet morbidity, *American Journal of Obstetrics and Gynecology*, 148, 1092, 1984.
3.   **Malm, J., Laurell, M., Dahlback,B .et al**, Changes in the plasma levels of vitamin K dependent protein C and S and of 4 b-binding protein during pregnancy and oral–contraception, *British Journal of Haematology*, 68, 437,1988.
4.   **Conard, J., Horellou, M.H., van Dreden,P. et al**, Thrombosis and pregnancy in congenital deficiencies in AT III protein C or protein S : study of 78 women, *Thrombosis and Haemostasis,* 63, 319, 1990.
5.   **Conard, J.**, Thrombophilia : diagnosis and management, in *Thrombosis and its Management*, Eds., Poller, L.and Thomse J.M., Churchill Livingstone 113, 1993.
6.   **Abildgaard, U.**, Antithrombin and related inhibitors of coagulation, in *Recent Advances in Blood Coagulation,* Ed.,Poll L.,Churchill Livingstone,151,1981.

7.   **Miletich, J., Sherman, L., Broze Jr.G.**, Absence of thrombosis in subjects with heterozygous protein C deficiency, *New England Journal of Medicine*, 317, 991,1987.

8.   **Winter, J.H., Fenech, A., Ridley, W. et al**, Familial antithrombin III deficiency, *Quarterly Journal of Medicine*, 51, 373, 1982.

9.   **Dahlman, T.C.**, Osteoporotic fractures and the recurrence of thromboembolism during pregnancy and the puerperium in 184 women undergoing thromboprophylaxis with heparin, *American Journal of Obstetrics and Gynecology*, 168, 1265, 1993.

10.   **Carter, C.J., Bellem, P.J.**, Management of protein C deficiency in pregnancy, *Fibrinolysis*, suppl 1,161,1988.

11.   **Trauscht-van Horn, J.J., Capeless, E.L., EasterlingT.R., B ovill, E.G.**, Pregnancy loss and thrombosis with protein C deficiency, *American Journal of Obstetrics and Gynecology*, 167, 968, 1992.

12.   **Manco-Johnson, M., Nuss, R.**, Protein C concentrate prevents peri-partum thrombosis, *American Journal of Hematology*, 40, 69, 1992.

13.   **Ogston, D.**, *Venous thrombosis.* Causation and prediction, Chester, Wiley,1987.

14.   **Goodnough, L.T., Saito,H., Ratnoff, O.D.**, Thrombosis or myocardial infarction in congenital clotting factor abnormalities and chronic thrombocythaemias : a report of 21 patients and a review of 50 previously reported cases, *Medicine*, 62, 248, 1983.

15.   **TenCate, J.W., Peters, M., Buller, H.**, Isolated plasminogen deficiency in a patient with recurrent thromboembolic complications, *Thrombosis and Haemostasis*, 50, 59, 1983.

16.   **Jorgensen, M., Mortensen, J.Z., Madsen, A.G. et al**, A family with reduced plasminogen activator activity in blood associated with recurrent venous thrombosis, *Scandinavian Journal of Hematology* , 29, 217, 1982.

17.   **Falconer, J., Pineo, G., Blahey W. et al**, Essential thrombocythemia associated with recurrent abortions and fetal growth retardation, *American Journal of Hematology*, 25, 345, 1978.

18.   **Jones, E.G., Mosesson, M.W., Thomason, G.L., Jackson, T.C.**, Essential thrombocythemia in pregnancy, *Obstetrics and Gynaecology*, 7, 501, 1988.

19.   **Chow, E.Y., Haley, L.P., Vickars, L.M.**, Essential thrombocythemia in pregnancy : platelet count and pregnancy outcome, *American Journal of Hematology*, 41, 249, 1992.

20.   **Randi, M.L., Barbone, E., Rossi, C., Girolami, A.**, Essential thrombocythemia and pregnancy : a report of six normal pregnancies in five untreated patients, *Obstetrics and Gynaecology*, 83, 915, 1994.

21.   **Birdsall, M.A., Pattison, N.S., Chamley, L.W.**, Antiphospholipid antibodies in pregnancy. *Australia and New Zealand Journal of Obstetrics and Gynaecology*, 32, 328, 1992.

HYPERCOAGULABILITY IN CHILDREN AND NEONATES

N. Schlegel

Service d'Hématologie Biologique, Hôpital Robert Debré, Paris

I. INTRODUCTION

Processes of high complexity, based on sophisticated cells and components, maintain blood fluidity and prevent thrombus formation. Procoagulant pathways are controlled at different levels[1]. The initiation phase of coagulation is controlled by Tissue Factor Pathway Inhibitor (TFPI) which inhibits the complex of tissue factor (TF), factor VIIa and factor Xa. The amplification phase is controlled by the protein C pathway which, through activated protein C and in the presence of its cofactor, protein S, inactivates factors Va and VIIIa. The propagation phase is controlled by antithrombin which forms a one-to-one complex to inactivate thrombin. Moreover, thrombosis formation is also regulated by the fibrinolytic system, mainly plasmin formation, which itself is regulated by several activators and inhibitors. Finally, platelets, vessel wall, and humoral agents, mainly nitric oxide (NO) play important roles in maintaining blood fluidity.

The hemostatic system of children and neonates is characterized by a maturation dynamic state, which allows an immature situation to develop to the adult stage[2-4]. The maturation duration is different from one component or one cell to another. Consequently, the equilibrium between pro- and anti-coagulants, and between coagulation and fibrinolysis, is constantly changing, and, for this reason, easily disrupted toward hemorrhagic manifestations or, at the opposite, hypercoagulable state and, as the case may be, thrombosis.

Thrombotic events are not frequent in children and neonates but can be fatal or associated with several sequelae such as the loss of a limb or an organ function. The peak incidence period for these thrombotic events is the neonatal period[5,6], and catheters are the main etiology.

We will first review the physiological developmental characteristics of the hemostatic system underlining which situations might induce a hypercoagulable state. Then we will focus on inherited or acquired pathological conditions which, in children and neonates, are able to lead to hypercoagulability and, subsequently, thrombosis.

II. PHYSIOLOGICAL PROTECTION OF CHILDREN AND NEONATES AGAINST HYPERCOAGULABILITY

Even though all the different components and cells involved in the hemostatic processes are already present at birth, they show quantitative and qualitative differences as compared to adults[2-4]. More the infant is pre-term, more the differences are important.

At birth, in healthy term newborns, vitamin K-dependent coagulant factors (F II, F VII, F IX, F X), and contact factors [F XII, F XI, prekallikrein (PK), high molecular weight fibrinogen (HMWF)], are approximately half of adult values. During development these two categories of factors increase toward adult values at about 6 months, but remain 20% below these values, until the late teenage years. On the other hand, concentrations of factors V, VIII, von Willebrand factor, factor XIII and fibrinogen are similar in neonatal and adult plasma. A fetal molecular form of fibrinogen present on the first days of the neonatal period, has been described[7-9] but seems to have the same response to thrombin as adult fibrinogen.

At birth, plasma concentration of thrombin inhibitors is approximately 50% of adult values for antithrombin (AT) and heparin cofactor II (HCII) but is increased 1.5 times for α_2 macroglobulin (α_2M). AT plasma concentration reaches adult values between 3 and 6 months but α_2M remains increased during childhood. HCII reaches adult values at 3 months, but remains at the lowest adult values during childhood.

There is some information about the protein C/protein S system. At birth, protein C level is approximately one third of adult level, and protein C is present in a fetal form[10] characterized by a two-fold increase in single chain protein C as compared to the adult form. During childhood, protein C plasma concentration increases slowly, reaches values higher than 60 per cent around 4-5 years, but remains lower than adult value during all this period. Protein S is at a very low concentration at birth, but completely in the free or active form, due to decreased C4B-binding protein in neonates[11]. Protein S reaches adult values at about 3 months. Plasma concentrations of thrombomodulin (TM) are increased at birth and gradually decrease during childhood[12]. The expression of TM at endothelial cell surface is not precisely known yet in neonates and children. Plasma concentration of TF and TFPI are not known yet at birth, and during childhood.

Thrombin generation, thrombin inhibition and fibrin generation reflect the consequences of the activity of the procoagulant proteins and their inhibitors. The differences between neonates, children and adults, as above mentionned, explain the pediatric characteristics of these three processes. In summary, after the birth process, which is characterized by an activation of coagulation, thrombin generation is both delayed and decreased (about 50 per cent)[13-14] in newborn plasma compared to adult plasma, at a level similar to plasma from adults receiving therapeutic doses of coumarin or heparin. Thrombin generation increases during childhood but remains reduced by approximately 20 per cent at the end of this period of life, compared to adult.

Thrombin inhibition rate is slower in neonatal than in adult plasma, due to decreased plasma levels of AT and HCII[15]. Furthermore, at birth thrombin inhibition by HCII is increased[16], due to the presence of a fetal circulating proteoglycan similar to dermatan sulphate[16], responsible for the catalyzation of thrombin inhibition by HCII. In addition, a larger amount of thrombin is inhibited in infant and children plasma due to a higher concentration of α_2M[17]. Fibrin generation, in relation to plasma concentration of prothrombin, has been found to be decreased at birth, as indicated by the decreased production of fibrinopeptide A obtained during the preparation of fibrin clots from cold plasma as compared to adult plasma.

Peculiarities of the fibrinolytic system have also been described for neonates and children[18]. At birth, plasma concentrations of plasminogen, the key molecule responsible for plasmin generation and clot lysis, are between 30 to 50 per cent of adult values[2,3,14,18,19]. A fetal molecular form of plasminogen has been described but is not demonstrated yet[20,21]. Interestingly, plasma concentrations of α_2 antiplasmin (α_2-AP), the major inhibitor of plasmin, are quite similar in neonates (80 per cent) and adults[14]. Plasma concentrations of tissue plasminogen activator (t-PA), an important activator of plasminogen, and Plasminogen Activator Inhibitor-1 (PAI-1), which are significantly lower in cord blood than in adult blood, are increased in the plasma of newborns on day one of life. Levels of plasminogen and α_2-AP reach adult values at six months, plasma concentrations of t-PA antigen remain decreased (50%) and PAI-1 activity increased (50%) throughout childhood[4].

During birth, the fibrinolytic system, as the coagulation system, is activated as indicated by the short euglobulin lysis time observed with neonatal plasma[22]. After birth, the ability of the newborn fibrinolytic system to generate plasmin in vitro is decreased compared to adults[23]. The most important cause of the impaired ability of the neonatal fibrinolytic system to lyse clots is probably the low concentration of neonatal plasminogen, but the quite adult concentration of α_2-AP might also contribute to the decreased fibrinolytic activity of neonatal plasma. The activity of the fibrinolytic system remains decreased during childhood, as a result of a decreased t-PA / PAI-1 ratio[4].

With the exception of birth stage, which is a very short period with very fast modifications of some components of both the coagulation and fibrinolytic systems, one can say that neonates and children are characterized by an enhanced thrombin regulation but a decreased plasmin generation and regulation. The enhanced thrombin regulation might contribute to a reduced risk of hypercoagulable states and thrombosis in neonates and children. At the opposite, the decreased fibrinolytic activity and plasmin generation might contribute to an increased risk. The balance between these two situations is well realized in normal full-term neonates and children, but can easily be disrupted either in pre-term infants and/or pathological situations.

As to peculiarities of platelets, vessel wall, and platelet/vessel wall interactions in children and neonates, they are not fully understood yet. It appears that, after the birth process characterized by a physiological activation of platelets[24], the neonatal platelets might present an hypofunction. The duration of these diminished platelet activities is not known. The platelet functions do not show consistent differences between children and adults. Among the main anti-thrombotic properties of vessel wall, i.e proteoglycans (eicosanoids), NO, protein C/Protein S system (including an endothelial cell receptor, the TM), and fibrinolysis (including two components produced by the endothelial cell, t-PA and PAI-1), several characteristics have been summarized above. Studies on human umbilical vessel endothelial cells showed an increased production of prostacyclin[25], but the maturation of the eicosanoids production and their activity are not known. Besides few recent reports[16] the development of vessel wall proteoglycans has to be studied more deeply.

NO (endothelium-derived relaxing factor, EDRF), is known to play an important role during the fetal period and during birth by regulating the lung vascular tone. NO is essential for the decrease of pulmonary resistance at birth.

III PATHOLOGICAL SITUATIONS RESPONSIBLE FOR HYPERCOAGULABILITY IN CHILDREN AND NEONATES

A. INHERITED PATHOLOGICAL HYPERCOAGULABLE STATES

Deficiencies of coagulation inhibitors, protein C, protein S and antithrombin are the most common inherited hypercoagulable states. They are usually inherited as autosomal dominant disorders. Interestingly, an acquired risk for thrombosis generally unveils the deficiency[6,26,27].

Hereditary protein C deficiency (homozygosity, compound heterozygosity and heterozygosity) is associated with a high thrombotic risk, mainly venous thrombosis (VT) and pulmonary embolism (PE). Two types of hereditary protein C deficiencies are described : type I, a quantitative deficiency, and type II a qualitative deficiency. Heterozygotes generally start to develop thrombosis during adulthood, but also in late childhood in a few cases. However, homozygotes or compound heterozygotes develop very severe thrombotic complications very early in their life, at birth or in the first months of life[28-31]. In most cases, the clinical manifestations are neonatal purpura fulminans, with large echymotic and necrotic lesions, mainly in the extremities. These manifestations can be associated with central nervous system thrombosis, already present in utero in some cases and responsible for hydroencephalia. Massive large vessel thrombosis, like vena cava, renal vein and iliac vein thrombosis have also been observed.

The diagnosis of hereditary protein C deficiency might be dificult to define in children and neonates. Homozygosity or double heterozygosity is generally discussed early in life in neonates with necrotic purpura and very low level of protein C. Severely diminished protein C concentrations can only reflect the association of the physiological low concentration of protein C[2] plus the pathologically decreased protein C level due to disseminated intravascular coagulation (DIC). In such a situation, it is important to eliminate carefully any other etiology of DIC, mainly infection, and also to study the protein C concentrations in the parents, searching for an heterozygous protein C deficiency. In these cases, the comparison between the protein C level and the other vitamin K dependent factors is obviously very helpful. The heterozygosity can be discussed not only in the neonatal period, in patients with protein C concentration below 20 per cent, but also later in childhood, taking in account the slow increase of protein C level during development (protein C concentration is only at 40 per cent of adult values at the age of eleven). However, if these assays are not available or not conclusive, molecular genetic studies might be proposed to identify the genetic anomaly[32].

Homozygous or compound heterozygous neonates or young children who develop thrombotic complications can now be treated with highly purified protein C concentrate[31], starting with doses of 20 to 40 U/kg every 6 hours, following with lower doses of 15 to 30 U/kg every 12 hours. The duration of the treatment with protein C concentrate is not definitively known yet. This treatment is then replaced by preventive coumarin therapy, itself initiated in association with protein C concentrate in order to prevent coumarin-induced skin necrosis[33,34]. A new concentrate of protein C in an activated form might be helpful for the treatment of such patients. The therapeutic management of heterozygotes consists of preventive anticoagulation with heparin or coumarin only in children who will have an increased thrombotic risk : disease with thrombotic risk (nephrotic syndrome or cancer), predisposing factor (surgery, prolonged immobilization), acquired anomaly (lupus anticoagulant). The treatment of acute thrombotic events includes both anticoagulation and purified protein C concentrate, as for homozygotes. After the treatment of the thrombotic event or a defined period of anticoagulant prophylaxis, a decision for long-term anticoagulation should consider the relative benefit of the therapy and the potential side-effects, which cannot be underestimated in children.

Hereditary protein S deficiency presents many clinical similarities with hereditary protein C deficiency. Heterozygotes generally start to develop thrombosis during adulthood, but some cases have been reported in children. A few cases of homozygous protein S deficiency have been reported : two neonates with purpura fulminans[35,36], two children with arterial thrombosis[37,38] and a family in which homozygotes have presented thrombotic complications after the age of 20[39].

The management of hereditary protein S deficiency is similar to the protein C deficiency treatment but there is no protein S concentrate available to day. Fresh frozen plasma can be used as substitutive therapy.

The recently described Activated Protein C Resistance (APCR) which is related to a genetic mutation of factor V (factor V Leiden, Arg 506 $\rightarrow$ Gln) delays the inactivation of factor V by activated protein C[40,41]. It has a prevalence of 2 to 7 per cent in the populations which have been studied[40,42,43]. Obviously, no modification of the mutation can be expected with age. However, this mutation might have time-changing effects during the dynamic developmental process of the coagulation system, even though the factor V level at birth is already similar to (even higher than) the adult one. These data remain to be studied. The prevalence of the factor V Leiden mutation in thrombotic children is now under evaluation. Even if this mutation might be considered as only one risk factor among others responsible for thrombosis, one can recommend inclusion of the detection of this mutation in children considered at risk of thrombosis.

Hereditary AT deficiency is also associated with a high risk of thrombosis, mainly VT and PE. Two types of hereditary AT deficiencies are described : the classical type I, characterized by a reduced synthesis of biologically normal AT molecule, and the type II produced by a discrete molecular defect within AT and characterized by a decreased functional activity of the molecule. Two different subcategories are described among type II : one with both diminished progressive AT activity and AT heparin cofactor activity and another with AT-heparin cofactor activity reduced at half of the normal and normal progressive AT activity. As for protein C and protein S deficiencies, heterozygotes start to develop thombosis during adulthood. A few cases have been reported during childhood or adolescence[44-47]. Homozygotes have a functional defect. Several mutations in heparin binding domains have been discovered in these homozygotes at a young age, in association with a very low heparin cofactor level. Among the homozygotes who have been reported, only one has presented thrombosis during childhood[48].

The diagnosis of hereditary AT deficiency is difficult early in life, till the age at which the maturation of AT is achieved, between 3 and 6 months. Before 6 months, or more if the infant is pre-term, the assays of AT in parents'plasma will be helpful, and, of course, the identification of the mutation.

The management of young patients with AT deficiency is comparable to the management of those with protein C or S deficiencies, including anticoagulation and, when necessary, substitutive therapy. Purified AT concentrates are available and must be infused in order to maintain plasma AT levels above 80 per cent generally necessary to obtain this cutoff value. The maintenance dose which is recommended is 50 to 60 per cent of the inital dose at 24 hour intervals[49].

For more details concerning the inherited deficiencies of coagulation inhibitors, one can refer to the state of art publications of Aiach et al[32], and Bauer[50].

The hereditary disorders of the fibrinolytic system associated with hypercoagulability and thrombosis are rare in adults and very rare in children. It has been reported in one 15-year-old child with abnormal plasminogen[51], and two adolescents with defective release of vascular plasminogen activator[52].

B. ACQUIRED PATHOLOGICAL HYPERCOAGULABLE STATES

A variety of etiologies can be responsible for acquired pathological hypercoagulable states in children and neonates.

Most commonly, such a state is iatrogenic, related to the presence of a catheter. Catheter related hypercoagulability has been reported to occur with a variety of catheter types, materials and placement techniques. Venous and arterial catheters may be responsible for hypercoagulability. Umbilical vessel catheterization is a special cause in neonates. Among venous catheter related hypercoagulability, two different situations are observed in infants, children and adolescents : long-term central lines usually placed for administering long-term total parenteral nutrition or for the treatment and supportive care of children with cancer. The most common localization of arterial catheter related hypercoagulability is the femoral artery, following cardiac catherization[53].

Catheter related hypercoagulability is at the origin of a large variety of thrombotic manifestations, since a silent aspect only suspected on biological markers of coagulation activation to extensive thrombosis from the extremity of the catheter, DIC and pulmonary embolism.

The approaches to prevention, non invasive diagnosis and treatment of catheter related hypercoagulability have been greatly improved this last decade. The single most important recommendation might be to remove the catheter at the first signs of related hypercoagulability, but it is not always feasible in very young patients with difficult vascular access. Heparin is commonly used as prophylaxis to maintain catheter patency but is not proved to be absolutely necessary[54]. Fibrinolytic therapy for catheter related hypercoagulability must be managed very carefully, due to the risk of dissemination of small thrombi in the systemic circulation and, consequently, pulmonary embolism.

Hypercoagulability can also be the consequence of different underlying disorders affecting children and neonates. As indicated for catheters, the hypercoagulability state is at the origin of a similar variety of thrombotic manifestations[55-57].

Several underlying disorders are common to neonates and children. Infection and inflammation are the most frequent causes, due in a number of cases to bacterial endotoxin, interleukin-1 and Tumor Necrosis Factor release. One can remember that the first descriptions of DIC were published more than twenty years ago in two pediatric journals[58,59]. A long list of other disorders responsible for hypercoagulability in children and neonates can be described, including acute intravascular hemolysis, liver failure, acute leukemias (mainly promyelocytic acute leukemia) and L-Asparaginase related therapy, tumors, multiple trauma, surgery, burns, major hyperthermia, cardiac diseases, nephrotic syndrome, Kasabach-Merritt syndrome and extra corporeal circulation technics.

Some underlying disorders are characteristic of the neonatal period, mainly : obstetrical complications (placenta praevia, eclampsia and pre-eclampsia), birth asphyxia and dehydration, birth trauma, hyperviscosity, respiratory distress syndrome, ulcero-necrotizing enterocolitis. More the infant is pre-term more the hypercoagulability risk is important.

Some underlying disorders are mainly observed after the neonatal period : sickle cell anemia, vasculitis, juvenile arthritis, homocystinuria, snake venom poisoning.

Acquired deficiencies in coagulation inhibitors, Protein C, Protein S, or antithrombin have been found to be associated with hypercoagulability in children and neonates. An acquired Protein C deficiency can reflect a liver failure or immaturity, or severe infection such as meningococcemia[60]. An acquired Protein S deficiency has been reported in DIC and idiopathic purpura fulminans in children[61]. An acquired antithrombin deficiency is associated with liver failure and is one of the most important thrombotic risk factors of children or neonates with nephrotic syndrome, due to urinary loss of antithrombin[62].

Lupus anticoagulant, more generally observed in late childhood, represents a risk of hypercoagulability, as in adults.

More recently, the development of transplantation is associated with hypercoagulability and thrombosis risk in the transplanted vessels. One of the underlying mechanisms in kidney and liver transplantation in children is related to the small size and lumen of the transplanted vessels. The veno-occlusive disease secondary to bone-marrow graft is associated with protein C deficiency, but other mechanisms are probably present.

The diagnosis of hypercoagulability in children and neonates is based on the same biological markers as those studied in adults : D-dimers, thrombin-antithrombin complexes, and prothrombin fragments 1+ 2. D-dimers are the markers most commonly studied in neonates and children, even though the absence of large series of systematic studies (which might be unfeasible in children and neonates).

The therapeutic management of hypercoagulability in children and neonates is based on antithrombotic therapy with heparin or coumarin, and in some cases, thrombolytic therapy. This management must take into account the influence of age on the response to the antithrombotic and fibrinolytic agents[63].

Newborns have been reported to be both sensitive and resistant to heparin compared to adults[64]. The higher sensitivity is related to the physiological prolonged APTT in neonates and the resistance is related to the low level of antithrombin. Furthermore, the heparin volume of distribution is probably larger in neonates than in adults[65], and plasmas from children generate 20% less thrombin than plasmas from adults in the presence of similar heparin concentrations. Generally, higher doses of heparin are necessary for neonates than for adults to obtain the same anticoagulation level. The optimal heparin doses remain to be established for neonates and children.

Coumarin requirements are dependent on the decreased capacity to generate thrombin throughout childhood, and, in very young children, the low plasma concentration of prothrombin. It has been reported that coumarin requirements are the highest in infants (0.32mg/kg), and the lowest in teenagers (0.09mg/kg)[66]. It has also been reported that, for a similar INR, the in vitro thrombin generation is delayed and decreased in childrens' plasma compared to adult plasma[67]. But the specific coumarin requirements in children and neonates are not fully understood yet.

The most important difficulty for thrombolytic therapy in neonates is the low level of plasminogen. The synthesis of recombinant plasminogen will be very helpful in such situations. If other mechanisms are responsible for different responses to thrombolytic agents in neonates and children compared to adults, they remain to be established.

REFERENCES

1.   **Roberts, H.R., Tabares, A.H.**, Overview of the coagulation reactions, in Molecular Basis of Thrombosis and Hemostasis, High KA. and Roberts H.R., Eds., Dekker, New York, 1995, chap.2.

2.   **Andrew, M., Paes, B., Milner, R., et al**, Development of the human coagulation system in the full-term infant, *Blood*, 70, 165, 1987.

3.   **Andrew, M., Paes, B., Milner, R., et al**, Development of the human coagulation system in the healthy premature infant, *Blood*, 72, 1651, 1988.

4.   **Andrew, M., Vegh, P., Johnston, M., Bowker, J., Ofosu, F., Mitchell, L.**, Maturation of the hemostatic system during childhood, *Blood*, 80, 1998, 1992.

5.   **Andrew, M.**, An approach to the management of infants with impaired haemostasis, *Baillière's Clinical Haematology*, 4, 251, 1991.

6.   **David, M., Andrew, M.**, Venous thromboembolism complications in children : a critical review of the literature, *J. Pediatr.*, 123, 337, 1993.

7. **Witt, I., Muller, H., Kunter, L.J.**, Evidence for the existence of fetal fibrinogen, *Thromb. Diath. Haemorrh.*, 22, 101, 1969.

8. **Hamulyak, K., Nieuwenhuiz, W., Devillee, P.P., Hemker, H.C.**, Re-evaluation of some properties of fibrinogen purified from cord blood of normal newborns, *Thromb. Res.*, 32, 301, 1983.

9. **Galanakis, D.K., Mosesson, M.W.**, Evaluation of the role of in vivo proteolysis (fibrinogenolysis) in prolonging the thrombin time of human umbilical cord fibrinogen, *Blood*, 48, 109, 1976.

10. **Greffe, B.S., Marlar, R.A., Manco-Johnson, M.**, Neonatal protein C : molecular composition and distribution in normal term infants, *Thromb. Res.*, 56, 91, 1989.

11. **Schwartz, H.P., Muntran, W., Watzke, H., Richter, B., Griffin, J.H.**, Low total protein S antigen but high protein S activity due to decreased C4B-binding protein in neonates, *Blood*, 71, 562, 1988.

12. **Aurousseau, M.H., Amiral, J., Boffa, M.**, Level of plasma thrombomodulin in neonates and children, *Thromb.. Haemostas.*, 65, 1232, 1991 (Abstract).

13. **Andrew, M., Schmidt, B., Mitchell, L., Paes, B., Ofosu, F.**, Thrombin generation in newborn plasma is critically dependent on the concentration of prothrombin, *Thromb. Haemostas.*, 63, 27, 1990.

14. **Andrew, M., Paes, B., Johnston, M.**, Development of the hemostatic system in the neonate and young infant, *Am. J. Pediatr.Hematol. Oncol.*, 12, 95, 1990.

15. **Schmidt, B., Mitchell, L., Ofosu, F., Andrew, M.**, Alpha-2-macroglobulin is an important progressive inhibitor of thrombin in neonatal and infant plasma, *Thromb. Haemostas*, 62, 1074, 1989.

16. **Andrew, M., Mitchell, L., Paes, B., et al**, An anticoagulant dermatan sulphate proteoglycan circulates in the pregnant woman and her fetus, *J. Clin. Invest.*, 89, 321, 1992.

17. **Andrew, M., Mitchell, L., Vegh, P., Ofosu, F.**, Thrombin regulation in children differs from adults in the absence and presence of heparin, *Thromb. Haemostas.*, 72, 836, 1994.

18. **Corrigan, J.J.**, Neonatal thrombosis and the thrombolytic system : pathophysiology and therapy, *Am. J. Pediatr. Hematol. Oncol.*, 10, 83, 1988.

19. **Corrigan, J.J., Sluth, J., Jeter, M., Lox, C.**, Newborn's fibrinolytic mechanism : components and plasmin generation, *Am. J. Hematol.*, 32, 273, 1989.

20. **Summaria, L.**, Comparison of human normal, full-term, fetal and adult plasminogen by physical and chemical analyses, *Haemostasis*, 19, 266, 1989.

21. **Edelberg, J.M., Enghild, J.J., Pizzo, S.V., Gonzalez-Gronow, M.**, Neonatal plasminogen displays altered cell surface binding an activation kinetics. Correlation with increased glycosylation of the protein, *J. Clin. Invest.*, 86, 107, 1990.

22. **Gibson, B.**, Neonatal haemostasis, *Arch. Dis. CHild.*, 64, 503, 1989.

23. **Andrew, M., Brooker, L., Paes, B., Weilz, J.**, Fibrin clot lysis by thrombotic agents is impaired in newborns due to a low plasminogen concentration, *Thromb. Haemostas.*, 68, 325, 1992.

24. **Suarez, C.R., Gonzalez, J., Menendez, C., Fareed, J., Fresco, R., Walenga, J.**, Neonatal and maternal platelets : Activation at time of birth, *Am. J. Hematol.*, 29, 18, 1988.

25. **Jacqz, E.M., Barrow, S.E., Dollery, C.T.**, Prostacyclin concentrations in cord blood and in the newborn, *Pediatrics*, 76, 954, 1985.

26. **Mannucci, P., Tripodi, A., Bertina, R.**, Protein S deficiency associated with "juvenile" arterial and venous thromboses, *Thromb. Haemostas.*, 55, 440, 1986.

27. **De Stefano, V., Leone, G., Carolis, M., et al**, Antithrombin III in full-term and pre-term newborn infants : three cases of neonatal diagnosis of AT III congenital defect, *Thromb. Haemostas*, 57, 329, 1987.

28. **Branson, H.E., Katz, J., Marble, R., Griffin, J.H.**, Inherited protein C deficiency and coumarin- response chronic relapsing purpura fulminans in a newborn infant, *Lancet*, 2, 1165, 1983.

29. **Sills, R.H., Marlar, R.A., Montgomery, R.R., Desphande, G.N., Humbert, J.R.**, Severe homozygous protein C deficiency, *J. Pediatr.*, 105, 409, 1984.

30. **Marciniak, E., Wilson, H.D., Marlar, R.A.**, Neonatal purpura fulminans : a genetic disorder related to the absence of protein C in blood, *Blood*, 65, 15, 1985.

31. **Dreyfus, M., Magny, J.F., Bridey, F., et al**, Treatment of homozygous protein C deficiency and neonatal purpura fulminans with a purified protein C concentrate, *N. Engl. J. Med.*, 325, 1565, 1991.

32. **Aiach, M., Gandrille, S., Emmerich, J.**, A review of mutations causing deficiencies of antithrombin, protein C and protein S, *Thromb. Haemostas*, 74, 81, 1995.

33. **Zauber, N.P., Stark, M.W.**, Successful warfarin anticoagulation despite protein C deficiency and a history of warfarin necrosis, *Ann. Int. Med.*, 104, 659, 1986.

34. **Bauer, K.A.**, Coumarin-induced skin necrosis, *Arch. Dermatol.*, 129, 766, 1993.

35. **Mahasandana, C., Suvatte, V., Marlar, R.A., et al**, Neonatal purpura fulminans associated with homozygous protein S deficiency, *Lancet*, 33 , 61, 1990.

36. **Pegelow, C.H., Ledford, M., Young, J.N., Zygeruelo, G.**, Severe protein S deficiency in a newborn, *Pediatrics*, 89, 674, 1992.

37. **Horowitz, J.N., Galvis, A.G., Gomperts, E.D.**, Arterial thrombosis and protein S deficiency, *J. Pediatr.*, 121, 934, 1992.

38. **Comp, P.C., Doray, D., Patton, D., Esmon, C.T.**, An abnormal plasma distribution of protein S occurs in functional protein S deficiency, *Blood*, 67, 504, 1986.

39. **Chafa, O., Fisher, A.M., Meriane, F., et al**, A new case of "type II" inherited protein S deficiency, *Brit. J. Haematol.*, 73, 501, 1989.

40. **Bertina, R.M., Koeleman, B.P.C., Koster, T., et al**, Mutation in blood coagulation factor V associated with resistance to activated protein C, *Nature*, 369, 64, 1994.

41. **Dahlbäck, B.**, Physiological anticoagulation. Resistance to activated protein C and venous thromboembolism, *J. Clin. Invest.*, 94, 923, 1994.

42. **Koster, T., Rosendaal, F.R., De Ronde, H., Briet, E., Vandenbroucke, J.P., Bertina, R.M.**, Venous thrombosis due to poor anticoagulant response to activated protein C Leiden thrombophilia study, *Lancet*, 342, 1503, 1993.

43. **Svensson, P.J., Dahlbäck, B.**, Resistance to activated protein C as a basis for venous thrombosis, *N. Engl. J. Med.*, 330, 517, 1994.

44. **Ambruso, D.R., Jacobson, L.J., Hathaway, J.E.**, Inherited antithrombin III deficiency and cerebral thrombosis in a child, *Pediatrics*, 65, 125, 1980.

45. **Leone, G., Valori, V.M., Storti, S., Myers, .J.**, Inferior vena cava thrombosis in a child with familial antithrombin III deficiency, *Thromb. Haemost.*, 43, 74, 1980.

46. **Mazza, J.J.**, Antithrombin III (AT III) deficiency spanning four generations, *Thromb. Haemost.*, 66, 737, 1991.

47.   **Vomberg, P.P., Breederveld, C., Fleury, P., Arts, W.F.M**, Cerebral thromboembolism due to antithrombin III deficiency in two children, *Neuropediatrics*, 18, 42, 1987.

48.   **Boyer, C., Wolf, M., Vedrenne, J., et al**, Homozygous variant of antithrombin III : AT III Fontainebleau, *Thromb. Haemost.*, 56, 18, 1986.

49.   **Schwartz, R.S., Bauer, K.A., Rosenberg, R.D., Kavanaugh, E.J., Davies, D.C., Bogdanoff, D.A.**, Clinical experience with antithrombin III concentrate in treatment to congenital and acquired deficiency of antithrombin, *Am. J. Med.*, 87, 53 S, 1989.

50.   **Bauer, K.A.**, Management of patients with hereditary defects predisposing to thombosis including pregnant women, *Thromb. Haemost.*, 74, 94, 1995.

51.   **Aoki, N., Moroi, M., Sakata, Y., et al**, Abnormal plasminogen. A hereditary molecular abnormality found in patient with recurrent thrombosis, *J. Clin. Invest.*, 61, 1186, 1978.

52.   **Stead, N.W., Bauer, K.A., Kinney, T.R., et al**, Venous thrombosis in a family with defective release of vascular plasminogen activator and elevated plasma factor VIII-von Willebrand's factor, *Am. J. Med.*, 74, 33, 1983.

53.   **Burrows, P.E., Benson, L.N., Williams, W.G., et al**, Iliofemoral arterial complications of balloon angioplasty for systemic obstructions in infants and children, *Circulation*, 82, 1967, 1990.

54.   **Smith, S., Dawson, S., Hennessey, R., Andrew, M.**, Maintenance of the patency of indwelling central venous catheters : is heparin necessary; *Am. J. Pediatr. Hematol. Oncol.*, 13, 141, 1991.

55.   **Bick, R.**, Disseminated Intravascular coagulation and related syndromes : a clinical review, *Semin Thromb. Hemost*, 14, 299, 1988.

56.   **Baker, W. F.**, Clinical aspects of disseminated intravascular coagulation : a clinician's point of view, *Semin Thromb. Hemost.*, 15, 1, 1989.

57.   **Bick, R.**, Coagulation abnormalities in malignancy ; a review, *Semin Thromb. Hemost.*, 18, 353, 1992.

58.   **Abilgaard, C.**, Recognition and treatment of intravascular coagulation, *J. Pediatr.*, 74, 163, 1969.

59.   **Feron, J.F., Saint Martin, J., Josso, F. et al**, Coagulopathies de consommation chez l'enfant, *Arch. Fr. Pediatr.*, 28, 5, 1971.

60.   **Peters, M., Funvandraat, K., Derk, B., et al**, Severely reduced protein C levels predict a high mortality in meningococcal shock, *Thromb. Haemost.*, 69, 1197, 1993 (Abstract).

61.   **Alessi, M.C., Ailleaud, M.F., Boyer-Neumann, C., et al**, Cutaneous necrosis associated with acquired severe protein S deficiency, *Thromb. Haemost.*, 69, 524, 1993.

62.   **Kauffman, R.H., Veltkamp, J.J., Van Tilburg, N.H., Van Es, L.A.**, Acquired antithrombin III deficiency and thrombosis in the nephrotic syndrome, *Am. J. Med.*, 65, 607, 1978.

63.   **Schlegel, N., Hurtaud-Roux, M.F., Beaufils, F.**, Anticoagulation for neonates, infants and children, in Anticoagulation, Doutremepuich, C., Ed, Springer-Verlag, New York, 1994, chap 11.

64.   **Vieira, A., Ofosu, A., Andrew, M.**, Heparin sensitivity and resistance in the newborn : an explanation, *Pediatr. Res.*, 25, 274, 1989.

65.   **Andrew, M., Ofosu, F., Schmidt, B., Brooker, L., Hirsh, J., Buchanan, M.**, Heparin clearance and ex vivo recovery in newborn piglets and adult pigs, *Thromb. Res.*, 52, 517, 1988.

66.   **Andrew, M., Marzinotto, V., Brooker, L., et al**, Oral anticoagulant therapy in pediatric patients : a prospective study, *Thromb. Haemost.*, 71, 265, 1994.

67.   **Massicotte, M., Marzinotto, V., Adams, M., Vegh, P., Mitchell, L., Andrew, M.**, Coumarin suppresses thrombin regulation to a greater extent in children compared to adults, *Thromb. Haemost.*, 1995, in press.

HYPERCOAGULABILITY AND DIABETES MELLITUS

S.C.L. Gough and C.R.M. Prentice
Division of Medicine - University of Leeds

I. INTRODUCTION

The major complications of both Type 1 (insulin-dependent) and Type 2 (non-insulin-dependent) diabetes mellitus are related to the occlusion of large and small arteries. The exact causes of vascular occlusion in diabetes mellitus remain unknown but are clearly multifactorial. Fibrin deposition is an important component of acute arterial thrombosis, and the incorporation of fibrin into the vessel wall may also be important in atherosclerotic plaque formation and in the development of microvascular disease in diabetic patients. Although many abnormalities of coagulation and fibrinolysis have been described in diabetics it is less certain whether these contribute to a hypercoagulable state and vascular complications.This chapter will review current literature on the activation of coagulation in diabetes mellitus and its relationship to the development of vascular disease and therapeutic interventions.

II. COAGULATION

A. DIABETES MELLITUS

Many studies describe abnormalities of coagulation factors and their inhibitors in patients with diabetes mellitus, suggesting the presence of hypercoagulability or "thrombophilia". However, standard clinical clotting assays, including prothrombin time, activated partial thromboplastin time and thrombin time are generally normal in diabetic subjects, irrespective of glycaemic control[1]. Using a modified plasma thrombin clotting time, designed to have increased sensitivity for hypercoagulability, Bannerjee found no difference between insulin-dependent diabetic (IDDM) subjects and controls, but evidence of hypercoagulability in patients with non-insulin dependent diabetes mellitus (NIDDM) [2,3].

However, a large number of studies have described abnormalities of at least one coagulation factor in patients with both IDDM and NIDDM. The results often conflict, but most of the differences can be explained by the heterogeneity of the disease and the small number of patients studied.

To examine the role of an increased "thrombotic tendency" in the development of vascular complications of diabetes a number of tests of haemostatic function were carried out in a mixed group of diabetic patients and compared to those of a similar age from the Northwick Park Heart Study[4]. Out of 154 patients, 111 had IDDM (72%). Fibrinogen, antithrombin III and coagulation factors VII and X were all higher in the diabetic group providing indirect evidence for activation of coagulation.

Although Factor VIII coagulant activity (factor VIII) was similar in controls and diabetics in Fuller's study, abnormalities of this clotting factor are those most frequently described in diabetic subjects. Factor VIII however increases significantly with age [5], and in most studies, particularly those investigating older patients with NIDDM, the controls are not age-matched.

Another confounding factor in the study of diabetic patients is the high incidence of atherosclerosis, which is also associated with abnormalities of coagulation. Increased factor VIII activity in patients with NIDDM [5-9] is particularly difficult to interpret since cardiovascular disease in these patients accounts for over 75% of all morbidity and mortality.

Abnormalities of both von Willebrand factor (vWF) antigen and activity have been described in young children with IDDM, in whom macrovascular complications were most unlikely. In a group of young IDDM subjects without evidence of microvascular complications those with longer duration of disease had elevated vWF antigen and factor VIII levels[10]. In those with poor glycaemic control and a short disease duration only elevated factor VIII was found, suggesting that increases in vWF develop over a longer period of time and that factor VIII is increased during poor metabolic control.

The same group[11] found increased levels of factor VIII but not vWF antigen in 75 patients with IDDM with poor glycaemic control. These results also suggest increased intravascular factor VIII during poor glycaemic control rather than increased endothelial production of vWF.

In a large study comparing 80 diabetic patients with 48 controls, fifteen coagulation and fibrinolysis parameters were measured[5]. Unfortunately, the type of diabetes present in individuals was not clear and controls were not age matched. Factor VIII was related to patient age and, not surprisingly therefore, factor VIII moieties were higher in the diabetic patients. In a further study, 36% of a group of 37 type 2 diabetic patients had elevated factor VIII compared to the "laboratory" normal range[6]. Unfortunately, the two groups were not age matched which, again, clouds results.

Despite the deficiencies in these studies they suggest that younger patients with IDDM have elevated levels of factor VIII in the absence of vascular complications. Factor VIII moieties are clearly elevated in most diabetic patients, but their relationship to the development of vascular disease is unclear.

Abnormalities of factor VII coagulant activity in diabetic subjects have been less frequently described. Some authors report increased levels in diabetic subjects[4,12,13] but not all[14]. The differences may result from coexistent micro- 4 or macro-vascular disease[15].

Increased plasma fibrinogen concentrations are found in patients with IDDM and NIDDM[2,4,14,16-19]. Although this in part could be due to the presence of vascular disease[15], it is clear that fibrinogen is elevated in the diabetic state and is affected by changes in glycaemic control[18,19].

The major inhibitor of thrombin, antithrombin III, has been described as increased[4,20-22], normal[5,23] and reduced[6,24] in diabetic patients. Ceriello reported a number of haemostatic abnormalities in diabetics[13,25,26] including those in a recent study of patients with IDDM in whom factor X and antithrombin III activity were reduced, and levels of fibrinopeptide A were increased[26]. However, levels of factor X and antithrombin III antigens were similar to the control group. In a study in which controlled hyperglycaemia was maintained by a glucose and insulin infusion, (a hyperglycaemic clamp) antithrombin III activity and factor X activity were inversely related to blood glucose. The authors suggested that increased thrombin activity in diabetic patients is in part due to a reduction in antithrombin III activity and that the differences between activity and antigen could be explained by non-enzymatic glycosylation of the proteins. However Patrassi reported no differences in levels of antithrombin III activity and antigen in thirteen patients with IDDM and fifteen patients with NIDDM compared to equivalent numbers of age and sex matched controls[27].

An indirect method for measuring thrombin generation involves the estimation of fibrinopeptide A (FPA), which is cleaved from fibrinogen by thrombin during fibrin formation, and also the prothrombin fragment 1+2 (F1+2). An increase in FPA[28] and F1+2[29] has been reported in diabetics. Jones reported plasma and urinary levels of FPA in thirty-two IDDM and sixteen NIDDM patients[30]. Compared to similar control groups, FPA levels were higher in the diabetic group suggesting increased thrombin production in diabetic patients. There was no difference in FPA levels between the two types of diabetes. Hyperglycaemia, induced by oral glucose challenge,increased FPA more in those with vascular complications than those without. Resting levels were not related to glycosylated haemoglobin. It is tempting to speculate that development of vascular complications in diabetic patients is related to acute fluctuations in glycaemic control and thrombin generation.

B. DIABETIC COMPLICATIONS

In Fuller's study described above, patients with either retinopathy or proteinuria had higher levels of factor VII, fibrinogen and antithrombin III than those without[4]. This association between abnormalities of coagulation and microvascular complications supports the theory of an increased thrombotic tendency in the development of vascular complications in diabetic patients. Increased factor VIII has been described in a mixed group of diabetic patients with microvascular complications, including nephropathy, compared to those without complications[5]. However such studies are unable to determine whether this is cause or effect or whether coagulation abnormalities precede vascular complications.

Retinopathy is easy to visualise and is good evidence of microvascular disease. Dornan investigated three groups of patients with IDDM; 12 with no retinopathy, 10 with background retinopathy and 10 with proliferative retinopathy. Factor VIII and vWF were significantly related to the degree of retinopathy[31]. The inhibitors of thrombin, alpha 2 macroglobulin and alpha 1 antitrypsin were highest in those with proliferative retinopathy although there was no difference in antithrombin III. C-reactive protein was similar in all groups. The authors concluded that the coagulation factors were not solely acute phase proteins due to diabetic tissue damage and that coagulation changes may promote retinopathy. Other studies confirm increased levels of factor VIII in diabetic patients with retinopathy[19,32] and higher levels of fibrinogen[19] and vWF[19,32,33] in patients with proliferative retinopathy. The highest levels of antithrombin III[21] were in patients with retinopathy. Prospective studies which would help determine whether these coagulation protein abnormalities are cause or effect are not available.

The cause of the increased incidence of cardiovascular disease in diabetic patients is unknown. Activation of coagulation causing increased fibrin deposition would be a prime candidate for the development of large vessel arterial occlusion. In a number of studies cited above coexistent atherosclerosis with NIDDM has been described as contributing to abnormalities seen in coagulation proteins, and as explaining some differences between younger IDDM patients unlikely to have atherosclerosis and older NIDDM patients in whom atherosclerosis is frequently present.

The relationship between diabetes mellitus, atherosclerosis and factor VIII was investigated by Bern et al[9] in five groups of patients: IDDM without retinopathy : IDDM and proliferative retinopathy; NIDDM and angiographically proven atherosclerosis; those with atherosclerosis but not diabetes mellitus and a group of normal controls. All factor VIII moieties were elevated in those with atheroma but only factor VIII and vWF in young patients with IDDM. This study demonstrates that factor VIII may be elevated in patients with atheroma. This should be taken into account when analysing studies of diabetic patients, particularly those with NIDDM for the reasons described above.

Unfortunately, similar problems cloud interpretation of antithrombin III data. Patients with NIDDM and silent myocardial ischaemia were found to have higher levels of glycosylated haemoglobin and antithrombin III than those without[34]. However mean antithrombin III levels were similar in the diabetic and control groups. Diabetic patients without silent ischaemia had lower levels of antithrombin III compared to controls. This study could not determine whether the difference in antithrombin III between the two groups was due to silent ischaemia or hyperglycaemia.

The complex formed between thrombin and antithrombin III can be measured and gives an indication of in vivo generation of thrombin. In a study of 18 diabetic patients (3 type 1 and 15 type 2 diabetics) with a mixture of retinopathy, nephropathy and coronary artery disease, thrombin-antithrombin III complexes were higher than in a group of normal non-diabetic controls without vascular disease (with a mean age almost half that of the diabetic group[8]. It is impossible to determine from this study of mixed diabetic patients whether the changes were due to diabetes, microvascular disease, macrovascular disease or age.

C . GLYCAEMIC CONTROL

Hyperglycaemia per se can influence plasma levels of coagulant activity. Changes in antithrombin III[26], Factor VII[13], Factor VIII[11] and Factor X coagulant activity[26], and plasma levels of fibrinogen[19] and FPA[30] appear to be more marked during poor glycaemic control. Unfortunately, few studies have addressed the effect of interventional therapy on coagulation. Interpretation of their results is difficult as changes seen in coagulation during the study may be due to either improved glycaemic control or the effect of the specific drug itself.

Gonzalez reported a reduction in factor VIII ristocetin - cofactor activity in a group of diabetic patients treated intensively with diet and insulin[35]. Paton treated fourteen newly diagnosed NIDDM patients for twelve months initially with diet and then added the sulphonylurea gliclazide to achieve glycaemic control [36]. Significant reductions in factor VIII and vWF were associated with reductions in blood glucose due to this regime. Toward the end of the study period factor VIII, blood glucose and weight increased despite continued compliance with gliclazide (assessed by drug levels), suggesting dietary failure. This study suggests that factor VIII levels are related to metabolic control. Gram et al studied patients with IDDM given gliclazide in addition to their usual insulin therapy[37]. Glycaemic control did not alter but levels of antithrombin III activity and alpha 2 antiplasmin increased. These returned to baseline levels when gliclazide was discontinued. Factor VIII levels were not documented in this study.

Thirty-seven patients with newly diagnosed NIDDM without retinopathy or vascular disease were treated for three months with diet and unspecified oral hypoglycaemic agents[6]. Initially high factor VIII levels normalised with glycaemic control. High antithrombin III levels did not change during. In contrast, elevated levels of FVIII in a group of type 2 diabetic patients with a high incidence of vascular disease were not affected by either insulin therapy or chloropropamide[16].

The results of these limited short term studies suggest that factor VIII is related to glycaemic control but the effects of specific agents on individual coagulation factors are not clear. Elevated fibrinogen levels in diabetic patients appear in part to be affected by metabolic control[4,19]. Elevated fibrinogen levels, found predominantly in patients with retinopathy, were related to the degree of glycaemic control.

D. SUMMARY

Coagulation abnormalities associated with the diabetic state include elevated levels of fibrinogen, vWF, factor VIII and factor VII. There is conflicting evidence concerning antithrombin III levels. Factor VIII and vWF levels may be affected by glycaemic control. The effect of disease duration on all clotting factors is unknown.

Abnormalities of vWF, factor VIII and antithrombin III are more pronounced in diabetic patients with microvascular disease.

Circumstantial evidence incriminates elevation of certain coagulation factors in the development of occlusive vascular disease in diabetic patients, in particular Factor VII and fibrinogen. Factor VII and fibrinogen are known as risk factors for cardiovascular disease in non-diabetic subjects. Indirect methods of thrombin production and newer methods of measuring thrombin generation may give us further insight into hypercoagulability and its role in vascular disease in diabetics.

III. FIBRINOLYTIC SYSTEM

A. DIABETES MELLITUS

Although large doses of fibrinolytic agents have been used clinically to dissolve thrombus, the fibrinolytic system in vivo is thought responsible for more controlled lysis of fibrin clot. Increased concentrations of naturally occurring inhibitors of the fibrinolytic system are largely responsible for the suppression of fibrinolytic activity seen in some disease states associated with increased thrombus formation.

Alterations in the fibrinolytic system have been described in patients with both IDDM and NIDDM. There is evidence to suggest that these abnormalities also have a role in the pathogenesis of vascular disease in both types of diabetes.

Over 30 years ago Fearnley demonstrated reduced fibrinolytic activity in patients with diabetes mellitus[38]. Subsequent reports describe conflicting findings on altered fibrinolytic activity in diabetics (review 39). However, much of the inconsistency can be removed by examining IDDM and NIDDM separately.

1. Insulin Dependent Diabetes Mellitus

In contrast to patients with NIDDM who have depressed fibrinolytic activity principally due to an increase in plasminogen activator inhibitor-1 (PAI-1)[40,41] patients with IDDM have reduced[42], normal[4,43] or even enhanced fibrinolytic activity[44]. Patients with IDDM are generally younger and less likely to have widespread vascular disease. It can be argued that changes in fibrinolysis seen in these individuals may be more representative of the diabetic state. However, the differing metabolic and clinical profiles of IDDM and NIDDM justify the need to analyse results from both groups separately.

In the absence of complications basal and post venous occlusion fibrinolytic activity are shown to be normal in patients with IDDM[45]. Although Auwerx et al reported increased t-PA antigen and PAI-1 activity in IDDM, they found no difference in the euglobulin clot lysis time (ECLT) when compared to a non-diabetic control group[43]. These results suggest activation of the fibrinolytic system without induction of fibrinolytic activity. In contrast, tPA activity was found to be elevated, both at rest and after venous occlusion, in IDDM[46]. There was a positive correlation between HbA_{1c} and the capacity to release tPA. Furthermore, global fibrinolytic activity, again using the ECLT, has been reported increased in 26 patients with IDDM, 36 patients with NIDDM, and 62 controls 44. A significant reduction in tPA was found in the patients with IDDM. This highlights a further confounding variable which should be taken into account when interpreting studies measuring fibrinolytic activity.

It is not known whether differences in fibrinolytic activity between male and female is a consistent finding. Normal clot lysis times in male patients with IDDM compared to significant reductions seen in a similar group of females demonstrates the need for careful sex matching [4] in all studies.

2. Non-insulin Dependent Diabetes Mellitus

A number of studies have shown that fibrinolytic activity is reduced in patients with NIDDM. Moreover exercise stimulated fibrinolytic activity, ie fibrinolytic capacity, is also attenuated in patients with NIDDM[47]. Schneider et al have shown that following 6 weeks of physical training, resting levels of fibrinolytic activity increased to that seen in a non-diabetic control control group. The response to exercise remained subnormal [47].

Specific assays of the individual components of the fibrinolytic system have confirmed that reduced fibrinolytic activity in NIDDM is the result of increased circulating plasma levels of PAI-1[40,42,43,48,49] rather than reduced t-PA. Moreover, plasma PAI-1 levels are closely related to the degree of hyperinsulinaemia seen (review 50). Due to clustering of risk factors for cardiovascular disease, NIDDM is frequently associated with obesity, coronary artery disease and hypertension, all of which are related (under the metabolic syndrome, Syndrome X), and may therefore be contributory to increased PAI-1 levels (review 51). However PAI levels have been found elevated in newly diagnosed normotensive patients with NIDDM, without clinical evidence of occlusive vascular disease[40]. Although PA1-1 levels are clearly related to coronary artery disease[52-54], obesity[55,56] hypertriglyceridaemia[52,53,55] and hypertension[57], increasing evidence from in-vivo and in-vitro studies suggest that hyperinsulinaemia and the associated lipoprotein changes may be involved in the regulation of PAI-1 levels (review 51).

B. COMPLICATIONS OF DIABETES MELLITUS

In-vitro studies have provided indirect evidence that poor metabolic control may inhibit clot lysis and favour vascular occlusion, as glycosylated fibrin is more resistant to plasmin digestion[58]. Clinical evidence from histological studies has shown that accumulation of fibrin occurs in tissues most affected by diabetic complications [59-62]. The functional properties of plasminogen activators and plasminogen improve with the normalisation of glycaemic control[63]. Fibrin is more resistant to fibrinolysis in diabetics. This explains some of the changes in the components of the fibrinolytic system in diabetics and suggests a mechanism for the development of micro- and macro vascular disease in these patients.

In Fearnley's 1963 study, fibrinolytic activity was reduced in patients with diabetes and evidence of ischaemia on electrocardiograms occurred twice as frequently in those with markedly reduced fibrinolytic activity[38]. These findings agree with those of Hamsten et al, who, in non-diabetic individuals, demonstrated high levels of t-PA inhibition in survivors of myocardial infarction compared with controls [52,53]. This reinforces the importance of abnormal fibrinolytic activity in the development of vascular disease.

Fibrinolytic activity has been examined in relationship to micro-vascular complications. In a mixed group of diabetic patients, those with retinopathy had lower spontaneous and post-venous occlusion activity compared to patients without complications[17]. Preservation of fibrinolytic activity in patients without complications may act to prevent the early vascular changes associated with retinopathy.

IDDM patients with retinopathy have been described as having higher levels of t-PA, both pre- and post-venous occlusion, with higher PAI-1 post venous occlusion than those without complications[64]. Walmsley et al confirmed higher levels of t-PA in such patients, but not differences in PAI-1[42]. Global fibrinolytic activity, assessed by fibrin plates, has been reported as normal in the resting state and reduced after venous occlusion in IDDM patients with retinopathy[45]. In contrast, patients with IDDM, retinopathy and hypertension have been reported to have higher levels of PAI-1 activity[65]. Post-venous occlusion fibrinolytic capacity, measured as tPA release, was reduced in patients with retinopathy, hypertension and peripheral vasculopathy. On the other hand, Rydzewski studied 31 patients with NIDDM and found that patients without retinopathy did not differ in fibrinolytic activity from controls[66]. However, patients with simple retinopathy had significantly higher levels of tPA than controls and those with proliferative retinopathy. Patients with simple retinopathy also had significantly higher levels of tPA/PAI-1 complex and PAI-1 antigen. These results indicate that fibrinolytic activity may be enhanced in patients with early diabetic microangiopathy but reduced in patients with more severe disease.

Microalbuminuria is a useful early predictor for the development of nephropathy in diabetic patients. It also predicts increased mortality due to cardiovascular disease in diabetic and non-diabetic subjects. In 12 patients with NIDDM and microalbuminuria, and 12 patients with normal albumin excretion compared with 12 non-diabetic controls, Collier et al[67] reported increased levels of t-PA in the group with microalbuminuria. However in larger study of patients NIDDM first examined at diagnosis the degree of microalbuminuria correlated with increased levels of PAI-1[40].

In a study designed to look specifically at fibrinolytic activity and the development of vascular complications, 20 diabetic patients with no complications, 17 with laser-treated retinopathy and 13 with neuropathy were compared with a group of 20 non-diabetic controls[42]. Patients with macrovascular disease, hypertension and smoking were excluded and assays of tPA and PAI-1 were assessed pre- and post-venous occlusion. Basal tPA inhibition was higher in the control group than in the diabetic patients and post-venous occlusion tPA antigen was higher in controls compared with neuropathic patients. These results indicate that patients with IDDM have enhanced fibrinolysis but a diminished response to venous occlusion in neuropathic patients. This would be consistent with an endothelial cell defect.

C. THE EFFECTS OF TREATMENT OF DIABETES

Unlike a large number of abnormalities of the coagulation system seen in diabetes mellitus, disturbances to the fibrinolytic system do not appear to be directly related to glycaemic control. The main abnormality seen in NIDDM, namely an increase in PAI-1, appears more closely related to the degree of insulin resistance than to the level of metabolic control[39,50]. Although long term studies designed to determine the effect of improvements in metabolic control on fibrinolytic activity do not exist, there are data which deserve mention.

Fibrinolytic activity measured by the ECLT was found to be reduced in 221 diabetics compared to 153 age and sex matched non-diabetic subjects[17]. This difference was largely due to significantly reduced fibrinolytic activity in 21 of the patients who received sulphonylureas. Diabetic patients on diet or insulin had activity similar to the control population. Overweight patients had lower fibrinolytic activity. The differences could not be attributed to the degree of glycaemic control and therefore raises the possibility of a specific action of sulphonylurea therapy.

In a study of 15 patients, Almer et al 68 compared fibrinolytic activity in patients initially on the sulphonylurea, chlorpropamide, who were then changed to gliclazide. Seven of 15 patients had abnormally low plasminogen activator activity on chlorpropamide but after 6 months on gliclazide all patients had normal plasminogen activator activity. After 24 and 48 months the results remained the same. At 48 months, only 8 patients remained in the study. The normalisation of fibrinolytic activity could not be explained by improvement in glycaemic control as this remained the same throughout the study. Increased levels of PAI-1 were monitored in 14 type 2 diabetic patients at diagnosis and after 3 months standard clinical dietary modification[69]. Over the period of study there was a significant fall in PAI-1. However this did not correlate with the improvement in HbA$_{1c}$ nor changes in BMI or triglyceride levels

Despite significant improvement in glycaemic control over a 12 month period in a group of patients with newly diagnosed NIDDM, fibrinolytic activity deteriorated as shown by a prolongation of the ECLT and an increase in the tPA/PAI-1 ratio[70]. However preservation of exercise stimulated fibrinolytic capacity over the 12 months. This suggests that in at least patients with NIDDM, suppression of fibrinolytic activity is independent of metabolic control.

The effects of weight reduction and metformin therapy in patients with NIDDM reinforce the relationship between hyperinsulinaemia and elevated PAI-1 levels. Weight reduction[56], exercise[71] and metformin[72] are all associated with improvement in insulin sensitivity and reduce PAI-1 levels[50].

D. SUMMARY

Reports of abnormalities of the fibrinolytic system in patients with diabetes mellitus are conflicting. Most studies point to reduced fibrinolytic activity in patients with NIDDM, mainly due to increased PAI-1 levels. The picture is less clear in patients with IDDM, in whom generally fibrinolytic activity is normal or even enhanced. It seems unlikely that abnormalities of fibrinolytic activity are related to glycaemic control although to date there are no long term studies available for analysis. The relationship between fibrinolytic activity and microangiopathy is not clear. Some reports suggest suppression of fibrinolytic activity while others describe normal or enhanced activity, particularly in early microangiopathy. The increase may represent a protective role. Whether such changes are cause or effect is uncertain. Depression of fibrinolysis in patients with venous and arterial thromboembolic disease and further depression in patients with NIDDM may contribute to the high incidence of vascular disease seen in this condition.

VI. CONCLUSIONS AND CLINICAL APPLICATION

When considering the biological aspects of hypercoagulability in patients with diabetes mellitus, four questions arise. First, do abnormalities of the coagulation and fibrinolytic systems exist ? Undoubtedly the answer to this question is yes. Altered levels of Factor VII, Factor VIII, vWF, Factor X and antithrombin III have been described. Elevated levels of thrombin-antithrombin III complexes, fibrinopeptide A and F1+2 provide indirect evidence for hypercoagulability in diabetes mellitus. Second, if abnormalities do exist, do they alter the fine balance between coagulation and fibrinolysis and favour fibrin deposition and vascular occlusion ? The answer here is less clear. Fibrin deposition is certainly increased in diabetic patients particularly in tissues most affected by complications, but dynamic tests demonstrating increased fibrin production due to increased coagulant activity and/or reduced fibrinolytic activity are not available. Third, are there any tests of hypercoagulability which should be routinely performed in the clinical management of diabetic patients ? There is currently no single test, or group of tests of hypercoagulability, which would help us treat or predict those individuals likely to develop vascular complications. Fourth and finally, do the results of research studies provide any theoretical advice, which, until the answer to question three becomes available, may help in the therapeutic management of patients ? The results of the recently published DCCT[73] show that microvascular complications in patients with IDDM can be considerably reduced by good glycaemic control. Some abnormalities of coagulation are clearly related to the degree of glycaemia, so in theory, the reduction in vascular complications in patients with good glycaemic control may be mediated via favourable changes in coagulant activity. Without the extrapolation of the DCCT data to patients with NIDDM, the exact relationship between glycaemic control and vascular disease remains unknown. Obesity and lack of physical exercise are known to be related to the development of cardiovascular disease. These risk factors are particularly important in the insulin resistant patient with NIDDM. Therefore, the recommendation of weight reduction, physical exercise and the use of biguanides in patients with NIDDM may reduce cardiovascular morbidity and mortality mediated in part by a reduction in PAI-1.

Although platelet alterations have not been discussed under "hypercoagulability" they deserve mention in this section. Increased platelet aggregation has been described in some[74,75] but not all[76] studies of diabetes mellitus with the greatest abnormalities in patients with poor control[77]. These changes also seem to be associated with platelet activation as evidenced by increased circulating levels of beta thromboglobulin[78] and platelet factor 4[79]. It is not clear whether these changes represent cause or effect although increased platelet aggregation has been described in young patients without vascular complications[80]. Aspirin inhibits platelet function[81] and its potential as an antithrombotic agent has been established in the treatment and prophylaxis of transient ischaemic attacks[82], unstable angina[83,84], and myocardial infarction[85]. Unfortunately its usefulness as an antiplatelet agent in the prevention of vascular complications is unknown. When considering the other potential antithrombotic effects of aspirin[86,87], it may be that a long term prospective study in patients with diabetes mellitus would provide a useful contribution to the prevention of vascular disease.

REFERENCES

1. **Jones, R.L., Peterson , C.M.** The fluid phase of coagulation and the accelerated atherosclerosis of diabetes mellitus, *Diabetes*, 30, (suppl 2), 33, 1981.
2. **Bannerjee, R.N., Kumar, V., Sahui , A.L.** Plasma thrombin clotting time and plasma fibrinogen in diabetes mellitus and atherosclerosis, *Indian J. Med. Res.*, 60, 1432, 1972.

3. **Bannerjee, R.N., Sahui, A.L., Kumar, V.** Fibrincoagulopathy in maturity-onset diabetes mellitus and atherosclerosis, *Thromb. Diath. Haemorrh.*, 30, 123, 1973.
4. **Fuller, J.H., Keen, H., Jarrett, R.J., Omer, T., Meade, T.W., Chakrabarti , R., North, W.R.S., Stirling, Y.** Haemostatic variables associated with diabetes and its complications, *Br. Med. J.*, ii, 964, 1979.
5. **Christe, M., Fritschi, B., Lammle, B., Tran, T.H., Marbet , G.A., Berger ,W.,Duckert, F.** Fifteen coagulation and fibrinolysis parameters in diabetes mellitus and in patients with vasculopathy, *Thromb. Haemostas.*, 52, 138, 1984.
6. **Hughes, A., McVerry, B.A., Wilkinson, L., Goldstone , A.H., Lewis, D., Bloom , A**. Diabetes a hypercoagulable state? Haemostatic variables in newly diagnosed type 2 diabetic patients, *Acta Haematol..*, 69, 254, 1983.
7. **Mayne,E.E., Bridges, J.M., Weaver, J.A.** Platelet adhesiveness, plasma fibrinogen and factor VIII in diabetes mellitus, *Diabetologia*, 6, 436, 1970.
8. **Takahashi, H., Tsuda, A., Tatewaki, W., Wada, K., Niwano, H., Shibata, A.**, Activation of blood coagulation and fibrinolysis in diabetes mellitus: evaluation by plasma levels of thrombin-antithrombin III complex and plasmin-alpha-2-plasmin inhibitor complex, *Thromb. Res.*, 55, 727, 1989.
9. **Bern,,M.M., Cassani, M.P., Horton, J., Rand, L., Davis, G.**, Changes of fibrinolysis and factor VIII coagulant, antigen, and ristocetin cofactor in diabetes mellitus and atherosclerosis, *Thrombosis Res.*, 19, 831, 1980.
10. **Borkenstein, M., Muntean, W.**, Elevated factor VIII activity and factor VIII related antigen in diabetic children without vascular disease, *Diabetes*, 31, 1006, 1982.
11. **Muntean ,W., Borkenstein, M.H., Haas, J.**, Elevation of factor VIII coagulant activity over factor VIII coagulant antigen in children without vascular disease, *Diabetes*, 34, 140, 1985.
12. **Valdorf-Hansen , F.** Thrombocytes and coagulability in diabetics, *Dan. Med. Bull.*, 14, 244, 1967.
13. **Ceriello, A., Giugliano, D., Quatraro, A. et al.**, Blood glucose may condition factor VII levels in diabetic and normal subjects, *Diabetologia*, 31, 889, 1988.
14. **Egeberg, O.**, The blood coagulability in diabetic retinopathy., *Scand. J. Lab. Invest.*, 15, 522, 1963.
15. **Meade, T.W., Mellows, S., Brozovic, M. et al.**, Haemostatic function and cardiovascular death : principle results of the Nothwick Park Heart Study, *Lancet*, ii, 533, 1986.
16. **Jones, R.L., Petersonn C.M.**, Reduced fibrinogen survival in diabetes mellitus: a reversible phenomenon, *J. Clin. Invest.*, 63, 485, 1979.
17. **Almer, L.O., Pandolfi, M., Nilsson, I.M.**, Diabetic retinopathy and the fibrinolytic system, *Diabetes*, 24, 529, 1975.
18. **Chakrabarti, R., Fearnley, G.R.**, Pharmacologic fibrinolysis in diabetes mellitus, *Diabetologia*, 10, 19, 1974.
19. **Coller, B.S., Frank, D.N., Milton, R.C. et al.**, Plasma co-factors of platelet function, Correlation with diabetic retinopathy and hemoglobins A1a+c, *Ann. Intern. Med.*, 88, 311, 1978.
20. **Corbella, E., Miraglitten, G., Masperi, R. et al.**, Platelet aggregation and antithrombin III levels in diabetic children, *Haemostasis*, 8, 30, 1979.
21. **Elder, G.E., Mayne, E.E., Daly, J.G., Kennedy , A.C. , Hadden, D.R., Montgomery, D.A.D., Weaver , J.A.**, Antithrombin and other coagulation changes in proliferative diabetic retinopathy, *Haemostasis*, 9, 288, 1980.
22. **Borsey, D.Q., Prowse, C.V., Gray, R.S., Dawers, J., James, K., Elton, R.A.**, Platelet and coagulation factors in proliferative diabetic retinopathy, *J. Clin. Pathol.*, 37, 659, 1984.
23. **Gandolfo, G.M., De Angelis, A., Torresi, M.V.**, Determination of antithrombin III activity by different methods in diabetic patients, *Haemostasis*, 9, 15, 1980.
24. **Bannerjee, R.N., Sahui, A.L., Kumar, V., et al.**, Antithrombin III deficiency in maturity onset diabetes and atherosclerosis, *Thromb. Diath. Haemorrh.*, 31, 339, 1974.
25. **Ceriello, A., Dello Russo, P., Zuccotti, C., et al.**, Decreased antithrombin III activity in diabetes may be due to nonenzymatic glycosylation. A preliminary report, *Thromb. Haemostas.*, 16, 458, 1986.
26. **Ceriello, A., Quatraro, A., Marchi, E., Barbanti, M., Dello Russo, P., Lefebvre, P., Giugliano, D.**, The role of hyperglycaemia-induced alterations of antithrombin III and factor X activation in the thrombin hyperactivity of diabetes mellitus, *Diabetic Med.*, 7, 343, 1990.
27. **Patrassi, G.M., Picchinenna, R., Vettor, R., Cappellato, G., Coccarielli,D., Girolami, A.**, Antithrombin III activity and concentration in diabetes mellitus, *Thromb. Haemostas.*, 54, 415, 1985.
28. **Rosove, M.H., Frank, H.S.L., Harving, S.S.L.**, Plasma beta thromboglobulin, platelet factor 4, fibrinopeptide A, and other hemostatic functions during improved short-term glycaemic control in diabetes mellitus, *Diabetes Care*, 7, 174, 1984.
29. **Ceriello, A., Giacomello, R., Colatutto, A., Taboga, C., Gonano, F.** , Increased prothrombin fragment 1+2 in type 1 diabetic patients, *Haemostasis*, 22, 50, 1992.
30. **Jones, R.L.**, Fibrinopeptide-A in diabetes mellitus. Relation to levels of blood glucose, fibrinogen disappearance, and hemodynamic changes, *Diabetes*, 34, 836, 1985.
31. **Dornan, T.L., Rhymes, I.L., Cederholm-Williams, S.A., et al.**, Plasma haemostatic factors and diabetic retinopathy, *Eur. J. Clin. Invest..*, 1983, 13: 231-235.
32. **Bennsoussan, D., Levy-Toledano, S., Passa, P.**, et al., Platelet hyperaggregation and increased levels of von Willebrand factor in diabetes with retinopathy, *Diabetologia*, 11, 307, 1975.
33. **Porta, M., Maneschi, F., White, M.C., Kohner, E.M.**, Twenty-four hour variations of von Willebrand factor and factor VIII-related antigen in diabetic retinopathy, *Metabolism*, 30, 695, 1981.
34. **Torrado, M.C., Garcia Frade, L.J., Lara, J.I., Rayo, I., Cuellar, L., Marin, E., Garcia Avello, A., de la Calle, H.**, Silent myocardial isçchaemia episodes in non-insulin dependent diabetes mellitus: relationship with haemostatic alterations, *Fibrinolysis*, 5, 121, 1991.
35. **Gonzalez, J., Colwell, J.A., Sarji, K.E., Nair, R.M.., Sagel, J.**, Effect of metabolic control with insulin on plasma von Willebrand activity (VIIIR:WF) in diabetes mellitus, *Thromb. Res.*, 17, 261, 1980.
36. **Paton, R.C., Kernoff, P.B.A., Wales, J.K., McNicol**, Effects of diet and gliclazide on the haemostatic system of non-insulin-dependent diabetics, *Br. Med. J.*, 283, 1018, 1981.
37. **Gram, J., Munkvad, S., KolD, A., Jespersen, J.**, Effects of an oral antidiabetic drug (Gliclazide) on inhibition of coagulation and fibrinolysis studied in insulin-treated diabetic patients (type 1), *Fibrinolysis*, 3, 153, 1989.
38. **Fearnley, G.R., Chakrabarti, R., Avis, P.R.D.**, Blood fibrinolytic activity in diabetes mellitus and its bearing on ischaemic heart disease and obesity, *Br. Med. J.* , i, 921, 1963.
39. **Gough, S.C.L., Grant, P.J.**, The fibrinolytic system in diabetes mellitus, *Diabetic Med.*, 8, 898, 1991.
40. **Gough, S.C.L., Rice, P.J.S., McCormack, L., Chapman, C., Grant, P.J.**, The relationship between plasminogen activator inhibitor-1 and insulin resistance in newly diagnosed type 2 diabetes mellitus, *Diabetic Med.*, 10, 638, 1993.
41. **Potter Van Loon, B.J., Kluft, K., Radder, J.K., Blankenstein, M.A., Meinders, A.E.**, The cardiovascular risk factor plasminogen activator inhibitor type I is related to insulin resistance, *Metabolism*, 42, 945, 1993.

42. **Walmsley, D., Hampton, K.K., Grant, P.J.**, Contrasting fibrinolytic responses in Type 1 (insulin dependent) and type 2 (non insulin dependent) diabetes, *Diabetic Med.*, 8, 954, 1991.

43. **Auwerx, J., Bouillon, R., Collen, Geboers J.**, Tissue-type plasminogen activator antigen and plasminogen activator inhibitor in diabetes mellitus, *Arteriosclerosis*, 8, 68, 1988.

44. **Sharma, S.C.**, Platelet adhesiveness, plasma fibrinogen and fibrinolytic activity in juvenile-onset and maturity onset diabetes mellitus, *J. Clin. Pathol.*, 34, 501, 1981.

45. **Haitas, B., Barnes, A.J., Cederholm-Williams, S.A., Moore J., Shogry , M.E.C. , Turner, R.C.**, Abnormal release of fibrinolytic activity and fibronectin in diabetic microangiopathy, *Diabetologia*, 27, 493, 1984.

46. **Nilsson, T.K., Lithner, F.**, Glycaemic control, smoking habits and diabetes duration affect the extrinsic fibrinolytic system in type 1 diabetic patients but microangiopathy does not, *Acta. Med. Scand.*, 224, 123, 1988.

47. **Schneider, S.H., Kim, H.C., Khachadurian, A.K., Ruderman, N. G.**, Impaired fibrinolytic response to exercise in type II diabetes : effects of exercise and physical training, *Metabolism*, 37, 924, 1988.

48. **Juhan-Vague, I., Roul , C., Alessi, M.C. , Ardissone, J.P., Heim, M., Vague, P.**, Increased plasminogen activator, inhibitor activity in non insulin dependent diabetic patients. Relationship with plasma insulin, *Thromb. Haemostas.*, 61, 370, 1989.

49. **Grant, M.B., Fitzgerald, C., Guay, C, Lottenberg, R.**, Fibrinolytic capacity following stimulation with desmopressin acetate in patients with diabetes mellitus, *Metabolism*, 38, 901, 1989.

50. **Juhan-Vague, I., Alessi, M.C. , Vague, P.**, Increased plasma plasminogen activator inhibitor 1 levels. A possible link between insulin resistance and atherothrombosis, *Diabetologia*, 34, 457, 1991.

51. **Gough, S.C.L., Juhan-Vague, I.**, Insulin resistance and alterations in the fibrinolytic system, *Cardiovascular Risk Factors*, 3, 387, 1993.

52. **Hamsten, A., Wiman, B., de Faire, U., Blomback, M.**, Increased plasma level of a rapid inhibitor of tissue plasminogen activator in young survivors of myocardial infarction, *N. Engl. J. Med.*, 313, 1557, 1985.

53. **Hamsten , A., Defaire, U., Walldius, G. , Dahlen, G., Szamosi, A., Landou, C., Blomback, M., Wiman, B.**, Plasminogen activator inhibitor in plasma : risk factor for recurrent myocardial infarction, *Lancet*, ii, 3, 1987.

54. **Mehta, J., Mehta, P., Lawson, D., Saldeen, T.**, Plasma tissue plasminogen activator inhibitor levels in coronary artery disease; correlation with age and serum triglyceride concentrations, *J. Am. Coll. Cardiol.*, 9, 263, 1987.

55. **Sundell, I.B., Nilsson, T.K., Hallmans, G., Nygren, C.**, The effect of body build, diet and endocrine factor on the extrinsic fibrinolytic system in healthy young women, *Scand. J. Clin. Lab. Invest..*, 48, 557, 1988.

56. **Vague, P., Juhan-Vague, I., Aillaud, M.F., et al.**, Correlation between blood fibrinolytic activity, plasminogen activator inhibitor level, plasma insulin level and relative body weight in normal and obese subjects, *Metabolism*, 35, 250,1986.

57. **Landkin, K., Tengborn, L., Smith , U.**, Elevated fibrinogen and plasminogen activator inhibitor (PAI-1) in hypertension are related to metabolic risk factors for cardiovascular disease, *J. Int. Med.*, 227, 273, 1990.

58. **Brownlee, M., Vlassara, H., Cerami, A.**, Nonenzymatic glycosylation reduced the susceptibility of fibrin to degradation by plasmin, *Diabetes*, 32, 680, 1983.

59. **Ireland, J.T., Viberti, G.C., Watkins, P.J.**, The kidney and renal tract. in Keen H., Jarrett J. eds., *Complications of Diabetes. London : Edward Arnold 1982*, 137-178.

60. **Cunah-Vaz, J.G.**, Pathophysiology of diabetic retinopathy, *Br. J. Ophthalmol.*, 62, 351, 1978.

61. **Timperly, W.R., Ward, J.D., Preston, et al.**, Clinical and histological studies in diabetic neuropathy, *Diabetologia*, 12, 237, 1976.

62. **Haust, M.D., Wyliss, J.C., Mor, R.H.**, Electron microscopy of in human atherosclerotic lesions, *Exp. Mol. Pathol.*, 4, 205, 1965.

63. **Geiger, M., Binder, B.R.**, Plasminogen activation in diabetes mellitus : normalisation of blood sugar levels improves impaired enzyme kinetics in vitro, *Thromb. Haemostat.*, 54, 413, 1985.

64. **McLaren, M , Jennings, P.E., Forbes, C.D., Belch, J.J.F.**, Fibrinolytic response to venous occlusion in diabetics with and without microangiopathy compared to normal age and sex matched controls, *Fibrinolysis*, 4, 95, 1990.ç

65. **Garcia Frade, L.J., de la Calle, H., Torade, M.C., Lara, J. I., Cuellar, L ., Garcia Avello, A.**, Hypofibrinolysis associated with vasculopathy in non-insulin dependent diabetes mellitus, *Throm. Res.*, 59, 51, 1990.

66. **Rydezewki, A., Kawamura, H., Watanabe, Y. , Takada, T.A.**, Plasminogen activators and plasminogen activator inhibitor (PAI-1) in type 1 diabetes mellitus, *Fibrinolysis*, 4, 183, 1990.

67. **Collier, A., Rumley, A., Leach, J.P., Lowe, G.D.O., Small, M.**, Abnormalities of haemostasis in type 2 diabetes with microalbuminuria (Abstract). *Diabetic Med.*, 8 (suppl): 36A, 1991.

68. **Almer, L.O.**, Effects of chlorpropamide and gliclazide on plasminogen activator activity in vascular walls in patients with maturity onset diabetes, *Thromb. Res.*, 35, 19, 1984.

69. **Bahru,Y., Kesteven, P., Alberti, K.G.M.M., Walker, M.**, Decreased plasminogen activator inhibitor-1 activity in newly diagnosed type 2 diabetic patients following dietry modification, *Diabetic Med.*, 10, 802, 1993.

70. **Gough, S.C.L., McCormack, Rice , P.J.S., Grant, P.J.**, The fibrinolytic response to exercise at diagnosis and after 12 months in patients with type 2 diabetes mellitus, *Fibrinolysis*, 8, 372, 1994.

71. **Rosenthal, M. , Haskell, W.L. , Solomon, R., Widstrom , A. , Reaven G. M.**, Demonstration of a relationship between the level of physical training and insulin stimulated glucose utilisation in normal humans, *Diabetes*, 32, 408, 1983.ç

72. **Jackson, R.A., Hawa, M.I., Jaspan, J.B., et al.**, Mechanism of metformin action in non insulin dependent diabetes, *Diabetes*, 36, 632, 1987.

73. **The Diabetes Control and Complications Trial Research Group**, The effect of intensive treatment of diabetes on the development and progression of long-term complications in insulin-dependent diabetes mellitus, *N. Engl. J. Med.*, 329, 977, 1993.

74. **Colwell, J.A., Halushka, P.V., Sarji, K. , et al.**, Altered platelet function in diabetes mellitus, *Diabetes*, 25, 826, 1976.

75. **Kwaan, H.C., Colwell, J.A., Cruz, S et al.**, Increased platelet aggregation in diabetes mellitus , *J. Lab. Clin. Med.*, 80, 236, 1972.

76. **Davis, J.W., Phillips, P.E., Yue, K.T. et al.**, Platelet aggregation. Adult-onset diabetes mellitus and coronary artery disease, JAMA, 239, 732,1978.

77. **Davis, J.W., Hartman, C.R., Davis, R.F., Kyner, J.L., Lewis, H.D., Phillips, P.E.**,Platelet aggregate ratio in diabetes mellitus, *Acta. Haemat.*, 67, 222, 1982.

78. **Davi, G., Rini, G.B., Averna, M. et al.**, Enhanced platelet release reaction in insulin-dependent and insulin-independent diabetic patients, *Haemostasis*, 12, 275, 1982

79. **Alessandrini, P, McRae, J., Feman, S., Fitzgerald, G.A.,** Thromboxane biosysnthesis and platelet function in type 1 diabetes mellitus, *N. Engl. J. Med.*, 319, 208, 1988.
80. **Winocour, P.D., Halushka, P.V., Colwell, J.A.**, Platelet involvement in diabetes mellitus, *In Longenecker GL (ed) The Platelets: physiology and pharmacology. Academic Press, New York,* pp 341-366.
81. **Weiss , H.J., Aledort, L.M.**, Impaired platelet connective-tissue reaction in man after aspirin ingestion, *Lancet*, ii, 495, 1967.
82. **UK-TIA Study Group**, United Kingdom transient ischaemic attack (UK-TIA) aspirin trial; interim results, *Br. Med. J.*, 296, 316, 1988.
83. **Results of a Veterans Administration Cooperative Study**. Protective effects of aspirin against acute myocardial infarction and death in men with unstable angina, *N. Engl. J. Med.*, 309, 396, 1983.
84. **Results of a Canadian Multicentre Trial**, Aspirin, Sulfinpyrazone, or both in unstable angina, *N. Engl. J. Med.*, 313, 1369, 1985.
85. **ISIS-2 collaborative group**, Randomised trial of intravenous streptokinase oral aspirin, both or neither amoung 17187 causes of suspected acute myocardial infarction, *Lancet*, ii, 349, 1988.
86. **Loew, D., Vinazzer, H.**, Dose-dependent influence of acetylsalicylic acid on platelet functions and plasmatic coagulation factors, *Haemostasis*, 5, 239, 1976.
87. **Moroz L.,** Increased blood fibrinolytic activity after aspirin ingestion, *N. Engl. J. Med.*, 296, 525, 1977.

HEMATOLOGICAL DISORDERS AND STROKE

M J Seghatchian*, T Baglin**, M M Samama***
*NBS, Colindale, London
** Addenbrooke's NHS Trust, Cambridge
*** Hôtel-Dieu, University Hospital, Paris

I. INTRODUCTION

The pathogenesis of stroke is multifactorial with major risk factors including hypertension, diabetes, atrial fibrillation and the so called "life style" syndrome. The balance between circulating levels of coagulant proteins and natural anticoagulants can influence thrombin generation but deficiency of natural anticoagulants is rarely implicated in the development of thrombotic stroke. Furthermore, no hereditary disorder of platelet function has yet been implicated in the aetiology of premature vascular disease and stroke. Nevertheless, among young patients 2 to 5% of strokes are associated with altered blood constituents. In fact the exact prevalence of hematological disorders that are related to strokes cannot be determined with accuracy for several reasons:

i.   The definition of stroke aetiology varies from study to study with only some including all hematological and coagulation abnormalities that predispose to thrombosis.
ii.   In only limited studies has hypercoagulability been assessed.
iii   Most of the evidence linking prothrombotic states to stroke is based on a small series of case reports inevitably subject to report bias.

This brief review summarises epidemiological and clinical laboratory aspects of various haematological disorders associated with ischemic stroke.

II. RED CELL ABNORMALITIES AND STROKE

A. PRIMARY PROLIFERATIVE POLYCYTHEMIA (PPP)

In PPP there is an increased risk of stroke due to increased blood[1,2]. Treatment with venesection to maintain the haematocrit below 45% reduces the risk of thrombosis. The contribution from associated thrombocytosis appears minimal if any with the use of aspirin increasing the risk of gastrointestinal bleeding without any apparent additional benefit to venesection alone[2-4]. Isovolaemic exchange may be preferable to venesection alone in the early stages of treatment of patients with haematocrits greater than 60% or in patients with neurological symptoms. Nevertheless caution is needed generally as repeated pheresis can be associated with thrombosis[5].

B. SECONDARY AND SPURIOUS POLYCYTHEMIA

An increased risk of cerebral thrombosis is observed frequently in association with secondary polycythemia due to kidney disease[6]. Similarly there is an association between stroke and spurious polycythemia (occurring in middle-aged, obese, smokers and hypertensive individuals) where the hematocrit is increased due to a reduced plasma volume. The role of the increased hematocrit in stroke in these patients is controversial as often a series of other risk factors coexist. Nevertheless, in the same aged-group of patients the risk of cerebral ischemic attack is greater in patients with an elevated hematocrit.

C. HEMOGLOBINOPATHY AND STROKE

Patients with sickle syndromes are prone to both primary cerebral infarction and secondary hemorrhagic stroke[7] :

1. Sickle Cell Anaemia (homozygous)

Between 8 and 17% of patients with homozygous sickle cell anaemia (HbSS) suffer stroke at some time. Cerebral infarction is almost always confined to children with hemorrhage occurring predominantly in adults. Recovery is usually incomplete and recurrence is common with approximately one third of patients having a recurrence each year over the next three years. This potential disaster usually occurs spontaneously and without warning, typically in children (median age 7 years). There is an increased risk in the siblings of affected children. Angiographic and post mortem examinations usually reveal more vessel involvement than anticipated on clinical grounds. Computed tomographic scanning or arteriography is required to rule out potentially treatable disorders (eg subdural hematoma, berry aneurysm or tuberculosis granuloma) all of which have been described in sickle patients[8]. Arteriography can also indicate stabilisation and smoothing of intimal lesions in transfused patients as opposed to progressive vessel damage in patients not receiving transfusions[8]. Long term transfusion therapy aiming to keep the HbS levels below 20-30% for more than 2 years reduces the risk considerably but the ideal HbS level and duration are unknown[9,10]. Other complications of long term transfusion include transmission of infection, red cell antigen sensitisation and iron overload. Furthermore, transient ischemic attacks can occur in patients on transfusion programmes.

Emergency treatment for stroke includes exchange transfusion to limit the extent of the ischemic damage and prepare the patient for arteriography.

2. Stroke in other sickle syndromes

Individuals with hemoglobin SA have an identical prevalence of stroke as that in the black population in general[11]. The frequency of stroke in thalassaemia major or intermedia is very low but hyperplasia of intracranial vessels and thrombosis, or fat embolism due to bone necrosis, have been described[8]. Thrombosis can occur in these patients in association with blood transfusion[12].

3. Stroke and severe anemia

Severe anemia associated with hyperthrombosis caused by bleeding has been suspected in exceptional cases of stroke in older patients without any known cause.

III. WHITE CELL ABNORMALITIES AND STROKE

Intracerebral thrombosis or hemorrhage may occur in association with all types of leukaemia. Hyperleucocytosis, thrombocytopenia, disseminated intravascular coagulation, vascular lesions, hepatic insufficiency and viral infection are possible contributory factors[13]. Stroke may also occur in the chronic hypereosinophilic syndrome[14,15]. In paroxysmal nocturnal hemoglobinuria (PNH) the risk of thrombosis is greater than hemorrhage even when patients are thrombocytopenic. Thrombosis typically occurrs in the abdominal venous system though the second most common site is the cerebral venous system. Thrombosis is unrelated to the duration or degree of hemolysis (see the chapter of Plessner on PNH).

IV. PLATELET ABNORMALITIES AND STROKE

A. THROMBOCYTOSIS

Thrombocytosis as a result of a myeloproliferative syndrome is associated with abnormalities of both the quantity and quality of platelets. Cerebrovascular disease accounts for one third of the thrombotic events. Transient ischemic attacks are frequent, and strokes occur in 3% to 9% of cases, usually due to small vessel occlusion. Hemorrhagic strokes are less common. Cerebral venous thrombosis is less frequent. The role of platelets in cerebral ischemic events is not well established. In patients with essential thrombocythaemia there is an increased risk of thrombotic events, including stroke, in patients over 60 years of age with a platelet count greater than $500x10^9$/L, particularly if they have suffered a previous event. Antiplatelet therapy appears to be of little if any value in preventing such events but reduction of the platelet count to less than $500x10^9$/L with hydroxyurea reduces the risk of all thrombotic events[16]. However, in this study there was only one stroke in each of the control and treatment groups and the benefit of platelet reduction on the risk of stroke has yet to be quantified.

Secondary thrombocytosis is not in itself associated with an increased risk of thrombosis[2]. This contrast between essential thrombocythaemia and reactive thrombocytosis is clearly a qualitative rather than a quantitative effect and may result from altered platelet-dependent thrombin generation as well as altered platelet-platelet and platelet-endothelial interactions[17].

B. THROMBOCYTOPENIA AND STROKE

Hemorrhagic stroke as a result of thrombocytopenia is usually associated with a platelet count less than $20x10^9$/L and platelet transfusion is indicated for patients with temporary thrombocytopenia to this degree[18]. The nature of the thrombocytopenia is also a critical determinant of bleeding risk. In alloimmune neonatal thrombocytopenia the risk of intracranial hemorrhage is approximately 25% in contrast to autoimmune thrombocytopenia where the risk is minimal[19].

Thrombotic stroke may complicate heparin induced thrombocytopenia and in such cases heparin therapy must be discontinued[20].

C. QUALITATIVE ABNORMALITIES OF PLATELETS

Platelet adhesiveness and aggregation may be diminished as a result of drug therapy (eg aspirin), in myeloproliferative disorders and paraproteinaemias, all of which may increase the risk of cerebral hemorrhage.

Elevated βTG and thromboxane B_2 are frequently observed in situations associated with acute thrombosis in cerebral arteries. Whilst these observations are indicative of platelet activation this is likely to be secondary to atherosclerosis and as yet a primary hereditary hyperactive platelet syndrome with primary arterial thrombosis has not been described. However, thrombotic thrombocytopenic purpura (TTP) the heparin induced thrombocytopenia/thrombosis syndrome (HIT) and paroxysmal nocturnal hemoglobinuria (PNH) illustrate how platelet activation can result in primary arterial thrombotic events.

It is noteworthy that homocysteinemias which are associated with qualitative abnormality of platelets can be responsible for stroke with fatal consequence in homozygous patients (see the chapter of Coccheri on homocysteinuria).

D. CHANGES IN PLATELET INDICES IN STROKE

In the acute phase of stroke platelet numbers are reduced with the count returning to the normal range 10 days from the onset of symptoms. The mean platelet count is significantly lower in the patients who die than in those who survive[21]. Recently measurement of platelet size by automated cell counters has been used to ascertain the relationship between cerebral infarction and mean platelet volume (MPV)[21]. Platelets obtained within 48 hours of cerebral infarction are on average 2.3 fl larger than normal platelet population (mean platelet volume). This returns to normal value within several weeks. The increased MPV may be a result of increased marrow production in reponse to increased platelet consumption. Formation of aggregates could also contribute to the increased MPV. Platelet accumulation in regions of low blood flow during the post-ischemic period together with changes in platelet survival may also contribute to the low platelet count and persistently high MPV[22]. Samples taken into EDTA to disperse reversible platelet aggregates may be of value in determining the nature of the increased MPV in this situation[23].

E. INFLUENCE OF SHEAR RATE

Apart from physiological agonists, physical shear stress, particularly at sites of vessel bifurcation and stenosis can promote platelet activation and enhance the response to biochemical stimuli, contributing to thrombogenesis in patients with ischemic stroke or transient ischemic attack[24]. Measurement of the effect of shear rate on platelet activation and the effect of various pharmacological agents on this parameter may provide further information on the role of platelets in cerebrovascular events and be useful in evaluating antiplatelet agents for the prevention of stroke in patients with atherosclerosis[25].

V. COAGULOPATHY AND STROKE

A. DEFICIENCY IN CLOTTING FACTORS

Intracranial hemorrhage is a major complication of severe congenital deficiency of coagulation factors, such as VIII or IX. Intracranial bleeding may follow minimal trauma and once localising signs are present hemorrhage is usually extensive. Prior to HIV infection intracranial hemorrhage was the most common cause of premature death in patients with severe deficiency of factor VIII or IX (<1%). Hemorrhagic stroke may complicate deficiency of other coagulation factors, eg; homozygous factor XI or VII deficiency.

B. DEFICIENCY OF ANTICOAGULANT PROTEINS

Congenital deficiency of Antithrombin[26], Protein C[27] and Protein S[28] has been reported anecdotally or in small series but there is still inconclusive evidence that deficiency is instrumental in the pathogenesis of arterial thrombosis. The recently described mutation in the factor V gene resulting in a resistance to the anticoagulant effect of activated protein C does not increase the risk of thrombotic stroke[29].

C. ANTIPHOSPHOLIPID ANTIBODY SYNDROME

The development of lupus anticoagulant or anticardiolipin antibody (in the context of SLE or the antiphospholipid syndrome) is associated with an increased risk of thrombosis, including stroke. A recent study indicates that anticoagulant therapy to maintain an INR in excess of 3.0 significantly reduces the risk of thrombosis[30] (see also the chapter on antiphospholipids by D. Triplett).

D. ELEVATION OF COAGULATION FACTORS

Elevated levels of Fibrinogen, factors VII & VIII and von Willebrand factor are risk factors for thrombosis[31]. These changes may be markers of atherosclerosis rather than being causative and as yet there is no evidence that intervention to lower the levels of these factors per se reduces the risk of thrombosis, including stroke.

D. ELEVATED ENDOGENOUS t-PA AND STROKE

Activation of the fibrinolytic system may occur years in advance of clinically apparent events in the cerebral circulation. Accordingly a high concentration of tissue plasminogen activity (tPA) may be associated with future risk of stroke. This is now substantiated by the study of Ridker et al[32] indicating the mean concentration of tPA antigen is significantly higher among men who later had strokes than in controls. Moreover the age adjusted relative risk was higher for thromboembolic stroke than for total stroke. High values of tPA activity were also found independent of an abnormal plasma lipid profile or of the other stroke risk factors.

VI. PARAPROTEINAEMIA AND STROKE

Patients with macroglobulinemia or multiple myeloma have an increasing tendency to develop both cerebral hemorrhage and ischemic stroke. Several factors such as hyperviscosity induced by high molecular weight paraproteins, erythrocyte rouleaux formation and disturbance of platelet function, thrombin generation and fibrin polymerisation may all contribute to the development of thrombotic or hemorrhagic stroke. Hyperviscosity is influenced by the concentration and class of immunoglobulin. The exponential increase in viscosity is greatest with IgM and thereafter IgA and then IgG3 [33]. Plasmapheresis is very effective at reducing viscosity as removal of a small proportion of paraprotein results in a major reduction in viscosity.

VII. HEMATOLOGICAL DISORDERS
AND CEREBRAL VENOUS THROMBOSIS (CVT)

The occlusion of cerebral veins by thrombosis is often associated with stasis in sites, causing ischemia and possibly hemorrhage. This makes the differential diagnosis of cerebral hemorrhagic infarction difficult in some cases. Such a distinction is important as the treatment of the two conditions are not essentially the same. The main causes of cerebral thrombosis are sepsis, paraneoplasia syndrome and some important unknown causes in which alterations in the haematological parameters need to be fully investigated. This is of particular relevance to patients with familial history of venous thrombosis, in particular ATIII deficiency. In this context, blood alterations responsible for CVT are very rare.

VIII. LABORATORY TESTS

According to Woimant and Bousser[34], from a practical point of view ; when a stroke occurs, especially in a young subject, the hematological tests of choice are : whole blood count and differential PT, APTT, fibrinogen, detection of a circulating anticoagulant and anticardiolipin measurement, eventually ATIII, Protein C, Protein S, plasminogen measurements and APC resistance diagnosis.

IX. CONCLUSION

The development of stroke is multifactorial involving vessel integrity and alterations of endothelial cell function. Nevertheless, alterations in the composition of the blood within the vessels may increase the risk of either thrombotic or hemorrhagic stroke. From the review of the current literature it is clear that although some improved differentiation of various aspects of stroke is now possible, which has improved the appropriate mode of therapy, much still remains to be achieved in this elusive field of clinical medicine. However, with the development of new markers of hypercoagulable states rapid advances in this direction are shortly expected. Nevertheless, the following hematological disorders are known to predispose to arterial ischemia, venous thrombosis and/or cerebral hemorrhage.

Table I : Hematological disorders and stroke from Woimant and Bousser [34]

Parameters	Arterial Ischemia	Cerebral Venous Thrombosis	Cerebral Hemorrhage
Red Cell			
Polycythemia vera	+	+	+
Renal polycythemia	+	?	-
Homozygote HbSS	+	+	+
β-Thalassemia	+	-	-
Anemia	+	+	-
PNH	+	+	+
Leucocytes			
Leukemia	+	+	+
Hypereosinophilic syndrome	+	-	+
Platelets			
Essential thrombocytopenia	+	+	+
Thrombocytopenia	-	-	+
Hyperactive platelets	?	?	-
Hypoactive platelets	-	-	+
Severe coagulation factor deficiency	-	-	+
Afibrinogenemia/dysfibriogenemia	?	?	+
ATIII-deficiency	-	+	-
Protein C/S deficiency	-	+	-
Activated protein C resistance	-	+?	-
Anti phospholipid syndrome	+	+	-
Paraproteinaemia	+	+	+

REFERENCES

1. **Massey E, Riggs J :** Neurologic manifestations of hematologic diseases. *Neurol Clin,* 7,549,1989.
2. **Schafer A,** Bleeding and thrombosis in the myeloproliferative disorders. *Blood,* 64,1,1984.
3. **Tartaglia A, Goldberg J, Berk O, Wasserman L :** Adverse effects of antiaggregating therapy in the treatment of polycythemia vera. *Semin in Haematol,* 33,172,1986.
4. **Berk P, Goldberg J, Donovan P, et al :** Therapeutic recommendations in polycythemia vera based on polycythemia vera study group protocols. *Semin Hematol* 23,132,1986.
5. **Ameri A, Bousser M :** Cerebral venous thrombosis. *Neurol Clin* 10,87,1992.
6. **Bogousslavsky J, Van Melle G, Regli, F :** The Lausanne Stroke Registry : analysis of 1000 consecutive patients with first stroke. *Stroke,* 19,1083,1988.
7. **Powers D, Wilson B, Imbus C, et al :** The natural history of stroke in sickle cell disease. *Am J Med* 65,461,1978.
8. **Russell M, Goldberg H, Hodson A, et al :** Effect of transfusion therapy on arteriographic abnormalities and on recurrence of stroke in sickle cell disease. *Blood,* 63,162,1984.
9. **Cohen A, Martin M, Silber J, et al :** A modified transfusion program for prevention of stroke in sickle cell disease. *Blood,* 79,1657,1992.
10. **Serjeant G :** The nervous system, in *Sickle Cell Disease,* G Serjeant (Editor), 1985, Osford University Press : Oxford.
11. **Hart R, Kanter M :** Haematologic disorders and ischemic stroke. A selective review. *Stroke* 21,1111,1990.
12. **Wong V, Yu Y, Liang R, et al :** Cerebral thrombosis in beta-thalasemia/hemoglobin disease. *Stroke,* 21,812,1990.
13. **Grauss F, Rogers L, Posner, J :** Cerebrovascular complications inpatients with cancer, *Medecine,* 64,16,1985.
14. **Moore P, Harley J, Fauci A :** Neurologic dysfunction in the idiopathic hypereosinophilic syndrome. *Ann Intern Med,* 102,109,1985.
15. **Roche S, Cross S, Kaufman B :** Intracranial hemorrhages occuring in the idiopathic hypereosinophilic syndrome. *J Neurol neurosurg Psychiatry,* 53, 440, 1990.
16. **Cortelazzo S, Finazzi G, Ruggeri M, et al :** Hydroxyurea for patients with essential thrombocythaemia and a high risk of thrombosis. *N Engl J Med* 332,1132,1995.
17. **Lee L, Baglin T :** Altered platelet phospholipid dependent thrombin generation in thrombocytopenia and thrombocytosis. *Br J Haem.* 89,131,1995.
18. **Beutler E :** Platelet transfusions : the 20,000/μl trigger. *Blood,* 81,1411,1993.
19. **Cohen D, Baglin T :** Assessment and management of immune thrombocytopenia in pregnancy and the neonate. *Arch Dis Childhood* 72,71,1995.

20. **Magnani H :** Heparin-induced thrombocytopenia (HIT) : an overview of 230 patients treated with Orgaran (Org 10172). *Thromb Haemostas* 70,554,1993.
21. **D'Erasmo E, Aliberti G, Celi F :** Platelet count, mean platelet volum and their relation to prognosis in cerebral infarction. *J Intern Med,* 227,11,1990.
22. **Obrenovitch T, Hallenbeck J :** Platelet accumulation in regions of low blood flow during the post-ischemic period. *Stroke,* 16,224,1985.
23. **Seghatchian M :** EDTA reveals the aggregation state and functional integrity of platelets. *Platelets* 5,219,1994.
24. **Goldsmith H, Marlow J, Yu S :** The effect of oscillary flow on the release rection andaggregation of human platelets. *Microvasc Res.* 11,335,1976.
25 **Fukuyama M, sukai K, Ftagaki I, et al :** Continuous measurement of shear-induced platelet aggregation. *Thromb Res,* 54,253,1989.
26. **Ueyama H, Hashimoto Y, Uchino M et al :** Progressing ischemic stroke in a homozygote with variant antithrombin III. *Stroke* 20,815,1989.
27. **Matsushita K, Kuriyama Y, Sawada T, Uchida K :** Cerebral infarction associated with protein C deficiency. *Stroke* 23,108,1992.
28. **Sacco R, Owen J, Mohr J, et al :** Free protein S deficiency : a possible association with cerebrovascular occlusion. *Stroke* 20,1657,1989.
29. **Ridker P, Hennekens C, Lindpaintner K et al :** Mutation in the gene coding for coagulation factorV and the risk of myocardial infarction, stroke, and venous thrombosis in apparently healthy men. *N Engl J Med* 332,993,1995.
30. **Khamashta M, Cuadrado M, Mujic F, et al :** The management of thrombosis in the antiphosphoipid-antibody syndrome. *N Engl J Med* 332,993,1995.
31. **Meade T, Mellows S, Brozovic M, et al :** Haemostatic function and ischemic heart disease : principle results of the Northwick Park Heart Sudy. *Lancet ii,* 533,1986.
32. **Ridker P, Hennekens C, Stampfer M, et al :** Prospective study of endogenous tissue plasminogen activator and risk of stroke. *Lancet ii* 940,1994.
33. **Somer T :** Rheology of paraproteinaemias and the plasma hyperviscosity syndrome. *Baillieres Clin Haematol* 1,695,1987.
34. **Woimant F, Bousser MG,** Affections hématologiques in *Accidents vasculaires cérébraux* Ed (Bogousslavsky J, Bousser MG, Mas JL) Doin,Paris,1993,324.

PAROXYSMAL NOCTURNAL HEMOGLOBINURIA
Pathogenesis and Clinical Manifestations of Thrombosis

T. Plesner, H. Birgens and N.E. Hansen
Herlev Hospital, University Hospital, Copenhagen

I. INTRODUCTION

Paroxysmal nocturnal hemoglobinuria (PNH) is a disease with a distinct propensity to vascular thrombosis. Although it is a rare disease its importance reaches beyond this rarity, mainly because recently the genetic defect and the biochemical abnormality have been described in detail opening up to a better understanding of mechanisms of hemolysis and thrombosis.

A. DEFINITION, OCCURRENCE DIAGNOSIS AND MOLECULAR BACKGROUND

PNH is an acquired, clonal stem cell disease which may be seen in all ages.[1-3] Although not definitely known it has been estimated to occur with a prevalence of 1:500,000 in the population. The principal clinical manifestation of PNH is a chronic hemolytic anemia with periodic exacerbations. The disease has a poorly understood relationship with aplastic anemia.[2] Thus, the PNH defect may sometimes be found in patients with aplastic anemia and PNH may develop into aplastic anemia. A novel development in this field was seen when it proved possible to treat patients with aplastic anemia successfully with immunosuppressive agents. Surprisingly, more than 20% of such patients develop PNH after regenerating from the aplasia, leading some to theorize that PNH, despite its membrane defect, confers a growth advantage to myeloid precursors in such circumstances.[4,5]

The diagnosis of PNH rests traditionally on the acidified serum test (Ham's test) or the sucrose hemolysis test, both of which demonstrate the enhanced sensitivity to complement lysis of PNH erythrocytes. With the recent knowledge of the basic membrane defect in PNH the diagnosis to-day should be confirmed by flow cytometry which will demonstrate the failure of blood cells to express phosphatidyl-inositol-glycan (PIG) anchored proteins.[6]

In recent years it has become clear that the common denominator behind the various clinical manifestations of PNH is a deficient expression of PIG-anchored proteins on blood cells (for reviews see ref. 2, 7). Genes encoding PIG-bound proteins (e. g. decay accelerating factor (DAF) and urokinase type plasminogen activator (uPAR)) are transcribed in PNH resulting in normal levels of mRNA for these proteins.[8,9] During the final processing of proteins destined for PIG-anchoring, a COOH-terminal hydrophobic fragment of 17-30 residues is removed and subsequently in normal cells the new COOH-terminus is condensed with a preassembled glycolipid moiety, possibly through the action of a transaminating enzyme.[10-13] PNH-affected cells are unable to synthesize the glycolipid anchor and as a consequence the proteins are not inserted into the plasma membrane. Murine cell lines exhibiting various defects in glycolipid anchor biosynthesis have been described and grouped into complementation classes.[14] The genetic defect in PNH has recently been traced to the PIG-A gene on the X-chromosome which is responsible for the first step in the biosynthesis of glycolipid anchors corresponding to the "group A" complementation class of the murine cell lines (Fig. 1).[15-18]

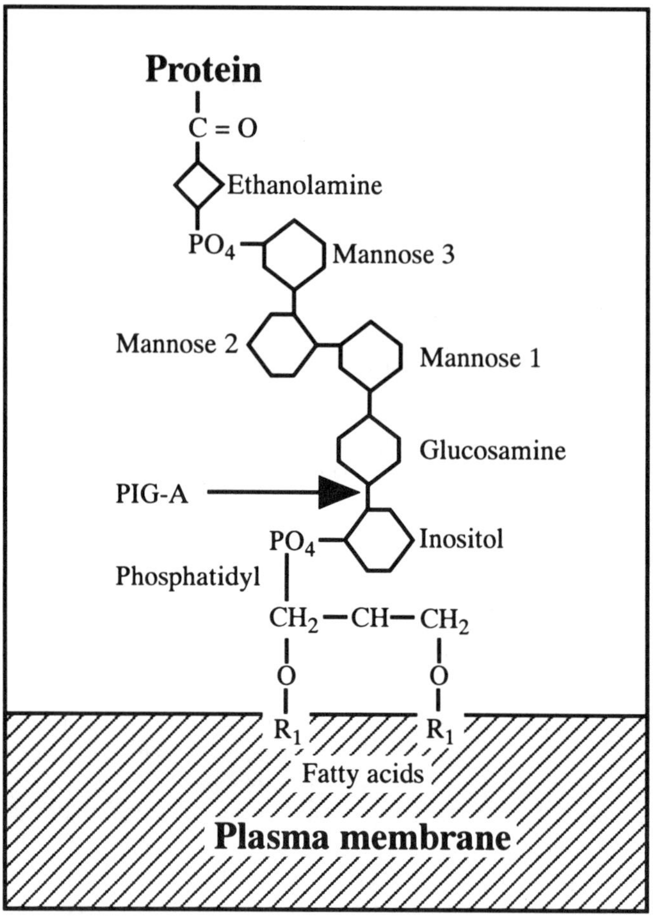

Figure 1: Diagram illustrating the basic structure of the phosphatidyl-inositol-glycan anchor. The genetic defect causing PNH has been traced to the PIG-A gene which is located to the X-chromosome and is responsible for the first step in the biosynthesis of the PIG-anchor (arrow).

B. CLINICAL MANIFESTATIONS

Although as a stem cell defect PNH affects all lineages of blood cell lines its main manifestation is due to hemolysis which is chronic with exacerbations during sleep (not necessarily associated with the night). Exacerbations of hemolysis are accompanied by hemoglobinuria and frequently also by bouts of abdominal pain. The combination of hemoglobinuria and abdominal pain may be misinterpreted as renal colic. The cause of the often intense and very disturbing attacks of abdominal pain is unexplained but may be due to mesenteric microthrombi. The pronounced hemoglobinuria often causes significant iron deficiency. Signs of bone marrow dysfunction with neutropenia and thrombocytopenia are frequently seen in PNH.[3,19,20]

II. THROMBOSIS IN PNH

Patients with PNH have a strong tendency for thrombotic events, mainly in the venous vasculature. Not seldom, these thromboses occur at rather extraordinary sites. Most frequent and serious are thromboses in the portal and hepatic veins.[21,22] Actually, hepatic vein thrombosis (the Budd-Chiari syndrome) might occur in 15-25 % of PNH patients and is a leading cause of death in PNH.[23] The Budd-Chiari syndrome in PNH may have an abrupt presentation with a painful enlarged liver and ascites. In some patients, however, the clinical course is more insidious, and the only clue to the presence of thrombosis in the hepatic veins is a slight elevation in liver enzymes such as aminotransferases. Ultrasonography seems to be the most sensitive of the non-invasive methods to detect hepatic vein thrombosis, and should be performed regularly (Fig. 2).[24]

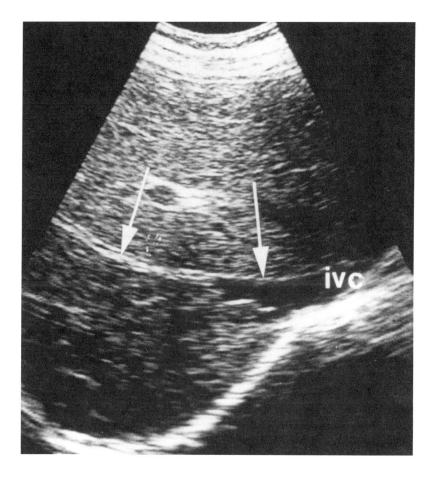

Figure 2 : Ultrasonogram demonstrating hepatic vein thrombosis in PNH (for details please see ref. 24). Reprinted with permission from Blackwell Scientific Publications Limited.

Thrombosis in the cerebral veins and dural sinus are well-described, and a severe sustained headache in a patient with PNH might be due to thrombosis in small cerebral veins.[25,26]

Thrombosis in the deep veins of the extremities is common. Also thrombotic skin lesions have been described in PNH.[27]

A. PATHOGENESIS OF THROMBOSIS

Human hemopoietic cells are usually protected from autologous activated complement by a series of proteins bound to the cell membrane by a PIG-anchor. Members of this family include decay-accelerating factor (DAF), which degrades or inhibits the assembly of C3 convertase, membrane-inhibitor of reactive lysis (MIRL) - an inhibitor of formation of the C5b-9 complex, and homologous restriction factor or C8-binding protein. Failure of erythrocytes to express these protective proteins will increase their susceptibility to complement components, shorten their life span (i.e. cause hemolysis) and, dependent on the capacity of the bone marrow to substitute the loss, result in variable degrees of anemia.

1. Platelets

The platelets in patients with PNH lack the same PIG-anchored membrane proteins as the red cells,[28] but the linkage between these findings and the pronounced tendency for thrombotic events in patients with PNH is not so clear-cut as the mechanism described in hemolysis.[29] The *in vivo* lifetime of PNH platelets is within the normal range, indicating that platelet lysis is not the cause of thrombosis in PNH.[30] Most likely the development of thrombosis in PNH is based on a multitude of abnormalities (Table I).

Table I

Factors which may Contribute to the Increased Thrombotic Tendency in Patients
with Paroxysmal Nocturnal Hemoglobinuria.

Increased sensitivity of platelets to complement :
> Lack of decay-accelerating factor (DAF) causes increased activation of classical C3 convertase leading to increased sensitivity of platelets to thrombin.
> Lack of membrane-inhibitor of reactive lysis (MIRL) causes increased assembly of the final C5b-9 polymer leading to exposure of membrane prothrombinase sites in platelets.
> Lack of homologous restriction factor causes enhanced formation of the final complement complex leading to increased platelet activation.

Impaired fibrinolysis:
> Lack of uPAR on PNH-leukocytes may impair the uPA-dependent plasminogen activation.
> Elevated plasma uPAR in PNH may competitively inhibit the binding of pro-uPA to the cell-associated uPAR.

Increased pro-coagulant activity:
> Increased liberation of "thromboplastic" material from hemolyzed PNH erythrocytes.

In normal platelets the susceptibility to aggregation after exposure to thrombin is increased in the presence of complement.[31] Platelets from patients with PNH are extraordinarily sensitive to thrombin.[29] They show increased C3 binding and platelet release reaction during activation of the alternative complement pathway.[32] This phenomenon may be due to lack of DAF in the platelet membrane, since the alternative pathway C3 convertase is not downregulated by DAF in this case. DAF however, is not the only molecule of importance for regulation of the alternative pathway C3 convertase. The platelet protein "factor H", which is released from thrombin-stimulated platelets, probably has a similar function as DAF with respect to anti-complementary effects, and may constitute a second mechanism, not impaired in PNH, to regulate surface-bound alterative pathway C3 convertase.[30]

The importance of DAF in regulating the classical pathway of complement activation is demonstrated by the increased susceptibility of the PNH platelet to lysis by antibody and complement.[33]

Thus, due to the rather more complex situation in the case of the alternative pathway for complement activation the biological consequences of the absence of DAF from the platelet membrane of PNH patients is still an open question.

MIRL inhibits the assembly of the final C5b-9 polymer by inhibiting the binding of C9 to the C5b-8 complex. The lack of MIRL, as seen on PNH platelets, might result in an enhanced production of this late-stage complement complex. Since the C5b-9 complement complex causes release of membrane vesicles from the platelet surface which contain receptors for factor Va and express prothrombinase activity, the consequence in PNH patients may be an increased tendency toward thrombotic complications.[34,35]

Also the lack of homologous restriction factor or C8 binding protein in the platelet membrane may, due to loss of the normal inhibition by this protein of terminal complement components, contributes to the enhanced platelet stimulation and thrombotic complications in PNH patients.[36]

2. Fibrinolysis

The fibrinolytic system is also partly impaired in PNH.[37] A key molecule in the urokinase dependent plasminogen activation is a specific cell surface receptor, uPAR, which is attached to the cell membrane by a glycolipid anchor in normal, but not in PNH affected leukocytes (Fig. 3).[9,37,39] The failure of PNH-leukocytes to express uPAR renders the cells incapable of supporting uPA-dependent plasminogen activation and may contribute to the development of clinically manifest thrombosis.[37,39] Neutrophils have been shown to accumulate rapidly in thrombi and contribute to the degradation of fibrin.[40,41] Theoretically, the failure of PNH leukocytes to activate plasminogen locally may tip the balance in favor of propagating a thrombus that will ultimately cause clinical symptoms. Membrane anchoring of uPAR is important for the biological activity of this molecule.[42] We have previously shown that uPAR is released in a water soluble form from PNH-cells and is present in PNH-plasma.[9] Elevated plasma uPAR may further impair the uPA-dependent fibrinolytic system in PNH by competitive inhibition of binding of circulating pro-uPA to cell associated uPAR. This may interfere with the conversion of pro-uPA to active enzyme, inhibit plasmin generation and thereby possibly contribute to the development of clinically manifest thrombosis in PNH.

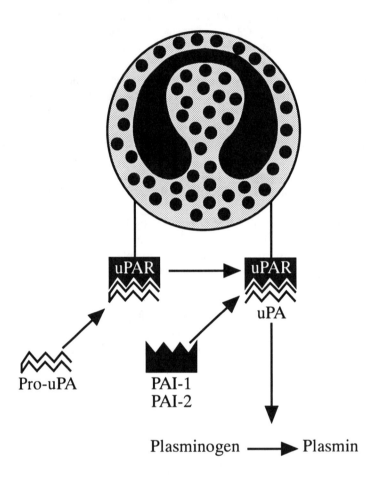

Figure 3 : Diagram illustrating the role of uPAR in cell-associated plasminogen activation. Enzymatically inactive pro-uPA is bound to a highly specific receptor and converted to enzymatically active uPA which subsequently activates plasminogen and thereby generates plasmin. Through the action of plasmin other proteolytic enzymes may be activated. The system is regulated by plasminogen activator inhibitors (PAI-1, PAI-2). uPAR is attached to the plasma membrane by a PIG-anchor. Leukocytes affected by PNH therefore do not express uPAR and cell-associated plasminogen activation by these cells is impaired (for review see ref. 39).

3. Miscellaneous

Liberation of "thromboplastic" material from hemolyzed erythrocytes has been proposed to be a contributing factor for the risk of thrombosis in PNH.[22,43]

The various factors that may contribute to thrombosis in PNH are summarized in Table I.

B. TREATMENT OF THROMBOSIS IN PNH

The only treatment that may cure PNH is allogeneic bone marrow transplantation from an HLA-identical donor, preferably an HLA-matched sibling donor.[44,45] The indication for this treatment modality may be obvious in the young patient, if PNH is associated with severe aplastic anemia, but in patients in whom the principal clinical manifestation is hemolytic anemia one must weigh the risk of complications from bone marrow transplantation against the severity of the hemolytic process and the risk of thrombosis.

Thrombotic complications may be treated with classical antithrombotic therapy including heparin and anticoagulants such as coumarin or warfarin. It has been postulated that some caution must be exercised in the use of heparin, since especially low-dose heparin may stimulate the alternative pathway of complement activation resulting in aggravation of the hemolysis, whereas high-dose heparin has anti-complementary properties.[46,47] Exacerbation of hemolysis has been described in PNH after treatment with low-dose heparin.[47] In fulminant hepatic vein or inferior vena cava thrombosis thrombolytic therapy with streptokinase and urokinase[48] or tissue plasminogen activator[49] may be indicated. In the latter paper, the thrombi were lysed successfully as long as 10-20 days after the presentation of the initial symptoms of hepatic vein thrombosis.

Whether PNH patients with or without earlier thrombotic complications should be kept on lifelong anticoagulant therapy is an unsolved question. We have treated one patient with manifest Budd-Chiari syndrome and two patients with asymptomatic thrombosis in the hepatic veins[24] with warfarin since 1985, and in this period we have not seen any signs of progression or development to manifest thrombosis. Women with PNH should probably refrain from the use of oral contraceptives in order to decrease the risk of thromboembolic complications.

REFERENCES

1. **Oni, S.B., Osunkoya, B.O. and Luzzatto, L.,** Paroxysmal Nocturnal Hemoglobinuria: Evidence for Monoclonal Origin of Abnormal Red Cells, *Blood,* 36, 145, 1970.
2. **Rotoli, B. and Luzzatto, L.,** Paroxysmal nocturnal hemoglobinuria, *Sem. Hematol.,* 26, 201, 1989.
3. **Ware, R.E., Hall, S.E. and Rosse, W.F.,** Paroxysmal nocturnal hemoglobinuria with onset in childhood and adolescence, *N. Engl. J. Med.,* 325, 991, 1991.
4. **Najean, Y. and Haguenauer, O.,** Long-term (5 to 20 years) Evolution of nongrafted aplastic anemias. The Cooperative Group for the Study of Aplastic and Refractory Anemias, *Blood,* 76, 2222, 1990.
5. **Tichelli, A., Gratwohl, A., Nissen, C., Signer, E., Stebler Gysi, C. and Speck, B.,** Morphology in patients with severe aplastic anemia treated with antilymphocyte globulin, *Blood,* 80, 337, 1992.
6. **Plesner, T., Hansen, N.E. and Carlsen, K.,** Estimation of PI-bound proteins on bloodcells from PNH patients by quantitative flow cytometry, *Br. J. Haematol.,* 75, 585, 1990.
7. **Rosse, W.F.,** Phosphatidylinositol-linked proteins and paroxysmal nocturnalhemoglobinuria, *Blood,* 75, 1595, 1990.
8. **Stafford, H.A., Tykocinski, M.L., Lublin, D.M., Holers, V.M., Rosse, W.F., Atkinson, J.P. and Medof, M.E.,** Normal polymorphic variations and transcription of the decay accelerating factor gene in paroxysmal nocturnal hemoglobinuria cells, *Proc. Natl. Acad. Sci. U. S. A.,* 85, 880, 1988.
9. **Ploug, M., Eriksen, J., Plesner, T., Hansen, N.E. and Dan0, K.,** A soluble form of the glycolipid-anchored receptor for urokinase-type plasminogen activator is secreted from peripheral blood leukocytes from patients with paroxysmal nocturnal hemoglobinuria, *Eur. J. Biochem.,* 208, 397, 1992.
10. **Low, M.G. and Saltiel, A.R.,** Structural and functional roles of glycosyl-phosphatidylinositol in membranes, *Science,* 239, 268, 1988.
11. **Bailey, C.A., Gerber, L., Howard, A.D. and Udenfriend, S.,** Processing at the carboxyl terminus of nascent placental alkaline phosphatase in a cell-free system: evidence for specific cleavage of a signal peptide, *Proc. Natl. Acad. Sci. U. S. A.,* 86, 22, 1989.
12. **Micanovic, R., Kodukula, K., Gerber, L.D. and Udenfriend, S.,** Selectivity at the cleavage/attachment site of phosphatidylinositol-glycan anchored membrane proteins is enzymatically determined, *Proc. Natl. Acad. Sci. U.S.A.,* 87, 7939, 1990.
13. **Doering, T.L., Masterson, W.J., Hart, G.W. and Englund, P.T.,** Biosynthesis of glycosyl phosphatidylinositol membrane anchors, *J. Biol. Chem.,* 265, 611, 1990.
14. **Fatemi, S.H. and Tartakoff, A.M.,** The phenotype of five classes of T lymphoma mutants. Defective glycophospholipid anchoring, rapid degradation, and secretion of Thy-1 glycoprotein, *J. Biol. Chem.,* 263, 1288, 1988.
15. **Miyata, T., Takeda, J., Iida, Y., Yamada, N., Inoue, N., Takahashi, M., Maeda, K., Kitani, T. and Kinoshita, T.,** The cloning of PIG-A, a component in the early step of GPI-anchor biosynthesis, *Science,* 259, 1318, 1993.
16. **Takeda, J., Miyata, T., Kawagoe, K., Iida, Y., Endo, Y., Fujita, T., Takahashi, M., Kitani, T. and Kinoshita, T.,** Deficiency of the GPI anchor caused by a somatic mutation of the PIG-A gene in paroxysmal nocturnal hemoglobinuria, *Cell,* 73, 703, 1993.

17. **Takahashi, M., Takeda, J., Hirose, S., Hyman, R., Inoue, N., Miyata, T., Ueda, E., Kitani, T., Medof, M.E. and Kinoshita, T.,** Deficient biosynthesis of N-acetylglucosaminyl-phosphatidylinositol, the first intermediate of glycosyl phosphatidylinositol anchor biosynthesis, in cell lines established from patients with paroxysmal nocturnal hemoglobinuria, *J. Exp. Med.,* 177, 517, 1993.
18. **Bessler, M., Mason, P. J., Hillmen, P., Miyata, T., Yamada, N., Takeda, J., Luzzatto, L. and Kinoshita, T.,** Paroxysmal Nocturnal Haemoglobinuria (PNH) Is Caused by Somatic Mutations in the Pig-A Gene, *EMBO J ,* 13, 110, 1994.
19. **Crosby, W.H.,** Paroxysmal nocturnal hemoglobinuria. Relation of the clinical manifestations to underlying mechanisms, *Blood,* 8, 769, 1953.
20. **Dacie, J.V. and Lewis, S.M.,** Paroxysmal nocturnal hemoglobinuria: Clinical manifestations, haematology, and nature of the disease, *Sem. Hematol.,* 5, 3, 1972.
21. **Grossman J.A. and Mc Dermont W.V.,** paroxismal nocturnal hemoglobinuria associated with hepatic and portal venous thrombosis. *Am. J. Surg.,* 127, 733, 1974.
22. **Peytremann, R., Rhodes, R.S. and Hartmann R.C.,** Thrombosis in paroxysmal nocturnal hemoglobinuria (PNH) with particular reference to progressive hepatic venous thrombosis. *Series haematologica* V, 115, 1972.
23. **Leibovitz, A.L. and hartmann R.C.,** The Budd-Chiari syndrome and paroxysmal nocturnal haemoglobinuria , *Br. J. Haematol.,* 48, 1, 1981.
24. **Birgens HS, Hancke S., Rosenklintt, A. and Hansen, N.E.,** Ultrasonic demonstration of clinical and subclinical hepatic venous thrombosis in paroxysmal nocturnal hemoglobinuria, *Br. J. Haematol.,* 64, 737, 1986.
25. **Johnson, R.V., Kaplan, S.R. and Blaibock, Z.R.,** Cerebral venous thrombosis in paroxysmal nocturnal hemoglobinuria, marchiafava-Micheli disease. *Neurology,* 20, 681, 1970.
26. **Donhowe, S.P. and Lazaro, R.P.,** Dural sinus thrombosis in paroxysmal nocturnal hemoglobinuria. *Clinical Neurology and Neurosurgery,* 86, 149, 1984.
27. **Rietschel, R.L., Lewis, C.W., Simmons, R.A. and Phyliky, R.L.,** Skin lesions in paroxysmal nocturnal hemoglobinuria, *Archives of Dermatology,* 114, 540, 1978.
28. **Nicholson-Weller, A., Spicer, D.B. and Austen, K.F.,** Deficiency of the complement regulatory protein, « decay-accelerating factor » on membranes of granulocytes, monocytes and platelets in paroxysmal nocturnal hemoglobinuria. *N. Engl. J. Med.,* 312, 1091, 1985.
29. **Rosse, W.F.,** paroxysmal nocturnal hemoglobinuria : the biochemical defects and the clinical syndrome. *Blood reviews,* 3, 192, 1989.
30. **Devine, D.V., Siegel, R.S. and Rosse, W.F.,** Interactions of the platelets in paroxysmal nocturnal hemoglobinuria with complement. *J. Clin. Invest.,* 79, 131, 1987.
31. **Polley, M.J. and Nachman, R.,** The human complement system in thrombin-mediated platele function. *J. Exp. Med.,* 147, 1713, 1978.
32. **Dixon, R.H., and Rosse, W.F.,** Mechanism of complement-mediated activation of human blood platelets in vitro. Comparison of normal and paroxysmal nocturnal hemoglobinuria platelets. *J. Clin. Invest,* 59, 360, 1977.
33. **Aster, R.H. and Enwright, S.E.,** A platelet and granulocyte membrane defect in paroxysmal nocturnal hemoglobinuria : Usefulness fo the detection of platelet antibodies. *J.Clin. Invest.,* 48, 1199, 1969.
34. **Sims, P.J., Faioni, E.M., Wiedmer, T. and Shattil, S. J.,** Complement proteins C5b-9 cause release of membrane vesicles from the platelet surface that are enriched in the membrane receptor for coagulation factor Va and express prothrombinase activity, *J. Biol. Chem.,* 263, 18205, 1988.
35. **Wiedmer, T., Hall, S.E., Ortel, T.L., Kane, W.H., Rosse, W.F. and Sims, P.J.,** Complement-Induced Vesiculation and Exposure of Membrane Prothrombinase Sites in Platelets of Paroxysmal Nocturnal Hemoglobinuria, *Blood,* 82, 1192, 1993.
36. **Blaas, P., Berger, B., Weber, S., Peter, H.H. and Hansch, G.M.,** Paroxysmal nocturnal hemoglobinuria. Enhanced stimulation of platelets by the terminal complement components is related to the lack of C8bp in the membrane, *J Immunol.,* 140, 3045, 1988.
37. **Ploug, M., Plesner, T., Ronne, E., Ellis, V., Hoyer-Hansen, G., Hansen, N.E. and Dano, K.,** The receptor for urokinase-type plasminogen activator is deficient on peripheral blood leukocytes in patients with paroxysmal nocturnal hemoglobinuria, *Blood,* 79, 1447, 1992.
38. **Ploug, M., Behrendt, N., Lober, D. and Dano, K.,** Protein structure and membrane anchorage of the cellular receptor for urokinase-type plasminogen activator, *Seminars In Thrombosis & Hemostasis,* 17, 183, 1991.
39. **Ellis, V., Ploug, M., Plesner, T. and Dano, K.,** Gene expression and function of the cellular receptor for uPA (uPAR), *Fibrinolysis in disease,* CRC Press, Inc. 1994.(In Press).
40. **Henry, R.L.,** Leukocytes and thrombosis, *Thromb. Diath. Haemorrhagica,* 13, 35, 1965.
41. **Murphy Ullrich, J.E. and Mosher, D.F.,** Localization of thrombospondin in clots formed in situ, *Blood,* 66, 1098, 1985.
42. **Ellis, V., Behrendt, N. and Dano, K.,** Plasminogen activation by receptor-bound urokinase. A kinetic study with both cell-associated and isolated receptor, *J. Biol. Chem.,* 266, 12752, 1991.
43. **Newcomb, T.F. and Gardner, F.H.,** Thrombin generation in paroxysmal nocturnal haemoglobinuria, *Br.J. Haematol., 9,* 84, 1963.
44. **Antin, J.H., Ginsburg, D., Smith, B.R., Nathan, D.G., Orkin, S.H. and Rappeport, J.M.,** Bone marrow transplantation for paroxysmal nocturnal hemoglobinuria: Eradication of the PNH clone and documentation of complete lymphohematopoietic engraftment, *Blood,* 66, 1247, 1985.
45. **Kawahara, K., Witherspoon, R.P. and Storb, R.,** Marrow transplantation for paroxysmal nocturnal hemoglobinuria, *American Journal of Hematology ,* 39, 283, 1992.
46. **Logue, G.L.,** Effect of heparin on complement activation and lysis in paroxysmal nocturnal hemoglobinuria red cells, *Blood,* 50, 239, 1977.
47. **Rosse, W.F.,** Treatment of paroxysmal nocturnal hemoglobinuria, *Blood,* 60, 20, 1982.
48. **Scholar, P.W. and Bell, W.R.,** Thrombolytic therapy for inferior vena cava thrombosis in paroxysmal nocturnal hemoglobinuria, *Ann. Int. Med.,* 103, 539, 1985.
49. **Mcmullin, M.F., Hillmen, P., Jackson, J., Ganly, P. and Luzzatto, L.,** Tissue Plasminogen Activator for Hepatic Vein Thrombosis in Paroxysmal Nocturnal Haemoglobinuria, *J Intern. Med.,* 235, 85, 1994.

SPINAL CORD INJURY: PATHOPHYSIOLOGY OF HYPERCOAGULABILITY AND CLINICAL MANAGEMENT

D. Green and D. Chen

Atherosclerosis Program, Rehabilitation Institute of Chicago, Illinois

I. PATHOPHYSIOLOGY OF HYPERCOAGULABILITY IN SPINAL CORD INJURY

In discussing the thrombotic tendency of patients with spinal cord injury (SCI), it is helpful to recall Virchow's Triad[1], which recognizes the contributions to thrombogenesis of the vessel wall, blood flow, and blood constituents. The blood vessel, and specifically the venous endothelium, may be injured by extrinsic pressure on the immobilized limbs of the paralyzed patient. In addition, the course of SCI patients is frequently complicated by inflammation and sepsis; exposure to free oxygen radicals or endotoxins may damage endothelium and provoke thrombosis. Reduced blood flow may be due to increased blood viscosity secondary to dehydration, transudation of fluid into the interstitial spaces of paralyzed limbs, and hyperfibrinogenemia; the latter is increased as a stress reactant.

Many profound changes occur in constituents of the hemostatic system. Not only is fibrinogen increased, but factor VIII and von Willebrand factor also rise[2] again as stress reactants. Several years ago, we measured factor VIII and von Willebrand factor levels in 37 patients with acute SCI not receiving thromboprophylaxis[3]. As shown in the lower panels of Figure 1, plasma levels of these hemostatic factors rose soon after injury, reaching maximum values two to three times normal about a week after injury. This coincided with the peak incidence of the diagnosis of venous thrombosis (Figure 2). When prophylaxis with calf compression boots with or without platelet function antagonists was implemented in the next 27 patients, both the frequency of thrombosis and the rise of factor VIII and von Willebrand factor were blunted.

We also performed serial determinations of platelet function, measuring their ability to aggregate in vitro (the platelet aggregate ratio[4] and platelet responsiveness to the aggregating activity of human collagen[5]. In untreated patients, both measures showed changes toward platelet hyperreactivity; with thromboprophylaxis there was a trend toward normalization of platelet function (Figure 1).

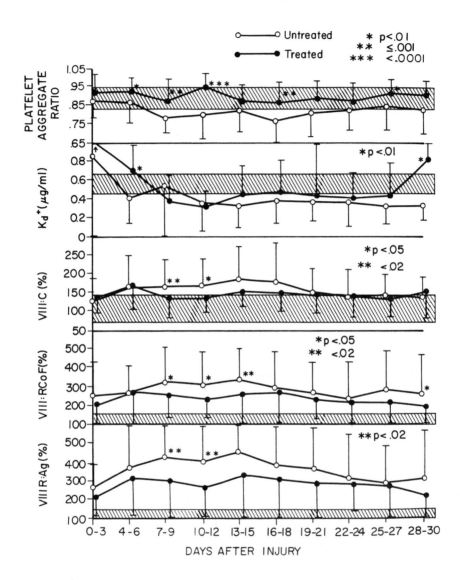

Figure 1 : Coagulation changes in acute spinal cord injury. Patients received no prophylaxis (untreated, n=37) or had external pneumatic calf compression (treated, n=27).

  Platelet aggregate ratio: varies inversely with affinity of platelets for each other.

  Kd: varies inversely with affinity of platelets for collagen

  VIII:C: Factor VIII coagulant activity

  VIII RCoF: functional activity of von Willebrand factor

  VIII RAg: von Willebrand factor antigen

  (Reproduced from (3) with permission)

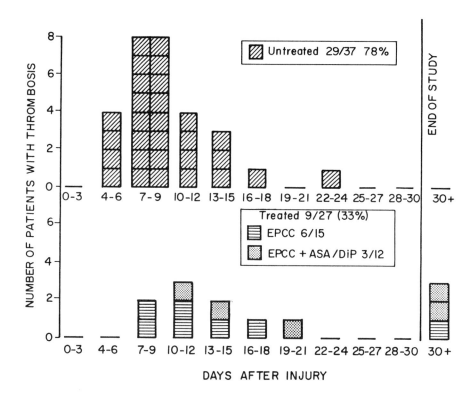

EPCC=external pneumatic calf compression
ASA/DiP=aspirin/dipyridamole (reproduced from (3) with permission)
Figure 2 : Deep vein thrombosis, detected by fibrinogen uptake test, in treated and untreated patients.

In addition to raised clotting factor levels and enhanced platelet function, other hemostatic changes in acute SCI affect inhibitors of coagulation and fibrinolysis. In the former category are decreases in antithrombin III, which may occur after trauma or surgery or associated with catabolic states. A reduction in the levels of proteins C and S is also possible, although these have yet to be measured in SCI. Diminished fibrinolysis may occur through three mechanisms; decreased release of tissue plasminogen activator due to lack of muscle contraction in paralyzed limbs[6,7], inhibition of plasminogen binding to fibrin by high ambient concentrations of fibrinogen[8] and increases in plasma levels of plasminogen activator inhibitor-1[9], a stress reactant. Impaired fibrinolysis is especially disabling as it may cause delayed recanalization of thrombosed vessels. We studied 50 patients with venographically confirmed lower limb venous thrombosis[10]. At three week intervals, venous ultrasound was performed to detect vein recanalization, which occurred by day 33 (mean value) in 26 non-paralyzed subjects (Figure 3). In contrast, recanalization was not observed until day 42 in hemiplegic patients and day 54 in para and quadriplegia ($p<0.04$ as compared with non-paralyzed subjects). This probably reflects the impaired fibrinolysis reported in such patients.

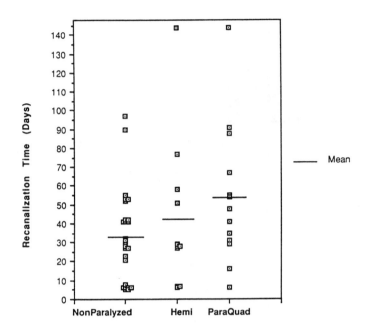

Figure 3 : Recanalization time in non-paralyzed and paralyzed subjects.
(Reproduced from (10) with permission)

II. INCIDENCE OF THROMBOEMBOLISM IN SPINAL CORD INJURY

Deep vein thrombosis (DVT) and pulmonary embolism (PE) are common complications of spinal cord injury, and are major causes of morbidity and mortality. Varying incidence figures for these complications have been reported. Unfortunately, the studies have not used uniform diagnostic techniques and/or criteria for assessment of thrombosis.

The earliest studies were based on autopsy findings and clinical criteria. Tribe[11] reported that pulmonary emboli were the cause of death in 37% of persons who died within three months of injury. In a review of 500 patients, Walsh and Tribe[12] reported a 13.2% incidence of thromboembolism in paraplegics. Watson[13] found an incidence of 12% for DVT and 5% for PE in 431 patients. In a later study, Watson[14] reported a 17% incidence of DVT and 10% of PE, and also noted that 85% of thrombotic episodes occurred within the first month after injury. Weingarden[15] summarized all studies in which the diagnosis of DVT and PE was based only on clinical criteria, and reported an incidence of 16.3%. Many of the patients with PE reported in these studies did not have clinical evidence of DVT.

In recent years, objective diagnostic techniques have improved the accuracy of DVT diagnosis. Using fibrinogen leg scanning, Todd et al[16] reported an incidence of 100% in SCI patients studied. It is important to note that in 40% of these patients the positive diagnosis was not confirmed by venography. Myllynen et al[17] also found a 100% incidence of DVT with the fibrinogen scanning method. Weingarden[15] summarized five studies that used fibrinogen scanning and impedance plethysmography. The incidence of DVT ranged from 47% to 100%.

Recently, duplex ultrasound imaging has become a popular non-invasive technique for diagnosing DVT. Unfortunately, the frequency of DVT in spinal cord injured persons as assessed by venous ultrasound has not been reported, nor has the sensitivity or specificity of this modality been validated using venography as the "gold standard." Nevertheless, whether such patients are studied by sensitive laboratory tests or simply examined at the bedside, they are very vulnerable to thrombosis, and effective, safe prophylactic measures are warranted.

III. PROPHYLACTIC MEASURES

A number of methods are available for the prevention of thromboembolism. They include physical modalities such as leg elevation and massage, compression stockings, and intermittent compression boots, and pharmacologic interventions such as antiplatelet agents, volume expanders, and anticoagulants. However, the prevention of thrombosis in patients with spinal cord injury poses a number of special problems. First, measures of proven efficacy such as early ambulation, which are used routinely in patients undergoing operations, cannot be applied to partially or completely paralyzed individuals with unstable spines. Second, there is great concern that even the slightest bleeding at the site of spinal cord injury will worsen the neurologic deficit; such bleeding could be provoked by antiplatelet or anticoagulant therapy. Third, the SCI patient is likely to remain at risk for thromboembolism for a protracted period, measured in weeks to months rather than days. Finally, the hospital course of the SCI patient may be punctuated by many acute interventions such as spine stabilization procedures, insertion of tracheostomy and enterostomy tubes, central lines, etc., so that rapid reversal of anti-hemostatic treatment must be readily achievable. For all these reasons, few trials of thromboprophylaxis have been undertaken in this patient population.

A . HEPARIN

A variety of studies have evaluated the effectiveness of heparin, oral anticoagulant agents, and physical modalities. Casas[18] compared two heparin doses (5,000 U or 7,500 U, subcutaneously (SC), every 12 hours) and found no cases of DVT by clinical examination in patients who remained in the study. Watson[19] compared a heparin treated group to an untreated control group from an earlier time period. He reported a 0% incidence of DVT in the treatment group and 17% in the control. Frisbie et al[20] compared low dose heparin (5,000 U SC every 12 hours) with placebo, and found a nearly equal incidence of DVT, 7.7% in the heparin group and 6.4% in the placebo group. These older studies suffered from many methodological inadequacies, including weak study design and insensitive endpoints.

B . ORAL ANTICOAGULANTS

The safety and efficacy of oral anticoagulants has also been examined. Hachen[21] compared the use of acenocoumaral with historical controls who had received heparin (10,000 U SC every 12 hours). He reported a 21% incidence of DVT in the oral anticoagulant group and 6.8% in the heparin group, with essentially equal rates of bleeding complications. Silver[22] evaluated another anticoagulant, phenindione, and found a 6% incidence of DVT in treated patients and 25% in untreated controls. Anticoagulant-associated bleeding was a significant problem. It should be noted that the treatment intensity given in 1974 when Silver's study was published was much greater than is currently used and could account for the increased bleeding. While a contemporary study of oral anticoagulants might clarify this issue, there is little enthusiasm for this approach because of inherent problems with warfarin therapy. These included delay in onset of therapeutic activity, difficulties in starting and stopping treatment because patients require frequent invasive procedures, and the confounding effects of other medications which potentiate or inhibit warfarin effect.

C. PHYSICAL MODALITIES

Various physical modalities used alone or in combination with pharmacologic agents have been studied. Becker et al[23] examined the use of rotating beds, comparing continuous rotation versus periodic rotation. With I^{125} fibrinogen leg scanning as the method of thrombus detection, they reported a 40% incidence of DVT in the continuous rotation group versus 80% in the periodic rotation group. Merli et al[24] compared the use of electrical stimulation of the calf muscles plus low dose heparin (5,000 U SC every 8 hours) with low dose heparin alone and placebo. DVT occurred in 6.7% of the electrical stimulation plus heparin group, 50% of the heparin alone group, and 47% of the placebo group. However, electical stimulation was labor-intensive and caused discomfort in some patients. Thus, it is unlikely that this treatment could be generally adopted. Nevertheless, Merli's study provides strong evidence that some combination of mechanical and pharmacologic modalities may be the most effective prophylaxis of thromboembolism in spinal cord-injured patients.

IV. CLINICAL MANAGEMENT-THE NORTHWESTERN EXPERIENCE

A. INTERMITTENT COMPRESSION BOOTS

Our initial studies utilized intermittent leg compression boots and antiplatelet agents[3]. Thrombi were detected by the by the I^{125} fibrinogen test. Twenty-eight patients were studied: fifteen were randomized to boots alone, and thirteen to a combination of boots, aspirin (600 mg daily), and dipyridamole (225 mg daily). Thrombi were detected in 6 of the boots alone group, and three of the boots plus antiplatelet agent group (difference not significant). The overall frequency of thrombosis, however, was significantly less than that observed in previously studied patients receiving no specific thrombo-prophylaxis (33% vs 78%, p<0.001). Furthermore, not only were fewer patients affected, but the onset of thrombosis was delayed and fewer of the thrombi were in proximal veins. Adverse effects were not observed in the boots only patients, but one subject receiving aspirin required urgent cervical fusion and bled extensively during the procedure. We concluded that compression boots were a partially effective means of preventing thromboembolism in SCI, but that the use of aspirin entailed too great a risk of bleeding in these very vulnerable patients.

Further experience with leg compression boots has revealed some important liabilities. The boots must be carefully applied to the leg; if the patient is having leg spasms, the boots may slide down the leg and become constricting. The intermittent compression is dependent on the integrity of the tubing connecting the boots to the compression pump; patient transfers, bedmaking, and careless housekeepers can all result in disconnection of the device. Excursions to the radiology suite or rehabilitation therapy room may interrupt leg compression for long periods. Finally, in patients with impaired lower limb sensation, boots may produce hematomas and skin abrasions. Therefore, we evaluated the use of anticoagulants as thromboprophylactic agents in SCI.

B. ANTICOAGULANTS
1. Unfractionated Heparin (UFH)

UFH may be used in a variety of ways to prevent thrombosis. Small, fixed doses of 5000 U given subcutaneously every 12 h have been found to be very safe and moderately efficacious in patients with medical illnesses and in those undergoing abdominal surgical procedures[25]. Heparin in these doses may be combined with leg compression boots to augment effectiveness. Heparin may be given in variable doses sufficient to prolong the activated partial thromboplastin time (aPTT) to the high normal or low anticoagulant range; this method has been used to advantage in patients undergoing hip replacement surgery[26]. We conducted a randomized clinical trial to evaluate fixed versus adjusted doses of UFH in patients with acute SCI[27]. Thrombosis was detected by venous Doppler examination and impedance plethysmography, and positive tests were confirmed by contrast venography. Seventy-five patients were randomized, and 58 (29 in each group) either remained in the study for more than seven weeks or had a thrombotic or hemorrhagic event. Of the patients receiving 5000 U every 12 hrs, nine (31%) had thromboembolism, as compared with only 2 (7%) of those receiving the adjusted doses (mean dose, 13,200 U every 12 hrs). On the other hand, while no patient getting the fixed dose had bleeding, seven of those on the adjusted doses bled. Thus, the overall number of patients with an event (bleeding or thrombosis) was the same in these groups. Based on this experience, we decided to investigate other heparins in these patients.

2. Low Molecular Weight Heparin (LMWH)

LMWHs are prepared by fractionating UFH, conserving those fragments that retain the pentasaccharide sequence necessary for binding antithrombin III, and potentiating its anticoagulant activity[28]. In clinical trials, they compare favorably with UFH of both efficacy and safety[29]. We selected a LMWH, Logiparin (Novo Nordisk, Denmark), for comparison with UFH in acute SCI[30]. The UFH was given in a dose of 5000 U every 8 hrs, intermediate between the two doses used in our previous trial. The LMWH dose administered was 3500 anti-factor Xa units once daily. 60 patients were planned for this trial, but the study was stopped when only 41 had been enrolled because a highly statistically significant difference had emerged between the two treatments. Of the 21 patients randomized to UFH, five had thrombotic events, including two fatal pulmonary emboli, and two others had bleeding (event rate, 34.7%). None of the 20 patients given LMWH had thrombosis or bleeding (p-value for the difference between groups= 0.006 by log-rank test)(Figure 4).

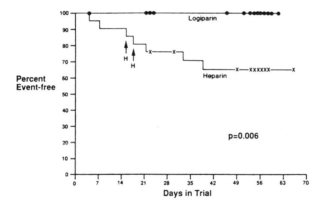

Figure 4 : Kaplan-Meier plot showing when hemorrhagic (H, arrows) or thrombotic events occurred. Times at which patients left the trial are shown by closed circles or crosses.
(Reproduced from (30) with permission)

Because of these results, during the next year all patients who would have met the eligibility criteria for the trial were given LMWH[31]. An additional 48 were enrolled, giving a total of 68 patients treated with LMWH. Events occurred in eight patients (11.8%); four had proximal vein thromboses, two had calf vein thromboses, and one suffered a fatal pulmonary embolism 39 days after injury. Only one patient had bleeding, which appeared within hours after a bowel resection. The estimated percentage of patients free of an event 56 days after injury was 85.9% (Figure 5).

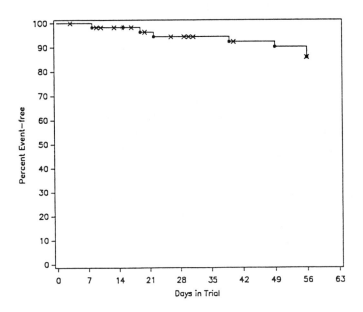

Figure 5 : Kaplan-Meier plot showing thrombosis-free survival for 60 patients treated with low molecular weight heparin. The estimated percentage of patients free of an event at 56 days is 85.9%. (Reproduced from (31) with permission)

We concluded that LMWH was significantly better than any UFH regimen studied in our previous trials (Table I).

Table I : The Northwestern Experience:
Low Molecular Weight Heparin(LMWH) vs Unfractionated Heparin(UFH)

	LMWH	UFH	p
Number of Patients	68	79	
Bleeding	1	9	0.04
Thrombosis	7	16	0.15
Total Events	8	25	0.007

V. DURATION OF THROMBOPROPHYLAXIS AFTER SPINAL CORD INJURY

An important question facing the clinician is how long to continue thromboprophylaxis. Prolonging anticoagulant administration increases the risk of bleeding and is costly. We studied this problem by discontinuing anticoagulant prophylaxis after eight weeks and then conducting weekly venous ultrasound examinations for the next four weeks[31]. Two of 33 patients (6%) developed thrombosis; one in the ileofemoral vein and one had a fatal pulmonary embolus. Both of these events occurred during the tenth week after spinal cord injury. To try to understand why certain patients might remain at risk for major thromboembolic events, we examined potential risk factors in patients with documented fatal pulmonary emboli[32]. As compared with 42 concurrently hospitalized SCI subjects without emboli, the nine patients who died of pulmonary emboli had a higher cord level of injury (fewer thoracic and lumbar injuries than in the controls, p=0.04), less spasticity (p=0.01), and a greater body mass index (p=0.01). There was also a trend toward more advanced age and more frequent serious infections. Thus, the patient at high risk of fatal embolism has a cervical spine injury and flaccid paralysis, is obese, older, and has had a more complicated hospital course. Such a patient should continue on LMWH prophylaxis for 12 or more weeks. On the other hand, persons who are walking or participating in rehabilitative therapies in an active rather than a passive role, and are making an accelerated recovery from their injury may cease thromboprophylaxis eight weeks after injury or even earlier if progress has been substantial.

VI. FUTURE INITIATIVES IN OPTIMIZING THROMBOPROPHYLAXIS

A multicenter trial is being conducted in North America to rigorously evaluate the safety and effectiveness of LMWH versus UFH in SCI. Approximately 350 patients will be fitted with leg and thigh compression leggings during the first two weeks following injury. All patients will also receive subcutaneous injections of either LMWH or UFH. At day 14, venography will be performed to compare the effectiveness of these two agents when combined with leggings in the initial management of SCI. Patients with negative venograms will then continue on either LMWH or UFH, without leggings, for eight weeks and then be restudied. This second phase of the study will determine which regimen is appropriate for the longer term management of these patients. This investigation should provide unambiguous guidelines for the prevention of thromboembolism in acute SCI.

REFERENCES

1. **Virchow R.** Phlogose und Thrombose in Gefabsystem, in *Gesammelte Abhandlungen zur Wissenschaftlicgen Medicin,* Virchow, R., Ed., Von Meidinger Sohn, Frankfurt, 1856, 458.
2. **Myllynen P, Kammonen M, Rokkanen P, et al.** The blood F VIII:Ag/ F VIII:C ratio is an early indicator of deep vein thrombosis during post-traumatic immobilization. *J Trauma* 1987;27:287.
3. **Green D, Rossi EC, Yao JST, Flinn WR, Spies SM.** Deep vein thrombosis in spinal cord injury: effect of prophylaxis with calf compression, aspirin, and dipyridamole. *Paraplegia* 1982;20:227.
4. **Wu KK, Hoak JC.** A new method for the quantitative detection of platelet aggregates in patients with arterial insufficiency. *Lancet* 1974;ii:924.
5. **Rossi EC, Louis G.** Kinetic parameters of platelet aggregation as an expression of platelet responsiveness. *Thromb Haemost* 1977; 37:283.
6. **Wiman B, Ljungberg B, Chmielewska J, Urden G, Blomback M, Johnsson H.** The role of the fibrinolytic system in deep vein thrombosis. *J Lab Clin Med* 1985; 105:265.
7. **Katz RT, Green D, Sullivan T, Yarkony G.** Functional electric stimulation to enhance systemic fibrinolytic activity in spinal cord injury patients. *Arch Phys Med Rehabil* 1987; 68:423.
8. **McDonagh J.** Suppression of plasminogen binding to fibrin by high fibrinogen: a mechansim for how high fibrinogen enhances the risk of thrombosis. *Bull Sanofi Assn Thromb Res* 1994; 4:2.
9. **Petaja J, Myllynen P, Rokkanen P, et al.** Fibrinolysis and spinal injury: relationship to post-traumatic deep vein thrombosis. *Acta Chir Scand* 1989; 155:241.
10. **Lim AC, Roth EJ, Green D.** Lower limb paralysis: its effect on the recanalization of deep-vein thrombosis. *Arch Phys Med Rehabil* 1992; 73:331.
11. **Tribe CR.** Causes of death in early and late stages in paraplegia. *Paraplegia* 1963;1:19.
12. **Walsh JJ, Tribe C.** Phlebo-thrombosis and pulmonary embolism in paraplegia. *Paraplegia* 1965;3:209.
13. **Watson N.** Anticoagulation therapy in prevention of venous thrombosis and pulmonary embolism in spinal cord injury. *Paraplegia* 1968;6:113.
14. **Watson N.** Anticoagulant therapy in the treatment of venous thrombosis and pulmonary embolism in acute spinal cord injury. *Paraplegia* 1974;12:197.
15. **Weingarden SI.** Deep venous thrombosis in spinal cord injury: overview of the problem. *Chest* 1992;102:636S-9S.
16. **Todd JW, Frisbie JH, Rossier AB, et al.** Deep venous thrombosis in acute spinal cord injury: comparison of 125 I fibrinogen leg scanning, impedance plethysmography and venography. *Paraplegia* 1976;14:50.
17. **Myllynen P, Kammonen M, Rokkanen P, et al.** Deep venous thrombosis and pulmonary embolism in patients with acute spinal cord injury: a comparison with non-paralyzed patients immobilized due to spinal fractures. *J Trauma* 1985;25:541.
18. **Casas E, Sanchez M, Arias C, et al.** Prophylaxis of venous thrombosis and pulmonary embolism in patients with acute traumatic spinal cord lesions. *Paraplegia* 1977-78;15:209.

19.   **Watson N.** Anticoagulant therapy in the prevention of venous thrombosis and pulmonary embolism in the spinal cord injury. *Paraplegia* 1978-79;16:265.
20.   **Frisbie J, Sasahara A.** Low dose heparin prophylaxis for DVT in acute spinal cord injured patients: a controlled study. *Paraplegia* 1981;19:343.
21.   **Hachen H.** Anticoagulant therapy in patients with spinal cord injury. *Paraplegia* 1974;12:176.
22.   **Silver J.** The prophylactic use of anticoagulant therapy in the prevention of pulmonary emboli in one hundred consecutive spinal injury patients. *Paraplegia* 1974;12:188.
23.   **Becker D, Gonzalez M, Gentili A, et al.** Prevention of deep vein thrombosis in patients with acute spinal cord injuries: use of rotating treatment tables. *Neurosurgery* 1987;20:675.
24.   **Merli G, Herbison G, Ditunno J, et al.** Deep vein thrombosis in acute spinal cord injured patients. *Arch Phys Med Rehabil* 1988;69:661.
25.   **National Institutes of Health Consensus Conference.** Prevention of venous thrombosis and pulmonary embolism . *JAMA* 1986; 256:744.
26.   **Leyvraz PF, Richard J, Bachmann F, et al.** Adjusted versus fixed-dose subcutaneious heparin in the prevention of deep vein thrombosis after total hip replacement. *N Engl J Med* 1983; 309:954.
27.   **Green D, Lee MY, Ito VY, et al.** Fixed- vs adjusted-dose heparin in the prophylaxis of thromboembolism in spinal cord injury. *JAMA* 1988; 260:1255.
28.   **Barrowcliffe TW, Johnson EA, Thomas DP.** *Low Molecular Weight Heparin.* John Wiley & Sons, New York, 1992, pp 6.
29.   **Green D, Hirsh J, Heit J, et al.** Low molecular weight heparin: a critical analysis of clinical trials. *Pharmacol Reviews* 1994; 46:89.
30.   **Green D, Lee MY, Lim AC, et al.** Prevention of thromboembolism after spinal cord injury using low-molecular-weight heparin. *Ann Intern Med* 1990; 113:571.
31.   **Green D, Chen D, Chmiel JS, et al.** Prevention of thromboembolism in spinal cord injury: role of low molecular weight heparin. *Arch Phys Med Rehabil* 1994; 75:290.
32.   **Green D, Twardowski P, Wei R, Rademaker AW,** Fatal pulmonary embolism in spinal cord injury. *Chest* 1994, 105,853.

HYPERCOAGULABILITY IN SURGICAL PATIENTS

G.D.O. Lowe

Department of Medicine, Royal Infirmary, Glasgow

I. INTRODUCTION

Hypercoagulability may exist even prior to the operation in surgical patients. This may be due to either congenital thrombophilias, or to acquired conditions such as antiphospholipid antibodies, trauma, infections, inflammatory bowel disease, nephrotic syndrome, recent venous thromboembolism, recent myocardial infarction or stroke, or cancer. Indeed, the indication for surgery may be one of the latter conditions. Surgery is a well-recognised precipitating factor for thrombosis in the presence of such congenital or acquired hypercoagulable states, many of which are reviewed in this volume.

Even in patients without such "background hypercoagulability" prior to surgery, surgery itself rapidly induces a state of acute hypercoagulability which may last for several weeks, especially if there are surgical complications such as haemorrhage or infection. Re-operation and prolonged immobility each intensify and prolong this acquired hypercoagulable state, and increase the risk of thrombosis.

Activation of the haemostatic system (endothelium as well as platelets and coagulation) and depression of fibrinolytic potential (by increases in both antiplasmin and plasminogen activator inhibitor type l) appear appropriate physiological responses to surgical trauma, in that they promote formation and persistence of haemostatic platelet-fibrin plugs to minimise post-traumatic bleeding. The post-operative increases in acute-phase plasma proteins such as fibrinogen may also play an important role in promoting margination of leucocytes in postcapillary venules (by increasing red cell aggregation) and hence in promoting delivery of leucocytes to injured tissues, removal of cell debris, limitation of wound infection, and tissue repair.[1] Unfortunately, such systemic hypercoagulability and rheological changes not only promote surgical haemostasis and wound repair, but also interact with immobility and venous stasis to induce venous thromboembolism. In some surgical patients (e.g. those undergoing orthopaedic surgery of the pelvis, hip or lower limb; pelvic or abdominal surgery for malignancy; or central venous cannulation), endothelial damage, as well as venous stasis, promotes venous thrombosis. Occasionally, postoperative arterial occlusion (myocardial infarction, cerebral infarction, critical limb ischaemia) may occur, due to hypercoagulability or sometimes hypotension, "paradoxical" venous thromboembolism through a patent foramen ovale, or disseminated intravascular coagulation (DIC).

Epidemiological studies have shown that up to 50 percent of cases of symptomatic deep vein thrombosis (DVT) or pulmonary embolism (PE) in the general population occur within a few months of hospital admission for trauma or other indications for surgery.[2-6] Furthermore, a major proportion of the 1 percent of patients admitted to hospital who die of PE while in hospital were admitted for surgery.[7,8] Many studies have shown that up to two-thirds of postoperative DVT and PE can be prevented by routine antithrombotic prophylaxis in patients at moderate or high risk, using either antithrombotic drugs such as low dose subcutaneous heparin,[9,10] low molecular weight heparins,[11,12] dextrans [9,13] or oral anticoagulants[14] or physical methods which reduce venous stasis in the lower limb such as graduated elastic stockings or intermittent pneumatic compression.[9,15] The efficacy of these measures, as well as the additive effect of heparins and mechanical devices in high risk patients,[16] strongly suggest that it is the combination of systemic hypercoagulability and leg venous stasis which induces DVT formation. The lesser, but definite, efficacy of aspirin or other antiplatelet agents in prophylaxis of DVT and PE[17-20] also supports a role for platelet-vessel wall interactions in pathogenesis.

In 1992, three consensus statements in the United Kingdom,[21] Europe,[22] and North America[23] reviewed the need for routine assessment of patients admitted for surgery for risk of venous thrombosis, the efficacy of antithrombotic agents, and the need for routine prophylaxis in patients at moderate or high risk. In 1994, the National Health Service in Scotland issued guidelines for assessment of risk of thromboembolism and for options in routine prophylaxis, which are now contractual obligations for purchasers and providers of health care in Scotland.[24] These developments emphasise the importance of surgery as a precipitant of venous thromboembolism, and the need for prophylaxis in surgical patients.

In this review, clinical risk factors for postoperative venous thromboembolism will first be reviewed: these can be readily defined by clinicians for routine risk stratification and prophylaxis. Secondly, perioperative changes in haemostatic and rheological variables and their relationships to postoperative thromboembolism will be reviewed. At present, such laboratory variables are used in studies of the pathogenesis of thrombosis and of the mechanisms of prophylactic methods, rather than for routine clinical risk prediction.

II. CLINICAL RISK PREDICTION OF POST-OPERATIVE THROMBOEMBOLISM

Clinical risk predictors for postoperative venous thromboembolism have been defined in several studies using necropsy findings, or routine screening with radiolabelled fibrinogen leg scans or venography, as endpoints (for reviews, see 21-25). "Background" factors include age, obesity, varicose veins, immobility (bed rest over 4 days), pregnancy or the puerperium, high dose oestrogen therapy, previous DVT or PE, congenital thrombophilias (deficiency of antithrombin, protein C or protein S; activated protein C resistance due to factor V Leiden; homocystinaemia) and acquired prothrombotic states (antiphospholipid antibodies, lupus anticoagulants, polycythaemias, paraproteinaemias, paroxysmal nocturnal haemoglobinuria, Behcet's disease, inflammatory bowel disease, nephrotic syndrome, recent myocardial infarction, heart failure, or lower limb paralysis). "Surgical" factors include the extent and length of the operation, trauma, infection, malignancy (especially pelvic, abdominal or metastatic), and operations on the pelvis, hip or lower limb.

A commonly-quoted risk stratification of nonobstetric surgical patients is one in which low-, moderate- and high-risk patients are defined. [26]

Low-risk patients have a risk of DVT by routine screening of under 10%, a risk of proximal DVT of under 1%, and a risk of fatal PE of about 0.01%. Such patients include those undergoing minor surgery (e.g. duration under 30 minutes) with no risk factors other than age; and those undergoing major surgery (e.g. duration over 30 minutes) who are aged under 40 years and who have no other risk factors noted above. In such low-risk patients, the costs and adverse effects of routine specific antithrombotic prophylaxis outweigh their benefits, and simple early mobilisation is employed.

Moderate-risk patients have a risk of DVT of 10-40%, a risk of proximal DVT of 1-10%, and a risk of fatal PE of 0.1-1%. They include those undergoing major general, urological, gynaecological, cardiothoracic, vascular, or neurological surgery; who are aged 40 years or over **or** who have other risk factors noted above. In such patients, routine prophylaxis is usually with low dose subcutaneous standard (or low molecular weight) heparin; or with graduated elastic compression stockings with or without intermittent pneumatic compression if heparins are contra-indicated (for example, because of a high risk of bleeding). In intracranial neurosurgery, mechanical methods are preferred due to the risk of intracranial bleeding with anticoagulants. In major trauma or burns patients, the balance of thromboembolic risk and bleeding (including major internal and intracranial bleeding) should be judged in the individual patient: intermittent pneumatic compression, low dose heparin or low molecular weight heparin, or adjusted-dose warfarin are possible options.

High-risk patients have a risk of DVT of 40-80%, a risk of proximal DVT of 10-30%, and a risk of fatal PE of 1-10%.

In **elective hip surgery**, there is a high risk of isolated, proximal DVT in the ipselateral femoral vein (and hence a high risk of PE), due to intraoperative damage to the femoral vein during joint manipulation[27] and local activation of blood coagulation.[28] Low molecular weight heparins[11,12], adjusted-dose standard heparin, adjusted-dose warfarin, or intermittent pneumatic compression appear more effective than low dose standard heparin in elective hip surgery.[21-24]

In **hip fracture surgery**, the risks of femoral DVT and PE are even higher, due not only to such local factors, but also to preoperative thrombogenesis as a result of the fracture, and to the higher mean age of hip fracture patients. Low dose standard heparin is ineffective; low molecular weight heparins, adjusted-dose oral anticoagulants[14], or intravenous dextran 70 are effective options.[21-24] It seems reasonable to advocate such prophylaxis in other patients with major lower limb fractures.

In **elective knee replacement surgery**, intermittent pneumatic compression, low molecular weight heparins, or adjusted-dose warfarin have been recommended. [21-24]

In patients undergoing **major pelvic/abdominal surgery for malignancy**, the high risk of DVT and PE may reflect injury to pelvic and abdominal veins (due to tumour invasion and/or extensive surgical dissection) as well as systemic hypercoagulability associated with malignant disease. In patients undergoing **major surgery who have a history of previous DVT, PE or thrombophilia**, the high risk of venous thromboembolism may reflect previous venous damage and/or chronic systemic hypercoagulability. In these groups of patients, prophylactic options include combining antithrombotic drugs (standard or low molecular weight heparin or dextran) with mechanical methods; adjusted-dose warfarin; or intermittent pneumatic compression and graduated elastic compression stockings if there is high risk of bleeding. **Spinal cord injury** is discussed later.

III. LABORATORY STUDIES OF HYPERCOAGULABILITY IN SURGICAL PATIENTS

As noted in the introduction, activation of the endothelium, platelets and coagulation; depression of fibrinolytic "potential", and rheological proinflammatory changes occur as "physiological" responses to surgical trauma, which may promote not only haemostasis and wound repair, but also postoperative thromboembolism, especially venous.

A. MECHANISMS OF HAEMOSTATIC ACTIVATION

The mechanisms by which such haemostatic, fibrinolytic and rheological changes occur are not fully understood, but include release of both systemic hormones (e.g. adrenaline, vasopressin and corticosteroids)[29] and cytokines (e.g. tumour necrosis factor or TNF, interleukin-1 or IL-1, and interleukin-6 or IL-6).[30] Release of endogenous vasopressin (which occurs especially during the manipulation of abdominal viscera) may be a major mechanism for release of factor VIII/von Willebrand factor (vWF) and tissue plasminogen activator (tPA) during surgery, promoting activation of coagulation and fibrinolysis.[29] Both septic shock and DIC (e.g. following endotoxin exposure) are associated with increases in TNF, IL-1 and IL-6 ; activation of blood coagulation and protein C; and increases in PAI-1.[30] Release of cytokines from activated monocytes and release of fibrin degradation products (FDP) at sites of surgical injury may be mechanisms for haemostatic activation and synthesis of acute phase proteins, including PAI-1 and fibrinogen.

The currently fashionable "keyhole" surgery, which involves small somatic wounds and earlier hospital discharge, has yet to be shown to carry a different risk of postoperative venous thromboembolism from conventional surgery. Haemostatic activation and cytokine formation does not appear to be reduced with "keyhole" surgery[31], possibly because they are triggered by visceral manipulation rather than somatic injury. Furthermore, earlier mobilisation and hospital discharge may be counterbalanced by impairment of perioperative venous drainage due to abdominal insufflation with air for organ visualisation during keyhole surgery.

The type of anaesthesia may also influence perioperative haemostatic activation, lower limb blood flow, and risk of venous thromboembolism. Spinal or epidural anaesthesia may have less thrombogenic effects on these processes than general anaesthesia in hip surgery [25] ; however the degree of thromboprophylactic effect (relative risk reduction 46-55%) is insufficient to recommend such anaesthesia as the sole form of prophylaxis; and there appears to be no effect of the type of anaesthesia in patients who receive specific thromboprophylaxis.[32]

B. ENDOTHELIAL FUNCTION

The endothelium plays a key role in regulation of haemostasis and fibrinolysis.[33] While in general morphological studies have not demonstrated local vessel wall damage in postoperative venous thrombosis[34], as discussed above it may play a role in the pathogenesis of thrombosis during hip surgery, major abdominal or pelvic surgery for cancer, or in central venous catheters. Likewise, local damage to the popliteal vein during knee replacement surgery may also play a role in thrombogenesis: this may be aggravated by application of a tourniquet.

More subtle endothelial disturbance might be the expression of tissue factor procoagulant activity in endothelial cells in morphologically normal veins, induced for example by cytokines such as IL-1 or TNF[30,34] or by thrombin.[35] Perioperative tissue factor procoagulant activity may also be expressed by activated monocytes which adhere to activated endothelium.

The relationship of endothelial function to surgery and postoperative venous thrombosis in man has been studied using plasma markers of endothelial disturbance such as vWF, tPA and PAI-1. Antigen levels of all three markers increase after trauma and surgery. In patients with spinal cord injury, increases in plasma vWF, associated with changes in platelet function, were observed prior to DVT formation.[36] Because vWF is an important cofactor in platelet adhesion and aggregation, elevated vWF levels may contribute to thrombogenesis: this hypothesis could be tested experimentally using anti-vWF antibodies. The roles of tPA and PAI-1 in postoperative venous thrombosis are discussed below.

C. PLATELET AND LEUCOCYTE FUNCTION

Platelets are activated after trauma and surgery, and postoperative increases in plasma levels of beta - thromboglobulin (a marker of platelet activation and release) have been associated with subsequent DVT formation.[37] Necropsy studies have shown platelet aggregates in venous valve cusps, and in the initial "white head" of deep vein thrombi.[38] A recent meta-analysis of randomised controlled trials of aspirin and other antiplatelet agents suggests that they may prevent about one-third of postoperative DVT and about two-thirds of postoperative PE.[17,19] While these findings were unexpected and controversial,[18,19] they are consistent with evidence that dextrans (whose antithrombotic properties include decreased platelet adhesion and aggregation) also prevent about one-third of postoperative DVT, and about two-thirds of postoperative PE.[9,13,39] It is possible that platelet inhibiting drugs are more effective in preventing postoperative PE than DVT by reducing thrombus extension (e.g. by reducing available activated platelet membrane for interaction of clotting factors) or by enhancing thrombolysis (e.g. by reducing platelet secretion of PAI-1). From a clinical viewpoint, other prophylactic methods are to be preferred to aspirin because they are twice as effective in prevention of DVT (which carries risks not only of embolisation, but also of recurrence as well as the post-thrombotic leg syndrome).

Leucocytes are also activated after trauma and surgery, and are also present in the initial "white head" of deep vein thrombi.[34,38] The possible role of monocytes in coagulation activation has been noted. Dextrans also inhibit leucocyte adhesion to venular endothelium, which may be another mechanism for thrombus prevention.

D. COAGULATION

Blood coagulation is also activated after trauma and surgery: the possible roles of hormones, cytokines, tissue factor expression on endothelium and monocytes, and platelet activation have been noted. Coagulation activation usually occurs via the tissue factor initiated extrinsic system.[40] Activation via the surface-initiated intrinsic system was thought to be possible during cardiopulmonary bypass[40]; however a recent study using activation markers suggested that activation occurred primarily via surgery itself, and via the tissue factor pathway.[40]

Fibrinogen, factor V and factor VIII are each positive acute phase reactants which increase after trauma and surgery; while factor VII, antithrombin and protein C are negative acute phase reactants which decrease (partly due to consumption). The postoperative increase in hepatic synthesis of fibrinogen may be stimulated by IL-6, FDP and corticosteroids.[41] There exist several mechanisms by which high fibrinogen levels may promote venous thrombogenesis including increased viscosity and platelet aggregability, and increased size and decreased deformability and lysability of fibrin thrombi; it is relevant that fibrinogen is also a predictor of arterial thrombosis.[41] Defibrination with ancrod prevented postoperative hyperfibrinogenaemia and hyperviscosity, and reduced the incidence and extent of DVT following hip fracture surgery.[42] A possible role for fibrinogen in venous thrombogenesis is also suggested by the association of plasma fibrinogen, plasma viscosity, and high-fibrinogen gene polymorphisms with previous DVT,[43,44] and by the predictive value of preoperative fibrinogen levels for postoperative DVT.[45]

The increases in factor Vc and factor VIIIc after surgery may partly reflect activation by thrombin. The possible role of vasopressin in factor VIII increase has also been noted.[29] The recent finding that a common procoagulant factor V polymorphism (factor V Leiden) which confers resistance to activated protein C, is strongly associated with previous DVT[46,47] raises the possibility that this polymorphism may be a preoperative risk factor for postoperative DVT. High factor VIIIc has been associated with previous DVT,[43,48] as well as predictive of postoperative DVT.[45] High VIIIc levels are also associated with increased plasma thrombin generation in vitro,[49] while the low risk of thrombosis in haemophilia A and the value of VIIIc for predicting arterial thrombosis[50] also support a role for factor VIIIc in postoperative hypercoagulability and thrombosis.

While DVT in congenital deficiencies of antithrombin, protein C or protein S is often precipitated by surgery, the role of the transient decrease in antithrombin and protein C after surgery in thrombogenesis is currently unclear.

Increased activation markers of coagulation such as fibrinopeptide A[37,51] and FDP[45,52] have also been associated with postoperative DVT, as well as with risk factors such as age, infection and malignancy. Finally, the efficacy of low-dose anticoagulant prophylaxis of postoperative DVT and PE supports a central role for coagulation activation.

E. FIBRINOLYSIS

Following trauma or surgery, there is an initial release of endothelial tPA, followed by a postoperative decrease in fibrinolytic "potential" due to increases in plasma levels of the acute phase reactants, PAI-l and antiplasmin. However there is no evidence for an absolute "shutdown" of fibrin lysis, as shown by elevated postoperative levels of plasmin degradation products of fibrinogen and fibrin,[37,51,52] and by the frequent lysis of postoperative DVT when studied by serial radiolabelled fibrinogen leg scanning. Thrombogenesis may however be promoted by a relative imbalance of coagulation over fibrinolysis,[51] and postoperative DVT has been associated in some studies with either increased preoperative clot lysis times or PAI-l levels[45,53] or with a greater postoperative rise in PAI-l levels.[54] However, several trials of stimulation of endogenous fibrinolysis with anabolic steroids (which reduce PAI-l levels) have shown negative results, and at present the relationship of endogenous fibrinolysis to postoperative DVT is uncertain.[55]

REFERENCES

1.   **Schmid-Schönbein H**. Robin Fahraeus and the way we see things in clinical hemorheology: 'Flow anomalies' as objects of scientific paradigms. *Clin Hemorheol* 1985;5:875.
2.   **Gjores JE**. The incidence of venous thrombosis and its sequelae in certain districts of Sweden. *Acta Chir Scand* 1956;206,Supplement.
3.   **Nylander G, Olivecrona H, Hedner U**. Earlier and concurrent morbidity of patients with acute lower leg thrombosis. *Acta Chir Scand* 1977;143: 425.
4.   **Anderson FA Jr, Wheeler HB, Goldberg RJ et al**. The prevalence of risk factors for venous thromboembolism among hospital patients. *Arch Intern Med* 1992;152:1660.
5.   **Kniffen WD Jr, Baron JA, Barrett J, Birkmeyer J D, Anderson FA Jr**. The epidemiology of diagnosed pulmonary embolism and deep venous thrombosis in the elderly. *Arch Intern Med* 1994;154:861.
6.   **Koster T, Rosendaal FR, Briet E, van der Meer FJM, Colly LP, Vandenbroucke JP**. Risk factors for deep vein thrombosis: L.E.T.S. interim analysis. *Thromb Haemostas* 1993;69:764.
7.   **Sandler DA, Martin JF**. Autopsy proven pulmonary embolism in hospital patients: are we detecting enough deep vein thrombosis? *J R Soc Med* 1989; 82:203.
8.   **Karwinski B, Svendsen E**. Comparison of clinical and postmortem diagnosis of pulmonary embolism. *J Clin Pathol* 1989;42:135.
9.   **Clagett GP, Reisch J**. Prevention of venous thromboembolism in general surgical patients. Results of meta-analysis. *Ann Surg* 1988;208: 227.
10.   **Collins R, Scrimgeour A, Yusuf S, Peto R**. Reduction in fatal pulmonary embolism and venous thrombosis by perioperative administration of subcutaneous heparin. *N Engl J Med* 1988;318: 1162.
11.   **Leizorovicz A, Haugh MC, Chapins FR et al**. Low molecular weight heparin in the prevention of perioperative thrombosis. BMJ 1992;305:913.
12.   **Nurmohamed MT, Rosendaal FT, Büller HR, Dekker E, Hommes DW, Vandenbroucke JP**. Low molecularweight heparins versus standard heparin in general and orthopaedic surgery: a meta-analysis. *Lancet* 1992;340:152.
13.   **Bergentz SE**. Dextran in the prophylaxis of pulmonary embolism. *World J Surg* 1978;2:19.
14.   **Sevitt S, Gallagher NG**. Prevention of venous thrombosis and pulmonary embolism in injured patients. *Lancet* 1959;ii:981.
15.   **Wells PS, Lensing AWA, Hirsh J**. Graduated compression stockings in the prevention of postoperative venous thromboembolism. *Arch Intern Med* 1994;154:67.
16.   **Wille-Jorgensen P**. Prophylaxis of postoperative thromboembolism. Copenhagen: *Laegeforeningens Forlag*, 1991.
17.   **Antiplatelet Triallists' Collaboration**. Collaborative overview of randomised trials of antiplatelet therapy. III. Reduction in venous thrombosis and pulmonary embolism by antiplatelet prophylaxis among surgical and medical patients. *BMJ* 1994;308:235.
18.   **Cohen AT, Skinner JA, Kakkar VV**. Antiplatelet treatment for thromboprophylaxis: a step forward or backwards? *BMJ* 1994;309:1213.
19.   **Collins R, Baigent C, Sandercock P, Peto R for the Antiplatelet Trialists' Collaboration**. Antiplatelet therapy for thromboprophylaxis: the need for careful consideration of the evidence from randomised trials. *BMJ* 1994;309:1215.
20.   **Powers PJ, Gent M, Jay R et al**. a randomized trial of less-intense warfarin or acetylsalicylic acid in the prevention of venous thromboembolism after surgery for fractured hip. *Arch Intern Med* 1989;149:771.
21.   **Thromboembolic Risk Factors (THRIFT) Consensus Group**. Risk of and prophylaxis for venous thromboembolism in hospital patients. *BMJ* 1992;305: 567.
22.   **European Consensus Statement**. Prevention of venous thromboembolism. *Intern Angiol* 1992;11: 151.
23.   **Clagett GP, Anderson FA Jr, Levine MN et al**. Prevention of venous thromboembolism. *Chest* 1992;102,Supplement:391S.
24.   **Scottish Office Home and Health Department**. Prophylaxis of venous thromboembolism. A national guideline for use in Scotland. Edinburgh: *HMSO* 1994.
25.   **Bergqvist D**. Postoperative thromboembolism. Frequency, etiology, prophylaxis. *Berlin: Springer Verlag*,1983.
26.   **Salzman EW, Hirsh J**. Prevention of venous thromboembolism. In: Colman RW, Hirsh J, Marder V, Salzman EW, eds. *Hemostasis and thrombosis: basic principles and clinical practice*. New York: Lippincott, 1982:986.
27.   **Stamatakis JD, Kakkar VV, Sagar S, Lawrence D, Nairn D, Bentley PG**. Femoral vein thrombosis and total hip replacement. *BMJ* 1977;ii:223.
28.   **Houghton GR, Papadekis EG, Rizza CR**. Changes in blood coagulation during total hip replacement. *Lancet* 1977;i:1336.
29.   **Grant PJ, Tate GM, Davies JA, Williams NS, Prentice CRM**. Intraoperative activation of coagulation - a stimulus to thrombosis mediated by vasopressin? *Thromb Haemostas* 1986;55:104.
30.   **Esmon CT**. Possible involvement of cytokines in diffuse intravascular coagulation and thrombosis. *Bailliere's Clin Haematol* 1994;7:453.
31.   **McMahon AJ, O'Dwyer PJ, Cruickshank AM et al**. Comparison of metabolic responses to laparoscopic and minilaparotomy cholecystectomy. *Br J Surg* 1993;80:1255.
32.   **Prins MH, Hirsh J**. A comparison of general anesthesia and regional anesthesia as a risk factor for DVT following hip surgery: a critical review. *Thromb Haemostas* 1990;64:497.
33.   **Pearson JD**. Vessel wall interactions regulating thrombosis. *Br Med Bull* 1994;50:776.

34.   **Thomas DP.** Venous thrombogenesis. *Br Med Bull* 1994;50:803.
35.   **Rabiet MJ, Plantier JL, Dejana E.** Thrombininduced endothelial cell dysfunction. *Br Med Bull* 1994;50:936.
36.   **Rossi EC, Green D, Rosen JS, Spies SM, Yao JST.** Sequential changes in factor VIII and platelets preceding deep vein thrombosis in patients with spinal cord injury. *Br J Haematol* 1980;45:14351.
37.   **Douglas JT, Blamey SL, Lowe GDO, Carter DC, Forbes CD.** Plasma betathromboglobulin, fibrinopeptide A and B~15-42 antigen in relation to postoperative DVT, malignancy and stanozolol treatment. *Thromb Haemostas* 1985;53:235.
38.   **Sevitt S.** The structure and growth of valvepocket thrombi in femoral veins. *J Clin Pathol* 1974;27:517.
39.   **Gruber UF, Saldeen T, Brokop T, Eklo'f B, Eriksson I, Goldie I.** Incidences of fatal postoperative pulmonary embolism after prophylaxis with dextran 70 and low-dose heparin: an international multicentre trial. *BMJ* 1980;280:69.
40.   **Boisclair MD, Lane DA, Philippou H et al.** Mechanisms of thrombin generation during surgery and cardiopulmonary bypass. *Blood* 1993;82:3350.
41.   **Lowe GDO, Fowkes FGR, Koenig W, Mannucci PM**, eds. Fibrinogen and cardiovascular disease. *Europ Heart J* 1995, supplement.
42.   **Lowe GDO, Campbell AF, Meek DR, Forbes CD, Prentice CRM, Cummings SW.** Subcutaneous ancrod in prevention of deep-vein thrombosis after operation for fractured neck of femur. *Lancet* 1978;ii:698.
43.   **Balendra R, Rumley A, Orr M, Lennie SE, McColl P, Lowe GDO.** Blood lipids, coagulation, fibrinolysis and rheology in spontaneous proven deep vein thrombosis. *Br J Haematol* 1991;77, supplement 1:83.
44.   **Koster T, Rosendaal FR, Reitsma PH, van der Velden PA, Briët E, Vandenbroucke JP.** Factor VII and fibrinogen levels as risk factors for venous thrombosis. *Thromb Haemostas* 1994;71:719.
45.   **Clayton JK, Anderson JA, McNicol GP.** Preoperative prediction of post-operative deep vein thrombosis. *BMJ* 1976;ii:910.
46.   **Koster T, Rosendaal FR, Ronde H de, Brie't E, Vandenbroucke JP, Bertina RM.** Venous thrombosis due to poor anticoagulant response to activated protein C: Leiden Thrombophilia Study. *Lancet* 1993;342:1503.
47.   **Svensson PJ, Dahlbäck B.** Resistance to activated protein C as a basis for venous thrombosis. *N Engl J Med* 1994;330:517.
48.   **Koster T et al.** The Leiden Thrombophilia Study (LETS): risk factors for venous thrombosis. Proceedings of the Meeting of the International Society for Haematology, *Cancun, Mexico, 1994.*
49.   **Ibbotson SH, Davies JA, Grant PJ.** The influence of infusion of l-desamino-8-D-arginine vasopressin (DDAVP) in vivo on thrombin generation in vitro. *Thromb Haemostas* 1992;68:37.
50.   **Meade TW, Cooper JA, Stirling Y, Howarth DJ, Ruddock V, Miller GJ.** Factor VIII, ABO blood group and the incidence of ischaemic heart disease. *Br J Haematol* 1994;88:601.
51.   **Owen J, Kvam D, Nossel HL, Kaplan KL, Kernoff PBA.** Thrombin and plasmin activity and platelet activation in the development of venous thrombosis. *Blood* 1983;61:476.
52.   **Rowbotham BJ, Whitaker AN, Harrison J, Murtaugh P, Reasbeck P, Bowie EJW.** Measurement of crosslinked fibrin derivatives in patients undergoing abdominal surgery: use in the diagnosis of postoperative venous thrombosis. *Blood Coag Fibrinolys* 1992;3:25.
53.   **Paramo JA, Alfaro MJ, Rocha E.** Postoperative changes in the plasmatic levels of tissue-type plasminogen activator and its fast-acting inhibitor - relationships to deep vein thrombosis and influence of prophylaxis. *Thromb Haemostas* 1985;54:713.
54.   **Kluft C, Jie AFH, Lowe GDO, Blamey SL, Forbes CD.** Association between postoperative hyperresponse in tPA inhibition and deep vein thrombosis. *Thromb Haemostas* 1986;56:107.
55.   **Prins MH, Hirsh J.** A critical review of the evidence supporting a relationship between impaired fibrinolysis and venous thromboembolism. *Arch Intern Med* 1991;151:1721.

HYPERCOAGULABILITY, INFLAMMATORY CYTOKINES, DISSEMINATED INTRAVASCULAR COAGULATION AND HYPERFIBRINOLYSIS

M.J. Seghatchian* and M.M. Samama **
* NBS, Colindale, London ;
** Hôtel-Dieu, University Hospital, Paris

I. INTRODUCTION

Normal haemostasis depends on healthy vasculature, functionally viable platelets and balanced components of the coagulation/fibrinolytic systems. These act together with other defence networks to maintain circulating blood in a fluid state in the vascular bed, while arresting bleeding after injury[1-3]. Any marked deviation in the hemostatic components, in particular, any alteration in the functional integrity of endothelium and certain components of biomodulation/bioamplification/bioattenuation systems[3] or the functional integrity of the fibrinolytic system as shown in chapter one, may induce a hypercoagulable state and a spectrum of thrombotic or haemorrhagic complications[4-11].

Several excellent reviews on this topic exist[1-3,6,10,11]. Therefore in this chapter, after a brief historical perspective, we focus on new developments in triggering mechanisms and accepted clinical and laboratory standpoints. The potential role of inflammatory cytokines, DIC versus hyperfibrinolysis and alteration in coagulation/fibrinolysis associated with cardiopulmonary bypass (CPB), chronic liver disease, and pregnancy will be briefly discussed.

II. DEFINITIONS

Disseminated intravascular coagulation (DIC) also referred to in earlier literature as "consumption coagulopathy" or "thrombohemorrhagic phenomena" or "defibrination syndrome" is an intermediate mechanism of the haemostatic disorder, with catastrophic life-threatening outcome. The term DIC is generally applied to describe a wide spectrum of intravascular clotting syndromes, characterised by the formation of microthrombi followed by clinical bleeding as a secondary process[11]. The essential event in DIC is intravascular soluble fibrin formation followed by formation of microclots in the microcirculation leading to organ failure if microclots are not spontaneously dissolved. This depends on the activation potential of the fibrinolytic system.

The currently proposed term by the subcommittee of ISTH on DIC is Disseminated Intravascular Fibrin Formation so called "DIFF"[12]. This is an acquired disease process associated with disseminated soluble fibrin oligomers formation within the microvasculature and an exaggerated degradation of fibrinogen-fibrin resulting from uncontrolled proteolytic enzymes in blood. DIC represents a special laboratory and clinical problem for several reasons. It may manifest as an acute life-threatening haemorrhage, diffuse thrombosis, localised thrombosis and/or any combination of the above[1,2]. In this group of patients, DIC has an appropriate synonym of "Death is Coming". DIC can be seen in many fields of clinical practice, regardless of speciality and in association with many pathophysiological states. It may manifest in acute, sub-acute or chronic forms each with differing laboratory and/or clinical manifestation[1-3,10,11]. The correct use of the term DIC is only accurate if the patient is not only bleeding but also severely thrombosing with attendant ischaemia and organ damage or necrosis. Unfortunately, despite many advances in the field of haemostasis, the etiology, pathophysiology, clinical/laboratory diagnosis and the optimal mode of therapy of DIC still remain controversial and rather confused. It would not be inappropriate to describe "Disseminated Intravascular Coagulation" by analogy as "Disseminated Intellectual Confusion"[1].

III. HISTORICAL PERSPECTIVE

The concept of haemostasis as a "cascade" is no longer compatible with the concept of hemostatic balance in which the vessel wall and cellular components of blood play major roles in modulating the activation of coagulation/fibrinolysis processes[1-3]. Today there is ample evidence that a large number of triggering mechanisms of cellular origin exist for local activation of coagulation leading to hypercoagulable states (see figure 1). These include changes in activation states and permeability of cells allowing leakage of biologically active substances; changes in cellular fragility leading to rupture and vasoconstriction (under local, neural and humeral controls) leading to occlusion; changes in the composition of the intima, media and adventitia subsequent to shock, acidosis, endotoxinemia and release of inflammatory cytokines capable of expressing tissue factor (TF) on the endothelium, monocytes and granulocytes, contributing indirectly to both thrombotic and haemorrhagic complications[10].

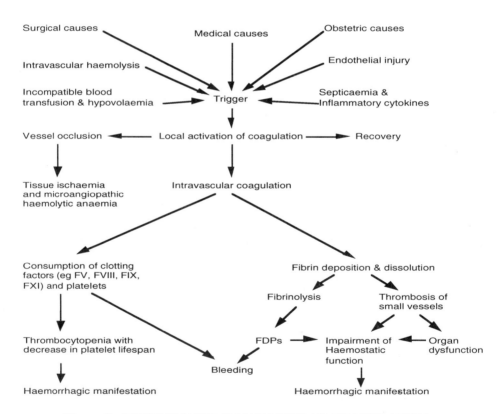

Figure 1 : DISSEMINATED INTAVASCULAR COAGULATION :
possible triggering mechanisms & laboratory/clinical findings.

The knowledge of tissue extract-induced instant death due to thrombosis is not new and, in fact, was reported in 1834 by de Blainville[13] to the French Academy of Medicine on the basis of animal studies. In 1950, Seegers[14] pointed out that in late pregnancy certain substances with "thromboplastin-like activities" may gain access to internal circulation and cause hemostatic difficulties resulting in the inactivation of factor V and the depletion of fibrinogen. In 1955, Ratnoff et al[15] reviewed the haemorrhagic states during pregnancy including the premature separation of the placenta, amniotic fluid embolisms, the presence of a dead fetus in utero and in pre-eclampsia or the generalised bleeding tendency seen in "criminal abortion", where hypofibrinogenemia accounted for the prolongation of clotting time despite the fact that the fibrinogen level was not always too low (see reference 1 for details). The development of secondary fibrinolysis subsequent to septicaemia is another in which fibrinolysis is directly involved in DIC as indicated by Ratnoff[16]. The concept of DIC, as an intermediate mechanism of disease with a self-perpetuating pathological cycle (generated by thrombin and plasmin) was redefined in 1964 by McKay[11]. It is only recently that the new concept involving the inflammatory cytokines as a major trigger of DIC in septicaemia became established[5,7,8].

IV. PATHOGENESIS AND MECHANISM OF DIC

The most likely cause of DIC is introduction of a procoagulant thromboplastin-like substance released from hypoxic or necrotic tissue or neoplastic cells into the circulation. Exposure of the collagen basement membrane in any invasive procedure or infection organisms that release endotoxin or invade endothelium and cause damage or decreased function of the reticulo-endothelial system can also lead to DIC.

Therefore DIC is usually triggered by continuous exposure of blood to clot-promoting factors of multiple pathogenic origins[5,10]. The possible sequence is indicated below :

i) Thrombus formation and occlusion/obstruction of the blood vessel. This may be associated with the activation and/or consumption of platelets as well as various coagulation factors (fibrinogen, factors V, VIII, IX and XI)[10]. Vessel obstruction causes tissue ischaemia and, when red cells manage to traverse the fibrin mesh, microangiopathic features can occur[10,11]. Furthermore, in response to the occlusion, the vessel wall releases a plasminogen activator which initiates secondary fibrinolysis through plasmin generation which leads to consumption coagulopathy and bleeding[5,6,10,11].

ii) Dissolution or lysis of microthrombi by plasmin can also lead to resumption of the blood flow and the development of variable amounts of fibrinogen/fibrin degradation products. These have diverse anticoagulant effects (antithrombin, anti-platelet aggregation, anti-fibrin polymerisation)[1-3]. If excess of plasmin is generated, a further consumption coagulopathy will ensue leading to severe bleeding[6,10].

iii) Once the mechanisms of thrombo-resistance of the vessel wall are compromised, a series of events take place with the consequence that antithrombin is consumed rapidly due to neutralisation of the serine proteases in the presence of heparan sulphate[10]. Prostacyclin generation (PGI_2) will occur leading to inhibition of platelet aggregation. Proteolysis of von Willebrand factor can occur enhancing its binding to platelet glycoprotein IIb/IIIa. Activation of the protein C pathway can occur on the thrombomodulin surface leading not only to the inhibition of factors V and VIII but also to the regulation of fibrinolysis through the neutralisation of type 1 plasminogen activation inhibitor (PAI-1)[5,7,8,10].

Based on the above DIC can be viewed as a disturbance of the hemostatic system in which the balance between the two integrated thrombin regulatory systems (anticoagulant, fibrinolytic) and effector systems (procoagulant, anti-fibrinolytic) which are activated by thrombin interaction is lost.

Thus, depending on the absolute and relative rate of fibrin formation and fibrinolysis, DIC may be asymptomatic (compensated by adequate   regulatory response) or lead to large or small vessel thrombosis or bleeding and/or simultaneous life threatening bleeding and thrombosis (i.e. uncompensated, in which the regulatory system is defective or overriden).

In the first case, enzyme inhibitor complexes comprised of components of the regulatory system such as TAT, PAP, tPA-PAI1, Xa-TFPI may appear in the circulation in absence of the excess consumption of fibrinogen or appearance of FDP and soluble fibrin monomers.

In the second case, these complexes may appear in conjunction with soluble fibrin monomers and FDP. The relative merit of the laboratory aspects will be adressed later in this chapter.

It is important to note that inflammatory stimuli (sepsis induced tissue factor expression and widespread deposition of fibrin in the small vessel) and some metabolic factors (i.e. diabetes) can disturb the above four integrated functional units that make up the haemostatic balance.

It is generally accepted that endotoxinemia is also associated with activation and subsequent inhibition of fibrinolysis. At the time of maximal coagulation activation fibrinolysis is completely inhibited[5]. This may promote intravascular fibrin deposition. The endotoxin-induced changes in fibrinolysis are not dependent on interaction of blood coagulation. Thus, the first priority in defining the severity of DIC is to establish the clinical relevance of markers proven specific for pre-DIC and various stages of DIC/DIFF. The latter should be correlated with development of well characterized clinical disorders in which there is a high risk of DIC.

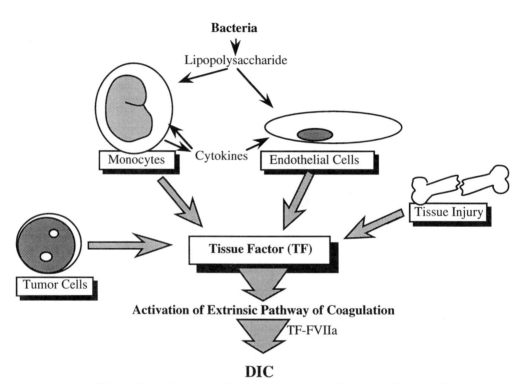

Figure 2 : Activation of intravascular coagulation leading to DIC
in various pathological conditions (modified from Uchiba et al [17]).

Moreover, neutrophil granulocytes are activated during sepsis and release aggressive mediators such as oxygen free radicals and elastase[7]. In the plasma elastase is inhibited by $\alpha 1$ antitrypsin and circulates as a complex. Plama levels of elastase-α_1 antitrypsin complexes are correlated with IL6 and some coagulation factors. Therefore, elastase as a neutrophil mediator is a good marker of DIC/DIFF in sepsis. Future developments in elastase specific peptides may prove useful in clinical diagnosis of various forms of DIC.

Infection (mainly gram negative), malignancies and trauma constitute the major causes of DIC syndrome. Obstetric problems appear relatively less frequent in the larger medical centres[10].

Various inducers of DIC involving factor XII activation, complement activation, endotoxin-induced tissue factor on leucocytes, and platelet microvesiculation[9] may have roles in generating DIC.

On the basis of recent findings, endotoxin-induced DIC thrombus formation through generation of tissue factor on the endothelium, monocytes, granulocytes and the release of several other mediators such as inflammatory cytokines (interleukin I and tumour necrosis factors) are believed to play a major role in septicaemia-induced DIC[7,8,17] (figure 2). Activation of the endothelial cells by cytokines is associated with the release of thrombomodulin further down-regulating the inhibitory capacity of the mechanism of endothelium thromboresistance[8].

Although in malignant diseases and in patients receiving infusion of activated factor IX concentrates, a direct activation of factor X occurs[18]. However, the role of the intrinsic pathway in the initiation of DIC seems to be rather limited, although in the presence of activated platelets, factor Xa does play a major role in the bioamplification/bioattenuation processes.

V. INFLAMMATORY CYTOKINES AND DIC

The potential role of inflammation and cytokines in thrombosis and DIC has been the focus of recent investigations[7,8] and there is now ample evidence to corroborate this concept :

First, the administration of tumour necrosis factor (TNF) to cancer patients increases by 2-3 fold the levels of fibrinopeptide A (FPA) and prothrombin fragment F1+2 (over baseline levels) with a concomitant fall in platelets to 60% of baseline[19]. Furthermore, monoclonal antibody to TNF reduces platelet consumption[19].

Second, TNF circulates in patients with septic shock and with DIC, who also have demonstrable levels of circulating non-adherent platelet microparticles, predisposing to thrombosis[9,10]. Massive activation of complement can occur with TNF. This in turn can lead to the formation of platelet microparticles[9].

Third, in gram negative and reperfusion injury, TNF is present and thought to down regulate the thrombomodulin-induced anticoagulant activity on the endothelial cell[8]. This is supported by finding that circulating thrombomodulin can be detected in plasma[20]. Finally, apart from cytokine-mediated transcriptional control of pro- and anti-coagulant activities, cytokines can also modulate the proteolytic processing of thrombomodulin through the activation of neutrophil and release of elastase. Activated leucocytes can damage the endothelium's thrombomodulin through oxidation further enhancing the development of DIC[7,8].

Inflammatory cytokines also increase C4bBP (an acute phase reactant) producing an increased level of free protein S, eliciting a massive thrombotic response by reducing the anticoagulant capacity of blood[21]. Since most of the protein C activation takes place in microcirculation where the thrombomodulin concentration is high, it is possible that the high prevalence of skin necrosis (1/300 in general population) is associated with this phenomenon[22]. It is known that the skin behaves as a potent inflammatory organ capable of releasing cytokines such as IL-1 and TNF which are involved in the biomodulation of haemostatic components[8].

Moreover *in vitro* evidence indicates that the rates of secretion of both tPA and fast-acting PAI-1 from endothelial cells are altered by cytokine treatment, which increases PAI-1 secretion with no change in tPA, a phenomenon implicated in the pathogenesis of DIC in septic shock[5,10]

Endothelial cells play critical roles in the control of vascular function. Although the procoagulant, anticoagulant, antithrombotic, and pro-anti-fibrinolytic balance of endothelium can be disturbed by circulating mediators in particular inflammatory cytokines, the levels of various responses differ. For example, tissue factor induction is transient and rapid (peaking at 2-4 hours) and thrombomodulin down-regulation is slow with a half-life of approximately 8 hours[8]. Although, inflammatory cytokines play an important role in DIC and thrombosis, they are insufficient in themselves in eliciting thrombotic complications without a secondary stimulus. A possible explanation is the fact that cytokine-induced down-regulation of thrombomodulin can be prevented by another cytokine, IL-4[23]. The possible mechanism of inflammatory cytokines in the development of DIC is shown schematically in figure 3.

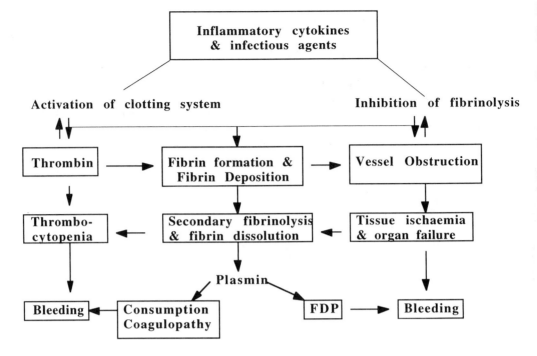

Figure 3 : Schematic representation of sequence of septicaemia and infection leading to thrombotic and hemorrhagic manifestations.

VI. CLINICAL AND LABORATORY ASPECTS OF DIC

A. CLINICAL ASPECTS

Recognising that patients in DIC are undergoing simultaneous haemorrhage plus severe thrombosis (usually manifested clinically by bleeding) efforts were focused in the following areas:

  i)   The effect of the underlying disease on the haemostatic mechanism.

  ii)   The identification of the eventual dynamic change in the parameters over the time of observation (i.e. chronic liver disease, leukaemia which may be unrelated to DIC).

  iii) The extent of the impairment of the different haemostatic parameters in conjunction with the extent of organ dysfunction.

DIC can occur in association with infection, neoplasia, leukemia, vascular disease, vasculitis, liver disease, sepsis and endotoxinemia, transfusion reaction, obstetric complications (septic abortion, retained dead fetus, retroplacental hematoma...), trauma, tissue injury, shock, respiratory distress and envenomation[1-3,10,11] (table I).

This list is by no means complete but the most frequent conditions associated with DIC are: malignancy including some forms of leukemia and prostatic cancer, diseases accompanied by severe bleeding and/or hypotension, acidosis and shock, sepsis and some obstetrical complications.

DIC occurs equally in both sexes at any age, but is more common in infants, children and the elderly. Almost 90% of the cases are acute and approximately 10% a chronic process.

The clinical general signs and symptoms of DIC are : fever, hypertension, acidosis, hypoxia, proteinuria. Specific signs of DIC symptoms are petechiae, purpura, haemorrhagic bullae, acral cyanosis, gangrene, wound bleeding, venepuncture bleeding and subcutaneous haematomas[1-3,10,11].

End organ dysfunction in DIC reflects microvascular thrombosis with resultant ischaemia and hypoxia rather than end organ haemorrhage. There is a high incidence of cardiac, pulmonary, renal and central nervous system dysfunction.

Table I : CLASSIFICATION OF THE MAIN CLINICAL CAUSES
ASSOCIATED WITH DIC

INFECTIONS
Bacterial, viral and parasital (protozoa) :
Gram negative or rarely positive bacteria, perfringens bacillus, mycobacterium tuberculosis, septicemia, viral infection (purpura fulminans), plasmodium falciparum

MALIGNANCY
Metastatic cancer (prostate, pancreas, intestine...)
Leukemia specially promyelocytic leukemia

MAJOR SURGERY
Thoracic, prostate, uterus, extracorporeal circulation

OBSTETRIC COMPLICATIONS
Abruptio placenta, septic abortion, uterine rupture, retained dead fetus
Toxemia of pregnancy, pre-eclampsia, eclampsia
Amniotic fluid embolism
Rh incompatibility

NEWBORN PERIOD
Respiratory distress syndrome, bacterial, viral infections, toxoplamosis, syphilis infection, purpura fulminans, giant hemangioma...

TRAUMA AND TISSUE INJURY
Brain injury and stroke
Burns-crush injury
Hyperthermia, hypothermia
Rhabdomyolysis
Fat embolism

ANAPHYLAXIS
Anaphylactic-shock
Transfusion reactions (ABO mismatch)

VASCULAR DISEASE
Kasabach-Merritt syndrome
Klippel-Trenaunay syndrome
Multiple telangectasia
Vascular tumors : cardiac and aortic, aneurysms

VARIOUS MEDICAL CAUSES
Liver cirrhosis - Polycythemia
Reye's syndrome, Respiratory distress syndrome, Envenomation

The laboratory investigations of DIC are highly variable. The results are often difficult to interpret unless the pathophysiology of this disorder is firmly understood.

The four selected pathocybernetic, self-perpetuating processes, in DIC are:

i) fibrinolytic activation as a consequence of factor XII generation leading to haemorrhage and biodegradation of haemostatic components[1-3,10,11].

ii) bradykinin activation leading to vasodilation and hypotension/shock[10,11].

iii) complement activation leading to cell lysis, vascular change and platelet release reaction[7].

iv) endothelial damage reaction due to viraemia, heat stroke, graft rejection, Ag-Ab complexes, shock, endotoxin and ongoing DIC[10].

It is noteworthy that the frequency of DIC seen in laboratory practice has been reduced possibly due to unproved patient management.

B. LABORATORY ASPECTS

The requests for laboratory diagnosis are generated by three observations :
- patient has a disease which is known to be a high risk for DIC condition
- patient has clinical bleeding similar to that seen in DIC
- patient has unexplained thrombocytopenia

The diagnosis of DIC should be based on accumulation of supportive laboratory tests in conjunction with the clinical picture. Objective laboratory diagnosis criteria are based on different tests which have been classified by R. Bick[1] in four groups:
- tests of fibrinogen depletion and of fibrinolytic activation : plamsa fibrinogen levels, D dimers, plasmin-antiplasmin complexes (PAP)
- markers of hypercoagulable states : F1+2, TAT
- tests indicating inhibitor consumption: decreased α_2-antiplasmin, AT III and/or elevated TAT and PAP
- tests reflecting end-organ failure or damage: elevated LDH, creatinine increase...

From a practical point of view, the laboratory approach should follow three consecutive steps
- confirming the existence of DIC : increased D dimers
- establishing the type of DIC : compensated DIC when fibrinogen plasma level is normal or even increased, or uncompensated DIC when hypofibrinogenemia is present
- evaluating severity based on altered laboratory findings

1. General laboratory indications

The diagnosis of DIC should be based on the accumulation of supportive laboratory tests in conjunction with the clinical picture. Formation of a small clot in a glass tube which could undergo lysis, a characteristic peripheral blood smear of fragmented red cells, decreased platelets and decreased plasma fibrinogen concentration are strong evidence for DIC. In DIC, soluble oligomers circulate in blood.Various sensitive methods for detection of soluble fibrin are now available such as Kabi test. Plasminogen activators are released into the blood and attached to soluble fibrin, causing widespread plasmin. The main characteristics of current laboratory approaches are described below :

i) Global coagulation tests

PT, APTT and TT are usually abnormal in approximately 50-75% of patients with DIC and considered unreliable for differential diagnosis of DIC. In fact, the presence of circulating activated factors can accelerate the rate of fibrin formation in the test system and early degradation products of fibrinogen are prone to gel more quickly leading to falsely normal or short clotting time. A normal PT or APTT should never be used to rule out the diagnosis of DIC as the presence of thrombin, activated factor V and/or factor VIII will produce falsely normal or short value.

In contrast, plasmin-induced biodegradation of factors V, VIII, IX and XI and low levels of fibrinogen (<100 mg/dl) prolong the APTT.

A prolonged thrombin or reptilase time should be expected in DIC because of circulating FDPs, their interference with fibrin monomer polymerisation and from the presence of hypofibrinogenemia.

A simple non quantitative tool is monitoring the clot lysis. Clinically significant fibrinolysis is unlikely to be present if the clot is not dissolved within 60 minutes.

ii) Specific factor assays

Since in most patients with fulminant DIC, circulating activated clotting factors, especially factors Xa, IXa and thrombin are present, specific coagulation factor assays provide little if any meaningful information. Factor VIII-like activity is usually high, though there may be limited amount of factor VIII present. Factor V is usually decreased.

iii) Thrombin-like activity (TLA)

Recently, a rapid global chromogenic test for the assessment of low grade proteolytic enzymes and their complexes with proteolytic inhibitors has been developed[24] to screen for hypercoagulability. TLA levels of plasma samples from patients with a clinical DIC were high in most cases as compared to the laboratory control and samples from individual who were predisposed to ischemic heart (figure 4).

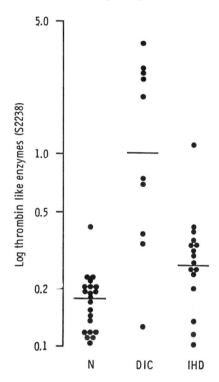

Figure 4. Plasma (100 μl) at 1/20 dilution is incubated at 37°C with 100μl of chromogenic substrate for thrombin (S2238m 1mg/ml). The reaction is stopped at 1h with 100 μl glacial acetic acid and optical density read either at 405 or at 540 after colour conversion[24]. The results are plotted on logarithmic paper.

2. Molecular markers of DIC

Fibrinog(en) degradation products (FDP) are also elevated in 85 to 100% of patients with DIC and are useful indicators of plasmin formation. A quantitative assay for fibrin monomer as mentioned previously, the FM-test (Chromogenix)[25], is now available and useful in the management of chronic DIC in patients with cancer. A new D dimer assay specific for fibrin degradation products as compared to the formation of fibrinolytic degradation products (X, Y; D, E fragments) is now available for clinical use, including DIC. The D dimer assay appears to be the most reliable test for patients with confirmed DIC (abnormal in 93%)[1]. However, certain interferences due to non specificity and the presence of an overwhelmining release of granulocyte enzymes such as collagenases and elastases which can further degrade all the avaible D and E fragments may lead to false-negative FDP titers in patients with acute DIC[1]. Despite these shortcomings FDP titers are elevated in most cases of DIC patients.

The assessment of an intermediate species, prethrombin2 which can generate FPA or combine with antithrombin, by ELISA assays, as well as the quantitation of F1+2 levels, TAT (thrombin-antithrombin) and other protease-protease inhibitor complexes such as PAP (plasmin-antiplasmin) as mentioned above might become useful in the assessment of the severity of DIC. These tests are useful in the early stages of development of DIC/DIFF. They are of interest in asymptomatic chronic forms of DIC, where a very low grade of activation occurred. A recent unexpected finding is the absence of factor VIIa increase in DIC[26].

C. CLINICAL MANAGEMENT OF DIC

Monitoring DIC therapy may be confusing and in some instances is controversial. To further complicate the situation, many new treatments are becoming available to assess appropriate therapy. However, not enough experience with the newer systems exists. The management of DIC is still based on clinical impressions and anecdotal evidence rather than unequivocal data based on controlled studies.

Despite the above shortcomings, the following generalised approaches are now accepted:

i) General supportive measures, counteracting shock, hypoxia, acidosis, volume depletion and organ dysfunction. A careful restoration of proper perfusion of the microcirculation may reactivate the mechanisms of vessel wall thrombo-resistance.

ii) Aggressive management of the DIC-inducer. Clearly the only way to halt the process of DIC is to prevent the inflow of the tissue factor or other components triggering DIC. Examples are debridement of crushed tissues in cases of trauma, intensive antibiotic treatment in septicaemia, aggressive chemotherapy in cancer patients or hysterectomy when appropriate.

iii) Since bleeding manifestation appears not to be greatly improved following heparin administration and, heparin can aggravate bleeding, it is therefore not advisable to universally use heparin in DIC patients, although a low dosage of heparin or LMW heparin in certain cases[27]. The critical point is to assess correctly whether the DIC process has been contained or not. This is hard to determine. Likewise, administration of antifibrinolytic agents is not recommended as these may block the compensatory secondary fibrinolysis, hence is extremely dangerous. Hemorrhagic episodes induced by heparin are relatively rare. They become rather frequent when invasive procedures, including surgery and child delivery, have occurred. Heparin for patients with DIC belonging to this high risk group is contraindicated.

Generally, if the DIC process is overcome, the coagulopathy will be corrected spontaneously by compensatory increased hepatic synthesis of clotting factors and thrombocytopenia will be rectified in a short period of time through increased thrombopoiesis by the bone marrow. However, replacement of clotting factors and cellular blood components to overcome low levels of fibrinogen and thrombocytopenia in DIC is definitely indicated when clinical bleeding is severe. The use of cryoprecipitate containing higher concentrations of fibrinogen factors V and VIII is preferred over fresh frozen plasma as it brings the fibrinogen level more quickly to about 15mg/ml. Administration of antithrombin III with favourable results has been reported in several uncontrolled trials although this mode of therapy has no effect on mortality in the controlled study performed by Blauhut *et al*[28]. A recent review has been devoted to antithombin concentrates and their clinical use in DIC[29].

The use of activated protein C concentrate is beneficial in alleviating endotoxin-induced DIC in monkeys[30] and tissue thromboplastin-induced DIC in rabbits[31] in which the effects of human APC (300-3000IU/Kg) were compared with heparin (100-300IU/Kg) on TF-induced DIC. Both products inhibited the fall in platelet count and fibrinogen level. APC improved the prolonged bleeding time but heparin aggravated bleeding. In APC-treated animals the fibrin deposition in glomeruli is less than in heparin-treated animals. Thus, at least in experimental DIC, administration of APC by exerting anticoagulant activity without exerting a bleeding tendency, could provide a very useful clinical treatment[30,31]. Recombinant human TFPI has been obtained and its administration may be of major importance in the defence against the development of DIC in severe shock[32].

Morbidity and mortality in DIC are usually due to the underlying disease rather than to DIC itself. Attempts should be made to eliminate the primary cause of DIC. Many patients with DIC require no specific therapy for the coagulopathy because it is self-limited or because it is not severe enough to present a major risk of bleeding or thrombosis. On the other hand, some patients may be in profound hyperfibrinolysis or hypercoagulability state. Then treatment of DIC can be life saving.

In common practice, the two accepted types of treatment of DIC include:

- drugs that block enzyme pathways responsible for coagulation and fibrinolysis

- blood products replacement therapy to correct the coagulation defects resulting from depletion of clotting factors, inhibitors of coagulation, fibrinolysis and platelets.

Although one unit of FFP (as mentioned earlier) can raise virtually all coagulation factors and inhibitors, some clinicians prefer to use cryosupernatant rather than FFP. This will keep just the circulation to flow. While providing all components of plasma free from cellular contaminants and factor VIII/fibrinogen at somewhat reduced levels. Patients with marked thrombocytopenia (plt< 10,000-20,000 µl) or moderate thrombocytopenia (plt< 50,000/µl) and active or high risk of bleeding should receive platelet concentrates (1-2 Units/10 kg per day).

The role of pharmacologic inhibitors of coagulation and fibrinolysis in the treatment of DIC is contoversial. Heparin might increase bleeding by virtue of its anticoagulant effect. However heparin therapy clearly benefits some DIC patients with cancer. There is presently no convincing evidence that giving heparin reduces morbidity or mortality in acute DIC. Antifibrinolytic drugs such as E-aminocaproic acid (EACA) and tranexamic acid which inhibit binding of plasmin, plasminogen and tPA to fibrin and fibrinogen may prove useful in diminishing bleeding caused by hyperfibrinolysis. However one should always bear in mind a potential thrombosis from unopposed fibrin formation. EACA has been used with favorable results in patients with DIC caused by prostate cancer and to prevent bleeding after cardiac bypass surgery and some other special cases. Concomitant administration of low dose heparin (100-150 IU/kg/24h) and EACA (8-10 mg/kg/h) are also found to be useful. Aprotinin, a natural inhibitor of trypsin, plasmin, kallikrein and genetically engineered mutant form of α1-antitrypsin that is a potent inhibitor of thrombin, factors XIa, XIIa appears useful in animal models against DIC and death due to gram-negative sepsis. Protein C concentrate is useful to treat purpura fulminans associated with acquired protein C deficiency. Monoclonal antibody to bacterial endotoxin led to a more rapid resolution of DIC in gram-negative sepsis in a large randomized trial. The potential activity of TFPI in DIC related to sepsis merits as already mentioned further investigation.The treatment of DIC in obstetric patients in discussed in paragraph VIII.

Finally, new therapeutic approaches include LMW heparin[27], recombinant hirudin[33], some chemical compounds such as nafamostat mesilate[17], a synthetic protease inhibitor which is used since a few years for the treatment of DIC. These new therapeutic approaches have been recently reviewed in a book devoted to DIC[34]. These developments offer new hope for improved treatment of DIC in the future.

VII. SIMILARITY BETWEEN CONDITIONS ASSOCIATED WITH HYPERFIBRINO(GENO)LYSIS OR DIC

Hyperfibrino(geno)lysis is commonly observed in cardiopulmonary bypass (CPB), liver disease and liver transplantation. Since a primary lysis manifests as a hemorrhagic syndrome without a thrombotic component, there is no major activation of coagulation factors or AT III consumption compared to DIC[1]. Furthermore, since in these conditions no fibrin monomer polymerisation occurs or is deposited in the microcirculation, the absence or presence of thrombocytopenia is a conventional differential diagnostic tool. The protamine sulphate (or ethanol gelation) test is nevertheless useful despite an occasional negative result in DIC.

Despite similarities in primary fibrinolysis and DIC, therapy for primary hyperfibrino(geno)lysis is markedly different from that of DIC. It is essential to quickly distinguish between these two syndromes from the clinical and laboratory standpoints[1].

The pathophysiology of altered haemostasis created by CPB, like DIC, remains confused. This precluded the development of uniform concepts of successful preventive measures and effective therapy. The most frequently cited abnormalities include inadequate heparin neutralisation, excess protamine, heparin rebound, thrombocytopenia, primary/secondary fibrinolysis, coagulation deficiencies and transfusion reactions (see reference 1 for details). The superficial similarities between DIC and hyperfibrinolysis render a clear-cut differential diagnosis, difficult in the absence of sophisticated and/or complete coagulation studies, a difficult task.

Likewise, thrombocytopenia, as a potential source of haemorrhage, is an inconsistent finding during CPB. A patient undergoing DIC develops a severe platelet function defect either due to coating of the platelet surface by FDP, platelet membrane damage or drug-induced bleeding. It is important to note that platelet activation is associated with microvesiculation[9], which may play a role in the development of DIC versus thrombotic events. As pointed out earlier, patients with DIC have demonstrable levels of circulating platelet microparticles[9]. This could be related to complement activation, an early event in bacterial infection. In today's concept, the haemostasis abnormalities associated with CPB are related to a combination of platelet function defect of unclear etiology occurring in all patients and a primary hyperfibrinolysis occurring in 80% of patients and with limited hemorrhagic significance.

Another patient group with superficial clinical similarity to DIC are those with chronic liver disease, which is also a multifaceted disorder with a complex etiology[1]. In the majority of patients with chronic liver disease "pseudo"-fibrinogenemia occurs due to the low clottability of fibrinogen sub-species which undergo a minimal cleavage by the plasmin, proteolysis of factors V, VIII, IX, XI and von Willebrand factor by circulating plasmin and platelet dysfunctioning due to FDP[1]. Haemorrhage in patients with chronic liver disease can no longer be attributed to a simple abnormality in the synthesis of Vitamin K dependent proteins. In regard to blood components therapy in these patients, factor IX concentrate and FFP are used to correct the hemorrhage associated with decrease/dysfunctional synthesis of II, VII, IX and X. The decrease in factor VII closely correlates with the prothrombin time, whereas the decrease/dysfunctional synthesis of factor IX and X relate well with clinical bleeding. Unsuccessful control of hemorrhage in these patients is usually due to the fact that while many defects are corrected primarily with the use of prothrombin complex factor, many others are left essentially unaltered. The imbalance may lead to further complications.

VIII. PREGNANCY, HYPERCOAGULABILITY AND DIC

Normal pregnancy may be regarded as a physiological hypercoagulable state[35] which carries special hazards for both mother and fetus[36]. Obstetric hemorrhage and blood loss, particularly childbirth is still one of the leading causes of maternal mortality. Knowledge of any family history of excessive bruising/bleeding and the awareness of the underlying inherited or acquired hemostatic defects is important. Rapid access to blood and blood products is essential for acceptable obstetric practice, as are appropriate laboratory facilities for blood grouping, compatibility testing and urgent haemostatic function testing[37].

The effect of pregnancy on hypercoagulability, as determined by the classical tests for hemostatic abnormality, is apparent from about the third month of gestation, when the prothrombotic tendency is at its peak. In principle, during pregnancy prothrombin, factor X, prekallikrein, factor IX and factor XII increase whereas factor XI tends to decrease[37]. Protein S appears to fall by 40-50% without associated changes in C4bBP[38-40]. Moreover, a reduction of 18% in AT III and approximately 10% in protein C (of the basal levels) of these proteins occur during pregnancy while the TFPI level increases in early labour[36,41]. (see the chapter of Bonnar : hypercoagulability and pregnancy).

DIC in pregnancy can occur in a wide variety of clinical conditions (Table I). Depending on the triggering event, DIC can manifest as a spectrum ranging from a chronic compensated state to an acute life-threatening hemorrhage. In many obstetric complications i.e. placental abruption, amniotic fluid embolism or septic abortion, there is an acute release of tissue thromboplastin into the circulation causing a pronounced depletion of some coagulation factors (factors V, VIII, IX and fibrinogen) and increased plasma fibrinolytic activity concomitant with a progressive increase in concentration of plasminogen activator inhibitor type 1 (PAI-I)[42]. Platelet consumption may also occur which can lead to severe clinical bleeding[43]. The chronic DIC which occurs in pre-eclampsia is associated with laboratory evidence of a very mild reduction of fibrinogen and an increased platelet turnover without excessive bleeding[36]. Various stages of severity of DIC in pregnancy are summarized in Table III along with the classical laboratory markers and clinical complications according to a recent review by Letsky[36].

Considering DIC in pregnancy is always a secondary process with a broad spectrum of hemostatic abnormalities, treatment should involve the removal of the triggering mechanism when this is known. The principles of management are usually the same whether massive bleeding is associated with DIC or not. Under certain conditions, it is very important to keep the circulation going with plasma replacement therapy until FFP and cross-matched packed red cells are available. Heparin is not indicated in these patients at high risk of bleeding except in dead fetus retention where subcutaneous heparin injections seem effective[44]. In premature separation of plasma, which is the most frequent cause of DIC in obstetrics therapy consists of emptying the uterus and supporting maternal circulation[44].

In amniotic fluid embolism, therapy is aimed at supporting the maternal circulation with transfusion of packed red blood cells, FFP and platelets while respiratory distress should be adressed by administration of oxygen and by ventilation with positive end-respiratory pressure[44].

TABLE III : The relationship between the severity of DIC spectrum, the specific tests and obstetric complications.

Severity of DIC	*In vitro* finding*	Obstetric condition commonly associated
Stage 1 : Low-grade compensated	FDPS Increased soluble fibrin complexes Increased ratio of <u>VWF</u> VIII:C	Pre-eclampsia Retained dead fetus
Stage 2 : Uncompensated but haemostatic failure	As above, plus fibrinogen factor V and VIII	Small abruptio Severe pre-eclampsia
Stage 3 : Rampant with haemostatic failure	Platelets Gross depletion of coagulation factors, particularly fibrinogen FDPs	Abruptio placenta Amniotic fluid embolism Eclampsia

* Notes : from Letsky Lecture at NLBTC, Clindale, 1994 (personal communication) ; see also ref. 36.
Rapid progression from stage 1 to stage 3 is possible unless appropriate action is taken.
The increased ratio of <u>VWF</u> and/or VIII:C correlate with increased low grade proteolytic enzymes assessed by Kallikrein
        VIII:C
or thrombin chromogenic substrates[24].

X. CONCLUSION

The etiology, pathophysiology, diagnosis and management of classical acute and chronic disseminated intravascular coagulation remain confused and controversial. DIC is thought to be synonymous with "Disseminated Intellectual Confusion"; the alternative is "Death is Coming" syndrome.

Another recently proposed term for DIC is disseminated intravascular fibrin formation so called "DIFF" as an acquired disease process accompanied by soluble fibrin oligomer formation and accelerated fibrinogen/fibrin degradation.

Considerable attention has been focused in the past on inter-relationships between disease states and DIC. The spectrum of confusing clinical and laboratory findings, makes it difficult to have consensus on DIC and many superficially related haematological syndromes.

The major focus of research on DIC is currently:

i)   to develop appropriate models to clarify the roles of inflammation, cytokines, infection, complement activation, platelet microvesiculation and hyperfibrinolysis in DIC.

ii)   to improve the differential diagnosis of DIC, hyperfibrinolysis and similar conditions. The development of new molecular markers such as a specific peptide released by elastase may help to differential diagnosis.

iii) to develop a safe and efficient therapy on a case specific basis.

The potential usefulness of activated protein C has been recently described as the most safe and efficient strategy in the management of DIC. The possible therapeutic advantages of recombinant hirudin or TFPI merits further investigations. Clearly DIC will still remain the focus of clinical and scientific interest for some time to come.

REFERENCES

1.   **Bick, R.L.** Disseminated Intravascular Coagulation. Objective laboratory diagnostic criteria and guidelines for management. in *Thrombosis and hemostasis for the clinical laboratory. Part I.* R. Bick, Edit. WB Saunders Company Philadelphia, 729, 1994.

2.   **Horellou, M.H. and Samama, M.M.** La coagulation Intravasculaire disséminée. *Encylopedie Medico-chirurgicale (Paris).*, 12, 2415, 1988.

3.   **Müller-Berghaus G.,** Pathophysiologic and biochemical events in disseminated intravascular coagulation : dysregulation of procoagulant and anticoagulant pathways. *Semin Thromb Haemost,* 15, 58, 1989.

4.   **Seghatchian, M.J.** Changes in the activation states of vitamin K dependent proteins in Hypercoagulability: some conceptual and methodological aspects. Shearer, M.J., and Seghatchian, M.J., Eds. *Vitamin K and Vitamin K dependent proteins*, CRC Press, Boca Raton, Florida, 9, 1993.

5.   **Semeraro N. and Colucci M.** Changes in the coagulation fibrinolysis balance of endothelial cells and mononuclear phagocytes: role of disseminated intravascular coagulation associated with infection disease. *Int. J. Clin. Lab. Res.*, 21, 214, 1992.

6.   **Fruchtman, S.M. and Rand, J.H.** Disseminated intravascular coagulation. Fuster, V, Verstraete, M. Eds. *Thrombosis in cardiovascular disorders*. W.B. Saunders Company, Philadelphia, London, Toronto, Montreal, Sidney, Tokyo 501, 1992.

7.   **Esmon, C.T.** Cell mediated events that control blood coagulation and vascular injury. *Review of Cell Biology*, 9, 1, 1993.

8.   **Esmon, C.T.** Possible involvement of cytokines in diffuse intravascular coagulation and thrombosis. *Baillières Clinical Haematology*, 7, 453, 1994

9.   **Holme, P.A., Solum, N.O. and Brosstad, F.** Clinical significance of platelet-derived microvesicles, demonstration of their presence in patients suffering from DIC. *Thromb. Haemostas.*, 69, 1198, 1993.

10. **Seligsohn, U.** Disseminated intravascular coagulation. in *William Haematology 5th Ed.* Eds (Beutler E, Lichtman MA, Coller BS, Kipps TJ) ; Mc Grow-Hill inc, New York, 1497,1995.

11. **McKay, D.G.** Disseminated intravascular coagulation (DIC). An Intermediary mechanism of diseases. *Harper and Row, New York*, 1964.

12. **Müller-Berghaus,G., Blombäck, M., ten Cate, J.W.** Attemps to define disseminated intravascular coagulation. In *DIC : Pathogenesis, Diagnosis and Therapy of Disseminated Intravascular Fibrin Formation*. Müller G, Madlener K, Blombäck M, ten Cate JW, Edit. Elsevier Science Publishers B.V.,3,1993

13. **de Blainville H.M.D.** Injections de tissu cérebral dans les veines. *Gaz Med. Paris (ser.2)*, 2, 524, 1934.

14. **Seegers, W.H.** Factors in the control of bleeding. *Cincinnati J. Med.*, 31, 395, 1950.

15. **Ratnoff, O.D., Pritchard, J.A and Colopy J.A.** Hemorrhagic states during pregnancy. *N. Engl. J. Med.*, 253, 63, 1955.

16. **Ratnoff, O.D. and Nebehay W.G.** Multiple coagulation defect in a patient with Waterhouse Friderichsen Syndrome. *Ann. Inter. Med.*, 56, 627, 1962.

17. **Uchiba, M., Okajima, K., Abe, H., Okabe, H., Takatsuki, K.,** Effect of nafamostat, a synthetic protease inhibitor, on the extrinsic pathway of coagulation. In *DIC: Pathogenesis, Diagnosis and Therapy of disseminated intravascular fibrin formation*. Müller-Berghaus et al Edit, Elsevier Science Publishers B.V.,243,1993.

18. **Gordon, S.G., Franks, J.J., Lewis, B.** Cancer procoagulant A: a factor X activating procoagulant from malignant tissue. *Thromb. Res.*, 6, 127 1975.

19. **Bauer, K.A., Ten Cate, H., Barzegar, S.** Tumor necrosis factor infusions have a procoagulant effect on the hemostatic mechanisms of humans. *Blood*, 74, 165, 1989.

20. **Aakano, S., Kimuras, O.H. Dama, S. and Aoki, N.** Plasma thrombomodulin in health and disease. *Blood*, 76, 2024, 1990.

21. **Dahlbäck, B.** Protein S and C4b-binding protein : complements involved in the regulation of the protein C anticoagulant system. *Thromb. Haemost.*, 66, 49, 1991.

22. **Colucci, M., Paramo J.A. and Collen D.** Generation in plasma of a fast-acting inhibitor of plasminogen activator in response to endotoxin stimulation. *J. Clin. Invest.*, 75, 818, 1985.

23. **Kaplotis, S., Besemer, J. Bevec, D, Valent, P, Bettelheim, P., Lechner, K. and Speiser, W.** Interleukin 4 counteracts pyrogen-induced down regulation of thrombomodulin in cultured human vascular endothelial cells. *Blood*, 78, 410, 1991.

24. **Seghatchian , M.J.** Low grade activated factors in plasma: a new approach for screening prethrombotic states. Ulutin, O.N., Vinazzer, H, Eds. *Thromboses and Hemorrhagic Diseases*, Gözlen Company, Istanbul, 165, 1986.

25. **Stibbe, J., Gomes, M., de Oude, A.,** The value of the FM-Test (Kabi) and thrombin-antithrombin III complexes (TAT) in the management of DIC and Cancer.*Thromb Haemost.* 65,1238 (abstract),1991.

26. **Saito, M., Asakura , H., Yoshida, T. et al.** Levels of activated factor VII in patients with disseminated intravascular coagulation. *Blood*, 85,3770,1995.

27. **Asakura, H., Jokaji, H., Saito M., et al.** The course of disseminated intravascular coagulation is predicted by changes in thrombin-antithrombinIII complex levels - Is there any difference between treatment with standard heparin or low-molecular-weight heparin ? *Blood Coag Fibrinol.* 2,623,1991.

28. **Blauhut, B., Kramar, H., Vinazzer, H., Bergmann, H.** Substitution of anti-thrombin III in shock and DIC: a randomized study. *Thromb. Res.*, 39, 81, 1985.

29. **Lechner K. and Kyrle P.A.** Antithrombin III Concentrates - Are they clinically Useful ? *Thromb. Haemostas.*, 73 (3) 340-348, 1995.

30. **Taylor, F.B., Chang, A., Esmon, C.T., d'Angelo, A., Vigano, D., d'Angelo, S., and Blick, K.E.** Protein C prevents the coagulopathic and lethal effects of Escherichia coli infusion in the baboon. *J. Clin. Invest.*, 79, 918, 1987.

31. **Katsuura, K., Aoki, H., Tanabe, M. et al.** Characteristic effects of activated human protein C on tissue thromboplastin-induced DIC in rabbits. *Thromb. Res.*, 76, 353, 1994.

32. **Creasey, A.A., Chang, A.C.K., Feigen, L., et al.**Tissue factor pathway inhibitor reduces mortality from *Escherichia coli* septic shock. *J.Clin. Invest.* 91 2850,1993.

33. **Saito, M., Asakura, H., Jokaji, H., et al.** Recombinant hirudin for the treatment of disseminated intravascular coagulation in patients with haematological malignancy. *Blood Coag Fibrinol* 6,60,1995.

34. **Müller-Berghaus, G., Madlener, K., Blombäck, M., ten Cate, J.W.** DIC: Pathogenesis, Diagnosis and Therapy of disseminated intravascular fibrin formation. Müller-Berghaus et al Edit, Elsevier Science Publishers B.V.,1993.

35. **Forbes, C.D., Greer, I.A.** Physiology of haemostasis and the effect of pregnancy. Greer, I.A., Turpie, A.G.G., Forbes, C.D., Eds. *Haemostasis and thrombosis in Obstetrics and Gynaecology*, London, Chapman & Hall, 1, 1992.

36. **Letsky, E.A.** Coagulation defects. de Swiet, M., Ed. *Medical disorders in obstetric practice* 3rd edition, Blackwells, 104, 1994.

37. **Stirling, Y., Wolf, L., North, W., Seghatchian, M.J., Meade, T.W.** Haemostatis in normal pregnancy. *Thromb. Haemostas.*, 52, 176, 1984.

38. **Pearson, J.D.** Endothelial cells function and thrombosis. The control of production and release of haemostatic factors in the endothelial cell. *Baillières Clinical Haematology*, 6, 629, 1993.

39. **Malm, J., Laurell, M., Dahlback, B.** Changes in the plasma levels of vitamin K dependent protein C and protein S and of C4b-binding protein during pregnancy and oral contraception. *Brit. J. Haematol.*, 68, 437, 1988.

40. **Comp, P.C., Thurnau, G.R., Welsh, J., et al.** Functional and immunologic protein S levels are decreased during pregnancy. *Blood,* 68,881,1986.

41. **Abildgaard, U., Sandset, D.M., Lindhal, U.,** Tissue factor pathway inhibitor. *Recent Adv Blood Coag.* L.Poller Ed 6,105,1993.

42. **Bonnar, J., Daly, L., Sheppard, B.** Changes in fibrinolytic system during pregnancy. *Semin. Thromb. Haemost.,* 16, 221, 1990.

43. **Chow, E.Y., Haley, L.P., Vickars, L.M.** Essential thrombocytopenia in pregnancy: platelet count and pregnancy outcome. *Am. J. Hematol.,* 41, 249, 1992.

44. **Ratnoff, O.D.** Disseminated intravascular coagulation during pregnancy. in *Haemostasis and Thrombosis in Obstetrics and Gynaecology,* London, Chapman & Hall, 117, 1992.

Acquired Disorders and Congenital Thrombophilia

B. Congenital Thrombophilia: Clinical Aspects, Diagnosis and Management

ANTITHROMBIN,
ITS DEFICIENCY AND VENOUS THROMBOEMBOLISM

D.A. Lane*, R.J. Olds** and S.L. Thein***

*Dept of Haematology, Charing Cross & Westminster Medical School, London, UK
**Dept of Pathology, University of Otago, Dunedin, New Zealand
***Institute of Molecular Medicine, John Radcliffe Hospital, Headington, Oxford, UK*

I. FUNCTION AND PHYSIOLOGICAL ROLE

Antithrombin, variously also known as antithrombin III and heparin co-factor, is the major physiological inhibitor of thrombin. It also plays a role in the inhibition of other serine proteinases, including factors Xa, IXa, XIa and XIIa. The mechanism of inhibition of proteinases by antithrombin involves two steps and is similar to that observed with other serpin-proteinase reactions. An initial weak association with a dissociation constant of 1.4×10^{-3} M is formed between antithrombin and proteinase, which is then converted to a stable complex at a rate constant of $10s^{-1}$. It is thought that the high dissociation constant of the initial complex is mainly responsible for the relatively long half-time (about 40 s) of inhibition of thrombin in plasma.[1]

The transformation of initial to final complex involves the formation of a highly stable bond between the reactive site (Arg393) and the Ser residue of the active site of thrombin. Initially, the reactive bond (P1-P1'; Arg393-Ser394) of the inhibitor acts as a substrate for the enzyme, but as cleavage of the reactive site bond takes place, a conformational change occurs that traps the enzyme. The conformational change appears to be associated with the incorporation of P14-P10 sequence into sheet A and may not be restricted to the region of the reactive P1-P1' bond.

Heparin has an appreciable accelerating effect upon the formation of antithrombin-proteinase complexes. The formation of the antithrombin-thrombin complex is accelerated at least 2000-fold under optimum conditions (rate constant of inhibition of 1.5×10^7 to 3×10^8 $M^{-1}s^{-1}$), and this reduces the half-time of inhibition of thrombin in plasma to about 10 ms.[1] Similar rate enhancements have been observed for the inactivation of factors Xa and IXa by antithrombin[2], but not for the coagulation proteinases participating in contact activation. The accelerating effect of heparin occurs in concentrations very much below those of antithrombin and the proteinases, each molecule accelerating the formation of many antithrombin-proteinase complexes.

Heparin promotes the formation of a ternary complex with antithrombin and proteinase[3-5], in which the active site of the proteinase is brought into close contact with the reactive site of antithrombin. Because of its high affinity for heparin, assembly of the ternary complex proceeds preferentially through formation of a heparin-antithrombin complex. The binding of heparin to antithrombin induces a conformational change in the protein that further enhances heparin binding. Thrombin, and other proteinases that bind with quite high affinity to heparin, will bind to the heparin chain adjacent to the antithrombin, on the relatively non-specific regions[6] of the polysaccharide chain that adjoin the antithrombin binding pentasaccharide sequence. In this circumstance, a crucial role of heparin seems to be the bringing together of inhibitor and proteinase ("approximation"), rather than just the induction of a conformational change.[7] It should be emphasised that in the case of thrombin, binding to the heparin chain and approximation are essential for its accelerated inhibition.[8] In contrast, factor Xa and other proteinases that bind only weakly to heparin are inhibited directly by the heparin-antithrombin complex, and approximation of antithrombin and proteinase on the heparin does not need to take place. Rather, the conformational change induced in the inhibitor by heparin appears to enable the inhibition reaction to proceed more rapidly. Recent work, using a reactive site labelled variant, and a monoclonal antibody that recognises the strand 1C/4B region, has confirmed that binding of heparin or its essential pentasaccharide to antithrombin results directly in perturbation of the environment of the reactive centre.[9,10] Once an acyl intermediate has formed between the reactive site of antithrombin and the active site of the proteinase (factor Xa or thrombin), the change in conformation in antithrombin results in a reduced binding affinity of the complex for heparin, enabling its release and participation in additional antithrombin-proteinase reactions.

The prime physiological role of antithrombin is the regulation of coagulation proteinase activity. While the reaction of heparin with antithrombin is clearly of clinical importance, it is unlikely to have an important physiological role as heparin is not found within the vasculature under normal circumstances. Nevertheless, evidence has been obtained for the presence of an analogous accelerating mechanism that operates through heparan sulphate proteoglycans, intercalated in the surface membranes of endothelial cells.[11-13]

II. PROTEIN STRUCTURE

Antithrombin is a single chain glycoprotein of molecular weight 58,200, whose primary structure has been elucidated by protein and cDNA sequencing.[14-17] The molecule is synthesized primarily in the liver with a signal peptide of 32 amino acids which contains the normal very hydrophilic region and is cleaved at a -1 Cys- +1 His bond prior to its secretion. This peptide is necessary for intracellular transport of the protein through the endoplasmic reticulum. Plasma antithrombin contains 432 amino acids, six of which are cysteines that form three intramolecular disulphide bonds linking Cys8-Cys128, Cys21-Cys95 and Cys247-Cys430. There are four glycosylation sites, Asn-96, Asn-135, Asn-155 and Asn-192, attached to which are oligosaccharide side-chains. A minor pool of normal antithrombin (10% of the total plasma concentration) is not glycosylated at Asn-135.[18,19] The heterogeneity of the molecule is apparent on isoelectric focusing, which reveals numerous major and minor bands within the pI range of 4.9-5.7.

A . SEQUENCE HOMOLOGY AND THE SERPIN SUPERFAMILY

Antithrombin shares structural and functional homology with other members of a family of proteins referred to as the serine proteinase inhibitors or serpin superfamily.[20] A close similarity between the primary structures of antithrombin and α_1-antitrypsin was noted by Petersen et al[14] and Carrell et al.[21] The two proteins share 33% homology at the amino acid level and 46% homology on comparison of cDNA sequences.[15-17,22] Hunt and Dayhoff [23] identified ovalbumin as another related protein and subsequently, numerous other serine proteinase inhibitors, including plasminogen activator inhibitor, α_1-antichymotrypsin, C1 inhibitor, angiotensinogen and heparin cofactor II have been identified. The family includes proteins that have retained their inhibitory role of serine proteinases, and proteins that have lost this role but have acquired other functional properties. Based on nucleotide sequence homologies, it has been suggested that the serpins probably evolved from a common ancestral gene more than 500 million years ago.[23]

The structure of the serpins was initially considered in terms of a prototypical model of α_1-antitrypsin derived from the pivotal work of Loebermann et al.[24] Their crystallographic studies demonstrated that α-antitrypsin is almost completely arranged in well-defined secondary structural elements, with 30% helical (nine helices, denoted A-I) and 40% β-sheet (three sheets, denoted A-C) regions. Subsequently, X ray structure determination of bovine and human antithrombins has validated the interpretation of antithrombin structure in terms of that of α_1-antitrypsin.[25-28] The validity of the model was also supported by the determination of the crystal structures of ovalbumin,[29] a non-inhibitory serpin, plakalbumin (its cleaved form) and of plasminogen activator inhibitor.[30]

When members of the serpin superfamily are aligned according to this model, consensus sequences are apparent throughout their structures, except at their N-terminal regions corresponding to the antithrombin sequence 1-50.[20] The structures of all the proteins generally conform to the helical/β-sheet model, except in the region of helices C and D. Here there is an extended insertion in placental plasminogen activator inhibitor (PAI) and smaller inserts in ovalbumin, chicken gene Y and angiotensinogen. Regions on either side of the reactive site which are directly involved in proteinase inhibition, are also well conserved particularly the sequences Gly-Thr-Glu-Ala (residues 379-382 in antithrombin) in sheet 4A and Pro-Phe-Leu-Phe (residues 407-410 in antithrombin) in sheet 4B. These sequences are believed to be essential for facilitating conformational changes and for the correct folding of the molecules. The importance of Ala-382 and Pro-407 in these sequences is illustrated by the impaired inhibitory activity of antithrombin and the thrombotic tendency in families with mutations affecting these sites (see below). The reactive sites themselves are not highly conserved, as might be expected, as these confer specificity on the inhibitory proteins.

B. THE REACTIVE SITE

The reactive site bond of antithrombin is located at the Arg-393-Ser-394 bond.[31,32] The inhibitor acts as a pseudosubstrate for its target proteinase with the reactive site bond being the site of attack. The proteinase cleaves the reactive site, but a conformational change in the inhibitor results in trapping of the proteinase in a highly stable inactive complex which is rapidly removed from the circulation. The presence of Arg-393 at the P1 position results in the rather broad specificity of antithrombin, enabling most of the coagulation proteinases to be inhibited but the most important of these is thrombin. Several other serpins contain Arg at their reactive site and this indicates the importance of the P1' (Ser in the case of antithrombin) and surrounding residues in contributing to specificity. The reactive bonds (P1-P1') of other Arg-serpins include Arg-Thr (C1 inhibitor) and Arg-Met (α_2-antiplasmin).[33]

The central role of the P1 residue in determining the specificity of the serpins has been illustrated by the study of natural and recombinant variants of these proteins. An interesting variant of α_1-antitrypsin was described by Owen et al.[34] A young child with a fatal bleeding disorder was found to have an inherited variant (α_1-antitrypsin Pittsburgh). The structural defect was identified as being an amino acid substitution at the reactive site, Met-358 to Arg. This substitution altered the specificity of α_1-antitrypsin, redirecting its main inhibitory action from elastase toward thrombin and proteinases that are involved in contact activation of blood coagulation.[35-37] Since α_1-antitrypsin is an acute phase protein, a rapid increase in the plasma concentration of the mutant inhibitor was stimulated by a bleeding episode, resulting in an excess of coagulation proteinase-inhibitory activity in plasma, exacerbating the bleeding problem which was fatal. Detailed consideration of inherited variants affecting the reactive site of antithrombin is given below.

The structural complexity of the thrombin reactive domain of antithrombin has yet to be fully defined. Studies of a series of recombinant α_1-antitrypsin variants have demonstrated that the specificity of that inhibitor is determined by the class of amino acid at the P1 position.[36,38,39] Alteration from an uncharged to a charged residue results in changes of inhibitor specificity and reactivity. Substitution of the P3 residue can additionally modify inhibitor reactivity. Studies with recombinant antithrombin mutants of the P1' position (Ser-394) have been described [40,41] (see below).

While the Loebermann et al[24] model of the structure of cleaved α_1-antitrypsin provided an excellent working model of the serpins, it could not be used for the structure of the reactive site loop, as the P1 and P1' residues of the cleaved molecule are widely separated by ~70A. Information on the reactive site region has been provided by the analysis of crystal structures of both ovalbumin (a non-inhibitory serpin),[29,42] of its cleaved form, plakalbumin,[43] and more recently of antithrombin.[27,28] Unlike cleaved α_1-antitrypsin and other inhibitory serpins, ovalbumin does not undergo a large conformational change extending beyond the reactive centre once it is cleaved [44] and, consequently, the P1-P1' residues remain in close proximity. The major difference between the two classes of cleaved serpins (inhibitory and non-inhibitory) is the incorporation of part of the reactive loop, containing the P14-P10 residues, into the sheet A, such that this structure then contains six rather than five strands. Stein and Chothia [42] have proposed a model to account for the conformational change that allows this insertion. They argue that a fragment of the protein, consisting of an α helix and three strands of β sheet, moves away from the rest of the molecule to make space for the new strand. A unique structural change allows this to happen: sheet 3A residues in the small fragment slide along grooves in the α helix B that belongs to the rest of the protein. Movement of the reactive loop from its surface to its sheet A location is supported by studies using synthetic peptides of α_1-antitrypsin and antithrombin that correspond to the sequence N-terminal to the reactive loop. These peptides are able to incorporate into the sheet structure of the uncleaved molecule, mimicking the insertion of the N-terminal arm of the reactive site loop into sheet A as strand 4, and render the inhibitor functionally inactive.[45-47] It is likely that this structural rearrangement in inhibitory serpins, such as antithrombin, is important in the formation and stabilization of the serpin-proteinase complex. This is further discussed below in the context of the effects of mutations in the P12-P10 sequence adjacent to the reactive centre of antithrombin.

The unexpected finding from the crystal structure determination of ovalbumin was that the counterpart of the reactive centre in inhibitory serpins could be an intact peptide loop taking the form of a protruding isolated helix.[29] In ovalbumin, this helix is formed by a 19 residue segment extending from P15 to P5'. A solvent channel runs between the helix and the rest of the molecule and the loop appears to be mobile. Recent structural investigation of intact human antithrombin has suggested that the reactive loop need not necessarily adopt a helical configuration.[27] Partial insertion of the intact reactive loop in the central sheet of the intact molecule results in the main reactive loop chain leaving the body of the molecule at a perpendicular angle. Residues in the P14-P10 sequence have weak electron density in this model, suggesting high mobility. Mobility of the reactive loop may facilitate interaction with the proteinase, and the insertion of the P14-P10 region into sheet A during stabilisation of the serpin-proteinase complex (see below). Residues 392-397 are well separated from the main body of the molecule and adopt a conformation not dissimilar to the Burman-Birk type inhibitors.[27]

C. THE HEPARIN BINDING DOMAIN

Early attempts at characterization of the interaction between heparin and antithrombin used heparin heterogeneous with respect to size and ability to interact with antithrombin. A major advance, therefore, was the finding that only a fraction of commercial heparin binds with high affinity to the protein.[48,49] The minimal binding sequence of heparin has been localised by a series of subsequent studies to a unique pentasaccharide sequence.[50-54] Heparin binds through this sequence to a single site on antithrombin with a dissociation constant of 2×10^{-8}M.[55-57] Binding depends strongly on ionic strength and pH, and it has been suggested that a maximum of five to six charged groups on each molecule is involved[58] with the negatively charged sulphates of the glycosaminoglycans interacting with positively charged residues (lysine and arginine) on antithrombin. Heparin binding alters the overall fluorescence spectrum of antithrombin, suggesting that the interaction has resulted in a conformational change.[55,59]

The heparin binding domain of antithrombin appears to consist of two regions encompassing amino acids 41 to 49, and amino acids 107 to 156. Both regions consist of clusters of basic amino acids and are localised at the amino-terminal end of the protein. The delineation of these regions was based on biochemical experiments and characterization of natural mutants affecting these sites. For instance, chemical or genetic modification of Trp49[55,59-61] results in impaired binding of heparin to antithrombin.[62] Using a combination of limited digestion with the enzyme proteinase V8 and quantitative N-terminal sequence analysis,[63] Liu and Chang suggested that cleavage of Glu34-Gly35, Glu42-Ala43 and Glu50-Leu51 was drastically inhibited by preincubation of antithrombin with heparin. The results suggest that Glu34-Leu51 may be involved in heparin binding. Further, studies of affected individuals has demonstrated that mutations at Arg-24, Pro41 and Arg47 interfere with heparin binding (see below).

The second heparin binding region has been proposed to be the positively charged amino acids, Lys107, Lys114, Lys125, Arg129, Arg132 and Lys133, at the surface of the antithrombin molecule.[64] Chemical modification studies of antithrombin with a water soluble reagent specific for lysine residues showed that Lys107, Lys114, Lys125 and Lys136 are involved in heparin binding.[65,66] Further evidence that the region encompassing residues 124-145 might be important in heparin binding comes from studies by Smith et al. They showed that polyclonal antibodies with specificity against a synthetic peptide comprising residues 124 to 145 block the binding of heparin to antithrombin.[67] As mentioned earlier, a minor pool of normal antithrombin exists without a carbohydrate side-chain at Asn135. This normal variant has an increased affinity for heparin.

A tertiary structure model, based on the crystal structure of cleaved α_1-antitrypsin, has also been used as a template to define the heparin binding domains of antithrombin. Borg et al[64] have proposed that seven basic residues are aligned to form a positive site stretching across the molecule from the A helix (Arg47) to the D helix (Lys125, Arg129, Arg132) and the adjacent Lys133. Thus the two putative heparin binding regions are adjacent to each other in this 3-dimensional structure. This interesting model appears to provide a partial explanation for many of the features of the heparin binding site of antithrombin. In this context, it is interesting that integrity of the Cys8-Cys128 (Cys128 is located within the second heparin binding domain) disulphide bond is important for binding heparin to antithrombin. It should be appreciated, though, that the proposed model is based on reactive site cleaved α_1-antitrypsin and neither reactive site cleaved antithrombin nor α_1-antitrypsin actually binds heparin with high affinity. Nevertheless, the crystal structures of both cleaved and intact antithrombin provide support for a surface orientated primary contact site comprised of elements of helices D, A and perhaps C.[27,28] From a consideration of the cleaved bovine antithrombin structure, it has been proposed that Arg13, Lys39, Arg46, Arg47, Arg129 and Arg132 comprise the primary pentasaccharide contact surface.[26]

While specific antithrombin residues are important in the heparin binding site providing the points of contact with the pentasaccharide, it is apparent that the overall conformation of the heparin binding domain must also be considered along with any structural changes that may occur in the heparin-induced conformational change. This is illustrated by results of the analysis of naturally occurring mutants, the so-called 'type Ib' or 'pleiotropic effect' antithrombin deficiencies, in which substitutions occur in strand 1C/4B near the C-terminus.[68] It appears that the hydrophobic region at the C-terminus is essential either for the maintenance of the 3D structure of the molecule or for propagation of heparin-induced conformation change. The substitution of essential amino acids in this region alters several properties of the molecule including its ability to bind heparin (see below). Similarly, Pro41, Leu99 Ser116 and Gln118 (see below) substituted in heparin binding variants, may not participate directly in binding but may be important to maintain secondary structure of the initial contact domain.

III. ANTITHROMBIN GENE STRUCTURE

Initial studies linked inherited antithrombin deficiency to Duffy blood group antigens on chromosome 1 [69-71] and the localisation to 1q was confirmed by analysis of somatic cell hybrids and by analysis of antithrombin deficient individuals with chromosomal deletions. In situ hybridisation has refined the localisation of the gene to 1q23-25. [72] Using DNA polymorphisms within the antithrombin gene, linkage studies in kindreds with antithrombin deficiency confirmed that the clinical phenotype was tightly linked to the antithrombin locus on 1q.[73,74]

The antithrombin gene occurs in a single copy on the haploid genome and contains seven exons spanning 13.4 kilobases of DNA from the transcription start site to the poly A signal. Initially it had been thought that there were only six exons but subsequent analysis revealed a 1 kilobase intron within exon 3.[75] Common usage now refers to these exons as 3A and 3B. The complete nucleotide sequence of the antithrombin gene has been determined; within the introns of the gene are located 9 full length and one partial length Alu repeat elements.[76] Alu repeats are the commonest members of the short interspersed family of DNA repeats. They are found at greater density within the antithrombin gene than is the average within the human genome. Two of the Alu repeats within the antithrombin gene, Alu 5 and Alu 8 within intron 4 have tails composed of (ATT) trinucleotide repeats which are polymorphic in copy number (see below). The Alu 8 polymorphism in particular has been useful, because of its high heterozygosity, in determining whether repeatedly identified mutations are of independent origin or represent founder effects.[77]

Expression of the antithrombin gene occurs in a regulated and tissue-specific manner; antithrombin being produced principally by the hepatocytes. Little is known of the cis-acting sequences or the trans-acting factors which control antithrombin gene expression. Commonly identified control regions such as the TATA box, the CCAAT box or GC elements are not found in the 5'-untranslated region of the gene. Two regions have been identified in the 5'-end of the gene which appear to act as regulatory elements, as shown either by in vitro expression studies [78] or by the presence of a sequence which bound a trans-acting factor.[79] While both these studies have identified regions of the 5' end of the antithrombin gene which apparently confer some tissue-specific control of expression, much remains to be learned about the regulation of antithrombin production.

The mRNA start site has been mapped by primer extension analysis of human liver RNA.[80] A single transcription start site was localised 72 base pairs 5' to the ATG initiation codon. The 3'-end of the gene contains the canonical poly A sequence, AATAAA, located 49 base pairs 3' to the termination codon. Normally the cleavage/polyadenylation site is located 24 base pairs downstream from the AATAAA sequence.[15,16,81]

Both wild type and variant forms of the antithrombin protein have been expressed using a variety of host cells, including E. coli,[16] HeLa, COS-1 and baby hamster kidney cells [10,40,41,80,82-84] and yeast cells.[85] Cell free expression has also been utilised.[86,87] A promising approach, allowing the expression of large quantities of functionally active inhibitor, is the use of baculovirus vectors in insect cells.[88]

The antithrombin gene contains a number of sequence polymorphisms. Several are readily detectable, including enzyme cutting site polymorphisms for PstI[89] (nucleotide 7626, codon 305 in exon 4), NheI[90] (nucleotide 7987, intron 4) and DdeI[91] (nucleotide 9893, intron 5), a 76bp length polymorphism located at the 5'-end of the gene [92] and (ATT) repeat polymophisms in the tails of Alu

5 and Alu 8 in intron 4.[76] Additionally, there is a sequence variation at nucleotide 7596, codon 295,[93] although this cannot be readily analysed except by sequencing. These polymorphisms can be used in the construction of antithrombin gene haplotypes for tracing a mutant gene in a family or in determining the origin of repeated mutations. The (ATT) trinucleotide repeat in the tail of Alu 8 has 10 alleles and a heterozygosity of at least 0.83 in Caucasian,[77] Asian-Indian and Jamaican Black populations (Olds et al, unpublished observations).

IV. ANTITHROMBIN DEFICIENT STATES

Antithrombin deficiency may be inherited or acquired; failure to maintain an adequate level of functional antithrombin in plasma results in an increased risk of thromboembolism. In this review we concentrate on the inherited antithrombin deficient states. For a discussion on the acquired antithrombin deficiencies see Lane et al.[94]

A. HEREDITARY DEFICIENCY
Patients with antithrombin deficiency have a high risk of developing venous thrombosis which rises with increasing age. However, there is still uncertainty regarding the prevalence of thromboembolism in affected individuals. Thaler and Lechner [95] reviewed the published reports and deduced that the median age of presentation was 24 years, with 67% having a first clinical episode between ages 10-35 years. This data is probably biased by the tendency to report clinical events; therefore asymptomatic individuals with antithrombin defects detectable by laboratory testing may well be under-represented. A study by Demers and colleagues[96] of a large family with a type II reactive site variant found that the incidence of confirmed venous thrombosis in affected individuals was less than 20%. Venous thrombosis is the usual mode of clinical presentation in antithrombin deficient individuals. The commonest sites for thromboses are the deep leg veins, the iliac, femoral and superficial leg veins. Other frequently encountered sites include the pelvic veins, inferior vena cava, mesenteric vessels, hepatic and portal veins (which may produce the Budd-Chiari syndrome[97]), renal, axillary, brachial, cerebral and retinal veins. Arterial thrombosis is uncommon, but has been reported.[98-100] The risk of thromboembolism depends on the type of antithrombin deficiency.[101-103] A consistent observation is that individuals heterozygous for an antithrombin variant with reduced heparin affinity have a low incidence of clinical thrombosis, whereas homozygous individuals exhibit a 100% frequency of thrombotic disease which may well be arterial.[100,104] Characteristics which may suggest an inherited thrombotic tendency include presentation at an early age, absence of any predisposing factor, recurrent venous thrombosis, thrombosis at an unusual site and a familial predisposition.[101] In 54% of cases it has been reported that the first thrombotic event is probably triggered by a known risk factor. The commonest were pregnancy or child birth; other-at-risk situations include prolonged immobilisation, oestrogen containing oral contraceptives and major trauma.[95]

B. INCIDENCE OF INHERITED DEFICIENCY
The incidence of hereditary antithrombin deficiency has been estimated at between 1:2000[105] and 1:5000[106] in the normal population. Recently, however, it has been reported that the actual incidence may be higher. In a survey of over 4000 Scottish blood donors,[107] using a sensitive heparin cofactor assay, an incidence of 1/350 was found, most of these individuals being clinically asymptomatic. These findings suggest that the "normal" population includes individuals who have biochemical antithrombin abnormalities, which for most do not represent a thrombotic risk according to our current understanding of venous thromboembolic disease.

A number of studies have examined the incidence of hereditary antithrombin deficiency in those presenting with venous thrombosis. In a review of the surveys of young (<45 years) patients with venous thrombosis the incidence of antithrombin deficiency was 4.5%.[101] In 210 consecutive patients presenting with venous thrombosis the incidence of antithrombin variants was around 4%,[108] while in another 204 patients with history of venous thrombosis only one patient was found with antithrombin deficiency.[109] In the latter study the overall incidence of either antithrombin, protein C, protein S or plasminogen deficiency was 4%. Another study examined the causes of acute, venographically proven deep vein thrombi in 277 consecutive patients in whom acquired deficiencies of natural anticoagulants had been excluded.[110] Overall, 8.3% had an identifiable inherited deficiency of either antithrombin

(1.1%), protein C (3.2%), protein S (2.2%) or plasminogen (1.4%). These surveys indicate that there is still uncertainty about the prevalence of antithrombin deficiency. Perhaps the most important observation that can be made is that the vast majority of venous thrombotic episodes occurred in the absence of any recognised biochemical abnormality. Undoubtedly many of these cases of venous thrombosis of undefined cause will now be found to be due to deficiency of the recently described activated protein C cofactor.[111,112]

C. CLASSIFICATION

A number of attempts have been made to classify all the cases of antithrombin deficiency [102,113,114] and none is completely satisfactory. This has been done with regard to their plasma levels and reported functional properties (rather than with regard to their molecular defects, which generally have not been available). Consequently, these classification schemes must remain tentative until the precise nature of more of the abnormalities is known. While a number of cases may well be placed in a wrong subgroup, these schemes have nevertheless been useful in providing a preliminary overview of the relationships between the functional abnormalities and the frequency of thrombosis. A system of classification that we have adopted[115] was subsequently revised[93] on the basis of groupings of known mutations and their effects upon the function of antithrombin. The revised classification is set out below:

Type I: Low functional and immunological antithrombin

Type II: Presence of variant antithrombin
   RS, effect on reactive site
   HBS, effect on heparin binding site
   PE, pleiotropic effect

For the purpose of the remainder of this chapter, the revised scheme only will be considered. Type I deficiency, the 'classical' antithrombin deficiency, has reduced levels (~50%) of immunologically and functionally determined antithrombin. Type II deficiency covers the cases in which the functionally determined antithrombin is reduced (~50%) and approximately half the antithrombin antigen is provided by a variant protein. The variant may have functional abnormalities of the reactive site (RS) or the heparin binding site (HBS). It has become apparent that in some cases with reduced immunological antithrombin small amounts of a variant can be identified. These were initially subtyped as type Ib, the original case being antithrombin Oslo.[114,116] Because recent functional characterisation of a group of such cases has suggested that they have multiple or "pleiotropic" functional abnormalities affecting the reactive site, the heparin binding site and the plasma concentration, these cases have now been assigned the subtype "pleiotropic effect".[68,93]

D. MOLECULAR BASIS OF INHERITED ANTITHROMBIN DEFICIENCY

Many mutations causing antithrombin deficiency have now been characterised. Type I deficiencies are produced by major gene deletions or point mutations, including small insertions or deletions which disrupt protein production from the affected allele. Single base substitutions within coding regions giving rise to variant antithrombins are the basis of all type II deficiencies identified to date. The nature of the amino acid substitution as well as its site in the antithrombin chain is a critical determinant of the resulting phenotype.

1. Type I Deficiencies

Most cases of type I deficiency are due to point changes, i.e. single base substitutions, minor insertions or deletions, within the antithrombin gene. The majority of these defects have been identified by systematically amplifying the coding regions and the intronic borders by the polymerase chain reaction and direct sequencing of the amplified DNA; for this reason most of the defects identified to date are contained within the exons. The mutations appear to cause a quantitative reduction in antithrombin synthesis by a variety of mechanisms: (i) minor insertions or deletions leading to frame shifts in translation and premature termination; (ii) nucleotide substitutions which produce a premature termination codon; (iii) mutations which affect RNA processing and (iv) mutations which produce unstable antithrombins which either are not exported efficiently or have shortened plasma half lives. The generation of unstable variant antithrombin protein has not been demonstrated experimentally, but can be inferred in cases where the mutation leads to single amino acid substitutions or deletions of intact codons and yet are associated with type I deficiency.

Most type I mutations identified to date have been unique to single families. Two of the exceptions are the CGA→TGA mutation in codon 129 and the deletion of 6 bp in codons 106-108. The mutation within codon 129(CGA→TGA) results in the replacement of the normal Arg residue by a STOP codon and has been described in at least 8 kindreds.[117] The base substitution occurs within a CpG dinucleotide, a recognised hotspot for single base mutations. Haplotype analysis of the mutant gene in six families suggested that the mutation had an independent origin in at least two families.[77] The six bp deletion within codons 106-108 has been identified in two kindreds, one of Norwegian origin and the other from New Zealand. The mutant antithrombin alleles in the two kindreds were associated with different antithrombin haplotypes and were therefore, probably, of independent origins.[118] The deletion site is flanked on both sides by a short sequence repeat (TTT) and the deletion removes one repeat and three intervening base pairs, compatible with a deletion mechanism that involves slippage and mispairing of the two DNA strands during DNA synthesis.

Major and partial gene deletion as a cause of type I deficiency is relatively uncommon. In a study of 45 kindreds with Type I deficiency, we identified four probands with a major deletion of the antithrombin gene.[119] In one case characterised at the sequence level a 2.8kb deletion affecting intron 4, exon 5 and intron 5 had arisen by homologous recombination between sequences of Alu 7 and Alu 10.[76] One other partial gene deletion has been the subject of a full report; the abnormality involved the deletion of the 5'-end of the gene, up to and including exon 2, but the basis for the deletion was not apparent. [120] A small number of other deletions affecting the gene have been reported but are otherwise uncharacterised.

2. Type II: Reactive Site (RS)

Type II RS variants are not able to inactivate proteinases; those that have been fully reported have amino acid substitutions in the vicinity of the reactive site (cases reported only as preliminary communications will not be discussed here). For convenience they can be classed as three subgroups. The first includes those with amino acid substitutions that directly impede the function of the reactive site. Substitutions at reactive site P1 position Arg393 to Cys, His and Pro in antithrombins Northwick Park, Glasgow and Pescara, respectively [121-123] and other similar cases [124-127] prevent any interaction with thrombin. A similar phenotype has been observed with a substitution at the P2 position, Gly392 to Asp, in antithrombin Stockholm.[128] The Arg-393 to Cys substitution is particularly interesting, as Cys393 is able to form a disulphide bond with albumin[121] circulating as a disulphide-linked heterodimer between albumin and antithrombin. Substitution at the P1' position, Ser394 to Leu (antithrombin Denver), reduces the inhibitory properties of antithrombin[83] but this depends upon the proteinase. Olson et al [57] have found that second order rate constants for antithrombin Denver reactions with thrombin, factor Xa and plasmin were reduced 430-fold, 7-fold and 45-fold, respectively, relative to normal antithrombin.

The second subgroup of reactive site variants include those with substitutions in the P12-P10 region, a region which is presently assuming some importance in terms of our understanding of antithrombin-proteinase complexes formation. A possible important functional role for this region is indicated by the serpin sequence alignment , which identified appreciable homology at least in the case of the P12 residue (Ala382), see above. This amino acid is conserved in all serpins that retain proteinase inhibitory activity. Initial studies suggested that substitution of Ala382 in antithrombin Hamilton[129] and Ala-384 in antithrombin Charleville[130] caused functionally inactive mutants. Closer examination, however, showed that these and similar variants (antithrombins Glasgow II and Vicenza) [131,132] are cleaved at their reactive site bonds following their interactions with thrombin but do not form inhibitory complexes with them. The cleavage causes a reduction in heparin binding affinity, as demonstrated by crossed immunoelectrophoresis. The transformation of these mutant inhibitors into substrates for the proteinase is not unique to antithrombin. Naturally occurring and engineered variants of several other serpins with substitutions in the same region also demonstrate substrate behaviour.[133-136] Because of the substrate behaviour of these variants, together with the structural transition observed in the crystallographic studies of cleaved serpins, Skriver et al[133] proposed a plausible model for stabilisation of the serpin-proteinase complex. They suggested that in the normal serpin-proteinase interaction, the conformational change required to trap the proteinase comprises a partial reactive loop insertion into sheet A structure. The rate of partial loop insertion must be fast enough to prevent reactive loop cleavage by the proteinase and the nature of the P12-P10 residues appears to be crucial in permitting rapid loop insertion. Substitution of P12 and P10 alanine residues must impair loop insertion and allows the proteinase cleavage reaction to proceed to completion.

3. Type II: Heparin Binding Site (HBS)

Type II HBS deficiency is characterized by the presence of variants with impaired heparin co-factor activity. Characterisation of the molecular basis has provided an unambiguous means of defining the heparin binding domain of antithrombin. The majority of the variants have mutations within the first putative heparin binding domain of heparin (residues 41 and 47). However, some of these variants have now been characterized with mutations affecting different residues. A variant, antithrombin Rouen III [137], with reduced heparin binding has been shown to have an Ile7 to Asn substitution. This substitution results in generation of a new potential glycosylation site at position 7. It is not clear whether the alteration in heparin binding arises from the amino acid substitution or the incorporation of the sugar side chain in the antithrombin. The substitution Arg24 to Cys (antithrombin Rouen IV)[138] involves the loss of a basic residue and the association with reduction in heparin binding affinity suggests that the residue is part of the primary contact site for the pentasaccharide.

A mutation Leu99 to Phe has been characterized in an individual who was homozygous for the defect. The variant alters heparin binding and interaction of the heparin binding domain with the pentasaccharide.[104] In the model of heparin binding that has been proposed on the basis of the serpin crystal structure, the binding domain is present as a region of high positive charge density, composed of basic residues of helices A and D. Leu99 is located on helix C, which lies beneath the heparin binding domain. It is assumed that the Leu99 to Phe substitution perturbs the geometry of the domain. Evidence for this has been obtained by demonstration of a small change in isoelectric point of this variant. A similar mechanism could explain the reduction in heparin affinity that occurs with the recently reported substitutions of Ser116 to Pro[139] Leu99 to Val[140] and Gln118 to Pro.[140]

An interesting type II HBS variant (antithrombin Geneva Arg 129→Gln) has been reported at position 129, the second heparin binding region of antithrombin. Church et al and Gandrille et al [141,142] propose that Lys125, Arg129, Arg132, Lys133, Lys136 and Lys139 are all on the same side of helix D and constitute an essential part of the primary heparin binding domain, a proposal well supported by the chemical modification studies and by the characterization of antithrombin Geneva.

Until recently, information regarding the affect of substitutions was of a qualitative nature and it might have been assumed that substitutions altering predicted primary pentasaccharide contact residues caused greatest alteration to heparin binding. The identification of a monoclonal antibody that competes with heparin and its pentasaccharide for binding to antithrombin has enabled such a prediction to be tested. Using a competitive binding assay, the dissociation constants between heparin and many of the known variant antithrombins were determined.[143] The dissociation constant between heparin and normal antithrombin was found to be 48.8nM and amino acid substitutions resulting in type II HBS variants resulted in a 10-1000 fold reduction in affinity, regardless of whether the substitution was in a predicted primary contact residue. Remarkably, the substitutions resulting in type II PE variants (see below) resulted in similar decrease in heparin affinity, ~200-1000 fold.

Haplotype analysis has again been utilised to examine the origin of some type II mutations that have been reported repeatedly. In four apparently unrelated kindreds with the mutation Leu99→Phe, due to a nucleotide substitution in a non-CpG dinucleotide, the mutant alleles were all associated with the same antithrombin haplotype, compatible with the presence of a founder effect.[77]

4. Type II: Pleiotropic Effect (PE)

Type II PE antithrombin mutants often present as "classical" or type I defects in that a reduced level of antithrombin is demonstrated both by functional and antigen assays. However, closer analysis of plasma reveals disproportionate higher antigen than activity levels and the presence of small quantities of the variant protein. The first of these variants characterised was antithrombin Utah, Pro 407 to Leu [75]. Subsequently, several similar cases have been identified prompting the classification of these antithrombin mutants as a separate group. The other variants of this subtype include those with amino acid substitutions at codons 402 (antithrombins Rosny, Torino, Maisons-Laffitte), 404 (antithrombins Oslo),405 (antithrombin La Rochelle),406 (antithrombin Kyoto) and 407 (antithrombin Budapest 5). [68] It is interesting that nearly all the variants in this subgroup involve substitutions in exon 6 in the region P9' to P14'. These variant antithrombins are not able to inactivate thrombin and have an associated reduction in heparin binding affinity. An explanation of the pleiotropic effect of these substitutions has been advanced[68] and uses the serpin crystal structure consensus features. Proximity of the reactive site makes loss of proteinase inhibitory function no surprise, given the predicted mobility of the reactive loop particularly in relation to the strand 1C/4B region.[9] An effect upon heparin binding can be explained, despite the distal localisation of the predicted pentasaccharide binding site to strand 1C, by the observation that the hydrophobic residues comprising strands 4B and 5B form much of an interface between the reactive site and the elements comprising the predicted primary heparin contact site. The substitutions may induce a conformational change in the heparin binding site, or may prevent the transmission of the heparin-induced conformational change to the reactive centre. Recent investigations of pentasaccharide binding to a series of N- and C-terminal substitution mutants with impaired heparin binding, favours the latter explanation.[144]

The substitution that has been found in the propositus with antithrombin Budapest (429 CCT→CTT Pro→Leu)[145] can also be included in this subgroup. Although the propositus is homozygous for the mutant antithrombin allele, two populations of antithrombin can be isolated from the plasma. The first binds strongly to heparin-Sepharose and has reduced ability (30%) to inactivate thrombin. The second binds only weakly to heparin and is devoid of inhibitory activity. The propositus has a reduced plasma concentration of antithrombin. It is proposed that the substitution may perturb the conformation of the reactive site in the first population, while a more profound alteration in structure may be present in the second. The reason for this unusual behaviour is not apparent at present.

The reduced levels of some of this group of variants can be seen within the context of the published work on the serpin-enzyme complex receptor recognition system. It appears that there is a hepatic receptor that specifically recognises serpins complexed to their proteinases.[146] An elegant series of experiments has shown that the serpin-proteinase complex is specifically bound to the surface of hepatocytes and that the receptor involved may mediate rapid clearance of serpin complexes from the circulation.[147-149] With regard to the variants presently under consideration, it has been shown that peptides with the highly conserved serpin sequence corresponding to amino acid sequence 408-412 in antithrombin can compete for the binding sites on the hepatocytes. This region may constitute a cryptic site on the antithrombin molecule, exposed during complex formation with proteinases and recognised by the receptor. The close proximity of these mutations to the recognition site suggests that they partially expose the hidden sequence, which the receptor falsely identifies as a complex. An alternative explanation for the reduced plasma concentration of strand 1C/4B variants is reduced synthesis or export from the hepatocytes.

ACKNOWLEDGEMENTS

The work of the authors reported in this article was supported by the British Heart Foundation, the Wellcome Trust and in part by the Health Research Council of New Zealand.

REFERENCES

1.   **Bjork I, Olson ST, Shore JD.** "Molecular mechanisms of the accelerating effect of heparin on the reactions between antithrombin and the clotting proteinases." *Heparin: Chemical and Biological Properties, Clinical Applications.* Lane DA and Lindahl U, eds. 1989 Edward Arnold. London.

2.   **Jordan RE, Oosta GM, Gardner WT, Rosenberg RD:** The kinetics of haemostatic enzyme-antithrombin interactions in the presence of low molecular weight heparin. *J Biol Chem*, 255, 10081, 1980.

3.   **Griffith MJ:** Kinetics of heparin enhanced antithrombin III/thrombin reaction. Evidence for a template model for the mechanism of action of heparin. *J Biol Chem*, 257, 7360, 1982.

4.   **Griffith MJ:** The heparin enhanced antithrombin III/thrombin reaction is saturable with respect to both thrombin and antithrombin III. *J Biol Chem*, 257,13899, 1982.

5.   **Pomerantz MW, Owen WG:** A catalytic role for heparin. Evidence for a ternary complex of heparin cofactor, thrombin and heparin. *Biochim Biophys Acta*, 535, 66, 1978.

6.   **Olson ST, Halvorson HR, Bjork I:** Quantitative characterisation of the thrombin-heparin interaction. Discrimination between specific and nonspecific binding models. *J Biol Chem*, 266, 6342, 1991.

7.   **Olson ST, Bjork I:** Predominant contribution of surface approximation to the mechanism of heparin acceleration of the antithrombin-thrombin reaction. Elucidation from salt concentration effects. *J Biol Chem*, 266, 6353, 1991.

8.   **Lane DA, Denton J, Flynn AM, Thunberg L, Lindahl U:** Anticoagulant activities of heparin oligosaccharides and their neutralization by platelet factor 4. *Biochem J*, 218, 725, 1984.

9.   **Dawes J, James K, Lane DA:** The conformational change in antithrombin induced by heparin, probed with a monoclonal antibody against the 1C/4B region. *Biochemistry*, 33, 4375, 1994.

10.   **Gettins P, Fan B, Crews B, Turko I, Olson S, Streusand V:** Transmission of conformational change from the heparin binding site to the reactive center of antithrombin. *Biochemistry*, 32, 8385, 1993.

11. **Marcum JA, Rosenberg RD**: Anticoagulantly active heparin-like molecules from vascular tissue. *Biochemistry*, 23, 1730, 1984.

12. **Marcum JA, Rosenberg RD**: Heparin-like molecules with anticoagulant activity are synthesized by cultured endothelial cells. *Biochem Biophys Res Comm*, 126, 365,1985.

13. **Marcum JA, Atha DH, Fritze LMS, Nawroth P, Stern D, Rosenberg RD**: Cloned bovine aortic endothelial cells synthesize anticoagulantly active heparan sulphate proteoglycans. *J Biol Chem*, 261, 7507, 1986.

14. **Petersen TE, Dudek-Wojciechowska G, Sottrup-Jensen L, Magnusson** S. "Primary structure of antithrombin III (heparin cofactor). Partial homology between α_1 antitrypsin and antithrombin III." The Physiological Inhibitors of Blood Coagulation and Fibrinolysis. Collen D, Wiman B and Verstraete M, eds. 1979 Elsevier Science Publishers. Amsterdam.

15. **Prochownik EV, Markam AF, Orkin SH**: Isolation of a cDNA clone for human antithrombin III. *J Biol Chem*, 258, 8389, 1983.

16. **Bock SC, Wion KL, Vehar GA, Lawn RM**: Cloning and expression of the cDNA for human antithrombin III. *Nucl Acids Res*, 10, 8113, 1982.

17. **Chandra T, Stackhouse R, Kidd VJ, Woo SLC**: Isolation and sequence characterisation of a cDNA clone of human antithrombin III. *Proc Natl Acad Sci USA*, 80, 1845, 1983.

18. **Peterson CB, Blackburn MN**: Isolation and characterisation of an antithrombin III variant with reduced carbohydrate content and enhanced heparin binding. *J Biol Chem*, 260, 610, 1985.

19. **Brennan SO, George PM, Jordan RE**: Physiological variant of antithrombin III lacks carbohydrate side chain at Asn 135. *FEBS Lett*, 219,431, 1987.

20. **Huber R, Carrell RW**: Implications of the three-dimensional structure of α_1-antitrypsin for the structure and function of serpins. *Biochemistry*, 28, 8951, 1989.

21. **Carrell RW, Owen M, Brennan S, Vaughan L**: Carboxy terminal fragment of human a1-antitrypsin from hydroxlamine cleavage: homology with antithrombin III. *Biochem Biophys Res Comm*, 91, 1032, 1979.

22. **Chandra T, Stackhouse R, Kidd VJ, Robson JH, Woo SLC**: Sequence homology between human α_1 antichymotrypsin, α_1-antitrypsin and antithrombin III. *Biochemistry*, 22, 5055, 1983.

23. **Hunt LT, Dayhoff MO**: A suprising new protein superfamily containing ovalbumin, antithrombin III and α_1-proteinase inhibitor. *Biochem Biophys Res Commun*, 95, 864, 1980.

24. **Loebermann H, Tokuoka R, Diesenhofer J, Huber** R: Human alpha 1-proteinase inhibitor. Crystal structure analysis of two crystal modifications, molecular model and preliminary analysis of the implications for function.*J Mol Biol*, 177, 531, 1984.

25. **Mourey L, Samama JP, Delarue M, Choay J, Lormeau JC, Petitou M, Moras D**: Antithrombin III: structural and functional aspects. *Biochimie* , 72, 599, 1990.

26. **Mourey L, Samama JP, Delarue M, Petitou M, Choay J, Moras D**: Crystal structure of cleaved bovine antithrombin III at 3.2A resolution. J Mol Biol, 232, 223, 1993.

27. **Schreuder HA, de Boer B, Dijkema R, Mulders J, Theunissen HJM, Grootenhuis PDJ, Hol WGJ**: The intact and cleaved human antithrombin III complex as a model for serpin-proteinase interactions. *Nature Structural Biology,* 1, 48, 1994.

28. **Carrell RW, Stein PE, Fermi G, Wardell MR**: Biological implications of a 3A structure of dimeric antithrombin. *Structure*, 2, 257, 1994.

29. **Stein PE, Leslie AGW, Finch JT, Turnell WG, McLaughlin PJ, Carrell RW**: Crystal structure of ovalbumin as a model for the reactive centre of serpins. *Nature,* 347, 99, 1990.

30. **Mottonen J, Strand A, Symersky J, Sweet RM, Danley DE, Geoghegan KF, Gerard RD, Goldsmith EJ**: Structural basis of latency in plasminogen activator inhibitor-I. *Nature,* 355, 270, 1992.

31. **Bjork I, Jackson CM, Jornvall H, Lavine KK, Nording K, Salsgiver WJ**: The active site of antithrombin. Release of the same proteolytically cleaved form of the inhibitor from complexes with Factor IXa, Factor Xa and thrombin. *J Biol Chem*, 257, 2406, 1982.

32. **Bjork I, Danielsson A, Fenton JW, Jornvall H**: The site in human antithrombin for functional proteolytic cleavage by human thrombin. *FEBS Letts* , 126, 257, 1981.

33. **Potempa J, Shieh BH, Travis J**: Alpha2-antiplasmin: a serpin with two separate but overlapping reactive sites. *Science*, 241, 699, 1988.

34. **Owen MC, Brennan SO, Lewis JH, Carrell RW**: Mutation of antitrypsin to antithrombin. a1-antitrypsin Pittsburg (358Met -Arg), a fatal bleeding disorder.*New Eng J Med*, 309, 694, 1983.

35. **Schapira M, Ramus MA, Jallat S, Carvallo D, Courtney** M: Recombinant alpha1-antitrypsin Pittsburgh (Met 358-Arg) is a potent inhibitor of plasma kallikrein and factor XII. *J Clin Invest* , 76, 635, 1985.

36. **Jallat S, Carvallo D, Tessier LH**: Altered specificities of genetically engineered alpha1 antitrypsin variants. *Protein Engineering*, 1, 29, 1986.

37. **Scott CF, Carrell RW, Glaser CB, Kueppers F, Lewis JH, Colman RW**: Alpha1 antitrypsin Pittsburgh. A potent inhibitor of human factor XIa, Kallikrein and factor XII. *J Clin Invest*, 77, 631, 1986.

38. **Travis J, Owen M, George P**: Isolation and properties of recombinant DNA produced variants of human alpha1-proteinase inhibitor. *J Biol Chem* , 260, 4384, 1985.

39. **Matheson NR, Gibson HL, Hallewell RA, Barr PJ, Travis** J: Recombinant DNA-derived forms of a1-proteinase inhibitor. *J Biol Chem* , 261, 10404, 1986.

40. **Stephens AW, Siddiqui A, Hirs CH**: Site-directed mutagenesis of the reactive center (serine 394) of antithrombin III. *J Biol Chem*, 263, 15849, 1988.

41. **Theunissen HJ, Dijkema R, Grootenhuis PD, Swinkels JC, de Poorter T, Carati P, Visser** A: Dissociation of heparin-dependent thrombin and factor Xa inhibitory activities of antithrombin-III by mutations in the reactive site. *J Biol Chem* , 268, 9035, 1993.

42. **Stein P, Chothia C**: Serpin tertiary structure transformation. *J Mol Biol*, 221, 615, 1991.

43. **Wright HT, Qian HX, Huber R**: Crystal structure of plakalbumin, a proteolytically nicked form of ovalbumin. Its relationship to the structure of cleaved alpha1-proteinase inhibitor. *J Mol Biol*, 213, 513, 1990.

44. **Gettins P**: Absence of large scale conformational change upon limited proteolysis of ovalbumin, the prototypic serpin. *J Biol Chem*, 264, 3781, 1989.

45. **Schulze AJ, Baumann U, Knof S, Jaeger E, Huber R, Laurell CB**: Structural transition of α_1-antitrypsin by a peptide sequentially similar to β-strand s4A. *FEBS Letts*, 194, 51, 1990.

46. **Carrell RW, Evans DL, Stein PE**: Mobile reactive centre of serpins and the control of thrombosis. *Nature*, 353, 576, 1991.

47. **Bjork I, Ylinenjarvi K, Olson ST, Bock PE**: Conversion of antithrombin from an inhibitor of thrombin to a substrate with reduced heparin affinity and enhanced conformational stability by binding of a tetradecapeptide corresponding to the P_1 to P_{14} region of the putative reactive bond loop of the inhibitor. *J Biol Chem*, 267, 1976, 1992.

48. **Hook M, Bjork I, Hopwood J, Lindahl U**: Anticoagulant activity of heparin: separation of high activity and low activity heparin species by affinity chromatography on immobilized antithrombin. *FEBS Letts*, 66, 90, 1976.

49. **Lam LH, Silbert JE, Rosenberg RD**: The separation of active and inactive forms of heparin. *Biochem Biophys Res Comm*, 69, 570, 1976.

50. **Lindahl U, Backstrom G, Thunberg L, Leder IG**: Evidence for a 3-O-sulfated D-glycosamine residue in the antithrombin-binding sequence of heparin. *Proc Natl Acad Sci USA*, 77, 6551, 1980.

51. **Casu B, Oreste P, Torri G**: The structure of heparin oligosaccharide fragments with high anti-(factor Xa) activity containing the minimal antithrombin III binding sequence. *Biochem J*, 80, 599, 1981.

52. **Thunberg L, Backstrom G, Lindahl U**: Further characterisation of the antithrombin-binding sequence in heparin. *Carbohydrate Res*, 100, 393, 1982.

53. **Choay J, Petitou M, Lormeau JC, Sinay P, Casu B, Gatti G**: Structure-activity relationship in heparin: a synthetic pentasaccharide with high affinity for antithrombin III and eliciting high anti-factor Xa activity. *Biochem Biophys Res Commun*, 116, 492, 1983.

54. **Atha DH, Stephens AW, Rosenberg RD**: Evaluation of critical groups required for binding of heparin to antithrombin. *Proc Natl Acad Sci USA*, 81, 1030, 1984.

55. **Nordenman B, Danielsson A, Bjork I**: The binding of low affinity and high affinity heparin to antithrombin. Fluorescence studies. *Eur J Biochem*, 90, 1, 1978.

56. **Jordan RE, Beeler D, Rosenberg RD**: Fractionation of low molecular weight heparin species and their interaction with antithrombin. *J Biol Chem*, 254, 2902, 1979.

57. **Olson ST, Sheffer R, Stephens AW, Hirs CHW**: Molecular basis of the reduced activity of antithrombin-Denver with thrombin and factor Xa. Role of the P'1 residue. *Thromb Haemostas*, 6, 670, 1991.

58. **Nordenman B, Bjork I**: Influence of ionic strength and pH on the interaction between high-affinity heparin and antithrombin. *Biochem Biophys Acta*, 672, 227, 1981.

59. **Blackburn MN, Sibley CC**: The heparin binding site of antithrombin III. Evidence for a critical tryptophan residue. *J Biol Chem*, 255, 824, 1980.

60. **Blackburn MN, Smith RL, Carson J, Sibley CC**: The heparin binding site of antithrombin III. Identification of a critical tryptophan in the amino acid sequence. *J Biol Chem*, 259, 939, 1984.

61. **Gettins P, Choay J, Crews BC, Zettlmeiss G**: Role of tryptophan 49 in the heparin cofactor activity of human antithrombin III. *J Biol Chem*, 267, 21946, 1992.

62. **Karp GI, Marcum JA, Rosenberg RD**: The role of tryptophan residues in heparin-antithrombin interactions. *Arch Biochem Biophys*, 233, 712, 1984.

63. **Liu CS, Chang JY**: Probing the heparin binding domain of human antithrombin III with V8 protease. *Eur J Biochem*, 167, 247, 1987.

64. **Borg JY, Owen MC, Soria C, Soria J, Caen J, Carrell RW**: Proposed heparin binding site in antithrombin based on arginine 47. A new variant Rouen-II, 47 Arg to Ser. *J Clin Invest*, 81, 1292, 1988.

65. **Chang JY**: Binding of heparin to human antithrombin III activates selective chemical modification at lysine 236. Lys-107, Lys-125 and Lys-136 are situated within the heparin binding site of antithrombin III. *J Biol Chem*, 264, 3111, 1989.

66. **Liu CS, Chang JY**: The heparin binding site of human antithrombin III. Selective chemical modification at Lys 114, Lys 125 and Lys 287 impairs its heparin cofactor activity. *J Biol Chem*, 262, 17356, 1987.

67. **Smith JW, Dey N, Knauer DJ**: Heparin binding domain of antithrombin III: characterization using a synthetic peptide directed polyclonal antibody. *Biochemistry*, 29, 8950, 1990.

68. **Lane DA, Olds RJ, Conard J, Boisclair M, Bock SC, Hultin M, Abildgaard U, Ireland H, Thompson E, Sas G, Horellou MH, Tamponi G, Thein SL**: Pleiotropic effects of antithrombin strand 1C substitution mutations. *J Clin Invest*, 90, 2422, 1992.

69. **Winter JH, Bennett B, Watt JL, Brown T, San Roman C, Schinzel A, King J, Cook PJL**: Confirmation of linkage between antithrombin III and Duffy blood group and assignment of AT3 to 1q22-25. *Annal Hum Genet*, 26, 29, 1982.

70. **Magenis RE, Donlon T, Parks M, Rivas ML, Lovrien EW**: Linkage relationships of dominant antithrombin III deficiency and the heterochromatic region of chromosome 1. *Cytogenet Cell Genet*, 22, 327, 1978.

71. **Lovrien EW, Magenis RE, Rivas ML, Goodnight S, Moreland R, Rowe S**: Linkage study of antithrombin III. *Cytogenet Cell Genet*, 22, 319, 1978.

72. **Bock SC, Harris JF, Balazs I, Trent JM**: Assignment of the human antithrombin III structural gene to chromosome 1q23-25. *Cytogenet Cell Genet*. 39, 67, 1985.

73. **Bock SC, Harris JF, Schwartz CE, Ward JH, Hersgold EJ, Skolnick MH**: Hereditary thrombosis in a Utah kindred is caused by a dysfunctional antithrombin III gene. *Am J Hum Genet.*, 37, 32, 1985.

74. **Sacks SH, Old JM, Reeders ST, Weatherall DJ, Douglas AS, Winter JH, Rizza CR**: Evidence linking familial thrombosis with a defective antithrombin III gene in two British kindreds. *J Med Genet*, 25, 20, 1988.

75. **Bock SC, Marrinan JA, Radziejewska E**: Antithrombin III Utah: proline-407 to leucine mutation in a highly conserved region near the inhibitor reactive site. *Biochemistry*, 2, 6171, 1988.

76. **Olds RJ, Lane DA, Chowdhury V, De Stefano V, Leone G, Thein SL**: Complete nucleotide sequence of the antithrombin gene: evidence for homologous recombination causing thrombophilia. *Biochemistry*, 32, 4216, 1993.

77. **Olds RJ, Lane DA, Chowdhury V, Sas G, Pabinger I, Auberger K, Thein SL**: (ATT) trinucleotide repeats in the antithrombin gene and their use in determining the origin of repeated mutations. *Human Mutation*, 4, 31, 1994.

78. **Prochownik EV**: Relationship between an enhancer element in the human antithrombin III gene and an immunoglobulin light-chain gene enhancer. *Nature*, 316, 845, 1985.

79. **Ochoa A, Brunel F, Mendelzon D, Cohen GN, Zakin MM**: Different liver nuclear proteins binds to similar DNA sequences in the 5' flanking regions of three hepatic genes. *Nucleic Acids Res*, 17, 119, 1989.

80. **Prochownik EV, Orkin SH**: In vivo transcription of a human antithrombin III "minigene". *J Biol Chem*, 259, 15386, 1984.

81. **Prochownik EV, Smith MJ, Markham A**: Two regions downstream of AATAAA in the human antithrombin III gene are important for cleavage-polyadenylation. *J Biol Chem*, 262, 9004, 1987.

82. **Fan B, Crews B, Turko I, Choay J, Zettlmeissl G, Gettins P**: Heterogeneity of recombinant human antithrombin III expressed in baby hamster kidney cells. Effect of glycosylation differences on heparin binding and structure. *J Biol Chem*, 268, 17588, 1993.

83. **Stephens AW, Thalley BS, Hirs CHW**: Antithrombin-III Denver, a reactive site variant. *J Biol Chem,* 262, 1044, 1987.

84. **Wasley LC, Atha DH, Bauer KA, Kaufman RJ**: Expression and characterization of human antithrombin III synthesized in mammalian cells. *J Biol Chem*, 262, 14766, 1987.

85. **Broker M, Ragg H, Karges HE**: Expression of human antithrombin III in Saccharomyces cerevisiae and Schizosaccharomyces pombe. *Biochim Biophys Acta,* 908, 203, 1987.

86. **Austin RC, Rachubinski RA, Fernandez RF, Blajchman MA**: Expression in a cell-free system of normal and variant forms of human antithrombin III. Ability to bind heparin and react with alpha-thrombin. *Blood* ,76, 1521, 1990.

87. **Austin RC, Rachubinski RA, Blajchman MA**: Site-directed mutagenesis of alanine-382 of human antithrombin III. *FEBS Letts*, 280, 254, 1991.

88. **Gillespie LS, Hillesland KK, Knauer DJ**: Expression of biologically active human antithrombin III by recombinant baculovirus in Spodoptera frugiperda cells. *J Biol Chem*, 266, 3995, 1991.

89. **Prochownik EV, Antonarakis S, Bauer KA, Rosenberg RD, Fearon ER, Orkin SH**: Molecular heterogeneity of inherited antithrombin III deficiency. *N Eng J Med*, 308, 1549, 1983.

90. **Bock SC, Radziejewska E**: A Nhe 1 RFLP in the human antithrombin III gene (1q23-25) (AT3). *Nucl Acids Res,* 19, 2519, 1991.

91. **Daly ME, Perry DJ**: Dde1 polymorphism in intron 5 of the ATIII gene. *Nucl Acids Res*, 18, 5583, 1990.

92. **Bock SC, Levitan DJ**: Characterisation of an unusual DNA length polymorphism 5' to the human antithrombin III gene. *Nucl Acids Res,* 11, 8569, 1983.

93. **Lane DA, Olds RJ, Boisclair M, Chowdhury V, Thein SL, Cooper DN, Blajchman M, Perry D, Emmerich J, Aiach M**: Antithrombin III mutation database: first update. *Thromb Haemostas,* 70, 361, 1993.

94. **Lane DA, Olds RJ, Thein SL**: Antithrombin and its deficiency states. *Blood Coag Fibrinol,* 3, 315, 1992.

95. **Thaler E, Lechner K**: Antithrombin III deficiency and thromboembolism. *Clin Haematol*, 10, 369, 1981.

96. **Demers C, Ginsberg JS, Hirsh J, Henderson P, Blajchman MA**: Thrombosis in antithrombin-III-deficient persons. Report of a large kindred and literature review. *Ann Intern Med*, 116, 754, 1992.

97. **Das M, Carroll SF**: Antithrombin III deficiency: an etiology of Budd-Chiari syndrome. *Surgery*, 97, 242, 1985.

98. **Coller BS, Owen J, Jesty J, Horowitz D, Reitman MJ, Spear J, Yeh T, Comp PC**: Deficiency of plasma protein S, protein C, or antithrombin III and arterial thrombosis. *Arteriosclerosis,* 7, 456, 1987.

99. **Johnson EJ, Prentice CR, Parapia LA**: Premature arterial disease associated with familial antithrombin III deficiency. *Thromb Haemost*, 63, 13, 1990.

100. **Chowdhury V, Lane DA, Auberger K, Gandenberger-Bachem S, Pabinger I, Olds RJ, Thein SL**: Homozygous antithrombin deficiency: report of two new cases (99Leu to Phe) associated with arterial and venous thrombosis. *Thromb Haemost*, 72, 166, 1994.

101. **Hirsh J, Piovella F, Pini M**: Congenital antithrombin III deficiency. Incidence and clinical features. *Am J Med*, 87 (suppl 3B), 34, 1989.

102. **Finazzi G, Caccia R, Barbui T**: Different prevalence of thromboembolism in the subtypes of congenital antithrombin III deficiency: review of 404 cases. *Thromb Haemost*, 58, 1094, 1987.

103. **Girolami A, Lazzaro AR, Simioni P**: The relationship between defective heparin cofactor activities and thrombotic phenomena in ATIII abnormalities. *Thromb Haemost*, 59, 121, 1988.

104. **Olds RJ, Lane DA, Boisclair M, Sas G, Bock SC, Thein SL**: Antithrombin Budapest 3: an antithrombin variant with reduced heparin affinity resulting from the substitution L99F. *FEBS Letts*, 300, 241, 1992.

105. **Rosenberg RD**: Actions and interactions of antithrombin and heparin. *N Eng J Med*, 292, 146, 1975.

106. **Abildgaard U**. "Antithrombin and related inhibitors of coagulation." Recent advances in blood coagulation. Poller L, ed. 1981 Churchill Livingstone. Edinburgh.

107. **Tait RC, Walker ID, Perry DJ, Carrell RW, Islam SIA, McCall F, Mitchell R, Davidson JF**: Prevalence of antithrombin III deficiency subtypes in 4000 healthy blood donors. *Thromb Haemost*, 65, 839, 1991.

108. **Harper PL, Luddington RJ, Daly M, Bruce D, Williamson D, Edgar PF, Perry DJ, Carrell RW**: The incidence of dysfunctional antithrombin variants: four cases in 210 patients with thromboembolic disease. *Brit J Haematol,* 77, 360, 1991.

109. **Tabernero MD, Tomas JF, Alberca I, Orfao A, Lopez Borrasca A, Vicente V**: Incidence and clinical characteristics of hereditary disorders associated with venous thrombosis. *Am J Hematol,* 36, 249, 1991.

110. **Heijboer H, Brandjes DP, Buller HR, Sturk A, ten Cate JW**: Deficiencies of coagulation-inhibiting and fibrinolytic proteins in outpatients with deep-vein thrombosis. *N Engl J Med,* 323, 1512, 1990.

111. **Dahlback B, Carlsson M, Svensson PJ**: Familial thrombophilia due to a previously unrecognised mechanism characterised by poor anticoagulant response to activated protein C. *Proc Natl Acad Sci USA* , 90, 1004, 1993.

112. **Bertina RM, Koeleman BPC, Koster T, Rosendaal FR, Dirven RJ, de Ronde H, van der Velden P, Reitsma PH**: Mutation in blood coagulation factor V associated with resistance to activated protein C. *Nature*, 369, 64, 1994.

113. **Sas G, Blasko G, Banhegyi D, Jako J, Palos LA**: Abnormal antithrombin III (Antithrombin III "Budapest") as a cause of a familial thrombophilia. *Thrombos Diathes Haemorr,* 32, 105, 1974.

114. **Hultin MB, McKay J, Abildgaard U**: Antithrombin Oslo: type 1b classification of the first reported antithrombin-deficient family with a review of hereditary antithrombin variants. *Thromb Haemost*, 59, 468, 1988.

115. **Lane DA, Ireland H, Olds RJ, Thein SL, Perry DJ, Aiach M: Antithrombin III**: a database of mutations. *Thrombos Haemostas,* 66, 657, 1991.

116. **Egeberg O**: Inherited antithrombin III deficiency causing thrombophilia. *Thromb Diath Haemorrhag,* 13, 516, 1965.

117. **Olds RJ, Lane DA, Ireland H, Finazzi G, Barbui T, Abildgaard U, Girolami A, Thein SL**: A common point mutation producing type 1a antithrombin III deficiency: AT129CGA to TGA (Arg to Stop). *Thromb Res*, 64, 621, 1991.

118. **Olds RJ, Lane DA, Beresford CH, Abildgard U, Hughes PM, Thein SL**: A recurrent deletion in the antithrombin gene, AT106-108(-6bp), identified by DNA heteroduplex detection. *Genomics*, 16, 298, 1993.

119. **Olds RJ, Lane DA, Chowdhury V, Samson D, De Stefano V, Leone G, Wiesel ML, Cazenave JP, Conard J, Thein SL**: Major rearrangements within the antithrombin locus: an unusual cause for inherited antithrombin deficiency. *Brit J Haematol ISH 24th Congress* Abstracts, 40, 1992.

120. **Fernandez-Rachubinski F, Rachubinski R, Blajchman M**: Partial deletion of an antithrombin III allele in a kindred with type I deficiency. *Blood*, 80, 1476, 1992.

121. **Erdjument H, Lane DA, Ireland H, Panico M, DiMarzo V, Blench I, Morris HR**: Formation of a covalent disulphide-linked antithrombin-albumin complex by an antithrombin variant, antithrombin Northwick Park. *J Biol Chem,* 262, 13381, 1987.

122. **Erdjument H, Lane DA, Panico M, DiMarzo V, Morris HR**: Single amino acid substitutions in the reactive site of antithrombin leading to thrombosis. Congenital substitution of arginine 393 to cysteine in antithrombin Northwick Park and to histidine in antithrombin Glasgow. *J Biol Chem,* 263, 5589, 1988.

123.   **Lane DA, Erdjument H, Thompson E, Panico M, Di Marzo V, Morris HR, Leone G, De Stefano V, Thein SL**: A novel amino acid substitution in the reactive site of a congenital variant antithrombin. Antithrombin Pescara, Arg 393 to Pro, caused by a CGT to CCT mutation. *J Biol Chem,* 264, 10200, 1989.

124.   **Erdjument H, Lane DA, Ireland H, Di Marzo V, Panico M, Morris HR, Tripodi A, Mannucci PM**: Antithrombin Milano, single amino acid substitution at the reactive site. *Thromb Haemost.,* 60, 471, 1988.

125.   **Erdjument H, Lane DA, Panico M, DiMarzo V, Morris HR, Bauer K, Rosenberg RD**: Antithrombin Chicago, amino acid substitution of arginine 393 to histidine. *Thromb Res,* 54, 613, 1989.

126.   **Lane DA, Erdjument H, Flynn A, diMarzo V, Panico M, Morris HR, Greaves M, Dolan G, Preston FE**: Antithrombin Sheffield: amino acid substitution at the reactive site (Arg 393 to His) causing thrombosis. *Brit J Haemat,* 71, 91, 1989.

127.   **Ireland H, Lane DA, Thompson E, Olds R, Thein SL, Hach-Wunderle V, Scharrer I**, Antithrombin Frankfurt I: arginine to cysteine substitution at the reactive site and formation of a variant antithrombin-albumin covalent complex. *Thromb Haemostas,* 65, 913, 1991.

128.   **Blajchman MA, Fernandez-Rachubinski F, Sheffield WP, Austin RC, Schulman S**: Antithrombin III Stockholm: a codon 392 (Gly to Asp) mutation with normal heparin binding and impaired serine protease reactivity. *Blood,* 79, 1428, 1992.

129.   **Devraj-Kizuk R, Chui DHK, Prochownik EV, Carter CJ, Ofosu FA, Blajchman MA**: Antithrombin-III-Hamilton: a gene with a point mutation (guanine to adenine) in codon 382 causing impaired serine protease reactivity. *Blood,* 72, 1518, 1988.

130.   **Mohlo-Sabatier P, Aiach M, Gaillard I, Fiessinger JN, Fischer AM, Chadeuf G, Clauser E**: Molecular characterisation of antithrombin III (AT III) variants using polymerase chain reaction. Identification of the ATIII Charleville as an Ala384 Pro mutation. *J Clin Invest,* 84, 1236, 1989.

131.   **Ireland H, Lane DA, Thompson E, Walker ID, Blench I, Morris HR, Freyssinet JM, Grunebaun L, Olds RJ, Thein SL**: Antithrombin Glasgow II: alanine 382 to threonine mutation in the serpin P12 position, resulting in a substrate reaction with thrombin. *Brit J Haematol,* 79, 70, 1991.

132.   **Caso R, Lane DA, Olds RJ, Thein SL, Panico M, Freyssinet JM, Aiach M, Rodeghiero F, Finazzi G**: Antithrombin Vicenza, Ala 384 to Pro (GCA to CCA) mutation, transforming the inhibitor into a substrate. *Brit J Haematol,* 97, 87, 1990.

133.   **Skriver K, Wikoff WR, Patston PA, Tausk F, Schapira M, Kaplan AP, Bock SC**: Substrate properties of Cl inhibitor Ma (A434E). Genetic and structural evidence suggesting that the 'P12-region' contains critical determinants of serpin inhibitor/substrate status. *J Biol Chem,* 266, 9216, 1991.

134.   **Rijken DC, Groeneveld E, Kluft C, Nieuwenhuis HK**: Alpha2-antiplasmin Enschede is not an inhibitor, but a substrate of plasmin. *Biochem J,* 255, 609, 1988.

135.   **Davis AE, Aulak K, Parad RB, Stecklein HP, Eldering E, Hack C E., Kramer J, Strunk RC, Bissler J, Rosen FS**: Cl inhibitor hinge region mutations produce dysfunction by different mechanisms. *Nature Genetics,* 1, 354, 1992.

136.   **Hopkins PCR, Carrell RW, Stone SR**: Effects of mutations in the hinge region of serpins. *Biochemistry,* 32, 7650, 1993.

137.   **Brennan SO, Borg JY, George PM, Soria C, Soria J, Caen J, Carrell RW**: New carbohydrate site in mutant antithrombin (7 Ile-Asn) with decreased heparin affinity. *FEBS Letts,* 237, 118, 1988.

138.   **Borg JY, Brennan SO, Carrell RW, George P, Perry DJ, Shaw J**: Antithrombin Rouen-IV 24 Arg→Cys. The amino-terminal contribution to heparin binding. *FEBS Letts ,* 266, 163, 1990.

139.   **Okajima K, Abe H, Maeda S, Motomura M, Tsujihata M, Nagataki S, Okabe H, Tatatsuki K**: Antithrombin III Nagasaki (Ser116-Pro): a heterozygous variant with defective heparin binding associated with thrombosis. *Blood,* 81, 1300, 1993.

140.   **Chowdury V, Mille B, Olds RJ, Lane DA, Pabinger I, Woodcock BE, Thein SL**: Antithrombin Southport (99Leu to Val) and Vienna (Gln 118 to Pro): two novel antithrombin variants which have abnormal heparin binding. *Brit J Haematol,* 89, 3, 602,1995.

141.   **Gandrille S, Aiach M, Lane DA, Vidaud D, Mohlo-Sabatier P, Caso R, de Moerloose P, Fiessinger JN, Clauser E**: Important role of arginine 129 in heparin-binding site of antithrombin III. *J Biol Chem* 265, 18997, 1990.

142.   **Church FC, Meade JB, Treanor RE, Whinna HC**: Antithrombin activity of fucoidan. The interaction of fucoidan with heparin cofactor II, antithrombin III and thrombin. *J Biol Chem,* 264, 3618, 1989.

143.   **Watton J, Longstaff C, Lane DA, Barrowcliffe TW**: Heparin binding affinity of normal and genetically modified antithrombin III measured using a monoclonal antibody to the heparin binding site of antithrombin III. *Biochemistry,* 32, 7286, 1993.

144.   **Mille B, Watton J, Barrowcliffe TW, Mani JC, Lane DA**: Role of N and C terminal amino acids in antithrombin binding to pentasaccharide. *J Biol Chem,* 269, 29435, 1994.

145.   **Olds RJ, Lane DA, Caso R, Panico M, Morris HR, Sas G, Dawes J, Thein SL**: Antithrombin III Budapest: a single amino acid substitution (429Pro to Leu) in a region highly conserved in the serpin super family. *Blood,* 79, 1206, 1992.

146.   **Mast AE, Enghild JJ, Pizzo SV, Salvesen G**: Analysis of the plasma elimination kinetics and conformational stabilities of native, proteinase-complexed, and reactive site cleaved serpins: comparison of alpha1-proteinase inhibitor, alpha1-antichymotrypsin, antithrombin III, alpha2-antiplasmin, and ovalbumin. *Biochemistry,* 30, 1723, 1991.

147.   **Perlmutter DH, Glover GI, Rivetna M, Schasteen CS, Fallon RJ**: Identification of a serpin-enzyme complex receptor on human hepatoma cells and human monocytes. *Proc Natl Acad Sci USA,* 87, 3753, 1990.

148.   **Perlmutter DH, Joslin G, Nelson P, Schasteen C, Adams P, Fallon RJ**: Endocytosis ans degradation of alpha1-antitrypsin-protease complexes is mediated by the serpin-enzme complex (SEC) receptor. *J Biol Chem,* 265, 16713, 1990.

149.   **Joslin G, Fallon RJ, Bullock J, Adams SP, Perlmutter DH**: The SEC receptor recognizes a pentapeptide neodomain of α_1-antitrypsin-protease complexes. *J Biol Chem,* 266, 11282, 1991.

ANTITHROMBIN III DEFICIENCY.
LABORATORY ASPECTS AND CLINICAL MANAGEMENT

M. J. Seghatchian*, M. M. Samama**, J. Conard**
* NBS, Colindale, London ; ** Hôtel-Dieu, University Hospital, Paris

I. INTRODUCTION

It is essential to differentiate between congenital and acquired deficiency of antithrombin (ATIII). We will also review briefly the basic principles and the clinical management of ATIII deficiencies. The biochemical aspects of AT III have been covered in the previous chapter.

A . BASIC PRINCIPLES

Antithrombin III is the most important overall physiological inhibitor of activated clotting factors.[1,2] A decreased concentration of ATIII below 80% is associated with an increased tendency of thromboembolism. Heparin can accelerate up to 2000 fold the rate of inhibition of thrombin by ATIII.[3] This results in 15 to 30% decrease in plasma ATIII concentration. The heparin-induced decrease in ATIII concentration is nevertheless reversed with cessation of heparin therapy.

The clearance of ATIII from plasma is biphasic.[4] The initial phase has a half life of approximately 10 minutes, possibly as the result of binding to a specific population of heparan sulphate proteoglycans synthesised by the microvascular and macrovascular endothelial cells. The acceleration of serine proteases inhibition is localised on surfaces where active enzyme generation takes place. The second phase has a half life of 3 hours as ATIII (like albumin) leaves the blood vessel and enters the extravascular space.[4]

Both familial and some acquired deficiencies of ATIII have been associated with an increased rate of venous thrombosis. Arterial thrombosis is less frequent. Compared to rare cases of congenital ATIII deficiency, the acquired states, in particular in the course of the shock syndrome and sepsis, are rather common and regularly observed in intensive care units.[5] There is a close correlation between the various phases of septic shock and alteration in the ATIII inhibitory system, where the initial hypercoagulability can rapidly lead to appearance of fibrin monomer complexes and formation of microclots in vital organs. It may trigger the fibrinolytic defence system by the release of the vessel wall activators. These activators then degrade fibrinogen as well as fibrin; some degradation products inhibit fibrin polymerisation and platelet adhesion, resulting in increased bleeding tendency. The initial hypercoagulability is transformed into full-fledged irreversible consumption coagulopathy with more or less complete depletion of fibrinogen, platelets and ATIII[5]. In view of heterogeneity in the triggering mechanism of sepsis (e.g. due to either gram positive, involving direct effect leucocyte elastase on ATIII, or gram negative, related to bacterial endotoxin attacks on endothelial linings ; or states of shock of any origin leading to stasis, hypoxia, acidosis and endothelial lesion-induced), the acquired deficiency of ATIII remains the focus of recurrent interest.

B. PHYSIOLOGICAL VARIATIONS

ATIII is synthesised by hepatocytes and endothelial cells.[6] The normal circulating level of human ATIII is about 15 mg/dL,[7] 50% of which can be traced in the extra vascular space.[8] The basal plasma level of ATIII varies in relation to gender, age and some other physiological conditions:

1. In healthy adult men there is a slight increase (10%) in ATIII as compared to women of the same age group (age 25-30).

2. In an oral contraceptive user there is 10-20% decrease in ATIII concentration.[9-11] This is related principally to the oestrogen content of oral contraceptives.

3. In post menopausal replacement therapy there is also a slight decrease in ATIII levels when oral 17β-estradiol or conjugated estrogens are used [12-14].

4. ATIII levels decrease by 10-15% during normal pregnancy as compared to the basal level in some individuals but remain within the normal range (80-120%).[15]

5. Average AT III level of 60% and 75% of normal have been reported after two hours and eight days postpartum.[2,16]

6. In infants the level of ATIII is approximately 50% of the normal adult values but reach within 6 months the normal adult value.[1,2] A greater reduction of ATIII concentration (20-40%) is found in preterm infants.[17] However, α_2-macroglobulin level is relatively higher in both full-term and premature infants on day one of life. Therefore, the decrease in ATIII in infancy can be compensated mainly by the increase in α_2-macroglobulin which is much higher in full term and premature infants as compared to adults.

7. A dysfunctional form of ATIII has been reported in sick, preterm infants with respiratory distress.[17]

C. ANALYTICAL AND METHODOLOGICAL ASPECTS

The level of ATIII is usually expressed as the percentage of a standard pool of normal plasma (80-120 %). This range is relatively narrower than that for some coagulant factors like factor VIII or factor IX which range from 50 to 150% of normal controls. This clearly demonstrates the importance of the circulating concentration of ATIII, which must remain above 70%. This is supported by the fact that heterozygotes for defective ATIII genes often have levels as high as 65% and yet suffer from repeated thrombosis.[1-3]

The diagnostic strategy for ATIII deficiencies requires a quantitative assay for its functional integrity in combination with the ATIII concentration. This is evaluated by immunological methods (Laurell rocket technique, Immunodiffusion or ELISA). The functional assays are usually based on measurement of residual factor Xa or factor IIa neutralisation by ATIII, in the absence or presence of heparin. The former, so called progressive antithrombin activity against factor Xa or factor IIa differentiates protease binding from heparin binding, hence can be used to characterise ATIII dysfunction. On the other hand the functional assay in the presence of heparin provides information on ATIII heparin cofactor function and is the assay to be prefered since it allows the detection of all types of ATIII deficiency. Both clotting and chromogenic assays are used. Rarely, dysfunctional ATIII will yield discrepant results on either assay.

Crossed immunoelectrophoresis is usually performed with heparin in the first dimension and can separate complexed ATIII from the native (non-complex forms). This methodology is used to detect the different molecular species with abnormal heparin binding. A gel cutting procedure based on parallel assay of ATIII by functional assay, after the first dimension and crossed immunoelectrophoresis has been successfully applied for screening various forms of ATIII, hence relating directly the functional activity to various molecular forms of ATIII, subsequent to electrophoresis (unpublished observation).

II. EPIDEMIOLOGICAL ASPECTS OF ATIII DEFICIENCY

Both congenital and acquired deficiencies of ATIII may predispose to thrombosis (see Blajchman[18] for recent review).

A. CONGENITAL DEFICIENCY OF ATIII

The first case of ATIII deficiency was reported in 1965 by Egeberg[19] in a Norwegian family with recurrent venous thrombosis and half the normal levels of progressive antithrombin and heparin cofactor. Inherited ATIII deficiency occurs at a frequency of 1:5000 in the general population[20] and in about 3% of all patients presenting a history of venous thrombotic disease.[1,2] The risk of thrombosis in heterozygous ATIII deficiency increased with age; 85% of these patients over the age of 50 will have experienced at least one thrombotic episode.[2] Demers et al[21], from their observation of a large kindred and a survey of literature concluded that a pooled prevalence of thrombosis in ATIII deficient subjects is 51% and in most recorded cases, a precipitating risk factor was present. Finazzi et al[22] reviewed 404 cases of ATIII deficiency and distinguished two types and five subgroups. New classification is proposed by Lane (see the previous chapter). The current molecular genetic analysis is providing useful information on many altered conformations of ATIII reactive sites.[1]

Rarely, abnormalities of both thrombin binding and heparin binding coexist. Rarely infants or children have presented with life threatening thrombosis.[23] The incidence of thrombosis before puberty is only about 10% but increases with age.[24] Cerebral thrombosis may be observed in young persons with ATIII deficiency.[25-27] In females, thrombosis often occurs with puberty; use of oral contraceptive, during pregnancy or in the postpartum period. Most ATIII deficient individuals require therapeutic anticoagulation with heparin and oral anticoagulants.[28]

B. ACQUIRED DEFICIENCY OF ATIII

ATIII measurement is considered to be the most important biological and diagnostic marker of thrombotic risk. Deficiency of ATIII can result from lack of sufficient synthesis, increased rate of consumption or clearance[29] in association with renal disease,[30,31] or hemodilution secondary to increased salt/water retention and/or in association with other clinical conditions. Some acquired ATIII deficiency (see Table I) can be very severe, with levels well below those seen in heterozygotic ATIII deficiency (35-75%).

Table I : Possible mechanisms of acquired ATIII deficiency

1. Altered function	Non-enzymatic glycosylation, hyperglycemia[32,33] hyperlipidaemia[34], sick newborn.
2. Proteolytic cleavage	Exaggerated deficiency during DIC[35] or due to release of neutrophil elastase or thrombin generation.
3. Increased external losses	Nephrosis[30,31], inflammatory bowel disease[29], plasmapheresis[36]
4. Increased elimination	Heparin therapy[1-8,37], surgery [38,39] and losses via vascular capillaries (sepsis, burns and acute thrombosis)[8]
5. Decreased production	L-Asparaginase chemotherapy [40,41]
6. Multiple factors	Liver disease (combined decreased synthesis and increased plasma disappearance)[1,2] ,oestrogen[9-11,42], preeclampsia[16] etc.

When low levels (e.g. below 80%) are discovered it is essential to distinguish their origin (whether congenital or acquired) as the mode of treatment may differ. A very low level of ATIII (<35%), though rare is usually related to acquired hepatic conditions, but a limited number of cases have been reported in infants with type II (low functional activity but normal level of antigen). Often levels in the regions of 35-75% are found during therapy with heparin, oestro-progestatives, L-asparaginase, tamoxifen or hepatic-nephrotic or septic shock. A small decrease in ATIII has also been observed in women on oestro-progestogen pill. Today the association of thrombosis with decreased ATIII in acquired deficiency states is suggested, but in most cases, the relationship of ATIII deficiency to thrombosis, including diabetes and sick newborn infants remains to be proven.

III. CLINICAL MANAGEMENT OF CONGENITAL ATIII DEFICIENCY

A. LABORATORY ASPECTS

The laboratory testing for diagnosis should be carried out when the patient is not receiving oral anticoagulants or prior to starting treatment. In some patients with congenital ATIII deficiency oral anticoagulant may increase ATIII levels to normal values; family studies may be necessary to exclude this possibility. Diagnostic tests should be repeated on at least two occasions, avoiding conditions that can cause a falsely low level.

A screening assay for antithrombin III deficiency is performed in the presence and absence of heparin to provide additional information on its cofactor activity. Chromogenic assays are superior to clotting assays. Tests of factor Xa inhibition may be better than assays of thrombin neutralisation in this setting because tests of thrombin inhibition may overestimate the levels of antithrombin III. This occurs because heparin cofactor II can inhibit the added thrombin when antithrombin III levels are decreased. One of two methods can be used to circumvent this potential problem. First, the use of factor Xa rather than thrombin for neutralisation purpose ; unlike antithrombin III, heparin cofactor II does not inhibit factor Xa. Alternatively, if a test of thrombin inhibition is used to measure antithrombin III activity, bovine thrombin should be used in place of human thrombin because the bovine enzyme is not readily neutralised by human heparin cofactor II.[43]

B. MANAGEMENT OF PATIENTS WITH HEREDITARY ATIII DEFICIENCIES

The treatment strategies vary according to the clinical settings: acute thrombosis, the need for long-term anticoagulant therapy, the role of anticoagulants in asymptomatic patients and the treatment of any high risk situation such as surgery or pregnancy[44]. It is important that the patient carries a medical certificate attesting his ATIII deficiency and stating that a prophylactic treatment is required in any condition medical or surgical, predisposing to venous thromboembolism.

1. Management of patients with acute thrombosis

Classically standard heparin therapy is given for 5 to 10 days and an oral anticoagulant is used for secondary prophylaxis after 24 to 48 hours using a regimen that produces an INR of 2 to 3. Heparin treatment is continued until the INR has remained at therapeutic level for two days consecutively and the two anticoagulants should overlap for at least 7 days. The same applies for patients with ATIII deficiency, but ATIII concentrates are sometimes administered simultaneously to heparin.

An APTT ratio during heparin treatment is used to monitor heparin therapeutic range. This requires strict standardization of laboratory procedures. Each laboratory should determine the therapeutic range in its own setting. Since heparin acts as an anticoagulant by catalysing antithrombin III, patients with antithrombin III deficiencies may be expected to be resistant to heparin. Although this can occur in rare individuals with marked antithrombin III deficiency, most such patients will have a satisfactory anticoagulant response to heparin, although they may require higher doses. The possibility of heparin resistance can be excluded by measuring the APTT 15 to 30 minutes after 5000 U of heparin is given intravenously as a bolus. If there is no prolongation of the APTT, antithrombin III concentrate should be given concomitantly with the heparin. An alternative approach is to determine the anti-Xa level on the mixture (50/50) of patient's plasma and control plasma. This would correct the low anti-Xa value indicating that the resistance is attributed to low ATIII level in patient. Infusion of antithrombin III concentrate at a dose of 50 U per kilogram will usually raise the plasma antithrombin III level to about 120 percent in a congenitally deficient individual with a baseline level at 50 percent of normal. Since the biologic half-life of antithrombin III is about 48 hours, daily infusions of antithrombin III concentrates are usually adequate. Thus, to maintain the plasma antithrombin III level above 80 percent, infusions of 40-60 percent of the initial dose are recommended at 24 hour intervals.

However, it has to be emphasized that this protocol is not based on clinical trials. Despite 15 years of clinical usage of ATIII concentrates, the benefit of this treatment has not been fully proven.[45-47]

Patients with documented episode(s) of thrombosis are candidates for lifelong anticoagulant therapy. This is particularly important for patients whose thrombosis occurred spontaneously or for those with recurrent thrombotic events. A possible exception may be those individuals with a single episode of thrombosis that occurred after a known predisposing condition that is no more present : pill, pregnancy, major surgery or trauma. Rather than subjecting these individuals to the possible side effects of long-term anticoagulant therapy, consideration should be given to vigorous prophylaxis at times of risk. In general, ATIII deficient patients respond well to oral anticoagulant therapy (INR of 2 to 3) , without recurrent thrombosis. A lower intensity (INR of 1.5-2) will reduce the risk of bleeding and may be reasonable for patients who remain free of recurrence for several years.

Heparin should be given to patients who develop documented recurrent thrombosis. Initially, full doses of heparin should be given intravenously. The patient can then be switched to subcutaneous heparin given twice daily in doses that produce a therapeutic APTT 6 hours after heparin injection. The heparin dose should be sufficient to achieve an anti-Xa level of 0.2 to 0.4U per millilitre as measured by protamine titration which corresponds to 0.3 - 0.6 anti-Xa IU when an amidolytic method is used. The usual mean daily dose needed to reach this heparin level is 30,000 to 35,000U. Long-term subcutaneous heparin in therapeutic doses can cause bruising and discomfort at the injection sites. Low molecular weight heparins appear to be preferable in patients with ATIII deficiencies as in contrast to unfractionated heparin, they induce less decrease in ATIII. The explanation for this phenomenon is unknown. The doses of LMWHs in patients with established DVT are approximatively 100 anti-Xa IU/kg bodyweight every 12 hours. Since long-term subcutaneous heparin is inconvenient and can produce osteoporosis, it may be reasonable to start oral anticoagulant after 6 to 8 weeks, aiming for an INR of 2 to 3.

2. Prophylaxis of thromboembolic episodes
a. Asymptomatic patients

There is considerable uncertainty as to the optimal management of asymptomatic individuals with deficiency of ATIII, as little information on the true risk of unprovoked thromboembolism in asymptomatic carriers is known. Moreover, it is not clear what proportion of thrombotic events are idiopathic and what percentage of events will be fatal. These are vital facts needed for rational risk/benefit decision making. However recognisable risk factors are identified in 30 to 70 percent of patients presenting with their first thrombotic event. Most of these events are likely to respond to therapy, and therefore, the frequency of fatal events is exceedingly low. Based on these considerations, it is reasonable to withhold anticoagulants until a thrombotic event occurs, sparing the patient the inconvenience and the potential complications of long-term anticoagulant therapy. Exceptions include patients with a family history of fatal thrombotic events or other serious thromboembolic problems. If a watch and wait approach is used, however, prophylaxis should be given whenever the patient is at risk for thrombosis.

b. High risk conditions

Patients with ATIII deficiency require vigorous prophylaxis preoperatively and during periods of immobilisation/bed rest and pregnancy which is also considered as a high risk factor for thrombotic event. Effective methods of prophylaxis include oral anticoagulants, adjusted dose of unfractionated heparin, and low molecular weight heparin at a dose which is not yet well defined

Patients on long-term anticoagulant therapy are more complicated to manage. For minor surgical procedures, such as dental extractions, the oral anticoagulant dose can be decreased preoperatively and the procedure done when the INR is between 1.5 and 1.8. The oral anticoagulant dose can then be increased postoperatively to achieve a therapeutic INR.

For major surgical procedures the oral anticoagulant will have to be discontinued, and reversal with vitamin K may be needed for those who require urgent surgery. Once oral anticoagulant is stopped, therapeutic doses of heparin can be given intravenously for anticoagulant coverage prior to surgery. The heparin should be discontinued 3 to 4 hours preoperatively and can be restarted 12 to 24 hours after surgery once hemostasis is obtained. It is reasonable to restart heparin at maintenance doses, without a bolus, to reduce bleeding risk. Oral anticoagulant can be restarted postoperatively, and the heparin can be discontinued when the INR has been therapeutic for several days. AT concentrates can be indicated during the perioperative period.

In patients with a history of thrombosis long term oral anticoagulant treatment is justified if careful monitoring in well informed patients can be conducted. A large European study EPCOT (European Prospective Cohort on Thrombophilia) has been organized recently to obtain more information on the management of these patients.

c. Pregnancy

Pregnancy is often a precipitating condition in patients with congenital thrombophilia.[2,48-50] In the absence of prophylactic treatment, the incidence of thrombosis during pregnancy is about 20% in ATIII deficiency, twice as frequent as in protein C or protein S deficiency. Episodes of thrombosis in the first trimester of pregnancy are not unusual in ATIII deficiency. Thrombotic episodes post-partum are twice as frequent as during pregnancy in patients with thrombophilia. Prophylactic treatment during pregnancy raises many problems because of the teratogenicity of oral anticoagulants during the first trimester and the risk of osteoporosis associated with long term heparin therapy. Some recommendations have been made regarding pregnant women with congenital ATIII deficiency[50,51], although general experience is still limited.

In contrast, a prophylactic treatment should be administered in the post partum period for at least six weeks in every woman with congenital thrombophilia. ATIII concentrates are often recommended in combination with heparin after delivery and during the first week of the post partum period. This topic is covered in more detail in Bonnar's chapter.

d. Other considerations

In general, oral contraceptives should not be used in asymptomatic patients with antithrombin III deficiency[52], although the thrombotic risks associated with oral contraceptives that contain low doses of oestrogen are unknown. However thrombosis may still occur in women taking pills with a low oestrogen content (20 micrograms). If the patient is receiving oral anticoagulant, it is probably safe to give oral contraceptives, even though this approach has never been evaluated in clinical trials. In any case, because of the potential teratogenic effects of oral anticoagulant, effective birth control is mandatory in women of childbearing potential who are receiving oral anticoagulants.

C. MANAGEMENT OF PATIENTS WITH ACQUIRED ATIII DEFICIENCY

The management of acquired ATIII deficiency consists of the treatment of the specific disease responsible for ATIII abnormality (eg liver disease, nephrotic syndrome). ATIII concentrates have been suggested to compensate for the deficiency state. ATIII concentrate has a plasma half life of 60 hours in normal and heterozygote ATIII deficient recipients during steady state conditions. One unit of ATIII per kilogram of body weight can as a rule achieve a 0.016 U/mL plasma rise.[45,46] Currently several human plasma derived, viral inactivated concentrates of ATIII are commercially available. This is reviewed by Menache et al[46] and more recently by Lechner et al [47]. ATIII therapy has been proposed in the treatment of DIC (sepsis, shock, newborn),[5,47,53,54] replacing losses (renal, liver disease, orthotopic liver, transplantation, apheresis), decreased production due to L-asparaginase therapy[40,41] and also to prevent thrombosis after surgery [55,56]. Replacement therapy in acquired conditions has not been a definitively proven therapeutic strategy. However, there is a rationale to replace ATIII to achieve normal concentration in deficient patients, with DIC or thrombosis, especially those who are refractory to conventional therapy. Equivocal results were observed in newborn infants with sepsis and renal transplant recipients.

IV. CONCLUSION

ATIII is an essential physiological serine protease inhibitor whose function is critical for maintaining hemostatic balance. A level of ≥80% must be maintained, in both congenital and acquired conditions to minimise thrombotic events. Human plasma derived ATIII concentrates are now available. Although the risk of viral contamination of these concentrates is probably extremely low, their administration should be restricted to well-documented indications (in congenitally deficient patients for instance). This administration to individuals with acquired deficiencies in state of shock and DIC is currently under investigation. Favourable effects of heparin in DIC can only be expected when there is sufficient circulating functional ATIII. This level must be kept in excess of 80%. Since in acute cases of DIC the recovery of ATIII is only ≈ 50% and its half life can be shortened, more frequent administration of ATIII might become essential. This should be based on the measured ATIII activity. The method employed should always be mentioned with the results and with the appropriate interpretation of the result obtained. Treatment with ATIII concentrates is an area where uncertainty still exists between optimistic expectations based on theoretical considerations or animal experiments and a lack of data based on large clinical trials. More information is needed to assess the clinical benefits of ATIII concentrate with regard to reduction of morbidity or mortality. Prognosis in individual cases is difficult.

REFERENCES

1. **Lane D.A., Olds R.R. Thein S.L.,** Antithrombin and its deficiencies states. *Blood Coag and Fibrinol.* 3, 315, 1992.
2. **Thaler E., Lechner K.,** Antithrombin III deficiency and thromboembolism *Clin Haematol.* 10, 369, 1981.
3. **Rosenberg R.D., Bauer K.A.,** The Heparin and Antithrombin System. A natural anticoagulant mechanism. In *Haemostasis and Thrombosis : basic principles and clinical practice* (Eds Colman R.W., Hirch J., Marden V.J., Salzman J.B., J.B. Lippincott Company, Philadelphia, 837, 1994.
4. **Carlson T.H., Simon T.L. and Atencio A.C.,** In vivo behaviour of human radio iodinated antithrombin III: distribution among three physiological pools. *Blood* 66, 13, 1985.
5. **Vinazzer H.A.** Antithrombin III in shock and disseminated intravascular coagulation. *Clin. Appl. Thrombosis/Hemostasis* 1, 62, 1995.
6. **Chan V., and Chan T.K.,** Antithrombin III in fresh and cultured human endothelial cells: a natural anticoagulant from the vascular endothelium. *Thromb Res.* 15, 209, 1979.
7. **Conard J., Brosstad F., Lie Larsen M., Samama M., Abildgaard U.,** Molar antithrombin concentration in normal human plasma. *Haemostasis,* 13, 363, 1983.
8. **Collen D., Schetz J., De Cock F. et al.,** Metabolism of antithrombin III (heparin cofactor) in man: Effect of venous thrombosis and of heparin administration. *Eur J of Clin Invest* 7, 27, 1977.
9. **Conard J., samama M., Salomon Y.,** Antithrombin III and the oestrogen content of combined oestro-progestagen contraceptives. *Lancet,* 1148,1972.
10. **Meade T.W., Brozovic M., Chakrabarti R. et al.,** Am epidemiological study of the haemostatic and other effects of oral contraceptives. *Brit J Haematol.* 34, 353, 1976.
11. **Jespersen J., Ingeberg S., and Bach E.,** Antithrombin III and platelets during the normal menstrual cycle and in women receiving oral contraceptives low in oestrogen. *Gynecol Obstet Invest.* 15, 153, 1983.
12. **Conard J., Samama M., Basdevant A., et al,** Differential ATIII-response to oral and parenteral administration of 17β-estradiol. *Thromb Haemost* 49,245,1983.
13. **Caine Y.G., Bauer KA, Barzegar S., et al.,** Coagulation activation following estrogen administration to postmenopausal women. *Thromb Haemost* 68,392,1992.
14. **Sporrong T., Matteson L.A., Samsioe G. et al.,** Haemostatic changes during continuous oestradiol-progestrogen treatment of post menopausal women. *Br J Obstet Gynaecol.* 97, 939, 1990.
15. **Stirling Y., Woolf L., North W.R., Seghatchian M.J.,** Haemostasis in normal pregnancy. *Thromb Haemost.* 52, 176, 1984.
16. **Owen J.,** Antithrombin III replacement therapy in pregnancy. *Seminars Hematol.* 28, 46, 1991.
17. **Andrew M., Massicotte-Nolan P., Mitchell L., et al.,** Dysfunctional antithrombin III in sick premature infants. *Pediatr Res.* 19, 237, 1985.
18. **Blajchman M.A., Austin R.C., Fernandez-Rachubinski F., et al.,** Molecular basis of inherited human antithrombin deficiency. *Blood* 80, 2159, 1992.
19. **Egeberg O.,** Inherited antithrombin deficiency causing thrombophilia. *Thromb Diath Haemorrh.* 13, 516, 1965.
20. **Odegard O.R., Abildgaard U.,** Antithrombin III : critical review of assay methods. Significance of variations in health and disease. *Haemostasis* 59,341,1977.
21. **Demers C., Ginsberg J.S., Hirsh J et al.,** Thrombosis in antithrombin III deficient persons. Report of a large kindred and literature review. *Ann Intern Med* 754, 1992.
22. **Finnazzi G., Gaccia R., Barbui T.,** Different prevalence of thromboembolism in the subtypes of congenital antithrombin III deficiency. Review of 404 cases. *Thromb Haemost* 58, 1094, 1987.
23. **Ellis D.,** Recurrent renal vein thrombosis and renal failure associated with antithrombin III deficiency. *Pediatr Nephrol* 6, 131, 1992.
24. **Simioni P., Zanardi S., Saracino A., et al.,** Occurrence of arterial thrombosis in a cohort of patients with hereditary deficiency of clotting inhibitors. *J Med* 23, 61, 1992.
25. **Martinez H.R., Rangel-Guerra R.A., Marfil L.J.,** Ischemic stroke due to deficiency of coagulation inhibitors. Report of 10 young adults. *Stroke* 24, 19, 1993.
26. **Graham J.A., Daly H.M., Carson P.J.,** Antithrombin III deficiency and cerebrovascular accidents in young adults. *J Clin Pathol.* 45, 921, 1992.
27. **Arima T., Motomura M., Nishiura Y., et al.,** Cerebral infarction in a heterozygote with variant antithrombin III. *Stroke* 23, 1822, 1992.
28. **Schulman S., and Tengborn L.,** Treatment of venous thromboembolism in patients with congenital deficiency of antithrombin III. *Thromb Haemost.* 68, 634, 1992.
29. **Buller H.R., Ten Cate J.W.,** Acquired antithrombin III deficiency: Laboratory diagnosis incidence, clinical implications and treatment with antithrombin III concentrate. *Am J Med.* 87, 44S, 1989.
30. **Lalch F.,** Hypercoagulability, renal vein thrombosis and thrombotic complications of nephrotic syndrome. *Kidney International* 28, 429, 1985.
31. **Igarashi M., Roy S., Stapleton F.B.,** Cerebrovascular complications in children with nephrotic syndrome. *Pediatr Neurol* 4, 362, 1988.
32. **Brownlee M., Vlassara H., and Cerami A.,** Inhibition of heparin-catalyzed human antithrombin III activity by nonenzymatic glycosylation. *Diabetes* 33, 532, 1984.
33. **Ducrocq R., Bachour H., Belkhodja R., et al.,** Evidence for nonenzymatic glycation of antithrombin III in diabetic patients. *Clin Chem.* 31, 338, 1985.
34. **Winter J.H., Bennett B., McTaggart F., et al.,** Lipoprotein fractions and antithrombin III consumption during clotting. *Thromb Haemostas.* 47, 236, 1982.
35. **Fourrier F., Chopin C., Goudemand J., et al.,** Septic shock, multiple organ failure and disseminated intravascular coagulation. Compared patterns of antithrombin III, protein C, and protein S deficiencies. *Chest* 101, 816, 1992.
36. **Toulon, P., Jacquot C., Capron L., et al.,** Antithrombin III and heparin cofactor II in patients with chronic renal failure undergoing regular hemodialysis. *Thromb Haemost.* 57, 263, 1987.
37. **Marciniak E., Gockerman J.P.,** Heparin induced clearance in circulating antithrombin III. *Lancet,* ii,581,1977.
38. **Sikorski J.M., Hampson W.G., Straddon G.E.,** The natural history aetiology of deep vein thrombosis after total hip replacement. *J Bone Joint Surg (Br)* 63, 171, 1981.
39. **Stulberg B.N., Insall J.N., Williams G.W. et al.,** Deep-vein thrombosis following total knee replacement. *J Bone Joint Surg (Am)* 66, 194, 1984.

40. **Conard J., Cazenave B., Maury J. Horellou M.H., Samama M.,** L-Asparaginase, antithrombin III and thrombosis. *Lancet,* 17, 1091, 1980.

41. **Anderson N., Lokich J.J., and Tullis J.L.,** L-asparaginase effect on antithrombin-III levels, *Med Pediatr Oncol.* 7, 335, 1979.

42. **Nagasawa H., Kim G.K., Steiner M. et al.,** Inhibition of thrombin-neutralising activity of antithrombin III by steroid hormones. *Thromb Haemost* 47, 157, 1982.

43. **Conard J., Bara L., Horellou M.H., Samama M.,** Bovine or human thrombin in amidolytic AT III assays. Influence of heparin cofactor II. *Thromb. Res.,* 41, 873, 1986.

44. **Samama M., Conard J. Horellou M.H.,** Hereditary thrombophilia: Management of patients. In *Haematology trends* 93, Eds (Lechner K & Gadner H.) Schattauer New York , 239, 1993.

45. **Tengborn L., Frohm B., Nilsson L.E. et al.,** Properties and catabolism of heat treated antithrombin III concentrate. *Thromb Res.* 48, 701, 1987.

46. **Menache D.,** Antithrombin III concentrate. *Haematol Oncol Clin North Am* 6, 1115, 1992.

47. **Lechner K., Kyrle P.A.,** Antithrombin III concentrates - Are they clinically usefull. *Thromb Haemostas,* 73, 340, 1995.

48. **Hellgren M., Tengborn L., and Abildgaard U.,** Pregnancy in women with congenital antithrombin III deficiency: experience of treatment with heparin and antithrombin. *Gynecol Obstet Invest.* 14, 127, 1982.

49. **Conard J., Horellou M.H., van Dreden P., Lecompte T., Samama M.,** Thrombosis and pregnancy in congenital deficiencies in ATIII, protein C or protein S : a study of 78 women. *Thromb Haemost* 63,319,1990.

50. **De Stefano V., Leone G., De Carolis S. et al.,** Management of pregnancy in women with antithrombin III congenital defect: report of four cases, *Thromb Haemostas* 59, 193, 1988.

51. **Samson D., Stirling Y., Seghatchian M.J., et al.,** Management of pregnancy in a patient with congenital antithrombin III deficiency. *Br. J. Haematol.* 56, 243 1984.

52. **Pabinger I., Schneider B., GHT study group of natural inhibitors,** Thrombotic risk of women with hereditary antithrombin III-, protein C- and protein S- deficiency taking oral contraceptive medication.*Thromb Haemost* 71,548,1994.

53. **Mammen E.F., Miyakawa T., Phillips T. et al.,** Human antithrombin concentrates and experimental disseminated intravascular coagulation. *Semin Thromb Hemost.* 11, 373, 1985.

54. **Maki M., Terao T., Ikenoue T., et al.,** Clinical evaluation of antithrombin III concentrate (BI 6.013) for disseminated intravascular coagulation in obstetrics. *Gynecol Obstet Invest.* 23, 230, 1987.

55. **Francis C.W., Pellegrini V.D., Marder V.J. et al.,** Prevention of venous thrombosis after total hip arthroplasty. *J Bone Joint Surg.* 71, 327, 1989.

56. **Francis C.W., Pellegrini V.D., Harris C.M. et al.,** Antithrombin III prophylaxis of venous thromboembolic disease after total hip or total knee replacement. *Am J Med* 87, 3B-61S, 1989.

HEREDITARY PROTEIN C AND PROTEIN S DEFICIENCY

I. Elalamy, J. Conard, M.H. Horellou, P. Van Dreden, and M.M. Samama
Service d'Hématologie Biologique, Hôpital Hôtel-Dieu, Paris

I. BRIEF HISTORICAL ASPECTS

The existence of familial venous thrombophilia has long been suspected but its importance has only recently been recognized.

The first discovery of a cause of hereditary thrombophilia was Antithrombin III (ATIII) deficiency by Egeberg[1] thirty years ago. It was the first example of a possible relationship between coagulation alteration and predisposition to venous thrombosis in accordance with the Virchow triad[2].

About fifteen years later using a dynamic flow system, the role of protein C (PC) in the anti-thrombogenicity of endothelial cells was demonstrated[3]. The role of protein C as a regulator of blood coagulation *in vivo* was confirmed by the discovery of the first family with hereditary protein C deficiency and thrombotic disease[4]. This initial observation was followed three years later by the discovery of families with venous thrombophilia and hereditary protein S (PS) deficiency[5]. Finally, in 1993, Dahlback et al[6] described a new cause of familial thrombophilia called Activated Protein C resistance (APC resistance) which is twice as frequent as the three other causes combined. This inherited resistance was linked to factor V gene mutation[7,8]. The prevalence of APC resistance in the normal population is high. A combined deficiency of APC resistance and PC or PS congenital deficiency seems to increase the risk of thrombosis (see below).

The main characteristics of PC and PS are summarized in Table I. The role of the system of PC/PS and thrombomodulin is to down regulate *in vivo* the amplification of coagulation (figure 1).

Table I. Main characteristics of protein C and protein S

	molecular weight Kd	synthesis site	protein characteristics	plasma level mg/l	chromosomal location	half-life hours
Protein C	62	liver endothelium	vitamin K dependent	5	2	6-8
Protein S	77	liver endothelium megakaryocytes	vitamin K dependent	25	3	60

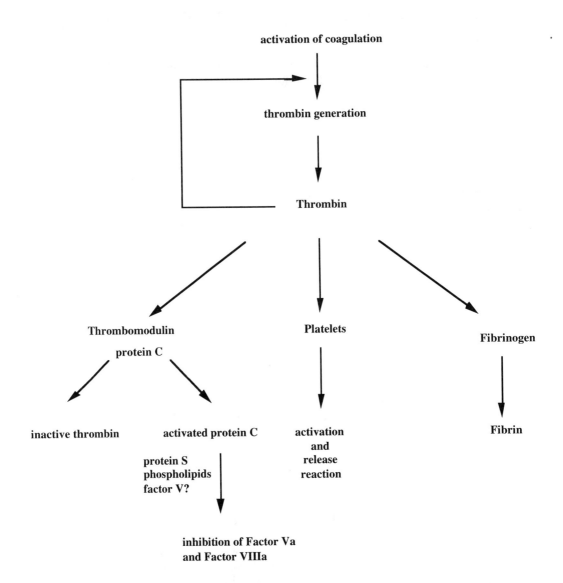

Figure 1. Simplified scheme of coagulation cascade focusing on protein C-protein S system

II. CLINICAL ASPECTS

Clinical aspects are clearly different in heterozygous and homozygous patients.

A. HETEROZYGOUS PATIENTS

We will describe the main characteristics of familial thrombophilia in PC and PS deficiency. This description is based on our own experience and on literature data. In a recent study, we described the clinical characteristics of these isolated deficiencies in 50 families including at least two affected members: 33 of PC and 17 of PS, comprising a total of 186 hereditary coagulation factor deficient patients[9].

The 50 families were identified from approximately 700 consecutive patients referred to our laboratory for biological investigation after either an initial or a reccurrent thrombotic episode. In this series of patients there was 21 families with ATIII deficiency.

Each patient was interviewed to establish the characteristics of the thromboembolic event (type, site, method of diagnosis, treatment, reccurrence, precipitating factors...). The main blood tests performed were whole blood cell count, prothrombin time, activated partial thromboplastin time, thrombin time, fibrinogen, detection of lupus anticoagulant, ATIII, PC, PS activities and antigens, total and free forms, plasminogen activity.

The test population consists of 186 patients, 50 propositi and 136 siblings with 105 symptomatic (56%) and 81 asymptomatic members (44%).

1. Prevalence

Prevalence of these deficiencies among patients with a history of thrombosis has been determined in various studies[10,15] (Table II). In our study, PC deficiency is more frequent than ATIII or PS deficiency since the prevalence was 4.7%, 3% and 2.4% respectively. Our results are rather similar to those of Heijboer et al[14] and Pabinger et al[15]. The incidence seems to be higher in Chinese than in Caucasians[16]. However, those numbers are probably overestimated due to bias in patient recruitment.

Table II. Prevalence of protein C and protein S congenital deficiency
in patients with a history of thrombosis (from ref.10)

First author	Protein C (%)	Protein S (%)
Engesser et al. 1987	7.8	8.0
Gladson et al. 1988	4.0	5.0
Conard et al. 1988	7.8	1.8
Ben-Tal et al. 1989	5.6	2.8
Heijboer et al. 1990	3.2	2.2
Pabinger et al. 1992	3.3	2.3

2. Clinical characteristics

An autosomal hereditary transmission was found in these families, corroborating the observations of others. PC deficiency affects men and women with similar frequency. We noted a male prevalence among PS deficient patients, as did Engesser[5] (table III).

A positive family history of thrombosis was found in about 80% of the propositi: this fact stresses the hereditary aspect of the biological defect. About 60% of deficient patients are symptomatic. Patients with ATIII and PS deficiency seem to be more severely affected than those with PC deficiency, with 70%, 71% and 48% of symptomatic patients respectively.

Table III. Clinical features of 186 hereditary heterozygous deficient patients in PC or PS

	Protein C	Protein S	Total
n families	33	17	50
deficient pts	117	69	186
symptomatic pts	56 (48%)	49 (71%)	105 (56%)
sex-ratio (M/F)	0.95	0.77	0.88
family history	26 (79%)	13 (77%)	78%
age of first episode			
≤ 15 y	2 (4%)	3 (6%)	5%
16 to 30 y	36 (64%)	27 (55%)	60%
31 to 40 y	12 (21%)	10 (21%)	21%
> 40	6 (11%)	9 (18%)	14%
first accident			
DVT	29 (52%)	28 (57%)	56%
PE ± DVT	23 (41%)	13 (27%)	34%
SVT	4 (7%)	6 (12%)	9%
CVT	0	1 (2%)	0.5%
AT	0	1 (stroke) (2%)	0.5%
recurrences	31 (55%)	32 (65%)	60%
out of treatment	27 (87%)	29 (91%)	89%
with treatment	4 (13%)	3 (9%)	11%
triggering factors			
pill	4 (7%)	4 (8%)	
pregnancy	16 (28%)	9 (18%)	
post-partum	11	6	
surgery	10 (18%)	2 (4%)	
immobilisation	6 (11%)	5 (10%)	
trauma or effort	9 (16%)	16 (34%)	
not evidenced	11 (20%)	13 (26%)	
asymptomatic pts	61 (52%)	20 (29%)	

pts : patients
DVT : deep vein thrombosis
PE ± DVT : pulmonary embolism associated or not to a DVT
SVT : superficial vein thrombosis
CVT : cerebral venous thrombosis
  AT : arterial thrombosis

In a recent case-control study of 474 consecutive outpatients, Koster et al[17] found an increase of thrombotic risk in PC or ATIII deficiency subjects with a gradient according to the inhibitor plasma level, but surprisingly, lowered PS levels were not associated with venous thrombosis.

The first episode of thrombosis occurs for all these deficiencies usually between 20 and 30 years of age (65% of cases under 30). It appears earlier and with a higher prevalence in ATIII deficiency (80% of cases under 30).

The most common clinical presentation is deep venous thrombosis, with or without symptomatic pulmonary embolism, in 90% of the cases. Superficial venous thrombosis (SVT) seems more frequent in PC and PS deficiency than in ATIII deficiency. The same is true for recurrences of SVT.

Some events occurred at an unusual site: mesenteric vein thrombosis in three cases of ATIII deficiency. Similar cases have also been reported with PC and PS deficiencies. Thromboses in cerebral, portal, axillary, inferior caval, renal vein and rare retinal vein occlusion have also been reported[4,8-10]. A recent review did not demonstrate a causal relationship between thrombophilia and retinal vein occlusion[18].

Clinical circumstances predisposing to the first episode of thrombosis were found in 75% of symptomatic patients.

Among women, *pregnancy* was the most frequent predisposing cause during the entire pregnancy in ATIII deficiency, but primarily post-partum for PC and PS deficiencies[19]. In the literature, the rate of thrombotic episodes during pregnancy was around 30%, 7% and 1% in ATIII, PC and PS deficiency, respectively[5,10,12]. During the post-partum period, the figures are higher except in ATIII deficiency, 23%, 21% and 23%, respectively[9].

Oral contraceptives are a precipitating factor in women with hereditary thrombophilia. This observation seems well documented in ATIII and probably in PC deficiency while it has been questioned for protein S deficiency by Pabinger et al[20]. Allaart mentioned that women with PC or PS deficiency did not have higher risk for thrombotic events than men[21]. Oral contraception by estroprogestative pill seems more often associated with thrombosis in ATIII than in PC or PS deficiencies[9,22].

Surgical events are also triggering factors. Even minor surgical interventions such as appendectomy were found (2 cases under 15 years old among 26 patients and 4 patients older than 15 years among 23 patients) to predispose to thromboembolic episodes.

Trauma (falls, strains, physical efforts...) or *prolonged immobilisation* (bed rest, car or plane travel, plaster cast...) are frequently reported.

These predisposing factors are found more often among young (<45 years) thrombophilic patients, while the first episode seems more often spontaneous above 45 years of age. It is important to point out that the spontaneous aspect of a thrombotic accident is not a specific criterion for screening for familial thrombophilia since it is present in only 25% of patients in our series.

Recurrences are common in patients with PC and PS deficiency. Recurrence rate is not influenced by sex or by age of the patient at the first episode of thrombosis. Two thirds of symptomatic patients have had at least one recurrence whatever the deficiency and the plasma level of the involved inhibitor. Interestingly, recurrences occurred mostly in the absence of anticoagulant treatment (89%) and after a triggering factor (75%).

Deep vein thrombosis and pulmonary embolism are the most frequent types of recurrence. SVT are more frequent in PC and PS deficiencies than in ATIII deficiency. That might illustrate the importance of the PC-PS-thrombomodulin system in microcirculation regulation.

When the first episode is precipitated, often the recurrence is as well (67%) and may be prevented by appropriate anticoagulant prophylaxis when a precipitating factor is present. But when the first episode seems "spontaneous", the recurrence also occurred "spontaneously" in 50% of cases. This suggests the necessity of long term prophylactic treatment in symptomatic thrombophilic patients when there was no recognized precipitating factor.

Arterial thromboses appear to be rare in our study (1% versus 90% of venous thromboembolism): 2 cases of stroke associated with vascular risk factors were observed (one ATIII and one PS deficient patient). There is evidence that PC deficiency may predispose to arterial thrombosis, particularly ischemic strokes in young deficient patients[23-26]. Similar results have been obtained in PS deficiency[27-29]. This problem has been recently discussed by Allaart et al[30]. Careful analysis of the literature, including the data of the Leiden group, led to the conclusion that heterozygous PS deficiency is associated with arterial thromboses. This observation is difficult to reconcile in the light of the new finding of the same group[17] who suggested the absence of a relationship between protein S deficiency and thrombosis.

The proportion of asymptomatic patients is higher in PC than in ATIII or PS deficiency, 52%, 30% and 29%, respectively. Although these patients (n=102) had similar triggering factors in about 50% at an age of high risk of thrombosis (mean age 30±16,4 years), they remained asymptomatic without any treatment.

Thus, there is heterogeneity of clinical characteristics among patients with congenital thrombophilia[31,32]. There is a greater prevalence of superficial vein thrombosis in PC and PS deficiency than in ATIII deficiency both for the first thrombotic episode and for recurrences. A higher risk of post-partum thrombosis exists in all three deficiencies and also during pregnancy in ATIII deficiency. The first thrombotic episode seems to occur later in the PC or PS deficient patient than those with ATIII deficiency.

Although *skin necrosis* has been reported among heterozygous PC and PS deficient patients at the initiation of oral anticoagulant therapy, no case of skin necrosis was observed in this series of heterozygous patients[33,34]. Combined acquired PS deficiency and increased antiphospholipids antibodies could increase the risk of cutaneous necrosis[35]. Transient PC and PS deficiencies have been reported in young children with varicella complicated by thrombotic complications and purpura fulminans[36].

In our series of patients, we have not noticed any relevant pathological state (hypertension, diabetes, hypercholesterolemia...) which was associated with the hereditary deficiency.

The severity of the clinical symptoms differs within each deficient family. Other factors are probably responsible for the occurrence of thrombosis, environmental factors or other blood alteration such as APC resistance. A relationship with the molecular defect has been also suspected but not demonstrated. Moreover, hypercoagulable states seem to result from " multigene " interactions[37] and clinical episodes of thrombosis are precipitated by acquired prothrombotic insults in patients with hereditary thrombophilia[38].

B. HOMOZYGOUS PATIENTS
1. Detection of neonatal manifestations:
In PC and PS homozygous deficiencies, purpura fulminans at birth has been reported[39-42]. This syndrome is characterized by a dermal vascular thrombosis and progressive hemorrhagic skin necrosis. The painful lesions have an irregular distribution of blue-black hemorrhagic necrosis. This disorder is often associated with disseminated intravascular coagulation. Cerebral, ophthalmic or renal thrombosis are suspected to occur in utero[40].

2. Detection in adults:
In some cases, onset of thrombosis was delayed and was associated with skin necrosis developed at the initiation of oral anticoagulant therapy in PC deficient patients[43]. We observed three homozygous PC deficient patients who experienced their first thrombotic episode at age of 17, 24 and 45 years, respectively, who had repeated skin necrosis at the beginning of treatment with vitamin K antagonists. Plasma PC levels varied between 10% and 23% and the homozygosity was confirmed by DNA analysis with mutations at positions 168, 267 and 301[43]. One of these three patients did not have a strong history of thrombosis in the absence of anticoagulant treatment. Heterozygous subjects of these families seem to have a low risk of thrombosis, suggesting that autosomal transmission might be recessive and other environmental factors play a part in the clinical expression of these deficiencies[44,45].

PS homozygous deficiency is more rare[42-46]. The clinical manifestations are similar to those of severe PC deficiency patients. It is interesting to note that there was no family history of thrombosis in these related cases.

C. Combined deficiencies
Several cases of combined familial deficiencies of these physiological inhibitors were reported. A protein C deficiency associated with different other causes of thrombophilia: ATIII deficiency[12,14,47], dysplasminogenemia[48], dysfibrinogenemia[49], PS deficiency[50], heparin cofactor II[51], Activated Protein C (APC) resistance[52]. PS deficiency combined with heparin cofactor II[53] and ATIII[15] deficiencies have

been also described. Inherited resistance to APC seems to be an additional genetic risk factor in hereditary deficiency of protein S[54].

III. LABORATORY DIAGNOSIS

The activity tests have the advantage of detecting both quantitative and qualitative deficiencies. PC determination is frequently performed by using the venom Protac® in an amidolytic method. Protac® is a convenient reagent for PC activation[55]. The clotting method may be of interest although it is somewhat more difficult to handle, and falsely low results may be obtained when factor VIII levels are elevated[56]. The diagnosis of congenital deficiency is often difficult during oral anticoagulant. It requires the simultaneous measurement of PC antigen and other vitamin K-dependent factors, such as factor II or X antigen, and comparing the results as a ratio[57]. In a recent work, the authors tried to improve the discrimination between deficient patients on oral anticoagulants and controls by the calculation of a best likelihood ratio[58]. The combination of protein C antigen by ELISA with factor VII activity gave the smallest overlap and the best discrimination between heterozygotes and controls. The combined protein C and factor X antigens assays were better than factor II antigen in the discriminant analysis. A calculated likelihood ratio favoring carriership for protein C deficiency may be used to express the uncertainty of the diagnosis and to calculate the genetic probability of deficiency with the pedigree analysis. Thus, a family study may also be helpful in this case. In some patients, substitution of subcutaneous heparin to oral anticoagulants for two weeks could be undertaken in order to reexamine the blood in the absence of the effect of vitamin K antagonists.

PS is usually measured by an immunological method as total and/or free PS after precipitation of the complex by treating the plasma with polyethylene glycol. Free PS may be measured with a monoclonal antibody. Free PS may be decreased if an inflammatory syndrome is present and is related to a higher plasma concentration of C4b binding protein. The same mechanism has been suggested during pregnancy or in women using oral contraceptives[59]. PS is the cofactor of activated PC and an interference exists in a PS functional assay giving spurious low results in the presence of an APC resistance[60,61]. The misdiagnosis can be prevented by performing the PS assay at several dilutions[62].

DNA analysis allows a reliable diagnostic test for the typing of the disease, and specially PC deficiency. It may be a great help when a patient has borderline values and/or when the diagnosis of congenital deficiency is not well ascertained[21]. This work has clearly shown that a low rate of false positive and false negative results is identified when the results of functional assay and those obtained by DNA analysis are compared (figure 2).

It is also essential to exclude an acquired deficiency of these inhibitors in different pathological conditions before asserting the congenital nature of the alteration: liver disease, disseminated intravascular coagulation, systemic lupus erythematosis or L-asparaginase treatment. During estroprogestogen intake or during pregnancy, protein S plasma levels are also decreased. Laboratory diagnosis of hereditary thrombophilia is discussed in more details in Preston's chapter.

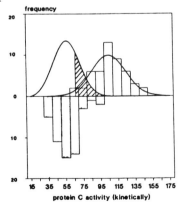

Figure 2: Distribution and expected distribution curves of the results of single protein C assay in 49 protein C deficient heterozygotes (dotted histograms) and 51 normal relatives (open histograms)[58].

Laboratory results are in percentage of normal. The shaded area represents the proportion of the heterozygotes misdiagnosed based on protein C activity values above this lower limit of normal.

IV. HETEROGENEITY OF MOLECULAR DEFECTS

Elucidation of the molecular basis of these deficiencies is critical for the understanding of their antithrombotic mechanisms[63]. It provides information on the structural features governing protein function and allows a classification based on genome abnormalities.

The PC gene maps to chromosome 2 (2q13-2q14) and includes 9 exons that have been sequenced[64,65]. A number of DNA sequence polymorphisms are known to occur within the mRNA of the PC gene and may or may not result in a change of amino-acid sequence. The PS genes are located near the centromere of chromosome 3 (3q11,1-3q11,2) and consist of an active gene PSα and a pseudogene PSβ[66], including 15 exons. A frequent polymorphism is reported in the PSα (Herlen polymorphism), and a polymorphic change in the PSβ, associated to PS deficiency is discussed[67].

Immunological and functional assays allow to identify two distinct phenotypes: quantitative or type I deficiency, characterized by a parallel decrease of the level and activity of the protein, and qualitative or type II deficiency involving the synthesis of an abnormal protein.

DNA analysis of nucleotide sequences of PC and PS genes became easier after the development of the polymerase chain reaction (PCR), followed by the direct sequencing of single-stranded DNA associated or not to the denaturing gradient gel electrophoresis (DGGE). Most of the genomic abnormalities observed in PC type I deficiencies are point mutations and exceptionally deletions. Several mutations have been described: nonsense mutation transforming a nucleotide triplet into a stop codon, frame shift produced by insertion or deletion of a small number of nucleotides in the coding sequence resulting in aberrant amino-acid sequences, mutations disrupting a known consensus sequence required for recognition of an intron/exon splice-site, missense mutation impairing the intracellular processing necessary for secretion and transport or stability of the protein[68]. Most type I and all type II mutations are of the missense variety. In type II, the defects are due to substitutions of amino-acids determining the functional domain of the protein at the cleavage site for thrombin or the Gla domain. Other mutations are described in the C terminal portion of the propeptide and in the N terminal part of the catalytic domain and in the promoter region. Mutations in the serine protease domain are common with more than 30 described[69].

The identification of amino-acid substitutions by sequencing of the purified protein has shown that a number of crucial amino-acids are responsible for protein function, secretion and stability. Mapping the genetic status may be useful to classify and identify deficient patients with risk of thrombosis[70]. Comparison of causal mutations with their clinical and biological phenotypes is important and the identification of molecular defects remains essential for understanding mechanisms acting *in vivo* and their physiological importance[71]. However, it is still restricted to research since molecular abnormalities are not similar and methods are time-consuming. Mutations associated with homozygous PC deficiency have been reported in different cases with deletion or missense mutation causing the synthesis of an abnormal protein that is either dysfunctional or not secreted into plasma[72-74]. Thus, molecular identification is a way to clarify the apparent heterogeneity of hereditary PC and PS deficiencies.

The PC mutation database currently contains more than 331 entries and about 132 different nucleotide substitutions have been noted within 32% occurring in CpG dinucleotides (hot spot mutations) (table IV and figure 3). Most type I mutations (85% at codons 132, 157, 306) and all type II mutations (majority in the Gla domain) are missense mutations.

Genetic abnormalities as splice-site, nonsense or missense mutations are also described in the PSa and PSb genes[75,76]. Two large deletions have been also reported[77,78]. A database created by the workshop group on familial thrombophilia will be updated annually.

In contrast to protein C and S mutation, the factor V gene mutation which is linked to APC resistance appears to be due to a single mutation of factor V (changing Arg506 to a Gln)[79].

Table IV: Examples of mutations in the protein C gene[69]

----

heterozygous deficiency type I	nucleotide position /mutation	amino acid	change
symptomatic	40 T-G	-29, W-G	signal peptide
symptomatic	41 G-A	-29, W-stop	signal peptide
symptomatic	1380-86 del 7 nt	del R-3/K-2	frameshift
asymptomatic	3172-89 del 18 nt	77-82 del SCDCRS	frame deletion
asymptomatic	3173-90 del 18 nt	78-83 del CDCRSG	frame deletion
recessive	6274 C-T	none	frameshift
type II			
symptomatic	1388 G-A	-1, R-H	
symptomatic	1414 C-T	9, R-C	
symptomatic	8886 G-A	391, G-S	
homozygous deficiency type I			
symptomatic	3217 G-T	92, E-stop	
symptomatic	6265 G-C	184, Q-H	splice donor

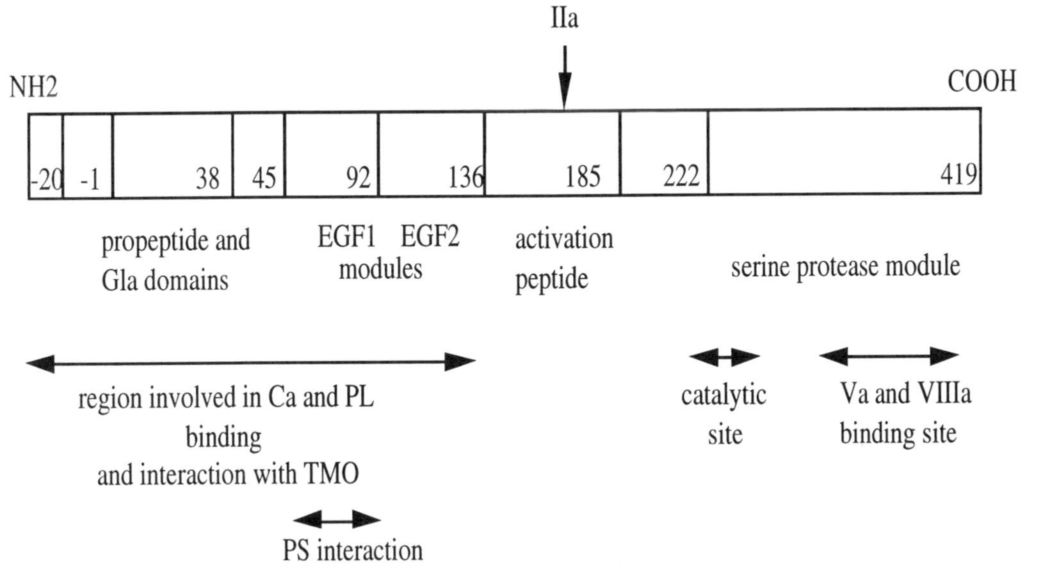

Figure 3 : Schematic model of human protein C and most frequent mutations inducing type I heterozygous deficiency

V. THE RULE OF THE "3 Cs"

Considering a blood alteration which could predispose to thrombosis, one has to take into account the rule of the "3 Cs"[80] (cause, consequence or coincidence of the thrombotic disease). For instance, in heparin cofactor II deficiency, after a clear suggestion of a causal relationship from two different groups, this relationship has been disputed (see chapter on Heparin cofactor II by Sie). The frequency of these abnormalities in individuals having a previous history of thrombosis is not greater than in those without such clinical events[81]. Thus, this decrease could be coincidental. An increase of PAI-1 activity in plasma is relatively frequent shortly after a thrombotic episode: this biologic alteration is a consequence rather than the cause of thrombosis.

In order to determine the causal relationship of the coagulation alteration and predisposition to thrombosis in a family, it is important to identify the siblings with the deficiency and among them those who have a history of thrombosis. Briet et al[82] have addressed this problem, very recently discussed by Tosetto et al[83]. At least two symptomatic first degree-relatives other than the propositus should be identified in a family in order to reach an acceptable specificity. Both groups have proposed a scoring system and/or a standardized questionnaire and an equation for a better approach to this difficult problem[84].

VI. MANAGEMENT OF PATIENTS

A. TREATMENT OF THROMBOTIC EPISODES

Intravenous heparin and oral anticoagulants are the treatment of thrombotic episodes, as in patients without hereditary thrombophilia. The only difference in therapeutic protocols is a more careful use of coumarin therapy in deficient patients to avoid the development of skin necrosis. In our experience, this accident has been only observed in patients with a PC homozygous deficiency[43,85-87]. Coumarin skin necrosis has also been observed in PS deficient patients but it is very rare[88-90]. The management of patients with skin necrosis is still disputed. The use of intravenous heparin is generally accepted. Concentrates of PC have been used with success in rare patients and their use may facilitate the introduction of oral anticoagulants[91,92]. In very rare patients, vitamin K1 has been given parenterally for a short period[93]. In order to minimize the risk of warfarin-induced skin necrosis, it has been advocated not to use a loading dose of oral anticoagulants and to continue heparin therapy until stable anticoagulation has been obtained[85]. In new-borns with purpura fulminans, heparin treatment may fail to prevent continuing skin necrosis[94,95]. Concentrates of PC or PS can be used and very rare cases have been published[96,97].

B. SECONDARY PREVENTION

The risk of recurrent thromboembolism is unknown, although it is likely to be higher in a triggering situation such as surgery, trauma or post-partum. All subjects with hereditary PC or PS deficiency should be provided with a medical certificate. This certificate should be renewed every year according to the evolution of our knowledge of the disease. Prophylaxis with subcutaneous unfractioned or low molecular weight heparin is indicated in asymptomatic patients when a prothrombotic circumstance such as immobilisation and/or severe trauma or surgery is present. Most thrombophilic patients with recurrent episodes at different and/or unusual sites are offered lifelong anticoagulant therapy. In patients with less than two episodes of venous thrombosis that followed an identifiable triggering factor, a shorter course of treatment may be proposed[98]. The benefit/risk ratio of a long term anticoagulant treatment has not been documented. Finally, when oral anticoagulant treatment is used as prophylactic prevention of venous thromboembolism the appropriate intensity of hypocoagulation is not well established. It has been suggested by the Leiden thrombosis group that the treatment should be adjusted at an INR ranging from 2 to 4[80]. Anabolic steroids have been used in PC type I deficiency: they can raise PC plasma concentration but are associated with side-effects in particular in the young women[99] and do not prevent thrombosis[100].

C. MANAGEMENT OF PREGNANCY

Pregnancy is often the precipitating condition in patients with congenital thrombophilia[19]. In the absence of prophylactic treatment, the incidence of thrombosis during pregnancy is about 10% in PC and PS deficiency particularly in the post-partum. Prophylactic treatment during pregnancy causes many problems: teratogenicity of oral anticoagulants during the first trimester and the risk of osteoporosis associated with long-term heparin-therapy.

The treatment must be considered in each individual, until more information is available in larger series of patients. In contrast to ATIII deficiency, it does not seem to be required to start a prophylactic treatment from the very begining of the pregnancy in protein C and protein S deficiency unless the patient was on life-long anticoagulant treatment before getting pregnant. Patients should receive special information from the angiologist regarding the use of graduable compression stockings during pregnancy and the Echo-Doppler monitoring of their legs. Subcutaneous unfractionated heparin is frequently used during the second and the third trimester of pregnancy at a prophylactic dose for instance 7500 anti-Xa International Units twice a day. The use of a Low Molecular Weight Heparin (LMWH) is attractive since it could be given in one injection per day. There is limited experience on the safety for the foetus of such treatment but encouraging results have been obtained[98,101]. There is convincing evidence that LMWH molecules with ATIII affinity do not cross the placenta since no anti-Xa activity has been detected in the blood of the foetus[102,103]. In the post-partum period, a prophylactic treatment is administered in every deficient woman for at least six weeks.

VII. CONCLUSION

The clinical profile of a heterozygous patient deficient in natural inhibitors of blood coagulation is:
- a man or a woman with a first thrombosis before the age of 40
- with a positive family history of thrombosis
- with a deep venous thrombosis associated or not with pulmonary embolism or thromboses at unusual sites (mesenteric, cerebral)
- with a high rate of recurrences in the absence of prophylactic treatment

A precipitating factor is frequently present and is not a criterion for exclusion of familial thrombophilia.

Despite several common features, deficiencies in ATIII, PC and PS show a clinical heterogeneity between the three deficiencies. This is also true for patients with a given deficiency and even between deficient patients from the same family. Combined deficiencies are also possible and must be documented. The single common ground is a thrombotic tendency. Minor differences such as the rate of superficial vein thrombosis which is higher in PC/PS than in ATIII deficient patients and skin necrosis restricted to PC and PS deficiencies have been well documented.

Finally, treatment is similar in these congenital deficiencies. The management of symptomatic and asymptomatic patients with familial thrombophilia is still controversial regarding the type and the duration of treatment.

REFERENCES

1. **Egeberg, O.** Inherited antithrombin III deficiency causing thrombophilia. *Thrombosis Diathesis Haemorrhagica.* 13, 516, 1965.
2. **Virchow, R.** Thrombose und embolie. Vol. Gesammelte Abhanlungen zur wissenschaftilchen medizin., Berlin: Verlag Maxirsch. 219, 1865.
3. **Esmon, NL., Owen, W., Esmond, CT.** Isolation of membrane bound cofactor for thrombin-catalyzed activation of protein C. *J. Biol. Chem.* 257, 859, 1982.
4. **Griffin, J.H., Evatt, B., Zimmerman, T.S., Kleiss, A.J., Wideman, C.,** Deficiency of protein C in congenital thrombotic disease. *J.Clin.Invest.,* 68, 1370, 1981.
5. **Engesser, L., Broekmans, A., Briet, E., Brommer, EJP., Bertina, RM.** Hereditary protein S deficiency: clinical manisfestations. *Ann. Intern. Med.* 106, 677, 1987.
6. **Dahlbäck, B., Carlsson, M., Svensson, P.** Familial thrombophilia due to a previously unrecognized mechanism characterized by poor anticoagulant response to activated protein C: prediction of a cofactor to activated protein C. *Proc. Natl. Acad. Sci. USA.,* 90, 1004, 1993.

7.   **Bertina, R.M., Koeleman, B.P.C., Koster, T., Rosendaal, F.R., Dirven, R.J., de Ronde, H., van der Velden, P.A., Reitsma, P.H.** Mutation in blood coagulation factor V associated with resistance to activated protein C.*Nature*, 369, 64, 1994.

8.   **Zöller, B., Dahlbäck, B.** Linkage between inherited resistance to activated protein C and factor V gene mutation in venous thrombosis. *Lancet.* 343, 1536, 1994.

9.   **Samama, MM., Conard, J., Horellou, MH., van Dreden, P., Elalamy, I.** The congenital deficiencies in antithrombin III, protein C and protein S: clinical aspects. in *International Congress of Angiology*. Paris (Abst.)1992.

10.   **Conard, J.** Thrombophilia: diagnosis and management. *Thrombosis and its management*, ed. Poller L. and Thomson JM., London, Churchill Livingstone. 113, 1993.

11.   **Thaler, E., Lechner, K.** Antithrombin III deficiency and thromboembolism. *prentice CRM* ed. Clinics in Haematology, London, WB Saunders. 369, 1981.

12.   **Broeckmans, AW., Conard, J.** Hereditary protein C deficiency. *Protein C and related proteins*, ed. R. Bertina. London, Churchill Livingstone. 160, 1988.

13.   **Finazzi, G., Barbui, T.** Different incidence of venous thrombosis in patients with inherited deficiencies of antithrombin III, protein C and protein S. *Thromb. Haemost.* 71, 15, 1994.

14.   **Heijboer, H., Brandjes, D., Buller, HR., Sturk, A., Cate, J.** Deficiencies of coagulation-inhibiting and fibrinolytic proteins in outpatients with deep vein thrombosis. *N. Engl. J. Med.* 323, 1512, 1990.

15.   **Pabinger, I., Brücker, S., Kyrle, PA., Schneider, B., Korninger, HC., Niessner, H., Lechner, K.** Hereditary deficiency of antithrombin III, protein C and protein S: prevalence in patients with a history of venous, thrombosis and criteria for rational patient screening. *Blood Coagulation Fibrinolysis.* 3, 547, 1992.

16.   **Liu, HW., Kwong, YL., Bourke, C., Lam, CK., Lie, AKW., Wei, D., Chan, LC.** High incidence of thrombophilia detected in chinese patients with venous thrombosis. *Thromb. Haemost.* 71, 416, 1994.

17.   **Koster, T., Rosendaal, FR., Briët, E., van der Meer, FJM., Colly, LP., Trienekens, PH., Poort, SR., Reitsma, PH., Vandenbroucke, JP.** Protein C deficiency in a controlled series of unselected outpatients: an infrequent but clear risk factor for venous thrombosis (Leiden Thrombophilia Study). *Blood*, 85, 2756, 1995.

18.   **Vine, AK., Samama, MM.** The role of abnormalities in the anticoagulant and fibrinolytic systems in retinal vascular occlusions. *Survey of ophtalmology.* 37, 283, 1993.

19.   **Conard, J., Horellou, MH., Van Dreden, P., Lecompte, T., Samama, MM.** Thrombosis and pregnancy in congenital deficiencies in Antithrombin III, protein C and protein S: a study of 78 women. *Thromb. Haemost.* 63, 319, 1990.

20.   **Pabinger, I., Kyrle, PA., Heistinger, M., Eichinger, S., Wittmann, E., Lechner, K.** The risk of thromboembolism in asymptomatic patients with protein C and protein S deficiency: a prospective study. *Thromb. Haemost.* 71, 441, 1994.

21.   **Allaart, CF., Briet, E.** Familial venous thrombosis. *Thrombosis and Haemostasis*, ed. Bloom and Thomas, New York: Churchill Livingstone. 1994.

22.   **Pabinger, I., Schneider, B.** Thrombotic risk of women with hereditary antithrombin III, protein C and protein S deficiency taking oral contraceptive medication. *Thromb. Haemost.* 71, 548, 1994.

23.   **van Kuijck, MA., Rotteveel, JJ., van Oostrom, CG., Novakova, I.** Neurological complications in children with protein C deficiency. *Neuropediatrics.* 25, 16, 1994.

24.   **Camerlingo, M., Finazzi, G., Casto, L., Laffranchi, C., Barbui, T., Mamoli, A.** Inherited protein C deficiency and non-hemorrhagic arterial stroke in young adults. *Neurology.* 41, 1371, 1991.

25.   **Chateil F, Baronnet R., Guerin V, Fontan D, Guillard JM,,** Cerebrovascular ischemic accident and congenital protein C deficiency in children: apropos of a case. *Pediatrie*, 43, 421, 1988.

26.   **Israels SJ, Seshia SS.,** Childhood stroke associated with protein C or S deficiency. *J. Pediatr.*, 111, 562, 1987.

27.   **Von Felten A, Schaefer HP,** Protein S deficiency in young patient with cerebral arterial thrombosis. *Thromb. Haemost.,.* 62, 12, 1989.

28.   **Burk M, Schottler B., Freund HJ,** Deficiency of both protein C and protein S in a family with ischemic strokes in young adults. *Neurology,.* 44.,1238, 1994 .

29.   **Horowitz IN, Galvis A.,** Gomperts ED, Arterial thrombosis and protein S deficiency. *J. Ped.,* 121, 934, 1992.

30.   **Allaart CF, Aronson DC, Ruys TH, Rosendaal FR, Van Boskel JH, Bertina RM, Briet E.,** Hereditary protein S deficiency in young adults with arterial occlusive disease. *Thromb. Haemost.*, 46, 54,1990.

31.   **Gouault-Heilmann M, Leroy-Matheron C., Levent M.,** Inherited protein S deficiency: clinical manifestations and laboratory findings in 63 patients. *Thromb. Res.*, 76, 269, 1994.

32.   **Conard J, Elalamy I, Horellou MH, Van Dreden P, Samama MM.,** Congenital deficiencies in antithrombin III, protein C and protein S: clinical heterogeneity in 71 families (255 patients). *Thromb. Haemost.*, 69, 575, 1993.

33.   **Friedman KD, Marlar R, Houston JG, Montgomery RR.,** Warfarin-induced skin necrosis in a patient with protein S deficiency. *Blood*, 68, 33A, 1986.

34.   **Goldberg SL, Orthner C, Yalisove BL, Elgart ML, Kessler CM.,** Skin necrosis following prolonged administration of coumarin in a patient with inherited protein S deficiency. *Am. J. Hematol.*, 38, 64, 1991.

35.   **Amster MS., Conway J, Zeid M., Pincus S.** Cutaneous necrosis resulting from protein S deficiency and increased antiphospholipid antibody in a patient with systemic lupus erythematosus. *J. Am. Acad. Dermatol.*, 29, 853, 1993.

36.   **Nguyen P, Reynaud J, Pouzol P, Munzer M, Richard O, François P.** Varicella and thrombotic complications associated with transient protein C and protein S deficiencies in children. *Eur. J. Pediatr.*, 153, 646, 1994.

37.   **Miletich, J.P., Prescott, S.M., White, R., Majerus, P.W., Bovill, E.G.** Inherited predisposition to thrombosis. *Cell*, 72, 477, 1993.

38.   **Schafer AI,** Hypercoagulable states: molecular genetics to clinical practice. *Lancet*, 344, 1739, 1994.

39.   **Gladson CL, Groncy P., Griffin JH.,** Coumarin necrosis, neonatal purpura fulminans and protein C deficiency. *Arch. Dermatol.*, 123, 1701a, 1987.

40.   **Marlar RA, Neumann A.,** Neonatal purpura fulminans due to homozygous protein C or protein S deficiencies. *Sem. Thromb. Haemost.*, 16, 299, 1990.

41.   **Seligsohn U, Berger A, Abend M, Rubin L, Attias D, Zivelin A, Rapaport SI.** Homozygous protein C deficiency manifested by massive venous thrombosis in the new born. *N. Engl. J. Med.*, 310, 559, 1984.

42.   **Mahasandana C, Suvatte V, Marlar RA, Manco-Johnson M, Jacobson L, Hataway WE.,** Neonatal purpura fulminans associated with homozygous protein S deficiency. *Lancet,.* 335, 61, 1990.

43.   **Conard J, Horellou MH, Van Dreden P, Samama MM.,** Homozygous protein C deficiency with late onset and recurrent coumarin-induced skin necrosis. *Lancet*, 1, 743, 1992.

44. **Reitsma PH, Poort SR, Bertina RM,,** Genetic abnormalities in the protein C genes of homozygous and compound heterozygotes for protein C deficiency. *Thromb. Haemost ,* 65, 808, 1991.

45. **Tsuda S, Reitsma PH., Miletich J,,** Molecular defects causing heterozygous protein C deficiency in three asymptomatic kindreds. *Thromb. Haemost.,* 65, 647, 1991.

46. **Pegelow CH, Ledford M, Young J, Zilleruelo G.** Severe Protein S deficiency in a new born. *Pediatrics,* 89, 674, 1992.

47. **Wolf M, Boyer-Neumann C., Mohlo-Sabatier P, Neumann C, Meyer D, Larrieu MJ.,** Familial variant of antithrombin III (ATIII Bligny 47 Arg to His) associated with protein C deficiency. *Thromb. Haemost.,* 63: 215., 1990.

48. **Manabe S, Matsuda M.,** Homozygous protein C deficiency combined with heterozygous dysplasminogenemia found in a 21-year old thrombophilic male. *Thromb. Res.,* 39, 333, 1985.

49. **Gandrille S, Priollet P., Capron L, Roncato M, Fiessinger JN, Aiach M.,** Association of hereditary dysfib, inogenemia with protein C deficiency in two patients with thrombotic tendency. *Thromb. Haemost.,* 58, 411, 1987.

50. **Samama MM,** personnel communication, 1990.

51. **Jobin F, Vu F., Demers M, Leblond PF, Lessard M.,** A case of inherited triple deficiency of antithrombin III, protein C and heparin cofactor II in a large kindred with functional antithrombin III deficiency. *Thromb. Haemost.,* 58, 1214, 1987.

52. **Koeleman BP, Reitsma PH., Allaart CF, Bertina RM.,** Activated protein C resistance as an additional risk factor for thrombosis in protein C-deficient families. *Blood,* 84, 1031, 1994.

53. **Bertina RM, A.T., Larsen ML, Abilgaard U.,** Low heparin cofactor II with abnormal crossed immuno-electrophoresis pattern in two norvegian families. *Thromb. Res.,* 47, 243, 1987.

54. **Zöller B., Berntsdotter A., Garcia de Frutos P., Dahlbäck B.** Resistance to activated protein C as an additional genetic risk factor in hereditary deficiency of protein S, *Blood,* 85, 3518, 1995.

55. **Stocker K, Fischer H, Meier J, Brogli M, Svendsen L.,** Protein C activators in snake venom. *Behring Institut Mitterlungen.,* 79, 37, 1986.

56. **De Moerloose P., Reber G, Bouvier CA.,** Spuriously low levels of protein C deficiency with a Protac activation clotting assay. *Thromb. Haemost.,* 59, 543, 1988.

57. **Bertina RM.** Assays for protein C. *Protein C and related proteins,* ed. Bertina. RM., 1988, London: Churchill Livingstone, 130.

58. **Allaart CF,** Hereditary deficiencies of protein C and protein S. 1994, *(Thesis),* Leiden, The Netherlands.

59. **Pabinger I, Lechner K.,** Acquired protein C and protein S deficiency. *Protein C and related proteins.,* ed. Bertina. RM., 1988, London: Churchill Livingstone. 213.

60. **Faioni EM, Franchi.F., Asti D, Sacchi E, Bernardi F, Manucci PM.,** Resistance to activated protein C in nine thrombophilic families: interference in a protein S functional assay.*Thromb. Haemost.,* 70, 1067, 1993.

61. **Cooper PC, Hampton K., Makris M, Abuzenadah A, Paul B, Preston FE.,** Further evidence that activated protein C resistance can be misdiagnosed as inherited functional protein S deficiency. *Br. J. Haematol.,* 88, 201, 1994.

62. **Faioni EM, Boyer-Neumann C., Franchi F, Wolf M, Meyer D, Manucci PM.,** Another protein S functional assay is sensitive to resistance of activated protein C. *Thromb. Haemost.,* 72, 648, 1994.

63. **Aiach M, Gandrille S., Emmerich J, Alhenc-Gelas M, Fiessinger JN.,** Molecular abnormalities responsible for thrombosis: genetic aspects. *Nouv. Rev. Fr. Hematol.,* 34, 279, 1992.

64. **Foster DC, Yoshitake S., Davie EW.,** The nucleotide sequence of the gene for human protein C. *Proc. Natl. Acad. Sci. USA.,* 82, 4673, 1985.

65. **Plutzky J, Hoskins JA, Long GL, Crabtree GR.,** Evolution and organisation of the human protein C gene. *Proc. Natl. Acad. Sci. USA.,* 83, 546, 1986.

66. **Ploos van Amstel JK, van der Zanden AL, Bakker E, Reitsma PH, Bertina RM.,** Two genes homologous with human protein S cDNA are located on chromosome 3. *Thromb. Haemost.,* 58, 982, 1987.

67. **Bertina RM, Ploos van Amstel JK, van Wijngaarden A, Bakker E, Reitsma PH.,** Heerlen polymorphism of protein S, an immunologic polymorphism due to dimorphism of residue 460. *Blood,* 76, 538, 1990.

68. **Tsay W, Greengard JS, Montgomery RR, McPherson RA, Fucci JC, Koerper MA, Coughlin J, Griffin JH.,** Genetic mutations in ten unrelated american patients with symptomatic type I protein C deficiency. *Blood Coagulation and Fibrinolysis,* 4, 791, 1993.

69. **Reitsma PH, Bernardi F, Doig R.G., Gandrille S, Greencard J.S., Ireland H., Krawczak M, Lind B, Long GL, Poort S.R., Saito H., Sala N, Witt I., Cooper DN.,** Protein C deficiency: a database of mutations.1995 update *Thromb. Haemost.,* 73, 876, 1995.

70. **Doig RG, Begley C., McGrath KM.** Hereditary protein C deficiency associated with mutations in exon IX of the protein C gene. *Thromb. Haemost.,* 72, 203, 1994.

71. **Greengard JS, Griffin JH, Fisher CL.** Possible structural implications of 20 mutations in the protein C protease domain. *Thromb. Haemost.,* 72, 869, 1994.

72. **Grundy CB, Chisholm M, Kakkar VV, Cooper DN.** A novel homozygous missense mutation in the protein C (PROC) gene causing recurrent venous thrombosis. *Hum. Genet.,* 89, 683, 1992.

73. **Sugahara Y, Miura O, Yuen P, Aoki N.** Protein C deficiency Hong Kong 1 and 2: hereditary protein C deficiency caused by two mutant alleles, a 5-nucleotide deletion and a missense mutation. *Blood,* 80, 126, 1992.

74. **Soria JM, Brito D, Barcelo J, Fontcuberta J, Botero L, Maldonado J, Estivill X, Sala N.** Severe homozygous protein C deficiency: identification of a splice site missense mutation (184, Q--->H) in exon 7 of protein C gene. *Thromb. Haemost.,* 72, 65, 1994.

75. **Gandrille S, Borgel D., Gufflet V, Aiach M and the french network INSERM on molecular abnormalities responsible for protein C and protein S deficiencies.** Identification of 14 novel mutations in the PSa gene of subjects with symptomatic protein S deficiency. *Thromb. Haemost.,* 69, 790, 1993.

76. **Hayashi T, Nishioka J, Shigekiyo T, Saito S, Suzuki K.** Protein S Tokushima: abnormal molecule with a substitution of Glu for Lys-155 in the second epidermal growth factor-like domain of protein S. *Blood,* 83, 683, 1994.

77. **Schmidel DK, Nelson RM, Broxson EH, Comp PC, Marlar RA, Long GL.** A 5,3 kb deletion including exon XIII of the protein Sa gene occurs in two protein S-deficient families. *Blood,* 77, 551, 1991.

78. **Ploos van Amstel HK, Huisman M., Reitsma PH, Ten Cate JW, Bertina RM,** Partial protein S gene deletion in a family with hereditary thrombophilia. *Blood,* 73, 479, 1989.

79. **Zöller B, Dahlbäck B.** "Linkage between inherited resistance to activated protein C and factor V gene mutation in venous trrombosis." *Lancet,* 343, 1536, 1994.

80. **Samama MM, Conard J., Horellou MH.,** Hereditary thrombophilia. *Haematology Trends'93,* ed. Lechner K.and.Gadner H. 1993, Vienna: Schattauer. 230.

81. **Bertina RM, van der Linden IK, Engesser L.,** Hereditary heparin cofactor II deficiency and the risk of development of thrombosis. *Thromb. Haemost.,* 57, 196, 1987.

82. **Briet E, van der Meer F., Rosendaal FR, Houwing-Duistermaat JJ, van Houwelingen HC.** The family history and inherited thrombophilia. *Br. J. Haematol.,* 87, 348, 1994.

83. **Tosetto A, Frezzato M., Rodeghiero F.** Family history and inherited thrombophilia. *Br. J. Haematol.,* 88, 227, 1994.

84. **Frezzato M, Tosetto A., Rodeghiero F.** Validation of a questionnaire for the diagnosis of previous thromboembolism. *Br. J. Haematol.,* 87, 79, 1994.

85. **Samama MM, Horellou MH, Soria J, Conard J, Nicolas G.,** Successful progressive anticoagulation in a severe protein C deficiency and previous skin necrosis at the initiation of oral anticoagulant treatment. *Thromb. Haemost.,* 51, 132, 1984.

86   **Pescatore, P., Horellou, M.H., Conard, J., Piffoux, M., van Dreden, P., Ruskone-Fourmestraux, A., Samama M.** Problems of oral anticoagulation in an adult with homozygous protein C deficiency and late onset of thrombosis. *Thromb. Haemost.,* 69, 311, 1993.

87. **Branson HE, Katz J, Marble R, Griffin JH,,** Inherited protein C deficiency and coumarin-responsive chronic relapsing purpura fulminans in a newborn infant. *Lancet,* 2, 1165, 1983.

88. **Friedman KD, Marlar RA, Houston JG, Montgomery RR.** Warfarin-induced skin necrosis in a patient with protein S deficiency. *Blood,* 68, 33A, 1986.

89. **Dettori AG, Quintavalla R., Manotti C, Pini P.** Warfarin-induced dermatitis and venous thrombosis in a patient with protein S deficiency. *Thromb. Haemost.,* 61, 1671, 1989.

90. **Grimaudo V, Gucissaz F, Hauert J, Sarraj A, Kruithof E, Bachmann F.** Necrosis of skin induced by coumarin in a patient deficient in protein S. *Br Med J,* 298, 233, 1989.

91. **Vukovich T, Auberger K, Weil J, Engelmann H, Knobl P, Hadorn HB.,** Replacement therapy for homozygous protein C deficiency-state using a concentrate of human protein C and S. *Br. J. Haematol.,* 70, 435, 1988.

92   **Conard, J., Bauer, K.A., Gruber, A., Griffin, J.H., Schwartz, H.P., Horellou, M.H., Samama, M.M., Rosenberg, R.D.** Normalization of markers of coagulation activation with a purified protein C concentrate in adults with homozygous protein C deficiency. *Blood,* 82, 1159, 1993.

93. **Marlar RA, Montgomery R, Madden RM,,** Homozygous protein C deficiency. *Protein C and related proteins,* ed. Bertina. RM. 1988, London: Churchill Livingstone. 182.

94. **Estelles A, Gracia-Plaza I, Dasi A.,** Severe inherited homozygous protein C deficiency in a newborn infant. *Thromb. Haemost.,* 52, 53, 1984.

95. **Marciniak E, Wilson.H, Marlar RA.** Neonatal purpura fulminans: a genetic disorder related to the absence of protein C in blood. *Blood,* 65, 15, 1985.

96. **Conard J, Bauer K, Gruber A, Griffin JH, Schwarz HP, Horellou MH, Samama MM, Rosenberg RD,,** Normalization of markers of coagulation activation with a purified protein C concentrate in adults with homozygous protein C deficiency,. *Blood,* 82, 1159, 1993.

97. **Dreyfus AM, Magny JF, Bridey F.** Treatment of homozygous protein C deficiency and neonatal purpura fulminans with a purified protein C concentrate, *N. Engl. J. Med.,* 325, 1565, 1991.

98. **Hirsh J, Martin H, Samama MM.,** Approach to the thrombophilic patient for hemostasis and thrombosis: basic principles and clinical practice. *Hemostasis and thrombosis basic principles and clinical practice,* ed. H.J. Colman RW Marder VJ, Salzman EW. 1993, Philadelphia: JB Lippincott Company.

99. **Broekmans AW, Conard J, van Weyenberg RG, Horellou MH, Kleift C, Bertina RM,** Treatment of hereditary protein C deficiency with stanazolol. *Thromb. Haemost.,* 57, 20, 1987.

100. **De Stefano V, Leone G, Mastrangelo S, Tripodi A, Rodeghiero F, Castaman G, Barbui T, Finazzi G, Bizzi B, Mannucci PM.** Clinical manifestations and management of inherited thrombophilia : retrospective analysis and follow up after diagnosis of 238 patients with congenital deficiency of antithrombin III, protein C, protein S. *Thromb. Haemost.,* 72, 352, 1994.

101. **Wahlberg TB, Kher A.** Low molecular weight heparin as thromboprophylaxis in pregnancy. A retrospective analysis from 14 european clinics. *Haemostasis,* 24, 55 (lett.), 1994.

102. **Forestier F, Daffos F, Capella-Pavlovsky M,,** Low molecular weight heparin (PK 10169) does not cross the placenta during the second trimester of pregnancy. Study by direct fetal blood sampling under ultrasound. *Thromb. Res.,* 34, 557, 1984.

103. **Bonnar J.** Management of venous thromboembolism in pregnancy and the puerperium. *Thrombosis and its management.,* ed. P.L.a.T. JM. 1993, Manchester: Churchill Livingstone. 47.

INHERITED RESISTANCE TO ACTIVATED PROTEIN C.
A Single Point Mutation in the Gene for Factor V as a Major Risk Factor for Venous Thrombosis

B. Dahlbäck

Clinical Chemistry, University of Lund, Malmö General Hospital

I. INTRODUCTION

In response to vascular injury, binding of factor VII to tissue factor initiates a cascade of reactions which leads to the formation of thrombin. Thrombin converts soluble fibrinogen to a fibrin network, activates platelets and stimulates coagulation by positive feed-back activation of factors V and VIII.[1-6] Within intact vessels, thrombin plays another role as initiator of the protein C anticoagulant system.[7-10] Thrombin binds to thrombomodulin (TM), a thrombin receptor which is present on the surface of intact endothelial cells. This leads to modulation of the functional properties of thrombin. Thrombin loses most of its procoagulant abilities and instead becomes a potent activator of protein C. Activated protein C (APC) inhibits coagulation by degrading the activated forms of factors V and VIII (Va and VIIIa). In contrast, the circulating, non activated forms of factors V and VIII are not affected by APC. The anticoagulant activity of APC is potentiated by two other plasma proteins, protein S and factor V. Protein S is a vitamin K-dependent plasma protein, which in human plasma circulates both as free protein (approximately 30%) and bound to the classical complement pathway regulatory protein C4b-binding protein (C4BP).[7,9,11-13] Binding of protein S to C4BP is associated with loss of its APC-cofactor activity.[14-16] The function of factor V as an anticoagulant cofactor in the protein C system was recently discovered.[17,18] Its mode of action is not yet fully understood but it appears to function in synergy with protein S . Thus, in a factor VIIIa degradation system, factor V stimulates the APC-cofactor activity of protein S and likewise protein S potentiates the anticoagulant effect of factor V.[17] Activation of factor V by thrombin is associated with loss of the APC-cofactor activity of factor V and gain of procoagulant activity because factor Va is a cofactor to factor Xa. This adds to the list of intriguing mechanisms which are involved in balancing pro- and anticoagulant forces. In vivo, APC is slowly neutralized by several proteinase inhibitors.[7,19-24] A long half-life of APC together with the highly specific proteolytic activity of APC provide the basis for the function of APC as a circulating anticoagulant.

Under physiological conditions, pro- and anticoagulant mechanisms are balanced in favour of anticoagulation. In contrast, at sites of vascular disruption, the anticoagulant system is down regulated and procoagulant forces prevail. This system maintains intravascular fluidity while it allows extravascular blood clotting to occur. Genetic or acquired molecular defects disturbing the delicate balance between pro- and anticoagulation may be associated with hypercoagulable states and increased risk of thrombosis.

II. RESISTANCE TO ACTIVATED PROTEIN C, A NOVEL MECHANISM FOR FAMILIAL THROMBOPHILIA

An observation made in our laboratory initiated the research that led to identification of inherited APC-resistance as a major cause of thrombosis. In a coagulation-assay based functional protein C assay, the dose-response of a sample from a thrombosis patient was found not to be parallel to that of the standard. At low dilution of the patient sample, the results of the analysis suggested the patient to have functional protein C deficiency, whereas normal values were obtained when the sample was tested at higher dilution. The plasma came from a middle-aged man who had experienced multiple episodes of deep venous thrombosis. Routine evaluation, including measurements of antithrombin III, protein C, protein S, plasminogen, and fibrinogen, was normal. Histories of recurrent venous thrombosis in several family members suggested the possibility of an inherited cause of the disease.[25]

The non-parallel dose-response curves in the functional protein C assay suggested that something in the patient plasma influenced the anticoagulant response to APC. To elucidate this in more detail, the APC-resistance test was developed. In this assay, the anticoagulant response to added APC is measured in an activated partial thromboplastine time (APTT) reaction. It was based on the idea that a poor response to APC could be a predisposing factor for thrombosis. We found the anticoagulant response to APC of the proband´s plasma was consistently found to be much smaller than that of control plasma (Figure 1). Several mechanisms could hypothetically explain a poor anticoagulant response to APC. They include the presence of autoantibodies against protein C, a lupus antibody inhibiting the APC function, a fast acting protease inhibitor to APC, functional protein S deficiency, mutations in the genes for factors VIII or V creating APC-resistant factors VIIIa or Va, and finally the involvement of previously unknown mechanisms or APC-cofactors.[25] An inherited defect was suggested by the observation that several of the family members were also APC-resistant. Although it was unlikely that inherited APC-resistance was due to an inhibitor of immunoglobulin type the proband´s plasma was again tested when depleted first of IgG, then IgA and finally IgM. Despite complete removal of respective immunoglobulin, the proband´s plasma still was APC-resistant. The possibility that APC-resistance was caused by another type of efficient APC-inhibitor was also excluded as APC was inhibited at a normal rate in the proband´s plasma.[25] The APC-resistance was not corrected by the addition of purified human protein S to the patients plasma, an observation which argued against the possibility of APC-resistance being caused by a functional protein S deficiency. Moreover, we now know that the APC-resistance test usually is normal in patients with protein S deficiency.[25,26]

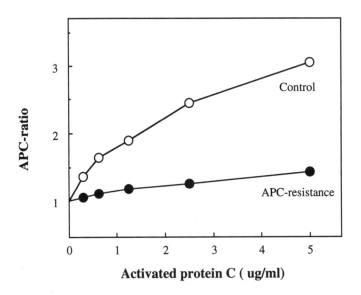

Figure 1 : APC-resistance in a patient with thrombosis. In the normal response, APC prolongs the activated partial thromboplastine time (APTT) (O). In contrast, plasma from a patient with recurrent thrombosis demonstrated APC-resistance (●). The APC-ratio is the APTT with APC divided by the APTT without APC. Modified from reference[25].

To further investigate the nature of APC-resistance, the anticoagulant response to APC was tested in clotting assays which were based on initiation of coagulation with factor IXa or factor Xa. In the factor Xa-based assay (sensitive to Va-degradation), the family members manifested significantly poorer anticoagulant response to APC than controls, although the difference was less pronounced than in the APTT-based assay. The factor IXa-based assay (sensitive to both Va- and VIIIa-degradation) was almost as efficient as the APTT-based assay in distinguishing APC-resistant family members from normal controls. The initial interpretation of these results was that a mutation in the factor V gene creating an APC-resistant factor Va was less likely. In retrospect it is obvious that this conclusion was premature because we now know that APC-resistance in a majority of cases indeed is caused by a mutation in the factor V gene which changes Arg506 in the APC-cleavage site to a Gln.[27-30] Corresponding mutation in the factor VIII gene (affecting Arg526), which is another possible cause of APC-resistance, was excluded after PCR-amplification and nucleotide sequencing of the factor VIII exons encoding the APC-cleavage sites.[25]

A. SINGLE POINT MUTATION IN THE FACTOR V GENE CAUSES APC-RESISTANCE

During efforts to elucidate the molecular nature of APC-resistance, we had made the observation that a protein fraction of normal plasma corrected the APC-resistance, whereas the corresponding fraction of plasma from an individual with severe APC-resistance was without effect. It was obvious that identification of this protein would lead to unravelling of the molecular cause of APC-resistance and we therefore decided to purify the protein. The protein, which corrected the APC-resistance in a dose-dependent manner, was isolated from normal plasma and to our surprise turned out to be identical to intact factor V.[18] This indicated APC-resistance to be caused by a genetic defect in the factor V gene. It also evoked the idea that factor V could function as an APC-cofactor (see above) and the initial working hypothesis was that APC-resistance was due to a defect in this novel anticoagulant activity. Other investigators also came to the conclusion that APC-resistance is caused by a molecular defect in the factor V gene.[27,31] They performed plasma mixing experiments and found APC-resistance to be corrected by all coagulation factor deficiency plasmas except that being deficient in factor V. Isolated factor V was then shown to correct the APC-resistance.[27] In addition, partially isolated factor V from an individual with heterozygous APC-resistance was found to transfer the APC-resistance phenotype.[31]

The concept that APC-resistance was caused by a factor V gene defect gained further support from linkage studies of two large families with inherited APC-resistance, one from The Netherlands and the other from Sweden (Figure 2).[27,29] The APC-resistance phenotype was found to be linked to a microsatellite marker located close to the factor V gene in one of the families, whereas in the other family, an intragenic polymorphism was perfectly linked to the phenotype. A G to A mutation in the factor V gene, at nucleotide position 1,691, was identified in the Dutch family and found to cosegregate with APC-resistance.[27] The mutation, which was subsequently found in the Swedish family[29], occurs in a CpG dinucleotide and predicts replacement of Arg506 in the APC cleavage site of factor Va with a Gln. Mutated factor Va is resistant to APC but expresses full procoagulant activity.[25,27,31] As a result, the prothrombinase complex is less sensitive to regulation by APC and this stabilization results in higher thrombin generation. The rate of activation of the coagulation cascade increases due to thrombin feed-back activation of factors VIII and V and concomitantly the factor V-dependent APC-cofactor activity is lost, which further potentiates the APC-resistance. Thus, the mutation of factor V indirectly leads to loss of APC-cofactor activity of factor V due to an imbalance between the pro- and anticoagulant properties of factor V (higher Va/V ratio). As a result, affected individuals have a life-long hypercoagulable state.

The mechanism by which purified factor V corrects APC-resistance is not yet understood. If mutated and normal factor V are activated equally well, addition of normal factor V may result in competitive inhibition of activation of mutated factor V. This could lead to correction of the APC-resistance because normal factor Va is degraded by APC. It may also be the result of increased APC-mediated degradation of factor VIIIa, because factor V is an APC-cofactor. If so, factor X activation will be inhibited and the activation rate of the coagulation cascade dampened. There are no data on record to support the third possibility of mutated factor Va being a competitive inhibitor to APC in degradation of factor VIIIa and normal factor Va.

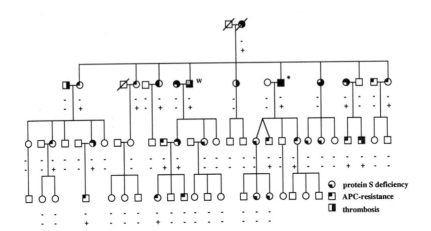

Figure 2 : Pedigree demonstrating linkage between APC-resistance and the Arg506 to Gln mutation in the factor V gene. This large kindred with thrombophilia was found to have independent inheritance of APC-resistance and protein S deficiency. The proband II:6 (indicated with an asterisk) had both defects and severe thromboembolism. Filled lower left quadrant denotes protein S deficiency and filled upper left quadrant APC-resistance. Filled right half of the symbol denote thrombosis. Individual II:4 was on oral anticoagulation (denoted with W) which made it difficult to diagnose APC-resistance. The + and - signs indicate presence or absence of the G to A mutation at nucleotide position 1691, changing Arg506 to Gln. Modified from reference[29]

B. APC-RESISTANCE IS A MAJOR CAUSE OF VENOUS THROMBOSIS

Thrombosis is often familial, demonstrating genetic factors to be involved in the pathogenesis. Before the discovery of APC-resistance and identification of the causative factor V gene mutation, well defined genetic defects were found in less than 10-15% of the patients. The most common genetic defects were deficiencies of protein C, protein S and antithrombin III, which together accounted for 5-10% of the thrombosis patients.[32-35] We studied a cohort of patients with thromboembolic disease (72 women and 32 men) to elucidate the prevalence of APC-resistance in this patient population.[26] The cohort was similar to a previously studied patient group in which the prevalence of other inherited deficiencies of anticoagulant proteins had been determined.[32] Histories of more than one thrombotic event were found in 31% of the patients and thrombotic events included deep venous thrombosis (n=83), pulmonary embolism (n=17) or thrombosis in cerebral vessels (n=4). Family histories of thrombosis were found in 45% of cases and in 60% predisposing factors for thrombosis were identified, the most common being pregnancy and the use of oral contraceptives. In the study population, no antithrombin III deficiency was identified, and none of the patients manifested signs of lupus anticoagulants. Two patients had protein C deficiency and another three had protein S deficiency. Patients on oral anticoagulation were excluded because APC-dependent prolongation of clotting time were excessive in individuals on oral anticoagulant therapy.

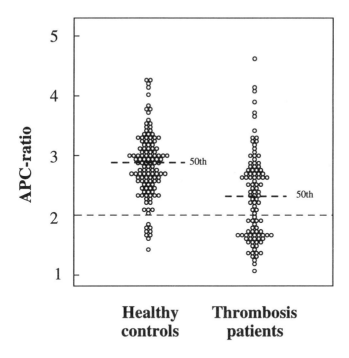

Figure 3 : APC-resistance in patients with thrombosis. APC-ratios of patients demonstrating a bimodal distribution, approximately 40% falling below the cut-off value of 2. In controls, corresponding value was 7%. Modified from reference [26].

In the patient cohort, the distribution of APC-ratios demonstrated a distinctly bimodal pattern (Figure 3). Also the control population showed a bimodal distribution but the number of individuals with low APC-ratios was smaller than in the patient group. With this kind of distribution of values in the control population it was not easy to determine the normal range. Using data from a large family study we came to the conclusion that an APC-ratio of <2.0 suggested inherited APC-resistance.[26] Recently, we have had the opportunity to test for the presence of the factor V gene mutation and found the cut-off of ≤2.0 to be appropriate. Individuals with APC-ratios below 2.0 usually have the factor V gene mutation, whereas most of those with APC-ratios above 2.0 are negative for the mutation. In this context it should be mentioned that the results of the APC-resistance test are affected by the choice of reagents as well as the instrumentation used.[26,36-38] We have recently started to use a commercially available kit for the APC-resistance test and in addition changed the instrumentation and under these conditions we find the cut-off value to be quite different from that obtained with our original method.[38] Combining results of the APC-resistance test and the factor V gene mutation analysis will help determine the cut-off value for different instruments.

Approximately 40% of the thrombosis patients had an APC-ratio of <2.0 and in patients with positive family history approximately 50% had APC-resistance. More than 95% of the APC-resistant cases carry the Arg506 to Gln mutation in the factor V gene.[39] In a control population, 7% demonstrated APC-resistance (APC-ratio ≤2.0) which suggests the factor V gene mutation to be rather common in the general population.[26] This is indeed the case and it was recently reported that approximately 3% of the Dutch population have APC-resistance due to the mutation.[27,37]

Family studies were initiated in 45 families in which the propositus had APC-resistance and thrombosis.[26] In 76% of the families, APC-resistance was found in at least one first degree relative. In total, 211 individuals (123 women and 88 men) were included and apart from the 34 propositi, 15 relatives from 13 families had had thrombosis. The APC-ratio was ≤2 in 45 of the 49 family members who had suffered from thrombosis. In approximately 45% of the relatives, an APC-ratio ≤2.0 was found, which was consistent with an autosomal dominant mode of inheritance. The probability of an APC-resistant individual in the families not to have suffered from thrombosis at the age of 45 was around 40%, whereas corresponding value for relatives without APC-resistance was 97% (Fig 4). Inclusion of the index cases into the analysis introduced a bias and the 34 index cases with APC-resistance were therefore excluded together with two protein S deficient cases with thrombosis among the non APC-resistant family members. Even after this exercise, the difference in survival curves was still significant (p=0.0015), suggesting individuals with APC-resistance to be at higher risk of thrombosis than those without the defect.[26] At the age of 50 years, 25% of relatives with APC-resistance had suffered a thrombotic event, which is higher than expected from population data and an estimated 5-10-fold increased thrombosis risk due to the APC-resistance. It would tend to suggest thrombosis-prone families with APC-resistance to be afflicted by more than one genetic defect, a concept which gained further support from more recent family studies.[39]

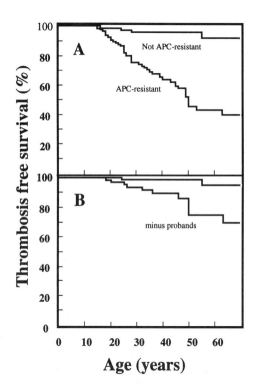

Figure 4 : Increased risk of thrombosis associated with inherited APC-resistance. A, Thrombosis-free survival curves of APC-resistant (n=104) and not APC-resistant (n=107) relatives. B, Thrombosis-free survival curves after exclusion of the 34 propositi from the group of APC-resistant individuals as well as 2 protein S-deficient individuals in the non-APC-resistant group. The difference in curves is highly significant in both A and B. Modified from reference [26].

The APC-resistance test is a satisfactory screening test and even though the APC-resistance test is not quantitative it is noteworthy that individuals with heterozygosity for the factor V gene mutation may have different severity of APC-resistance. This was particularly obvious in a recently performed study of 50 families with APC-resistance in which we obtained results to suggest that a combination of the APC-resistance test and the factor V gene mutation analysis is most useful in evaluation of the thrombosis risk.[39] It also appeared that several of the APC-resistant, thrombosis-protein families that we studied carried more than one genetic defect, which contributed both to a low APC-response and to the increased risk of thrombosis. In this respect, it is interesting to note that both families used for the linkage studies also had independent inheritance of yet another genetic defect; protein S deficiency in the Swedish family and protein C-deficiency in the Dutch.[27,29] Individuals having both genetic defects had more severe thrombotic disorder than those with a single defect.

Protein S did not influence the APC-resistance test to any significant degree and the plasma levels of protein S did not correlate with the APC-ratio. However, the factor V gene mutation has been found to influence available functional assays for protein S. Faioni and colleagues in re-evaluating nine families in which they had previously suspected functional protein S deficiency, came to the conclusion that these families did not suffer from functional protein S deficiency but rather from APC-resistance.[40]

Our conclusion that APC-resistance is the most prevalent cause of thrombosis yet identified has been confirmed by several other laboratories.[37,40-42] A 52-64% prevalence of APC-resistance was reported in patients with juvenile and/or recurrent venous thromboembolism unexplained by other causes.[42] Koster et al[37] found APC-resistance in 21% of unselected, consecutive thrombosis patients (n=301), whereas Faioni and colleagues[40] reported approximately 33% of their thrombosis patients to have APC-resistance. The differences in prevalence in the different studies are presumably due to different selection criteria. In the patient cohort (n=301) studied by Koster et al[37], the factor V gene mutation was found in heterozygous state in 47 of the APC-resistant individuals, in homozygous form in 6, and in approximately 3% of controls.[27] This suggests that heterozygosity for the factor V gene mutation is associated with a 5 to 10-fold increased thrombosis risk, whereas homozygosity gives an almost 90-fold increased risk. The Dutch study suggested a founder effect to be involved[27], but it is not known whether this applies for all different ethnic groups or if APC-resistance is the effect of different mutational events. The Arg506 to Gln mutation in the factor V gene is to my knowledge the most prevalent well defined genetic defect associated with disease so far described. The high prevalence indicates positive genetic selection pressure to have been involved in maintaining it in the population. A slight hypercoagulable state may have conferred an advantage in situations like traumatic injury and pregnancy during evolution. Moreover, it should be borne in mind that many of the circumstantial risk factors for thrombosis are products of modern life.

The Arg506 to Gln mutation inflicts a life-long risk of venous thrombosis and some preliminary reports suggest that APC-resistance may also be associated with arterial thrombosis.[41,43,44] However, unless the factor V gene mutation is associated with other genetic defects or circumstantial risk factors, thrombosis may not present until advanced age or not at all. The prevalence in Europe of the factor V gene mutation appears to be 3-5% and from this it follows that 0.2 to 0.6 per 1000 people is expected to be homozygous and the risk for thrombosis is quite high in these individuals.[27,39] Moreover, the factor V mutation may also be present in individuals with other single gene defects, e.g. protein C or protein S deficiency, and such combinations of genetic defects have increased risk of thrombosis.

The high prevalence of APC-resistance due to the factor V gene mutation raises the question whether it is worthwhile to screen for APC-resistance before surgery, during pregnancy and before the use of oral contraception. In this respect it is interesting to note that APC-resistant individuals had significantly shorter APT-times than individuals with high APC-response[26] and that a short APT-time has been found to be a significant risk factor for postoperative thrombosis.[45] The large number of APC-resistant cases that are going to be found in such screening procedures will evoke the question how to handle these individuals. I believe that demonstration of APC-resistance in a person calls for analysis of the factor V gene mutation. Heterozygous individuals without personal or family history of thrombosis, and with no other anticoagulant defect, should probably be given prophylactic anticoagulant therapy only in situations known to provoke thrombosis, e.g. major surgery. In the case they have already had thrombosis they should be treated like people with thrombosis associated with other anticoagulant protein deficiencies. Thus, at risk situations they should be given preventive anticoagulation therapy and if thrombosis is recurrent, anticoagulant medication for more extended time should be considered. Homozygous cases, and patients having two genetic defects should be given prophylactic anticoagulant therapy liberally at risk situations and extended anticoagulation therapy should probably be given after a thrombotic event.

REFERENCES

1. **Davie, E.W., Fujikawa, K. and Kisiel, W.** The coagulation cascade: Initiation, maintainance, and regulation, *Biochemistry*, 30, 10363, 1991.
2. **Furie, B. and Furie, B.C.** The molecular basis of blood coagulation, *Cell*, 53, 505, 1988.
3. **Edgington, T.S., Mackman, N., Brand, K. and Ruf, W.** The structural biology of expression and function of tissue factor, *Thromb.Haemost.*, 66, 67, 1991.
4. **Nemerson, Y.** The tissue factor pathway of coagulation, *Semin.Hematol.*, 29, 170, 1992.
5. **Jenny, R.J., Tracy, P.B. and Mann, K.G.** The physiology and biochemistry of factor V, In *Haemostasis and Thrombosis*, 3rd Ed. Bloom, A.L., Forbes, C.D., Thomas, D.P. and Tuddenham, E.G.D. Eds. Churchill Livingstone, 1994, 465.
6. **Kane, W.H. and Davie, E.W.** Blood coagulation factors V and VIII: Structural and functional similarities and their relationship to hemorrhagic and thrombotic disorders, *Blood*, 71, 539, 1988.
7. **Dahlbäck, B. and Stenflo, J.** The protein C anticoagulant system, In, *The molecular basis of blood diseases*, Stamatoyannopoulos, G., Nienhuis, A.W., Majerus, P.W. and Varmus, H. Eds. W.B. Saunders, Philadelphia, 1994, 599.
8. **Esmon, C.T.** Cell mediated events that control blood coagulation and vascular injury, *Annu.Rev.Cell.Biol.*, 9, 1, 1993.
9. **Esmon, C.T.** Molecular events that control the protein C anticoagulant pathway, *Thromb.Haemost.*, 70, 29, 1993.
10. **Dittman, W.A. and Majerus, P.W.** Structure and function of thrombomodulin: A natural anticoagulant, *Blood*, 75, 329, 1990.
11. **Esmon, C.T.** The Protein C Anticoagulant Pathway, *Arterioscler.Thromb.*, 12, 135, 1992.
12. **Dahlbäck, B.** Protein S and C4b-binding protein: Components involved in the regulation of the protein C anticoagulant system, *Thromb.Haemost.*, 66, 49, 1991.
13. **Dahlbäck, B. and Stenflo, J.** High molecular weight complex in human plasma between vitamin K-dependent protein S and complement component C4b-binding protein, *Proc.Natl.Acad.Sci.USA*, 78, 2512, 1981.
14. **Dahlbäck, B.** Inhibition of protein C_a cofactor function of human and bovine protein S by C4b-binding protein, *J.Biol.Chem.*, 261, 12022, 1986.
15. **Bertina, R.M., van Wijngaarden, A., Reinalda-Poot, J., Poort, S.R. and Bom, V.J.** Determination of plasma protein S - the protein cofactor of activated protein C, *Thromb.Haemost.*, 53, 268, 1985.
16. **Comp, P.C. and Esmon, C.T.** Recurrent thromboembolism in patients with a partial deficiency of protein S, *N.Engl.J.Med.*, 311, 1525, 1984.
17. **Shen, L. and Dahlbäck, B.** Factor V and protein S as synergistic cofactors to activated protein C in degradation of factor VIIIa, *J.Biol.Chem.*, 269, 18735, 1994.
18. **Dahlbäck, B. and Hildebrand, B.** Inherited resistance to activated protein C is corrected by anticoagulant cofactor activity found to be a property of factor V, *Proc.Natl.Acad.Sci.USA*, 81, 1396, 1994.
19. **Marlar, R.A., Kressin, D.C. and Madden, R.M.** Contribution of plasma proteinase inhibitors to the regulation of activated protein C in plasma, *Thromb.Haemost.*, 69, 16, 1993.
20. **van der Meer, F.J., van Tilburg, N., van Wijngaarden, A., Van Der Linden, I.K., Briët, E. and Bertina, R.M.** A second plasma inhibitor of activated protein C: α_1-antitrypsin, *Thromb.Haemost.*, 62, 756, 1989.
21. **Heeb, M.J. and Griffin, J.H.** Physiological inhibition of human activated protein C by alpha-1-antitrypsin, *J. Biol. Chem.*, 263, 11613, 1988.
22. **Heeb, M.J., Espana, F. and Griffin, J.H.** Inhibition and complexation of activated protein C by two major inhibitors in plasma, *Blood*, 78, 2283, 1988.
23. **Hoogendoorn, H., Toh, C.H., Nesheim, M.E. and Giles, A.R.** α_2-macroglobulin binds and inhibits activated protein C, *Blood*, 78, 2283, 1991.
24. **Heeb, M.J., Gruber, A. and Griffin, J.H.** Identification of different metal ion-dependent inhibition of activated protein C by alpha 2-macroglobulin and alpha 2-antiplasmin in blood and comparisons by inhibition of factor Xa, thrombin and plasmin, *J.Biol.Chem.*, 266, 17606, 1991.
25. **Dahlbäck, B., Carlsson, M. and Svensson, P.J.** Familial thrombophilia due to a previously unrecognized mechanism characterized by poor anticoagulant response to activated protein C: Prediction of a cofactor to activated protein C, *Proc.Natl.Acad.Sci.USA*, 90, 1004, 1993.
26. **Svensson, P.J. and Dahlbäck, B.** Resistance to activated protein C as a basis for venous thrombosis, *N. Engl. J. Med.*, 330, 517, 1994.
27. **Bertina, R.M., Koeleman, B.P.C., Koster, T., Rosendaal, F.R., Dirven, R.J., de Ronde, H., van der Velden, P.A. and Reitsma, P.H.** Mutation in blood coagulation factor V associated with resistance to activated protein C, *Nature*, 369, 64, 1994.
28. **Greengard, J.S., Sun, X., Xu, X., Fernandez, J.A., Griffin, J.H. and Evatt, B.** Activated protein C resistance caused by Arg506Gln mutation in factor Va, *Lancet*, 343, 1362, 1994.
29. **Zöller, B. and Dahlbäck, B.** Linkage between inherited resistance to activated protein C and factor V gene mutation in venous thrombosis, *Lancet*, 343, 1536, 1994.
30. **Voorberg, J., Roelse, J., Koopman, R., Büller, H., Berends, F., ten Cate, J.W., Mertens, K. and van Mourik, J.A.** Association of idiopathic thromboembolism with single point mutation at Arg506 of factor V, *Lancet*, 343, 1535, 1994.
31. **Sun, X., Evatt, B. and Griffin, J.H.** Blood coagulation factor Va abnormality associated with resistance to activated protein C in venous thrombophilia, *Blood*, 83, 3120, 1994.
32. **Malm, J., Laurell, M., Nilsson, I.M. and Dahlbäck, B.** Thromboembolic disease - critical evaluation of laboratory investigation, *Thromb.Haemost.*, 68, 7, 1992.
33. **Tabernero, M.D., Tomas, J.F., Alberca, I., Orfao, A., Borrasca, A.L. and Vicente, V.** Incidence and clinical characteristics of hereditary disorders associated with venous thrombosis, *Am.J.Hematol.*, 36, 249, 1991.
34. **Gladson, C.L., Scharrer, I., Hach, V., Beck, K.H. and Griffin, J.H.** The frequency of type I heterozygous protein S and protein C deficiency in 141 unrelated young patients with venous thrombosis, *Thromb.Haemost.*, 59, 18, 1988.
35. **Heijboer, H., Brandjes, D., Büller, H.R., Sturk, A. and ten Cate, J.W.** Deficiencies of coagulation-inhibiting and fibrinolytic proteins in outpatients with deep-vein thrombosis, *N. Engl. J. Med.*, 323, 1512, 1990.
36. **Koster, T. and Rosendaal, F.R.** Activated protein C resistance in venous thrombosis, *Lancet*, 343, 541, 1994.
37. **Koster, T., Rosendaal, F.R., de Ronde, F., Briët, E., Vandenbroucke, J.P. and Bertina, R.M.** Venous thrombosis

due to poor response to activated protein C: Leiden thrombophilia study, *Lancet*, 342, 1503, 1993.

38.   **Rosén, S., Johansson, K., Lindberg, K. and Dahlbäck, B**. Multicenter evaluation of a kit for activated protein C resistance on various coagulation instruments using plasmas from healthy individuals, *Thromb.Haemost.*, 72, 255, 1994.

39.   **Zöller, B., Svensson, P.J., He, X. and Dahlbäck, B.** Identification of the same factor V gene mutation in 47 out of 50 thrombosis-prone families with inherited resistance to activated protein C, *J.Clin.Invest.*, 94, 2521, 1994.

40.   **Faioni, E.M., Franchi, F., Asti, D., Sacchi, E., Bernardi, F. and Mannucci, P.M.** Resistance to activated protein C in nine thrombophilic families: Interference in a protein S functional assay, *Thromb.Haemost.*, 70, 1067, 1993.

41.   **Halbmayer, W.M., Haushofer, A., Schön, R. and Fischer, M.** The prevalence of poor anticoagulant response to activated protein C (APC resistance) among patients suffering from stroke or venous thrombosis and among healthy subjects, *Blood.Coagul.Fibrinol.*, 5, 51, 1994.

42.   **Griffin, J.H., Evatt, B., Wideman, C. and Fernandez, J.A**. Anticoagulant protein C pathway defective in a majority of thrombophilic patients, *Blood*, 82, 1989, 1993.

43.   **Lindblad, B., Svensson, P.J. and Dahlbäck, B.** Arterial and venous thromboembolism with fatal outcome in a young man with inherited resistance to activated protein C, *Lancet*, 343, 917, 1994.

44.   **Holm, J., Zöller, B., Svensson, P.J., Berntorp,E., Erhardt,L., and Dahlbäck, B**. Myocardial infarction in two young women associated with homozygous resistance to activated protein C. *Lancet*, 344, 952,1994.

45.   **Gallus, A.S., Gent, M. and Hirsh, J.** Relevance of preoperative and postoperative blood tests to postoperative leg-vein thrombosis, *Lancet*, ii, 805, 1973.

HEPARIN COFACTOR II

P. Sié

Laboratoire d'Hématologie, Université Paul-Sabatier, Toulouse

The anticoagulant activities of glycosaminoglycans are partly mediated by two plasma proteins: antithrombin III (AT) and heparin cofactor II (HCII). HCII shares similarities with AT and other members of the SERin Protease Inhibitors (SERPIN) superfamily. HCII and AT both inhibit thrombin by forming covalent 1:1 molar complexes with it. The rate of complex formation is greatly accelerated by low concentrations of heparin in purified systems.[1,2] Unlike AT, HCII does not inhibit the other proteases of the coagulation cascade. HCII is not readily activated by heparin at pharmacological concentrations in plasma and therefore plays a limited role, if any, in the antithrombotic effect of heparin.[3] HCII is preferentially activated by dermatan sulfate (DS) rather than heparan sulfate.[4] As DS-containing proteoglycans are abundant in subendothelial vascular tissues and in extravascular spaces, it has been suggested that HCII helps control thrombin activity on the injured vessel wall and in the interstitial fluids.[5,6]

The importance of AT as a naturally occurring antithrombotic is well established, but the physiological significance of HCII remains unknown. Two observations suggest that HCII plays a physiological role. First, it is highly conserved among species and seems to have been perserved through evolution.[7] Second, although heterozygous moderate HCII deficiency is relatively frequent in asymptomatic people (see below), severe homozygous deficiency has not been reported, indicating that the latter may be incompatible with life. This chapter will examine the possible role of plasma HCII in the prevention of vascular thrombosis and consequently the risk factor associated with HCII deficiency.

Determination of functional levels of HCII in citrated or EDTA plasma is measured by its ability to inhibit human thrombin in the presence of DS.[8-13] To reduce the interference of AT present in the test plasma, because it could react with traces of heparin in commercial preparations of DS, the test plasma is treated with anti human AT antiserum or immunoabsorbed on an anti-AT Sepharose column. Alternatively, the DS is treated with $NaNO_2$/acetic acid, or polybrene is added to the buffers to neutralize heparin. The concentration of HCII antigen is measured by immunoelectrophoresis using a monospecific antiserum, which may be produced in house or commercially purchased.

The normal range in a "healthy" adult population is relatively wide. The distribution of values is assumed to be normal around 1 U/mL and the lower limit (m - 2SD) is usually around 0.6 U/mL. The largest study, performed in 379 subjects selected randomly from a blood donor population in Norway,[12] describes a gradual increase of HCII activity with age between 20 and 60 years, but no significant differences between men and women. HCII levels do not vary during pregnancy,[14] Similar changes in HCII-antigen were found by the Leiden group.[15] HCII activity increases slightly (by about 0.2 U/mL) during early acute deep venous thrombosis (DVT), suggesting that HCII behaves as an acute phase reactant.[16] This hypothesis however is questionable, since in healthy volunteers HCII levels are not correlated with those of another acute phase reactant, orosomucoïd.[15] To avoid misinterpretation of results, the measurement of HCII levels in patients with thrombosis should preferably be performed some weeks after the acute episode. Neither heparin nor oral anticoagulants influence HCII levels.[17]

Low levels of HCII are found in various clinical conditions: liver failure, disseminated intravascular coagulation and severe pre-eclampsia are the most common[8-11,18-20] since the protein is synthesized by the hepatocytes and forms inhibitory complexes with thrombin. Unlike AT, plasma HCII is not decreased in patients with nephrotic syndrome.[21,22] HCII levels are reduced in patients with chronic renal failure undergoing regular hemodialysis. [23] This is presumably due to the accumulation of a DS proteoglycan in the plasma of these patients[24]. HCII levels may be significantly reduced during the acute phase of pancreatitis due, at least in part, to the formation of serpin-enzyme complexes with pancreatic proteinases.[25] Finally, HCII levels are frequently reduced in patients infected with the human immunodeficiency virus.[26] It does not appear that acquired HCII deficiencies in any of the above conditions are related to a thrombotic tendency.

Inherited HCII deficiency associated with thrombosis was first described simultaneously in 1985 by Sie *et al*[27] and Tran *et al.*[28] Several groups have since reported additional cases. The hereditary nature of the condition has been suspected by family study in some instances ; usually it has been suspected on the basis of persistently low levels of HCII in an individual, in the absence of any known cause of acquired deficiency.

The prevalence of suspected HCII deficiency in patients with previous DVT or pulmonary embolism is shown in Table I. The average HCII is about 1.06%. Using comparable laboratory criteria, the prevalence of the deficiency in the general, healthy population is close to 1.5% (10 subjects out of 649 without history of thrombosis), compiled from ref 12,15,19 and 29.

Table I : Prevalence of Suspected Inherited HCII Deficiency (Quantitative Type) in Patients with a history of DVT

References	N of Patients with Thrombosis	N of Patients with HCII deficiency
10	105	0
11	31	0
15	277	3
18	74	0
19	274	6
27	74	1
29	264	4
30	233	1
31	70	0
Total	1402	15 (1.07%)

Seven families with hereditary HCII deficiencies have been reported in detail [15,27,28,32,33]. Five probands had DVT (first episode between the ages of 18 and 47 years), and one each had cerebrovascular disease, spontaneous abortion and suspected but non-confirmed calf vein thrombosis. Among 17 relatives with HCII deficiency, 14 were asymptomatic, one had DVT during pregnancy and one after knee surgery. One had a transient ischemic attack at the age of 66 years.

A qualitative deficiency in HCII has been reported in two related asymptomatic blood donors who had about 50% of normal HCII activity determined by functional assay, and a double peak demonstrated by crossed immunoelectrophoresis in the presence of DS.[31] This pattern suggested the presence of approximately equal amounts of normal HCII and of a variant form, unable to bind DS. The variant from one family, called HCII Oslo was studied further.[34] A single point mutation was found, namely substitution of His for Arg in position 189. It is interesting that Arg 189 can be aligned with Arg 129 in

AT, which is also known to be important for the interaction of AT with heparin.[35] The same mutation has been reported in two other families.[36-37] Of the 10 individuals heterozygous for HCII Oslo, only 2 have a history of DVT. A similar functional deficiency, defined by a low activity and normal antigen value but not characterized further, has been described in two other unrelated patients with a history of previous thrombosis[38] and in several members of a large kindred.[39] In this family both types of HCII deficiency (qualitative and quantitative) were found and some individuals also had additional defects in protein C, S or AT.

Combined inherited deficiencies of HCII and other clotting proteins have been described: Protein S-HCII deficiency in 3 families,[15,39,40] Protein C-HCII deficiency and a triple deficiency AT-HCII-Protein C or S in one family.[40,41] In these families, the defects segregated separately. Three of 7 members of these 3 families experienced a thrombotic episode at a young age, but the majority of the deficient individuals who remain asymptomatic are still under 40 years old. Whether HCII deficiency combined with deficiency in other antithrombotic proteins increases thrombotic risk is not determined.

There are several case reports of patients with hereditary HCII deficiency associated with arterial thrombosis[42], of which the first was published by Tran *et al.*[28] Vinazzer *et al*[19] found 19 cases of HCII deficiency, 10 of them confirmed by family study, among a group of 557 patients with arterial obstruction (3.4%). Unfortunately the description of these patients was poor. Although this proportion is low and the finding should be confirmed prospectively, the possibility that HCII deficiency is an additional risk factor for arterial thrombosis cannot be ruled out.

Finally, although this short review deals primarily with the relationship between HCII deficiency and hypercoagulable states, the occurrence of spontaneous abortions in affected females with HCII deficiency should be mentioned.[33-36] As it is unlikely that such a history will come to the attention of most authors, its association with HCII deficiency may be underestimated. This deserves attention in the future, in view of the possible importance of the HCII-DS proteoglycan system during pregnancy.[41]

To sum up:

1) Available data do not indicate that a moderate heterozygous HCII deficiency either quantitative or qualitative, is in itself a risk factor for venous thrombosis. Laboratory screening of HCII deficiency is not mandatory in symptomatic patients. Should HCII deficiency be recognized in such patients, it would not require special management..

2) A higher prevalence of low HCII levels in patients with arterial thrombosis compared with healthy subjects has been reported by one group. This remains to be confirmed.

3) It is possible, under certain conditions such as combined with a defect in another regulatory protein, e.g. protein C, S, AT or aPC resistance), that HCII deficiency is an additional risk factor for thrombosis. It will, however, be difficult to prove or disprove this hypothesis since these combinations are probably very rare.

REFERENCES

Tollefsen, D.M. and Blank, M.K., Detection of a new heparin-dependent inhibitor of thrombin in human plasma, *J. Clin. Invest.,* 68, 589,1981.

Tollefsen, D.M., Majerus D.W. and Blank M.K., Heparin cofactor II. Purification and properties of a heparin-dependent inhibitor of thrombin in human plasma, *J. Biol. Chem.,* 257, 2162,1982.

Sie, P., Ofosu, F., Fernandez, F., Buchanan, M.R., Petitou, M. and Boneu B., Respective role of antithrombin III and heparin cofactor II in the in vitro anticoagulant effect of heparin and of various sulphated polysaccharides, *Br. J. Haematol.,* 64, 707,1986.

Tollefsen, D.M., Pestka, C.A. and Monafo, W.J., Activation of heparin cofactor II by dermatan sulfate, *J. Biol. Chem,* 258, 6713,1983.

McGuire, E.A. and Tollefsen, D.M., Activation of heparin cofactor II by fibroblasts and vascular smooth muscle cells, *J. Biol. Chem.,* 262, 169, 1987 .

Pasche, B., Swedenborg, J., Frebelius, S. and Olsson, P., Heparin cofactor II significance for the inhibition of thrombin at the injured vessel wall, *Thromb. Res.,* 62, 409,1991.

Sheffield, W.P., Schuyler, P.D. and Blajchman, M.A., Molecular cloning and expression of rabbit heparin cofactor II: a plasma thrombin inhibitor highly conserved between species, *Thromb. Haemost.,* 71, 778, 1994.

Tran, T.H. and Duckert, F., Heparin cofactor II determination. Levels in normals and patients with hereditary antithrombin III deficiency and disseminated intravascular coagulation, *Thromb. Haemost.,* 52, 112, 1 984.

9.   **Abildgaard, U. and Larsen, M.L.,** Assay of dermatan sulfate cofactor (heparin cofactor II) activity in human plasma, *Thromb. Res.,* 35, 257, 1984.

10. **Tollefsen, D.M. and Pestka, C.A.,** Heparin cofactor II activity in patients with disseminated intravascular coagulation and hepatic failure, *Blood,* 66, 769, 1985.

11. **Ezenagu, L.C. and Brandt, J.T.,** Laboratory determination of heparin cofactor II, *Arch. Pathol . Lab. Med.,* 110, 1149, 1986.

12. **Andersson, T.R., Larsen, M.L., Handeland, G.F. and Abildgaard, U.,** Heparin cofactor II activity in plasma: application of an automated assay method to the study of a normal adult population, *Scand. J. Haematol.,* 36, 96, 1986.

13. **Nakhleh, E., Vogt, J.M. and Edson, J.R.,** Heparin cofactor II assay. Elimination of heparin and antithrombin III effects, *Am. J. Clin. Pathol.,* 89, 353, 1988.

14. **Sandset, P.M., Hellgren, M., Uvebrandt, M. and Bergstrom, H.,** Extrinsic coagulation pathway inhibitor and heparin cofactor II during normal and hypertensive pregnancy, *Thromb. Res.,* 55, 665,1989.

15. **Bertina, R.M., van der Linden, I.K., Engesser, L., Muller, H.P. and Brommer, E.J.P.,** Hereditary heparin cofactor II deficiency and the risk of development of thrombosis, *Thromb. Haemost.,* 57,196,1987.

16. **Toulon, P., Vitoux, J.F., Fiessinger, J.N., Sicard, D. and Aiach,** M., Heparin cofactor II: an acute phase reactant in patients with deep vein thrombosis, *Blood Coag. Fibrinol.,* 2, 435,1991.

17. **Toulon, P., Vitoux, J.F., Capron, L., Roncato, M., Fiessinger, J.N. and Aiach,** M., Heparin cofactor II in patients with deep venous thrombosis under heparin and oral anticoagulant therapy, *Thromb. Res.,* 49, 497, 1 988.

18. **Chuansumrit, A., Manco-Johnson, M.J. and Hathaway, W.E.,** Heparin cofactor II in adults and infants with thrombosis and DIC, *Am. J. Hematol.,* 31,109, 1989.

19. **Vinazzer, H. and Stocker, K.,** Heparin cofactor II: experimental approach to a new assay and clinical results, *Thromb. Res.,* 61, 235,1991.

20. **Langley, P.G. and Williams, R.,** Physiological inhibitors of coagulation in fulminant hepatic failure, *Blood Coag. Fibrinol.,* 3, 243,1992.

21. **Grau, E., Oliver, A., Felez, J., Barcelo, P., Fernandez, C., Ballarin, J.A., Fontcuberta, J. and Rutllant, M.L.,** Plasma and urinary heparin cofactor II levels in patients with nephrotic syndrome. *Thromb. Haemost.,* 60, 137, 1988.

22. **Sié, P., Meguira, B., Bouissou, F., Boneu, B. and Barthe, Ph.,** Plasma levels of heparin cofactor II in nephrotic syndrome of children, *Nephron,* 48, 175, 1988.

23. **Toulon, P., Jacquot, C., Capron, L., Frydman, M.O., Vignon, D. and Aiach, M.,** Antithrombin III and heparin cofactor II in patients with chronic renal failure undergoing regular hemodialysis, *Thromb. Haemost.,* 57, 263, 1987.

24. **Delorme, M.A., Saeed, N., Sevcik, A., Mitchell, L., Berry, L., Johnston, M. and Andrew, M.,** Plasma dermatan sulfate proteoglycan in a patient on chronic hemodialysis, *Blood,* 82, 3380,1993.

25. **Toulon, P., Chadeuf, G., Bouillot, J.L., Amiral, J., Cambillau, M., Sultan, Y. and Aiach, M.,** Involvement of heparin cofactor II in chymotrypsin neutralization and in the pancreatic proteinase-antiproteinase interaction during pancreatitis in man, *Eur. J. Clin. Invest.,* 21, 303, 1991 .

26. **Toulon, P., Lamine, M., Ledjev, 1., Guez T., Holleman, M.E., Sereni, D. and Sicard, D.,** Heparin cofactor II deficiency in patients infected with the human immunodeficiency virus, *Thromb. Haemost.,* 70, 730, 1993.

27. **Sié, P., Dupouy, D., Pichon, J. and Boneu,** B. Constitutional heparin cofactor II deficiency associated with recurrent thrombosis, *Lancet,* ii, 414, 1 985.

28. **Tran, T.H., Marbet, G.A. and Duckert, F.,** Association of hereditary heparin co-factor II deficiency with thrombosis, *Lancet,* ii, 413, 1985.

29. **Toulon, P., Vitoux, J.F., Fiessinger, J.N. and Aiach, M.,** Heparin cofactor II deficiency: a risk factor for thrombophilia in *Angiologie,* ed., Boccalon, H., John Libbey Eurotext, Eds, Paris, 1988, 475.

30. **Conard, J., Horellou, M.H. and Samama, M.,** Incidence of thromboembolism in association with congenital disorders i coagulation and fibrinolysis, *Acta. Chir. Scand.,* suppl 543, 15, 1988.

31. **Andersson, T.R., Larsen, M.L. and Abildgaard, U.,** Low heparin cofactor II associated with abnormal crosse immunoelectrophoresis pattern in two Norwegian families, *Thromb. Res.,* 47, 243,1987.

32. **Weisdorf, D.J. and Edson, J.R.,** Recurrent venous thrombosis associated with inherited deficiency of heparin cofactor II, *Br. J. Haematol.,* 77, 125, 1991.

33. **Simioni, P., Lazzaro, A.R., Coser, E., Salmistraro, G. and Girolami, A.,** Hereditary heparin cofactor II deficiency an thrombosis: report of six patients belonging to two separate kindreds, *Blood Coag. Fibrinol.,* 1, 351, 1990.

34. **Blinder, M.A., Andersson, T.R., Abildgaard, U. and Tollefsen, D.M.,** Heparin Cofactor II Oslo. Mutation of ARG-18 to His decreases the affinity for dermatan sulfate, *J. Biol. Chem.,* 264, 5128,1989.

35. **Gandrille, S., Aiach, M., Lane, D.A., Vidaud, D., Molho-Sabatier, P., Caso, R., de Moerloose, P., Fiessinger, J.N. ar Clauser, E.,** Important role of arginine 129 in heparin-binding site of antithrombin III. Identification of a novel mutatic arginine 129 to glutamine, *J. Biol. Chem.,* 265,18997, 1990.

36. **Borg, J.Y., Perry, D., Vasse, M. and Carrell, R.W.,** Molecular characterization (ARG 189 -> His) of a hereditary cofactor II (HCII) variant with low affinity for heparin and dermatan sulfate (DS), *Thromb. Haemostas.,* 65, 785,1991.

37. **Toulon, P., Gandrille, S., Mathiot, C. and Aiach, M.,** Hereditary heparin cofactor II (HCII Toulouse), *Nouv. Rev. F Hematol.,* 31, 292, 1989 (abstract).

38. **Marbet, G.A., Zbinden, B. and Duckert, F.,** Konstitutionelle dysfunktion von heparin-kofaktor II mit venos thromboseneigung, *Schweiz. Med. Wschr.,* 118, 1586, 1988.

39. **Jobin, F., Vu, L. and Lessard, M.,** Two cases of inherited triple deficiency in a large kindred with thrombotic diathes and deficiencies of antithrombin III, heparin cofactor II, proteinC and protein S, *Thromb. Haemost.,* 66, 295, 1991.

40. **Simioni, P., Zanardi, S., Prandoni, P. and Girolami, A.,** Combined inherited protein S and heparin co-factor deficiency in a patient with upper limb thrombosis: a family study, *Thromb. Res.,* 67, 23, 1992.

41. **Jobin, F., Vu, L. and Bigonesse, J.M.,** Follow-up: A young man with three deficiencies of antithrombotic protein asymptomatic unitl now, spontaneously develops pulmonary embolism, *Thromb. Haemost.,* 67, 730, 1992.

42. **Matsuo, T., Kario, K., Sakamoto, S., Yamada, T., Miki, T., Hirase, T. and Kobayashi, H.,** Hereditary heparin cofact II deficiency and coronary artery disease, *Thromb. Res.,* 65, 495, 1992.

43. **Andrew, M., Mitchell, L., Berry, L., Paes, B., Delorme, M., Ofosu, F., Burrows, R. and Khambalia, B.,** / anticoagulant dermatan sulfate proteoglycan circulates in the pregnant woman and her fetus, *J. Clin. Invest.,* 89, 3. 1992.

HEREDITARY DYSFIBRINOGENEMIA, AFIBRINOGENEMIA, HYPOFIBRINOGENEMIA AND THROMBOSIS

M.M. Samama*, F. Haverkate**
* Service d'Hématologie Biologique - Hôtel-Dieu - Paris
** Gaubius Laboratory, TNO - Leiden

I - HEREDITARY DYSFIBRINOGENEMIA

Familial dysfibrinogenemia has been reported in over 250 cases[1]. Approximately 20% are presented with thrombophilic dysfibrinogenemia,[1] 25% with (mild) bleeding,[2] and 55% is asymptomatic [2]. The prevalence of dysfibrinogenemia in patients with a history of venous thrombosis is low i.e. 0.8%.[1]

It is not easy to establish an association between familial dysfibrinogenemia and thrombophilia due to the small number of families (only 5) with sufficient relatives to establish a convincing association. Moreover, in contrast to the cases with a bleeding tendency, there is no clear rationale for an association between an impaired clotting function of fibrinogen and the occurrence of thrombotic episodes.

A recent study[1] shows that an association between dysfibrinogenemia and thrombophilia is indicated by studies on relatives of 26 probands (Table I), who fulfilled arbitrary criteria for familial dysfibrinogenemia and for thrombophilia. Analysis of 187 investigated family members revealed that thrombophilia affected 20 persons exclusively in the group of 99 relatives with dysfibrinogenemia while no thrombosis was reported in the group of 88 relatives without the defect. Convincing evidence for such an association became apparent for only five individual probands of whom at least 2 relatives had both the defect and thrombotic episodes at a young age i.e. Caracas V, Frankfurt IV / Vlissingen, Melun, Naples and Paris V.[1]

The 26 probands in Table I with thrombophilic dysfibrinogenemia had the following characteristics[1] :
- homozygosity was established by DNA analysis in two cases (Marburg and Naples);
- the mean age of the first episode of thrombosis was approximately 30 years;
- venous thrombosis highly predominates over arterial thrombosis;
- severe bleeding is rare and limited to bleeding post-partum in only 2 cases (Bethesda III and Marburg);
- hypodysfibrinogenemia (< 1.50 mg/ml) was reported in 5 cases with thrombophilia i.e. Bethesda III, Fuenlabrada, Malmö, Marburg and New York I;
- a high incidence of pregnancy related problems was observed, amongst the 15 women with thrombophilic dysfibrinogenemia, in particular thrombosis post-partum and spontaneous abortions.

At present, the molecular defect of the abnormal thrombophilic fibrinogens has been elucidated mostly by DNA sequencing in 16 cases. Why a particular defect leads to malfunction of fibrin(ogen) is still unknown. However, it is intriguing that most of the defects found are localized in the C-terminal parts of the Aα- and γ-chain, and in the N-terminal part of the Bß-chain (figure 1).

493-5804-3/96/$0.00+$.50
1996 by CRC Press

One would expect that the same molecular defect in different probands is associated with the same disease, in this connection with the risk of thrombosis. This is not easy to check as the number of probands with equal molecular defects is limited. Moreover, patients reported as asymptomatic may reveal the first episode of thrombosis at a later stage. The data available show :

- The Aα 16 Arg→Cys mutation is associated with thrombophilia in Frankfurt V (Table I) and with mild bleeding in Homburg III [2], Ledyard [2], and Metz[2].
- The Aα 554 Arg→Cys mutation causes thrombophilia in Chapel Hill III and Paris V (Dusart) (Table I).
- The Bß 14 Arg→Cys mutation is associated with thrombosis in IJmuiden (Table I), with mild bleeding (epistaxis) in Christchurch II[2], and is asymptomatic in Seattle I[2].
- The γ 275 Arg→His mutation causes thrombophilia in Bergamo I and Haifa (Table I), and is asymptomatic in Essen,[2] Perugia,[2] and Saga.[2]
- The γ 275 Arg→Cys mutation is associated with thrombophilia in Bologna (Table I), and is asymptomatic in 5 other probands. [2]

FIBRINOGEN MOLECULE (half)

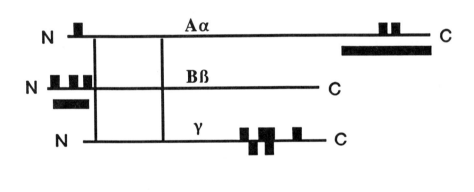

Figure 1 : Vertical lines represent disulphide bridges. N = N-terminalsite ; C = C-terminal site of the amino acid chains. Mutation are point mutations, fibrinogen Frankfurt IV/Vlissingen has a deletion of 2 amino acids (γ 319 + 320) which is represented as a bar

These data show that one and the same mutation i.e. the Aα 16 Arg→Cys, or the Bß 14 Arg→Cys can be associated with thrombophilia in one proband and with mild bleeding in the other. It can, however, not be excluded that the mild bleeding is caused by other mechanisms than dysfibrinogenemia.

Table I. Cases of congenital dysfibrinogenemia
associated with thrombophilia according to arbitrary criteria (1).

Name (country)	Sex	Thromb.*	Localization defect**	Ref.
Baltimore I (USA)	F	VEN (1)	γ 292 Gly→Val	21
Bergamo II (Italy)	F	VEN	γ 275 Arg→His	22
Bethesda III (USA)	F	VEN (1)		23
Bicêtre II (F)	M	VEN (1)	γ 308 Asn→Lys	24
"Bologna" (Italy)	F	VEN	γ 275 Arg→Cys	-
Caracas V (Ven)	F	VEN/ART	Aα 532 Ser→Cys	10
Chapel Hill III (USA)	M	VEN	Aα 554 Arg→Cys	14
Charlottesville (USA)	F	VEN		25
Copenhagen I (DK)	F	ART		26
Frankfurt IV (FRG)	M	ART		-
Vlissingen (NL)	F	VEN (1)	γ 319/320 del	27
Frankfurt V (FRG)	M	VEN	Aα 16 Arg→Cys	-
"Fuenlabrada" (Esp)	M	VEN		-
"Giessen IV" (FRG)	F	VEN	γ 318 Asp→Gly	-
Haifa (Israel)	F	ART	γ 275 Arg→His	28
IJmuiden (NL)	M	VEN/ART	Bß 14 Arg→Cys	18
Irvine (USA)	M	VEN		29
Malmö (S)	F	VEN		6
Mannheim II (FRG)	M	ART		30
Marburg (FRG)	F	VEN	Aα 461 Lys→Stop	31
"Melun" (F)	F	VEN	γ 364 Asp→Val	31a
Nancy (F)	M	VEN		32
Naples (Italy)	M	VEN (1)	Bß 68 Ala→Thr	12
New Orleans II (USA)	F	VEN		33
New York I (USA)	F	VEN	Bß 9-72 del	13
Pamplona II (Esp)	F	VEN (1)		9
Paris V (F) (Dusart)	M	VEN	Aα 554 Arg→Cys	19

*Thrombosis (1) = one episode of thrombosis; others multiple episodes.
**11 of the 16 defects mentioned were elucidated during the study period by J. Koopman, J. Grimbergen and F. Haverkate, Gaubius Laboratory TNO-PG, Leiden, NL, in cooperation with Dr. P. Reitsma, Academic Hospital, Leiden, NL.

An association between thrombosis and dysfibrinogenemia is not easy to explain, except for Oslo I. This abnormal fibrinogen is the only case known, not with a prolonged but a shortened thrombin time[3]. Moreover, it has a more efficient action on ADP induced platelet aggregation.[4] Both observations could explain the thrombophilia. Unfortunately this defect was found in only one single member of a large family[4]. All other abnormal fibrinogens in Table I were discovered by a prolonged thrombin clotting time which seems contradictory to the risk of thrombosis. Besides an abnormal platelet function, two other possible mechanisms may explain thrombosis on the basis of malfunctions of the fibrin part of the abnormal fibrinogens. The first one, suggested by Liu et al.[5] , may be a defective binding of thrombin to the abnormal fibrin leading to an excess of thrombin in the circulation which may stimulate processes such as platelet aggregation. Indeed, defective thrombin to fibrin binding has been established for Malmö[6], Naples[7], New York I[8] and Pamplona II[9] and mentioned for Caracas V[10]. Also Poitiers[11] not fulfilling the criteria of the Working Party, had a decreased thrombin binding. Naples and Pamplona II showed a normal clotting by reptilase, indicating a normal binding to fibrin of this snake venom enzyme. A defective interaction between thrombin and fibrin(ogen)s Naples and New York I causes a delayed release of fibrinopeptides A and B by the action of the enzyme. In these two abnormal fibrinogens the molecular defect was localised in the Bß-chain of fibrinogen at amino acid Bß 68 (Ala→Thr)[12] and Bß 9-72 (deletion)[13] , respectively, showing a defective binding of thrombin to the anion-binding exosite, a site in fibrin independent of the catalytic site [5].

An alternative proposed mechanism to explain thrombosis is a decreased lysis of abnormal fibrin. Resistance against lysis of fibrin by plasmin was reported for Argenteuil[11], Chapel Hill III[14], and Pamplona II[9]. A defective role of fibrin in stimulating the activation of plasminogen by tissue plasminogen activator (t-PA) was more specifically explained by a defective binding of t-PA to fibrin Date[15], New York I[8] and Nijmegen[16], or by a defective binding of plasminogen (Paris V or Dusart[17]). Molecular defects elucidated so far reveal that abnormal t-PA binding is associated with defects at the N-terminal site of the fibrin ß-chain, i.e. a deletion of Bß 9-72 for New York I[13] and a mutation Bß Arg 44→Cys for Nijmegen[18]. Defective binding of plasminogen (Paris V) is associated with a defect at the C-terminal end of the Aα-chain (554, Arg→Cys)[19]. Both Paris V and Fibrinogen Chapel Hill III with the same defect show abnormally thin fibrin fibers and resistance to fibrinolysis[14].

The t-PA mediated stimulation of fibrinolysis has been reported to be associated with the fibrinogen regions Aα 148-160 and γ 311-379[20]. Although the defects in the fibrinogens Vlissingen, Giessen IV and Melun are localized in the γ-chain between amino acids 311 and 379, an abnormal binding of t-PA or plasminogen to the corresponding abnormal fibrins has not been demonstrated.

II - SEVERE HYPOFIBRINOGENEMIA AND AFIBRINOGENEMIA

In 1964, two independent reports were published in France by Caen et al. [34] and by one of the authors of this paper, Marchal et al [35]. In these two cases acute arterial thrombosis of the limbs with ischemic necrosis of the toes in the former case and amputation of a limb in the later one were considered to be related to hereditary fibrinogen alteration.

In 1966 a case of severe hypofibrinogenemia associated with fatal pulmonary embolism was described by Ingram et al [36] and a patient with hypofibrinogenemia associated with massive thrombosis was reported [37].

In these patients a possible congenital dysfibrinogenemia rather than severe hypofibrinogenemia was not ruled out.

More recently, we are aware of five other cases of such an association in two french patients[38,39], one originated from Alger[40] and two from North America[41,42]. In these patients dysfibrinogenemia was ruled out and the five patients were well documented as having afibrinogenemia.

These anecdotal reports are very puzzling since they demonstrate at least that massive venous thrombosis and severe arterial thrombosis can occur in patients with an extremely low plasma fibrinogen level since only traces of fibrinogen can be detected in their plasma, with sensitive immunologic methods. Another patient with arterial thrombosis, and afibrinogenemia associated with protein C deficiency has been reported [43]. In three cases [36,41,42] thrombosis occurred as a complication of fibrinogen concentrate infusion but in the other patients thrombosis was observed independently of substitutive therapy.

The mechanism of this paradoxical association is unknown. Two hypotheses have been suggested : one is related to the existence of platelet hyperaggregation probably mediated by von Willebrand factor[38]. The second one which seems very interesting relies on the observation that thrombin generation in an afibrinogenemic or in a hypofibrinogenemic plasma is increased[40] since the excess of thrombin formed during coagulation is normally adsorbed by fibrin. As reported very recently in a study[44] the forming clot withdraws thrombin from solution and in the absence of fibrin the lag time before thrombin generation is reduced and the amount of thrombin formed is increased.

In conclusion, the association of afibrinogenemia or severe hypofibrinogenemia and thrombosis is very intriguing. The very rare cases reported in the literature demonstrate that thrombosis may occur in patients with an extremely low fibrinogen plasma level and that infusion of fibrinogen concentrates may be hazardous in these patients. A causal relationship between fibrinogen alteration and thrombosis is suspected but its mechanism remains obscure.

Predisposition to thrombosis in patients with hereditary dysfibrinogenemia is also very rare and is limited to few families, with sufficient siblings establish a convincing evidence. At this stage, the link between some cases of dysfibrinogenemia and thrombosis remain to be fully established.

REFERENCES

1.   **Haverkate F, Samama M.** Familial dysfibrinogenemia and thrombophilia. Report on a study of the SSC Subcommittee on Fibrinogen. *Thromb Haemost* 1995; 73: 151.
2.   **Ebert R.** Index of variant human fibrinogens. *CRC*, Boca Raton, Ann Arbor, Boston, USA, 1991.
3.   **Egeberg O.** Inherited fibrinogen abnormality causing thrombophilia. *Thromb Diath Haemorrh* 1967; 17: 176.
4.   **Thorsen LI, Brosstad F, Solum NO, Storkorken H.** Increased binding to ADP-stimulated platelets and aggregation effect of the dysfibrinogen Oslo I as compared with normal fibrinogen. *Scand J Haematol* 1986; 36: 203.
5.   **Liu CY, Nossel HL, Kaplan KL.** The binding of thrombin by fibrin. *J Biol Chem* 1979; 254: 10421.
6.   **Soria J, Soria C, Hedner U, Nilsson IM, Bergquist D, Samama M.** Episodes of increased fibronectin level observed in a patient suffering from recurrent thrombosis related to congenital hypodysfibrinogenemia (fibrinogen Malmoe). *Brit J Haematol* 1985; 61: 727.
7.   **Haverkate F, Koopman J, Kluft C, d'Angelo A, Cattaneo M, Mannucci PM.** Fibrinogen Milano II: a congenital dysfibrinogenemia associated with juvenile arterial and venous thrombosis. *Thromb Haemost* 1986; 55: 131.
8.   **Liu CY, Wallén P, Handley DA.** Fibrinogen New York I: the structural, functional and genetic defects and an hypothesis of the role of fibrin in the regulation of coagulation and fibrinolysis. In: *Fibrinogen, Fibrin Formation and Fibrinolysis.* Lane DA, Henschen A, Jasani MK (Eds). Walter de Gruyter, Berlin, New York 1986; 4: 79.
9.   **Fernandez J, Paramo JA, Cuesta B, Aranda A, Rocha E.** Fibrinogen Pamplona II. A new congenital dysfibrinogenemia with abnormal fibrin-enhanced plasminogen activation and defective binding of thrombin to fibrin: In: *Fibrinogen and its Derivatives. Biochemistry, Physiology and Pathophysiology.* Müller-Berghaus G, Scheefers-Borchel U, Selmayr E, Henschen A (Eds). Excerpta Medica, Elsevier Science Publishers, Amsterdam, New York, Boston 1986; 25.
10.   **Arocha Piñango CL, Torres A, Marchi R, Rodriguez S, Camarillo H, Muller-Soyano A, Bosch NB.** A new thrombotic dysfibrinogenemia present in several members of a Venezuelan family. *Thromb Haemost* 1987; 58: 149 (Abstr 541).
11.   **Gandrille S, Priollet P, Capron L, Roncato M, Fiessinger JN, Aiach M.** Association of inherited dysfibrinogenemia and protein C deficiency in two unrelated families. *Brit J Haematol* 1988; 68: 329.
12.   **Koopman J, Haverkate F, Lord ST, Grimbergen J, Mannucci PM.** Molecular basis of fibrinogen Naples associated with defective thrombin binding and thrombophilia. Homozygous substitution of Bß 68 Ala→Thr. *J Clin Invest* 1992; 90: 238.
13.   **Liu CY, Koehn JA, Morgan FJ.** Characterization of fibrinogen New York I. A dysfunctional fibrinogen with a deletion of Bß (9-72) corresponding exactly to exon 2 of the gene. *J Biol Chem* 1985; 260: 4390.
14.   **Wada Y, Lord ST.** A correlation between thrombotic disease and a specific fibrinogen abnormality (Aα 554 Arg→Cys) in two unrelated kindred Dusart and Chapel Hill III. *Blood* 1994; 84: 3709.
15.   **Ieko M, Sawada KI, Sakurama S, Yamagishi I, Isogawa S, Nakagawa S, Satoh M, Yasukouchi T, Matsuda M.** Fibrinogen Date: congenital hypodysfibrinogenemia associated with decreased binding of tissue-plasminogen activator. *Am J Haematol* 1991; 37: 228.
16.   **Engesser L, Koopman J, De Munk G, Haverkate F, Nováková I, Verheijen JH, Briët E, Brommer EJP.** Fibrinogen Nijmegen: Congenital dysfibrinogenemia associated with impaired t-PA mediated plasminogen activation and decreased binding of t-PA. *Thromb Haemost* 1988; 60: 113.
17.   **Lijnen HR, Soria J, Soria C, Collen D, Caen JP.** Dysfibrinogenemia (fibrinogen Dusard) associated with impaired fibrin-enhanced plasminogen activation. *Thromb Haemost* 1984; 51: 108.
18.   **Koopman J, Haverkate F, Grimbergen J, Engesser L, Nováková I, Kerst AFJA, Lord ST.** Abnormal fibrinogens IJmuiden (Bß Arg 14→Cys) and Nijmegen (Bß Arg_{44}→Cys) form disulfide-linked fibrinogen-albumin complexes. *Proc Natl Acad Sci USA* 1992; 89: 3478.
19.   **Koopman J, Haverkate F, Grimbergen J, Lord ST, Mosesson MW, DiOrio JP, Siebenlist KS, Legrand C, Soria J, Soria C, Caen JP.** The molecular basis for fibrinogen Dusart (Aα 554 Arg --> Cys) and its association with abnormal fibrin polymerization and thrombophilia. *J Clin Invest* 1993; 91: 1637.
20.   **Yonekawa O, Voskuilen M, Nieuwenhuizen W.** Localization in the fibrinogen γ-chain of a new site that is involved in the acceleration of the tissue-type plasminogen activator-catalysed activation of plasminogen. *Biochem J* 1992; 283: 187.
21.   **Bantia S, Mane SM, Bell WR, Dang CV.** Fibrinogen Baltimore I: polymerization defect associated with a γ 292 Gly→Val (GGC→GTC) mutation. *Blood* 1990; 76: 2279.
22.   **Reber P, Furlan M, Henschen A, Kaudewitz H, Barbui T, Hilgard P, Nenci GG, Berrettini M, Beck EA.** Three abnormal fibrinogen variants with the same amino acid substitution (γ 275 Arg→His): Fibrinogens Bergamo II, Essen and Perugia. *Thromb Haemost* 1986; 56: 401.
23.   **Gralnick HR, Coller BS, Fratantoni JC, Martinez J.** Fibrinogen Bethesda III: a hypodysfibrinogenemia. *Blood* 1979; 53: 28.
24.   **Grailhe P, Boyer-Neumann C, Haverkate F, Grimbergen J, Larrieu MJ, Anglés-Cano E.** The mutation in Fibrinogen Bicêtre II (γ Asn 308→Lys) does not affect the binding of t-PA and plasminogen to fibrin. *Blood Coag Fibrinol* 1993; 4: 679.
25.   **Laugen RH, Bithell TC.** Hereditary dysfibrinogenemia characterized by slow fibrinopeptide release and competitive inhibition of thrombin. *Acta Haematol (Basel)* 1984; 71: 150.
26.   **Sandbjerg Hansen M, Clemmensen I, Winther D.** Fibrinogen Copenhagen; an abnormal fibrinogen with defective polymerization and release of fibrinopeptide A, but normal adsorption of plasminogen. *Scand J Clin Lab Invest* 1980; 40: 221.
27.   **Koopman J, Haverkate F, Briët E, Lord ST.** A congenitally abnormal fibrinogen (Vlissingen) with a 6-base deletion in the γ-chain gene, causing defective calcium binding and impaired fibrin polymerization. *J Biol Chem* 1991; 266: 13456.
28.   **Siebenlist KR, Mosesson MW, DiOrio JP, Tavori S, Tatarsky I, Rimon A.** The polymerization of fibrin prepared from fibrinogen Haifa (γ_{275} Arg --> His). *Thromb Haemost* 1989; 62: 875.
29.   **Lehmer RR, Elias AN, Capdeville MJ, Brown DR, Branson HE.** Fibrinogen Irvine: a qualitatively abnormal fibrinogen associated with the predisposition to recurrent visceral and peripheral venous thrombosis. *J Natl Med Ass* 1985; 78: 561.

30.   **Dempfle CE, Kirschstein W, Watzlawick H, Brossmer R, Simianer S, Harenberg J, Heene DL.** Hypodysfibrinogenemia with impaired fibrin polymerization associated with excessive postpartum bleeding: Fibrinogen Mannheim II. *Thromb Haemost* 1989; 62: 159 (Abstr 473).

31.   **Koopman J, Haverkate F, Grimbergen J, Egbring R, Lord ST.** Fibrinogen Marburg: a homozygous case of dysfibrinogenemia, lacking amino acids Aa 461-610 (Lys 461 AAA→Stop TAA). *Blood* 1992; 80: 1972.

31a.   **Bentolila S, Samama MM, Conard J, Horellou MH, Ffrench P** : Association dysfibrinogénémie et thrombose. A propos d'une famille (fibrinogène Melun). *Ann Med Intern.* in press.

32.   **Streiff F, Alexandre P, Vigneron C, Soria J, Soria C, Mester L.** Un nouveau cas d'anomalie constitutionnelle et familiale du fibrinogène sans diathese hémorragique. *Thromb Diath Haemorrh* 1971; 26: 565.

33.   **Andes WA.** Fibrinogen New Orleans II: a new dysfibrinogenemia with venous thrombosis. *Thromb Haemost* 1983; 50: 337 (Abstr 1060).

34.   **Caen J, Faur Y, Inceman S, Chassigneux J, Seligmann M, Anagnostopoulos T, Bernard J.** Nécrose ischémique bilatérale dans un cas de grande hypofibrinogénémie congénitale. *Nouv Rev Fr Hématol* 1964; 4: 321

35.   **Marchal G, Duhamel G, Samama M, Flandrin G.** Thrombose massive des vaisseaux d'un membre au cours d'une hypofibrinémie congénitale. *Hémostase* 1964; 4: 81.

36.   **Ingram DIC, McBrien DJ, Spencer H.** Fatal pulmonary embolus in congenital fibrinopenia : Report of two cases. *Acta Haematol.* 1966, 35: 56.

37.   **Nilsson IM, Niléhn JE, Cronberg S, Nordén G.** Hypofibrinogenaemia and massive thrombosis. *Acta Med Scand* 1966; 180: 65.

38.   **Molho-Sabatier P, Soria C, Legrand CH, Belluci S, Dupuy E, Laurian C, Tobelem G.** Fibrinogen-independent platelet aggregation responsible of arterial thrombosis in an afibrinogenemic patient. *Thromb Haemost* 1991; 65: 850

39.   **Drai E, Taillan B, Schneider S, ferrari E, Bayle J, Dujardin P.** Thrombose portale révélatrice d'une afibrinogénémie congénitale. *Presse Med* 1992; 21: 1820-1821.

40.   **Fischer AM.** Personal Communication.

41.   **Cronin C, Fitzpatrick D, Temperley I.** Multiple pulmonary emboli in a patient with afibrinogenemia. *Acta Haematol* 1988; 79: 53.

42.   **MacKinnon HH, Fekete JF.** Congenital afibrinogenemia vascular changes and multiple thromboses induced by fibrinogen infusions and contraceptive medication. *Can Med Assoc J* 1971; 140: 597.

43.   **Hanano M, Takahashi H, Itoh M, Shibata A.** Coexistence of congenital fibrinopenia and protein C deficiency in a patient. *Am J Hematol* 1992; 41: 57.

44.   **Kumar R, Béguin S, Hemker HC.** The influence of fibrinogen and fibrin on thrombin generation - evidence for feedback activation of the clotting system by clot bound thrombin. *Thromb Haemost* 1994; 72 (5): 713.

PLASMA FIBRIN GEL ARCHITECTURE
AND THROMBOTIC DISORDER

J.P. Collet*,**, J. Soria**, M. Mirshahi**, Z. Mishal***,
M. Vasse*, J.P. Caen**** and C. Soria*.
* Diféma, Faculté de Médecine et de Pharmacie, Rouen
** Laboratoire Sainte-Marie, Hôtel-Dieu, Paris
*** Laboratoire de Cytométrie, CNRS, Villejuif
**** IVS, Hôpital Lariboisière, Paris

I. INTRODUCTION

High levels of fibrinogen in blood have been associated independently with increased risk for development of ischemic heart disease and stroke by numerous epidemiological studies.[1,2] However there is no rational explanation despite the fact that fibrinogen is involved in various pathophysiological processes such as blood coagulation, blood rheology and platelet aggregation. Presently, there is no evidence whether fibrinogen might be considered as a simple marker or a real cause of vascular lesions. The common feature of arterial and venous thromboembolic disease is the presence of occlusive events mostly due to the presence of fibrin clot, whose properties should be important to consider. It has been hypothesized that abnormal plasma fibrin gel network architecture could be associated with thrombotic disorders (arterial or venous) when developed *in vivo*. This may explain the thrombogenicity of fibrinogen.[3]

II. CHARACTERISTICS OF FIBRIN GEL NETWORK ARCHITECTURE

A. FIBRINOGEN ACTIVATION AND FIBRIN FORMATION

Fibrinogen, a dimeric molecule with a molecular mass of 340 kDa, consists of three pairs of polypeptide chains Aα, Bβ and γ linked together by symmetrical disulfide bonds. The molecule has two fold axis of symmetry. Fibrin monomer, produced by cleavage of the pairs of A and B fibrinopeptides from fibrinogen by the serine protease enzyme thrombin, aggregates to yield two stranded protofibrils and then a network of fibers.

After removal of fibrinopeptide A from the N terminal end of the Aα chain, the polymerization site «A» interacts with a complementary site, «a», located in the C terminal part of another fibrin(ogen) molecule. Then the molecules aggregate in a half staggered fashion to form linear polymers (called protofibrils) which are stabilized by covalent bonds induced by the action of factor XIIIa. These structures grow up in different directions creating nuclei of growth and form the fibrin gel with hydrated fibers and branch points.[4] Removal of fibrinopeptide B from the N-terminal part of the Bβ chain increases the reactivity of the molecules (additional calcium binding and conformational changes) and induces interaction between a second set of polymerization sites. The delay of fibrinopeptide B cleavage appears to be necessary for both normal protofibril and fiber assembly in an ordered fashion.[5] The timing of the different steps of fibrin gel formation has a great influence on the final architecture of the gel. This has crucial consequences on the susceptibility of fibrin to fibrinolytic drugs.

B. FACTORS INFLUENCING FIBRIN GEL ARCHITECTURE

It has been shown by Blombäck et al. that the structure of the fibrin gel is mainly determined by kinetic factors, ie the clotting potential (thrombin concentration) and the fibrinogen concentration under otherwise constant conditions (ionic strength, calcium concentration).[3] Increasing thrombin concentration and/or fibrinogen concentration leads to the formation of a tight structure with thin and short fiber strands, numerous branch points and small pores. On the contrary, a decrease of the clotting potential or fibrinogen concentration favours formation of coarse structure with thick and long fiber strands, large pores and fewer branch points. The former structure is rigid and less permeable to the flow than coarse ones which are plastic and easily give way to flow. Many other factors may influence the fibrin architecture, especially in the plasma milieu. Plasma proteins such as albumin and fibronectin, but also calcium ions, favour formation of coarse structure. On the other hand, lipoproteins lead to the formation of tight gels.

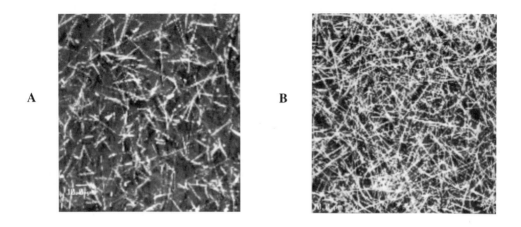

A   B

Figure 1 : 3D reconstruction of fibrin gel networks obtained by confocal microscopy from normal plasma. Plasmas were recalcified (20 mMol $CaCl_2$) and clotted with thrombin at 0.1 (A) and 1 (B) IU/mL respectively. Gels were labeled with FITC (Fluorescein isothiocyanate).

C. FIBRIN ARCHITECTURE AND THROMBOLYSIS

Fibrin gel architecture is important because the rate of fibrinolysis can be altered by changes in slow flow pattern through the clot resulting in a decreased aviability of fibrinolytic enzymes in the fibrin network. Moreover, the fibrin structure contributes to the regulation of the fibrinolyic rate as reported by Don Gabriel.[6] Thin fiber strands have a lower rate of conversion of plasminogen to plasmin by t-PA and are lysed more slowly by plasmin than thick fibers. This could be accounted for by decrease of plasminogen binding which is in contrast to t-PA highly dependent on the fibrin structure. It decreased as fibrinogen and fibrin I concentration increased in the clot, and plasmin interaction with these gels is similarly inhibited as a consequence.[7]

III. FIBRIN GEL ARCHITECTURE IN THROMBOTIC DISORDERS

The correlation that exists between fibrin structure and fibrin lysis on one hand and the presence of occlusive events in thrombotic processes on the other hand prompt us to support the concept that altered fibrin gel architecture rather than small increases of fibrinogen level in blood is more important in vascular disease.

A. VENOUS THROMBOEMBOLIC DISEASE

The major role of fibrin architecture in venous thrombosis process has been well illustrated with the Dusart syndrome (fibrinogen Paris V) described by Soria and Caen in 1983.[8] It was related to a dysfibrinogenemia with an abnormal fibrin polymerization (translucent clot) due to defective lateral aggregation of fibrin polymers. The molecular defect is a substitution of cysteine for arginine at position 554 in the Aα chain with binding of albumin. This abnormal fibrinogen was responsible for a severe thrombotic disorder with a high incidence of pulmonary embolism. It was first attributed to defective clot thrombolysis with reduced binding of plasminogen to fibrin and defective plasminogen activation by tissue plasminogen activator. The architecture of fibrin Dusart is highly abnormal with a less ordered structure made up of thin and short fibers which are highly branched and numerous displaying small pores. Pharmacological modulation of clot structure using dextran prior to clotting restored both the fibrin architecture and fibrinolysis to normal. This shows that both thrombolysis resistance and abnormal rigidity of the fibrin Dusart are related to the abnormal architecture, which reduces access of fibrinolytic enzymes to the fibrin and then breaks up the brittle clot resulting in a high incidence of pulmonary embolism.[9]

Other abnormal fibrinogen molecules associated with defective gelling and thrombotic disorder have been reported, eg fibrinogens Chapel Hill III,[10] Tampere and Laconia[3] although the mechanism accounting for formation of tight gel networks may be different.

B. ARTERIAL DISEASE

Elevated plasma fibrinogen level is associated with arterial disease (ischemic heart disease, stroke and peripheral arterial disease) but a causal relationship is unclear. Fibrinogen is a component of atherosclerotic lesions at every stage of evolution. The fibrin-degradation product stimulates smooth muscle cell proliferation and migration. The question arises whether this elevation is a cause or a consequence of the vascular lesions or their thrombotic complications ?

Fibrinogen genotyping may be a useful investigation to better understand the role of fibrinogen in vascular disease. Variations at the fibrinogen β locus (which controls the formation of the Bβ chain, the rate limiting step in fibrinogen synthesis) have been shown to be linked with an increased risk of peripheral atherosclerosis.[11] This significant influence of the fibrinogen genotype was clearly independent from the plasma fibrinogen level (haplotype had a small effect on it). The authors assume that haplotype may influence some structural variants of fibrinogen which could account for the development of peripheral arterial disease. These former variants could be responsible for alteration of fibrin architecture.

This is supported by Blombäck et al. who have found alteration of fibrin gel architecture in patients suffering from a first myocardial infarction before the age of 45 years.[12] These patients had abnormal fibrin gel with decreased porosity and heterogeneity of fiber size. The author suggests that it might be important in the formation of coronary lesions in man. Modifications of the fibrin gel structure toward tight gels were not entirely explained by variation in plasma fibrinogen concentration.

Platelets should be taken into account in arterial thrombogenesis. There is substantial evidence for their involvement in fibrin matrix stabilization, rendering it less sensitive to degradation by fibrinolysis.[13] Several mechanisms may explain this resistance, especially fibrin clot architecture modifications. First, platelet secretion product modifies fibrin formation toward tight conformation.[14] This is important *in vivo* because platelet activation occurs just before or during fibrin polymerization Second, platelets bind to fibrin through specific interactions mediated by the membrane receptor GPIIb/IIIa promoting clot retraction. This effect may have significant contribution for fibrin resistance to thrombolysis despite unclear molecular mechanisms.[15]

IV. CONCLUSION

Modification of fibrin clot architecture toward tight gels may be part of the pathogenesis of vascular disease and may explain the role of fibrinogen in their development. Furthermore, this may have therapeutic implications. It remains important to study the effect of lowering fibrinogen concentration on fibrin gel properties and the evolution of vascular lesions.

REFERENCES

1.   **Meade TW, Mellows S, Brozovic M, Miller GJ, Chakrabati RR, North WRS, Haines AP, Stirling Y, Imeson JD, Thomson SG,** Haemostatic function and ischemic heart disease: Principal results of the Northwick Park heart study. *Lancet II*, 533, 1986.
2.   **Kannel WB, Woll PA, Castelli WP, D'agostino RB**. Fibrinogen and risk of cardiovascular disease. *JAMA,* 258, 1183, 1987.
3.   **Blombäck B, Barnerjee D, Carlsson K, Hamsted A, Hessel B, Zarchaski L.** Native fibrin gel networks and factors influencing their formation in health and disease, in Liu CY, Chien S (Eds): *Fibrinogen, Thrombosis, Coagulation and Fibrinolysis*. New-York, NY, Plenum, 1992,1.
4.   **Blombäck B,** Fibrinogen structure, activation, polymerization and fibrin gel structure. *Thromb. Res.* 75, 327, 1994.
5.   **Weisel JW, Veklich Y, Gorkun O,** The sequence of cleavage of fibrinopeptides from fibrinogen is important for protofibril formation and enhancement of lateral agregation in fibrin clots. *J Mol Biol,* 232, 285, 1993.
6.   **Don A Gabriel, Muga K, Boothroyd EM**. The effect of fibrin structure on fibrinolysis. *J Biol Chem,* 267, 34, 24259,1992.
7.   **Mc Donagh,** Suppression of plasminogen binding to fibrin by high fibrinogen: A mechanism for how fibrinogen enhances the risk of thrombosis. *Thrombosis.* Sanofi Association for Thrombosis Research 1994, 4, 1, I.
8.   **Soria J, Soria C, Caen JP**. A new type of congenital dysfibrinogenemia with defective fibrin lysis: Dusart syndrome, a possible relation to thrombosis. *Br J Haematol,,* 53, 575, 1983.
9.   **Collet JP, Soria J, Mirshahi Mc, Hirsh M, Dagonnet FB, Caen J, Soria C**. Dusart syndrome: a new concept of the relationship between fibrin clot architecture and fibrin clot degradability: Hypofibrinolysis related to an abnormal clot structure. *Blood*, 82, 8, 1993.
10.   **Carrell N., Don A Gabriel , Blatt PM, Carr ME, Mc Donagh J,** Hereditary dysfibrinogenemia in a patient with thrombotic disease. *Blood* 62, 439, 1983.
11.   **Fowkes FGR, Connor JM, Smith FB, Wood J, Donnan EM, Lowe GDU.** Fibrinogen genotype and risk of peripheral atherosclerosis. *Lancet*, 339, 693, 1992.
12.   **Fatah K, Hamsten A, Blombäck B, Blombäck M.** Fibrin gel network characteristics and coronary heart disease: relations to plasma fibrinogen concentration, acute phase protein, serum lipoproteins and coronary heart disease. *Thromb Haemost*, 68, 130, 1992.
13.   **ISIS-2 (Second International Study of Infarct Survival) Collaborative Group,** Randomized trial of intravenous streptokinase, oral aspirin, both or neither among 17,187 cases of suspected acute myocardial infarction: ISIS 2. *J Am Coll Cardiol* , 12, 3A, 1988.
14.   **Dhall TZ, Shah GA, Fergusson IA, Dhall DP,** Fibrin network structure: modification by platelets. *Thromb Haemost,* 49, 42, 1983.
15.   **Sabovic M, Lijnen HR, Keber D, Collen D,** Effect of clot retraction on the lysis of human clots with fibrin specific and non specific plasminogen activators.*Thromb Haemost*, 62, 1083, 1989 .

PLASMINOGEN ALTERATION

T. Koyama and N. Aoki

The First Department of Internal Medicine, Tokyo Medical and Dental University

I. ABNORMAL PLASMINOGEN

A.CLINICAL ASPECTS

1. Clinical manifestations

In 1978, a Japanese patient with recurrent thrombosis was found to have a hereditary nonfunctioning plasminogen (designated plasminogen Tochigi) due to a molecular defect.[1] This report was followed by the discoveries of several cases with abnormal plasminogen (dysplasminogenemia) associated with recurrent thrombosis.[2-9] Thrombi were restricted to the venous side and included superficial as well as deep vein thrombosis, intracranial sinus vein thrombosis, mesenteric venous thrombosis and pulmonary embolism.

These cases of abnormal plasminogen suggest that once the initial thrombotic event has occurred, low fibrinolytic activity caused by the low level of plasminogen activity predisposes an individual to a thrombotic tendency. However, there seems to be only a weak association between thrombotic tendency and low plasminogen activity due to the presence of an abnormal plasminogen molecule because almost none of the family members (heterozygotes with ~50% activity) other than the propositi experienced any thrombotic events. Surprising was the fact that a small girl (aged 6) in the family (plasminogen Tochigi) who had less than 10% of normal plasminogen activity and was considered to be a homozygote had experienced no thrombotic event.[1] She is now 23 years old and has thus far had no thromboembolic episode. On the other hand, a recent study[10] has reported that in 72 consecutive patients with deep vein thrombosis (DVT) 12.5% were diagnosed having dysplasminogenemia. The mean ages of the genetically normal patients and patients with dysplasminogenemia were 52±15 and 40±15 years, respectively ($p<0.05$), indicating an earlier onset of DVT in patients with dysplasminogenemia. These findings suggest that dysplasminogenemia is related to the development of DVT, and that abnormality of the fibrinolytic system is one of the major etiologic factors in DVT.

2. Gene frequency and polymorphism

The frequency distributions of abnormal plasminogen were studied using electrofocusing coupled with immunofixation and zymography to screen plasma samples and a racial difference was found.[11] The gene frequency of the abnormal variant (plasminogen Tochigi or PLG V) in a Japanese population was 0.018, whereas the abnormal variant was not detected in an American Caucasian population, suggesting the very rare occurrence of this variant in Caucasian. The discovery of an abnormal plasminogen of the same type in France,[5] however, excludes a possibility that the distribution of the gene is localized to Japan.

In 1984, at a plasminogen symposium in Munich, a unified nomenclature for plasminogen alleles was adopted.[12] The two most commonly observed phenotypes found in all races were called plasminogen A (PLG A) (A for acidic pI) and PLG B (B for basic pI). Variants with intermediate pI were designated as PLG M. Alleles were designated with an asterisk (e.g. PLG*A). A marked difference of PLG gene frequencies was observed in different ethnic groups. Predominantly high frequency of PLG*A and very low frequency of PLG*B are typically observed in Mongoloids including Japanese, Chinese, Amerindians and Eskimos.[11,13-15] Some rare alleles exist only in limited populations. Functionally abnormal plasminogen variant (e.g. PLG M5) appears to be identical with plasminogen Tochigi (PLG V) and was found only in Japanese[11,14] and Chinese populations.[15] PLG*M5 might be the specific genetic marker of the Mongoloids.[15]

0-8493-5804-3/96/$0.00+$.50

3. Association between abnormal plasminogen and thrombophilia

It has been indicated that plasminogen activity as low as 50% of normal would not induce a thrombotic tendency itself, but would be merely one of the risk factors of thrombosis.[16] It is natural to assume that a deficiency of a protective mechanism against development of thrombosis cannot cause thrombosis by itself. This is also the case in antithrombin III deficiency, which is well known to induce a thrombotic tendency, although not all individuals who have the defect develop thrombosis. The affected individuals developed thrombosis after adolescence only after such triggering events as child birth, surgery or trauma.

Recently a new assay for defects in the action of activated protein C has been discovered.[17] Following studies have clearly shown that a mutation at Arg-506 in factor V gene gives rise to activated protein C resistance with a striking increase in thrombotic risk and that this mutation is by far the commonest abnormality detectable in thrombophilia.[18,19] In fact, the mutation is common not only in thrombophilia but also in the normal Dutch population (2-4%).[18] Interactions of this mutation with other known genetic and environmental risk factors including plasminogen alteration (abnormal plasminogen as well as plasminogen deficiency) are intriguing subjects to be studied. Moreover, the racial or geographic distribution of the gene as well as the comparison of the occurrence rates of thrombosis between populations with or without the abnormal factor V and plasminogen are interesting subjects.

B. BIOLOGICAL ASPECTS AND DIAGNOSIS

1. Identification of abnormal plasminogens

In addition to determining plasma plasminogen antigen and functional levels, the determination of plasma plasmin generation rates with plasminogen activators and structural polymorphisms of plasminogen detected by isoelectric focusing-immunofixation/zymography methods have become useful tools in the identification of plasminogen variants.[11] Most important is the isolation of plasminogen from the patient's plasma and the characterization of the plasminogen molecule, using a variety of physical and biochemical parameters. The plasma yield and the specific activity of the isolated plasminogen give useful information. The abnormal or slow generation of plasmin with catalytic amounts of different types of plasminogen activators (such as tissue plasminogen activator, urokinase as well as streptokinase and its complexes) indicates that the molecule is a variant. A classification of abnormal plasminogens (dysplasminogenemia) has been proposed.[8,9] Two types, Type 1 dysplasminogenemias and Type 2 dysplasminogenemia-hypoplasminogenemia have been suggested. In a revised form of the classification, the type 1 class is subdivided into three kinds of defects. a) active center defect, e.g., Tochigi I,[20] II, III, Nagoya,[21] Paris I[5] and Tokyo,[3] b) active center defect and charge mutant, e.g., Frankfurt I[6] and San Antonio[7] and c) active center and kinetic defects, e.g., Chicago I, II,[2] III[4] and Marywood.[9] Type 2 has only one kind, a) active center defect, e.g., Frankfurt II.[8] Structural changes of the molecules leading to abnormal functions, however, have not been elucidated except for plasminogen Tochigi. Furthermore, type 1 and 2 usually designate quantitative or qualitative deficiencies (abnormal molecules present in plasma) respectively, and the use of this kind classification for dysplasminogenemia may be misleading.

A single point mutation was found in plasminogen Tochigi in the initial Japanese family whose affected member had an increased tendency for venous thrombosis.[20,21] The Ala residue at position 601 from the NH_2 terminus (Ala-601) was replaced by a Thr residue (in this article, a new numbering system has been used for amino acid position above 65 by the observation that an additional Ile was present at position 65). The replacement appears to be responsible for the loss in catalytic activity, since amino acid residues of the active site catalytic triad, namely, His-603, Asp-646 and Ser-741 are intact. Ala-601 is located very close to the active site residues Asp and His, as inferred from making the reasonable assumption of a polypeptide chain conformation similar to that of trypsin.[22] It can be seen from the crystallographic data for the bovine trypsin-pancreatic trypsin- inhibitor complex[23] that the side chain CH_3 group of the Ala in the trypsin molecule is located just behind the imidazole ring of the active site residue His (Fig 1). Therefore it was proposed that the replacement of the Ala by Thr found in the plasmin light chain alters the properties of the side chain of Asp-646 or the side chain of His-603, perhaps inducing a change in charge distribution in the His residue, and thus leads to the loss of the enzyme activity.

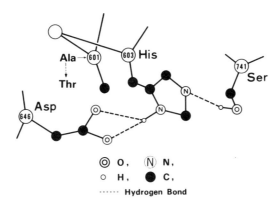

Figure 1. Schematic representation of active site structure of a serine proteinase. Replacement of Ala-601 by Thr in the abnormal plasminogen. Modified from Aoki.[16]

2. Analysis of the abnormal genes for plasminogen

The structure organization of the gene coding for human plasminogen have been established by nucleotide sequencing employing DNA segments obtained by *in vitro* amplification of leukocyte DNA and isolation of λ phage from genomic libraries.[24] These data have made it possible to prepare primers for *in vitro* amplification and sequence analysis of the abnormal genes for plasminogen.[25] The gene coding for plasminogen has been compared with several abnormal genes from Japanese patients by the polymerase chain reaction (PCR) and DNA sequence analysis. In Tochigi-type plasminogen, a guanosine in GCT coding for Ala-601 near the active site His was replaced by an adenosine resulting in ACT coding for Thr. This mutation is readily shown by the loss of a cleavage site for Fnu4HI endonuclease. In the other type of mutation, a guanosine in GTC coding for Val-355 was replaced by a thymidine resulting in TTC coding for Phe. This change is easily shown by the digestion with AvaII. No other dysplasminogenemias have been elucidated for their gene abnormalities.

II. PLASMINOGEN DEFICIENCY (HYPOPLASMINOGENEMIA)

A. CLINICAL ASPECTS

There have been several reports of plasminogen deficiency found in patients with thrombosis.[26-33] Their plasminogen levels were 30-50% of normal by both functional and immunological methods. Previous reports suggest that the pattern of inheritance for this disorder is autosomal dominant[27-30,32,33], and that patients with half-normal plasminogen levels are heterozygotes. However, a correlation between congenital/acquired plasminogen deficiency and thrombosis has not been confirmed, since the propositus is often the only symptomatic family member.[31,33,34] Certain triggering events or other causes of thrombosis in patients who suffered from thrombosis should be considered as described above for dysplasminogenemia.

B. BIOLOGICAL ASPECTS AND DIAGNOSIS

The purified plasminogen of the propositus was indistinguishable from normal plasminogen in terms of several functional parameters, suggesting that low concentrations of a functionally intact plasminogen are the pathophysiological basis of the inherited defect.[26-28,31] There was no evidence for an accelerated in vivo activation, and it was suggested that a low level of plasminogen was due to a decreased rate of synthesis. Alternatively, a low level of plasminogen may be due to delayed intracellular transport and excretion as stated below.

All 19 exons of the plasminogen gene in a Japanese patient with congenital plasminogen deficiency[33] and her family members were analyzed using PCR strategy and restriction fragment polymorphism analysis.[35] Sequence analysis following amplification of each exon and its flanking regions showed a single thymine to cytosine transition in exon 14, which changed a Ser-572 codon (TCC) to Pro-572 codon (CCC).[35] This mutation generates a new FokI site. While this mutation is the first reported genetic abnormality in patients with congenital plasminogen deficiency, the mechanism by which the Ser-572 to Pro-572 substitution elicits the phenotype seen in the propositus has not been defined.

The most probable explanation is that the mutation may disrupt the protein's conformation and result in the impaired secretion of the mutant protein. Alternatively, the mutant plasminogen molecules, if they are secreted, may be cleared faster and more selectively than the normal molecules in the circulation. An increasing number of mutant genes coding abnormal proteins have recently been reported in various congenital deficiencies of factors involved in coagulation and fibrinolysis. We previously analyze genes from two families with hereditary deficiency of α_2-plasmin inhibitor (α_2-PI).[36,37] To investigate molecular and cellular mechanisms of how the mutations cause the near absence of α_2-PI in the plasma, we expressed the mutated genes in cultured cells and analyzed the synthesis and cellular processing of the expressed glycoproteins. It was revealed that these mutants were delayed in transport from the rough endoplasmic reticulum to the Golgi apparatus, where oligosaccharide chains of glycoprotein are processed to become endoglycosidase H-resistant forms.[36,38] They were degraded while they were retained in the cells. Recently, we and others have also disclosed five mutations expected to lead to molecular abnormalities of protein C in three families affected with the deficiency of this regulatory factor of coagulation.[39-41] Expression of the mutant proteins in cultured cells again suggested an impairment of secretion as the cause of the absence of protein C in the plasma. These results suggest that the impaired intracellular transport may be one of the prevalent causes for the deficiencies of these factors. Moreover, available protein-sequence data reveal that plasminogen has strong homology to other serine proteases such as protein C, prothrombin and tissue plasminogen activator in the region of Ser-572. The residue in plasminogen molecule is conserved among all of these proteins. It has also been shown that normal plasminogen molecules are cleared from the circulation mainly by binding to endothelial cells.[42] A fully glycosylated plasminogen molecule cannot extensively bind to endothelial cells, but a partially glycosylated plasminogen molecule or a non-glycosylated plasminogen molecule expressed in *Escherichia coli* can efficiently bind to endothelial cells and can be cleared faster than a fully glycosylated form.[42] These results suggest that a receptor-recognition site on the plasminogen molecule may be masked and can be exposed by conformational changes. Transfection experiments in mammalian cells with plasmids containing normal or mutant plasminogen cDNA should be used to clarify the mechanism of plasminogen deficiency.

C . MANAGEMENT

Warfarin was effective in the prophylaxis and treatment of thrombosis in individuals with dysplasminogenemia.[1-7,9,10] Lifelong anticoagulant therapy is probably indicated in affected individuals with recurrent thrombosis. However, as mentioned above, it has not been established that familial plasminogen variant or deficiency is always a thrombophilic disorder. Management of such asymptomatic persons has not been defined and lifelong anticoagulant therapy would not be indicated. Plasminogen levels appear to rise to within normal range during pregnancy and return to low levels after delivery.[30] While an anabolic steroid stanozolol[29] or an attenuated androgenic steroid danazol[43] may increase depressed levels of plasminogen, it is uncertain if it results in clinical benefit.

REFERENCES

1.   **Aoki, N., Moroi, M., Sakata, Y. and Yoshida, N.** Abnormal plasminogen : A hereditary molecular abnormality found in a patient with recurrent thrombosis. *J. Clin. Invest.*, 61, 1186, 1978.

2   **Wohl, R. C., Summaria, L. and Robbins, K. C.** Physiological activation of the human fibrinolytic system : Isolation and characterization of human plasminogen variants, Chicago I and Chicago II. *J. Biol. Chem.*, 254, 9063, 1979.

3.   **Kazama, M., Tahara, C., Suzuki, Z., Gohchi, K. and Abe, T.** Abnormal plasminogen, a case of recurrent thrombosis. *Thromb. Res.*, 21, 517, 1981.

4.   **Wohl, R. C., Summaria, L. Chediak, J., Rosenfeld, S. and Robbins, K. C.** Human plasminogen variant Chicago III. *Thromb. Haemostas.*, 48, 146, 1982.

5.   **Soria, J., Soria, C., Bertrand, O., Dunn, F., Drouet, L. and Caen, J. P.** Plasminogen Paris I : Congenital abnormal plasminogen and its incidence in thrombosis. *Thromb. Res.*, 32, 229, 1983.

6.   **Scharrer, I. M., Wohl, R. C., Hach, V., Sinio, L., Boreisha, I. and Robbins, K. C.** Investigation of a congenital abnormal plasminogen, Frankfurt I, and its relationship to thrombosis. *Thromb. Haemostas.*, 55, 396, 1986.

7.   **Liu, Y., Lyons, R. M. and McDonagh, J.**, Plasminogen San Antonio: An abnormal plasminogen with a more cathodic migration, decreased activation and associated thrombosis. *Thromb. Haemostas.*, 55, 396, 1988.

8.   **Robbins, K. C.** Classification of abnormal plasminogens: Dysplasminogenemias. *Semin. Thromb. Hemostas.*, 16, 217, 1990.

9.   **Robbins, K. C., Boreisha, I. G. and Godwin, J. E.**, Abnormal plasminogen Maywood I. *Thromb. Haemostas*, 66, 575, 1991.

10. **Kawasaki, T., Kambayashi, J., Uemura, Y., Sakon, M., Shiba, E., Suehisa, E., Amino, N. and Mori, T.**, Involvement of dysplasminogenemia in occurrence of deep vein thrombosis. *Int. Angiol.*, 14,65, 1995.

11. **Aoki, N., Tateno, K. and Sakata, Y.** Differences of frequency distributions of plasminogen phenotypes between Japanese and American populations : New methods for the detection of plasminogen variants. *Biochem. Genet.*, 22, 871, 1984.

12. **Skoda, V., Bertams, J., Dykes, D., Eiberg, H., Hobart, M., Hummel, K., Kuhnl, P., Mauff, G., Nakamura, S., Nishimukai, H., Raum, D., Tokunaga, K. and Weidinger, S.**, Proposals for the nomenclature of human plasminogen (PLG) polymorphism. *Vox Sang.*, 51, 244, 1986.

13. **Dykes, D., Nelson, M. and Polesky, H.**, Distribution of plasminogen allotypes in eight populations of the Western Hemisphere. *Electrophoresis*, 4, 417, 1983.

14. **Yamaguchi, M., Doi, S. and Yoshimura, M.**, Plasminogen phenotypes in a Japanese population. *Hum. Hered.*, 39, 356, 1989.

15. **Yiping, H., Qing, G. and Meiyun, W.**, Genetic polymorphism of human plasminogen (PLG) in a Chinese population. *Eur. J. Immunogen.*, 20, 91, 1993.

16. **Aoki, N.**, Genetic abnormalities of the fibrinolytic system. *Semin. Thromb. Hemostas.*, 10, 42, 1984.

17. **Dahlback, B., Carlsson, M. and Svensson, P. J.**, Familial thrombophilia due to a previously unrecognized mechanism characterized by poor anticoagulant response to activated protein C. *Proc. Natl. Acad. Sci. USA*, 90, 1004, 1993.

18. **Bertina, R. M., Koeleman, B. P. C., Koster, T., Rosendaal, F. R., Dirven, R. J., de Ronde, H., van der Velden, P. A. and Reitsma, P.H.**, Mutation in blood coagulation factor V associated with resistance to activated protein C. *Nature*, 369, 64, 1994.

19. **Voorberg, J., Roelse, J., Koopman, R., Buller, H., Berends, F., ten Cate, J. W., Mertens, K. and van Mourik, J. A.**, Association of idiopathic venous thromboembolism with single point-mutation at Arg 506 of factor V. *Lancet*, 343, 1535, 1994.

20. **Miyata, T., Iwanaga, S., Sakata, Y. and Aoki, N.**, Plasminogen Tochigi: Inactive plasmin resulting from replacement of alanine-600 by threonine in the active site. *Proc. Natl. Acad. Sci. USA* , 79, 6132, 1982.

21. **Miyata, T., Iwanaga, S., Sakata, Y.Aoki, N., Takamatsu, J. and Kamiya, T.**, Plasminogen Tochigi II and Nagoya: Two additional molecular defects with Ala-600--->Thr replacement found in plasmin light chain variants. *J. Biochem.*, 96, 277, 1984.

22. **Stroud, R. M., Kay, L. M. and Dickerson, R. E.**, The structure of bovine trypsin: Electron density maps of the inherited enzyme at 5 and at 2.7 resolution. *J. Mol. Biol.*, 83, 185, 1974.

23   **Huber, R, Kukla, D., Bode, W., Schwager, K., Bartels, K., Deisenhofer, J. and Steigemann, W.** Structure of the complex formed by bovine trypsin and bovine pancreatic trypsin inhibitor. *J. Mol. Biol.*, 89, 73, 1974.

24. **Petersen, T. E., Martzen, M. R., Ichinose, A. and Davie, E. W.** Characterization of the gene for human plasminogen, a key proenzyme in the fibrinolytic system. *J. Biol. Chem.*, 265, 6104, 1990.

25. **Ichinose, A., Espling, E. S., Takamatsu, J., Saito, H., Shinmyozu, K., Maruyama, I., Petersen, T. E. and Davie, E. W.**, Two types of abnormal genes for plasminogen in families with a predisposition for thrombosis. *Proc. Natl. Acad. Sci. USA*, 88, 115, 1991.

26. **Lottenberg, R., Dolly, F. R. and Kitchens, C. S.**, Recurring thromboembolic disease and pulmonary hypertension associated with severe hypoplasminogenemia. *Am. J. Hematol.*, 19, 181, 1985.

27. **Girolami, A., Marafioti, F., Rubertelli, M. and Cappellato. M. G.**, Congenital heterozygous plasminogen deficiency associated with a severe thrombotic tendency. *Acta. Haematol.* (Basel), 75, 54, 1986.

28. **Mannucci, P. M., Kluft, C., Traas, D. W., Seveso, P. and D'Angelo, A.**, Congenital plasminogen deficiency associated with venous thromboembolism: therapeutic trial with stanozolol. *Br. J. Haematol.*, 63, 753, 1986.

29. **Tengborn, L., Johannessen, M. and Hedner, U.**, Family with hypoplasminogenemia. *Thromb. Haemostas.*, 58, 93 (Abstract), 1987.

30. **Dolan, G., Greaves, M., Cooper, P. and Preston, F. E.** Thrombovascular disease and familial plasminogen deficiency: a report of three kindreds. *Br. J. Haematol.*, 70, 417, 1988.

31. **Hach-Wunderle, V., Scharrer, I. and Lottenberg, R.**, Congenital deficiency of plasminogen and its relationship to venous thrombosis. *Thromb. Haemostas.*, 59, 277, 1988.

32. **Leebeck, F. W. G., Knot, E. A. R., Ten Cate, J. W. and Traas, D. W.**, Severe thrombotic tendency associated with a type I plasminogen deficiency. *Am. J. Hematol.*, 30, 32, 1989.

33. **Shigekiyo, T., Uno, Y., Tomonari, A., Saitoh, K., Hondo, H., Ueda, S and Saito, S.**, Type I congenital plasminogen deficiency is not a risk factor for thrombosis. *Thromb. Haemostas.*, 67, 189, 1992.

34. **Tait, R. C., Walker, I. D., Conkie, J. A., Islam, S. I. A. M., McCall, F., Mitchell, R. and Davidson, J. F.**, Plasminogen levels in healthy volunteers- Influence of age, sex, smoking and oral contraceptives. *Thromb. Haemostas.*, 68, 506, 1992.

35. **Azuma, H., Uno, Y., Shigekiyo, T. and Saito, S.**, Congenital plasminogen deficiency caused by a Ser 572 to Pro mutation. *Blood*, 82, 475, 1993.

36. **Miura, O., Sugahara, Y. and Aoki, N** Hereditary α_2-plasmin inhibitor deficiency caused by a transport-deficient mutation (α_2-PI-Okinawa). Deletion of Glu 137 by a trinucleotide deletion blocks intracellular transport. *J. Biol. Chem.*, 264, 18213, 1989.

37. **Miura, O., Hirosawa, S., Kato, A. and Aoki, N.**, Molecular basis for congenital deficiency of α_2-plasmin inhibitor. A frameshift mutation leading to elongation of the deduced amino acid sequence. *J. Clin. Invest.*, 83, 1598, 1989.

38. **Miura, O. and Aoki, N.**, Impaired secretion of mutant α_2-plasmin inhibitor (α_2-PI-Nara) from COS-7 and HepG2 cells : molecular and cellular basis for hereditary deficiency of α_2-plasmin inhibitor. *Blood*, 75, 1092, 1990.

39. **Sugahara, Y., Miura, O., Yuen, P. and Aoki, N.**, Protein C deficiency Hong Kong 1 and 2: Hereditary protein C deficiency caused by two mutant alleles, a 5-nucleotide deletion and missense mutation. *Blood* , 80, 126, 1992.

40.   **Yamamoto, K., Tanimoto, M., Emi, N., Matsushita, T., Takamatsu, J. and Saito, H.**, Impaired secretion of the elongated mutant of protein C (Protein C- Nagoya): molecular and cellular basis for hereditary protein C deficiency. *J. Clin. Invest.*, 90, 2439, 1992.

41.   **Sugahara, Y., Miura, O., Hirosawa, S. and Aoki, N,** Compound heterozygous protein C deficiency caused by two mutations Arg-178 to Gln and Cys-331 to Arg, leading to impaired secretion of mutant protein C. *Thromb. Haemostas.*, 72,814, 1994.

42.   **Gonzalez-Gronow, M., Grenett, H. E., Fuller, G. M. and Pizzo, S. V**.The role of carbohydrate in the function of human plasminogen : comparison of the protein obtained from molecular cloning and expression in *Escherichia coli* and COS cells. *Biochim. Biophys. Acta*, 1039, 269, 1990.

43.   **Al-Momen, A. K., Gader, A. M. A., Shamena, A.-R., Daif, A. K. and Ajarim, D.**, Significant elevation of protein C and protein S levels in thrombotic disorders by low dose danazol. *Blood Coagul. Fibrinolysis*, 2, 495, 1991.

HYPERHOMOCYSTEINEMIA AND VASCULAR DISEASE

G. Palareti, C. Legnani, and S. Coccheri

Chair and Dept. Angiology and Blood Coagulation, University Hospital S. Orsola, Bologna, Italy

I. INTRODUCTION

Homocystinuria refers to the presence in urine of normally undetectable homocystine, the disulfide of homocysteine (HCY), secondary to increased blood levels of the latter (hyperhomocysteinemia). This condition was first described by Carson and Neill in 1962 in two siblings in a survey on mentally retarded children[1]. The homozygous enzyme defect of cystathionine β-synthase was identified by Mudd et al.[2] in 1964 as the most common cause of homocystinuria. Other rarer genetic enzyme deficiencies leading to hyperhomocysteinemia were identified later.[3]

Among the main symptoms which affect homocystinuric patients (including skeletal, ocular, neurological and vascular abnormalities), arterial and venous thrombotic complications together with premature arteriosclerosis are of predominant importance.[4] The association between hyperhomocysteinemia and vascular disease is so strong that a "homocystinuria theory of arteriosclerosis" has been suggested by McCully and Wilson since 1975.[5]

In the last fifteen years several clinical studies have shown that even mild to moderate elevations of homocysteinemia are associated with a markedly increased risk of premature vascular disease, both arterial and venous. Moderately elevated levels of plasma HCY may be found in heterozygotes for homocystinuria, and also in patients with various acquired pathologic conditions, such as vitamin B_{12} or folic acid deficiencies. The number of individuals with mild hyperhomocysteinemia, and subsequent increased risk of premature vascular disease, is thus much greater than that of patients with congenital homocystinuria, a rare disease. The attempt to identify the high number of individuals at risk and prevent or treat the vascular consequences, given that it is possible to pharmacologically modulate blood HCY levels, accounts for the large number of studies devoted to this issue in recent years.

II. BIOCHEMISTRY OF HOMOCYSTEINE

A. HOMOCYSTEINE METABOLISM

HCY is a sulfhydryl amino-acid formed as intermediate in the metabolic conversion of methionine to cysteine, and constitutes a point of juncture between the transmethylation cycle and the transsulfuration pathway[3] (Figure 1). It is produced by demethylation of methionine, an essential amino-acid derived from dietary intake. Methionine is first converted to S-adenosylmethionine, which is demethylated to form S-adenosylhomocysteine, and then hydrolyzed to adenosine and HCY; this reaction in particular conditions may also be reversible.

Via the transsulfuration pathway, approximately 50% of HCY formed from methionine condenses irreversibly with serine forming cystathionine (reaction 1), which in turn is transformed to cysteine. This reaction is catalyzed by the enzyme cystathionine β-synthase, with pyridoxal 5-phosphate (vitamin B_6) as coenzyme.

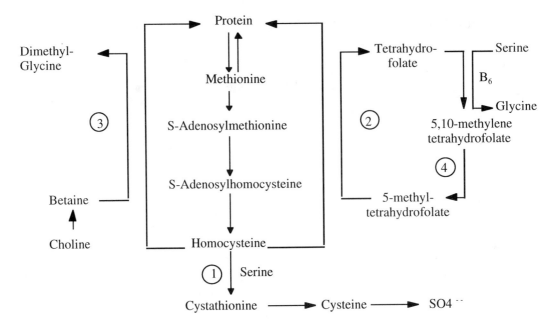

Figure 1. Pathways of methionine-homocysteine metabolism and interrelationship with folate and cobalamin;

(1) Cystathionine β-synthase (CBS) (coenzyme: vitamin B_6);

(2) 5-Methyltetrahydrofolate-homocysteine methyltransferase (methionine synthase) (coenzyme: vitamin B_{12});

(3) Betaine-homocysteine methyltransferase;

(4) 5,10-Methylenetetrahydrofolate reductase (5,10 MTHFR)

The remaining HCY is conserved by remethylation to methionine through the following reactions:
a) HCY + 5-methyltetrahydrofolate (as a methyl donor) ---> methionine + tetrahydrofolate, reaction 2 in Figure 1, which is regulated by the widely distributed 5-methyltetrahydrofolate-homocysteine methyltransferase (methionine synthase) enzyme which has vitamin B_{12} (Methyl B_{12}) as coenzyme;
b) HCY + betaine ---> methionine + dimethylglycine, reaction 3, regulated by an enzyme found only in liver tissue and probably of limited importance *in vivo*.

B. FORMS OF HOMOCYSTEINE IN PLASMA

HCY has a free reactive -SH group; it therefore readily oxidizes forming disulfides[6]. Approximately 70-80% of total HCY in plasma is protein-bound (mainly to albumin) by a covalent mixed disulfide bond[7]. The remainder consists of oxidized forms with other sulfhydryls present in plasma, mainly mixed disulfide with cysteine (MDS) or homodisulfide (homocystine); only a small portion is present as HCY[8-11]. The sum of these nonprotein-bound forms is referred to as free homocysteine. Total HCY is defined as the sum of protein bound and free HCY forms.

C. MEASUREMENT OF HOMOCYSTEINE

To measure free HCY, plasma should first be deproteinized (with sulfosalicylic or perchloracetic acid) immediately after collection since a larger proportion of HCY would become protein-bound ex vivo; this redistribution takes place in samples either kept at room temperature or frozen at -20°C[6]. The supernatant is treated with a reducing agent (usually dithiothreitol or 2-mercaptoethanol) to cleave the disulfide bonds present in mixed disulfide with cysteine (MDS) and homocysteine; free HCY is then measured.

Most of the methodologies recently used to quantitate plasma HCY, however, measure the total HCY. For this purpose plasma samples are first treated with the reducing agent in order to liberate HCY from all oxidized forms (protein-bound, MDS, homocystine); deproteinization is then performed followed by HCY measurement. Various methods have been adopted, including standard amino acid analyzers, ion-exchange chromatography[12], radio-enzymatic assays[7], gas chromatography[13], gas chromatography-mass spectrometry[14], and fluorescence detection with HPLC[10]. The total HCY concentration in fasting normal individuals has been reported as being between 6-14 μmol/L.[7,15]

HCY measurement may be affected by pre-analytical factors which should be given due consideration, such as specimen collection, processing, and storage[16]. As mentioned above, the difference in intervals between blood sampling and sample deproteinization constitutes a factor of variability in the measurement of free HCY. Total HCY determination is clearly unaffected by this factor. Since HCY is released from cells in blood left at room temperature[7], it is generally recommended that plasma be obtained by immediate centrifugation of blood (within 30-60 min from sampling), preferably anticoagulated with EDTA and collected in chilled tubes left on ice. Following these guidelines for specimen handling, it has been found that total plasma HCY is stable and can be measured in up to 10 year old frozen plasma samples[17].

As regards the enzyme cystathionine β–synthase, its activity may be specifically measured in cultured fibroblasts[18,19].

D. METHIONINE LOADING

Methionine ingestion induces a transient increase in plasma HCY levels; the increase is greater if the transsulfuration pathway is less efficient in metabolizing methionine because of reduced cystathionine β-synthase activity. Oral methionine loading is a test used mainly to identify cystathionine β-synthase deficiency heterozygotes[20], who have normal or slightly elevated concentrations of fasting plasma HCY. In these subjects, ingestion of 0.1 g/kg body weight of L-methionine (or of the almost equivalent dose of 3.8 g/m^2 body surface area, adopted to reduce the effect of body weight[21]) induces plasma HCY levels that are higher and more sustained than in normal controls. The test is usually given early in the morning to overnight fasting subjects: immediately after basal blood sampling, methionine is given diluted in 200 ml of fruit juice; a further blood sample is drawn after a fixed time period, usually 4 hours[20]. While it has been suggested that the most accurate way to evaluate the methionine loading test is to measure the area under the curve of HCY elimination[15], it has been observed that peak HCY levels at 4 hours after ingestion correlate well with the area under the curve values[22].

Since there is an overlap in post-methionine loading HCY values between heterozygotes and normal subjects, it is not easy to establish when a methionine loading test should be considered abnormal (a condition that has been referred to as "methionine intolerance"). Different criteria have been proposed: values above the upper limit of the control group, greater than the mean plus 2 SD[23], or above 95th percentile for comparable control group[24]. Brattström et al.[21] use as criterion the post-load HCY increase above basal level rather than the absolute level reached.

III. HOMOCYSTINURIA

A. INHERITED CAUSES

Homocystinuria is a genetically determined inborn error of metabolism which leads to increased HCY levels in plasma (reaching concentrations as high as 200-400 μmol/L in fasting non-treated patients) and presence of large amounts of homocystine in urine (for comprehensive reviews of the disease see references 3,4,25). The most common form of homocystinuria arises from a deficiency in cystathionine β-synthase, resulting from the presence of homozygous gene inherited in autosomal recessive fashion, and presenting a marked genetic heterogeneity. About 50% of the patients, with a residual enzyme activity, respond to treatment with large doses of vitamin B_6, precursor of pyridoxal 5'-phosphate[3]. In responsive patients, this treatment achieves a reduction in plasma and urinary HCY levels in fasting state but not after methionine loading[26]. This form is biochemically characterized by increased plasma HCY and methionine and decreased cysteine.

The prevalence of homocystinuria is about 1/200,000 worldwide though it varies greatly in different areas, being as high as 1/40,000 in New South Wales, 1/57,000 in Ireland, and only 1/1,052,000 in Japan[3,27].

In recent years it has been shown that even heterozygosity for cystathionine β-synthase deficiency may result in a condition of mild hyperhomocysteinemia. The incidence of heterozygosity has been estimated to be between 0.3 and 1% in the general population[3].

Other less common forms of homocystinuria are caused by congenital deficiencies of enzymes involved in the remethylation of HCY. These include the deficiency of the enzyme 5,10-MTHF reductase[28] (reaction 4 in Figure 1), and other deficiencies of any of the enzymes leading to the synthesis of Methyl-B_{12}[3,29,30]. In these forms, plasma and urinary HCY is increased due to reduced remethylation; methionine, however, is low or normal and cysteine normal. A thermolabile mutant of methylenetetrahydrofolate reductase has recently been described[31], resulting in moderate hyperhomocysteinemia[32] and associated with increased risk for coronary artery disease[33] (CAD).

B. VENOUS AND ARTERIAL THROMBOEMBOLISM IN HOMOCYSTINURIA

Among the major clinical manifestations of this disease, including marfanoid habitus, dislocation of optic lenses, mental retardation, seizures, and osteoporosis with skeletal abnormalities, a strong association with thromboembolic complications is of paramount importance (the clinical features are comprehensively reviewed elsewhere[3,4,34]).

Thrombotic disease is markedly premature in these patients, sometimes arising in the first decade of life, involves both arterial and venous systems, and is the most conspicuous cause of complications and death[3,4]. Thrombosis may, albeit infrequently, be the single/first clinical feature leading to investigation for homocystinuria[35-37]. This possibility should be considered in order to avoid such cases being misdiagnosed as idiopathic thrombosis.

C. THE SURVEY OF MUDD ET AL. ON THE NATURAL HISTORY OF HOMOCYSTINURIA

In 1985, Mudd et al.[4] reported the results of an international survey on clinical manifestations and natural evolution of the disease in 629 patients with homocystinuria due to cystathionine β-synthase deficiency. Thromboembolic complications were recorded in 158 (25%) of these patients who had experienced a total number of 253 thrombotic events: 51% thrombosis of peripheral veins (complicated by pulmonary embolism in about 25% of cases), 32% cerebrovascular accidents, 11% peripheral arterial obstructions and 4% myocardial infarctions.

Occurrence of thromboembolic events was age-dependent, the chances of being affected being about 25% by age of 16 and 50% by age of 29. The rate of thromboembolic events was lower in B_6-responsive patients, though untreated, than in untreated B_6-unresponsive patients. Patients with a first thrombotic event were at higher risk of suffering further thrombotic episodes than patients of the same age and B_6-responsiveness but not yet affected by thrombosis. After the 586 major surgical procedures or eye operations performed in the patients, clinically overt postoperative thromboembolic events were recorded in 25 (4.3%) cases (six fatal), thus confirming earlier reports suggesting that these patients are at higher risk of postoperative thromboembolic complications[38]. Thromboembolic events were either the direct cause or a major contributing factor for death in 47 (73%) out of the 64 deceased patients in the survey.

D. OTHER REPORTS ON THROMBOEMBOLISM IN HOMOCYSTINURIA

A large number of studies have reported on the occurrence of thrombotic disease in homocystinuria. Venous thrombosis is particularly frequent in these patients; the deep veins of the legs are especially affected but also renal veins and vena porta[38-41]. Cerebrovascular events are common, sustained by thrombosis of both extra- and intra-cranial arteries, and of sinuses[34,37,42-46]. Symptomatic stenosis or occlusion of peripheral arteries has often been reported, leading to intermittent claudication, trophic lesions of the legs, and reno-vascular hypertension[39,47-50]. Early signs of premature peripheral artery disease were detected by non-invasive methodology (Duplex scanner) in still asymptomatic homocystinuric patients and in obligate heterozygotes[51]. Fatal myocardial infarction due to coronary artery occlusion has been described in very young patients[39,47,52].

Vascular complications have also been reported in the rarer forms of homocystinuria due to inborn defects of HCY remethylation. Though many of these patients died at a very young age, autopsy studies showed in some of them signs of a prominent vascular involvement with presence of cerebral or pulmonary thrombosis and widespread arterial lesions[53-57]. Severe recurrent strokes have also been reported in adult patients as the first symptom of homocystinuria due to 5,10-MTHF[58].

IV. INHERITED AND ACQUIRED CONDITIONS OF MODERATE HYPERHOMOCYSTEINEMIA

A number of conditions have been recognized as being associated with moderate hyperhomocysteinemia or methionine intolerance (for review see ref. 15). Heterozygosity for cystathionine β-synthase deficiency should be considered along with several acquired conditions. Fasting HCY values - measured either as free or total - may be only moderately raised[59] and not higher than in controls[21,60], with a wide overlapping of results with the controls[61]. Measurement after methionine loading improves efficiency in identifying heterozygotes[62] and detecting cases with methionine intolerance.

First, we should consider sex- and age-related variations of HCY levels. Men have higher fasting HCY plasma levels than women[10,12,63]. It has been reported that premenopausal women have lower levels than men[8]; after menopause, however, this difference is no longer detectable[64]. Moreover, post-methionine loading levels have been reported to be higher in post- than in pre-menopausal women[64]. Even though a recent study[63] was not able to completely confirm these data, it has been suggested that a greater efficiency in methionine metabolism is a protective factor against vascular disease in women during reproductive age[65]. Recently, increased fasting HCY levels in relation to age have been found in a large number of healthy subjects[63] together with reduced cystathionine β-synthase activity[66].

Deficiencies in vitamin B_{12}, folate or vitamin B_6, or even their low-normal values have been found to be associated with high HCY levels[14,60,67]. Cobalamin deficiency and/or elevated HCY levels have been recorded in a high proportion (14.5%) of a large number of elderly outpatients; these alterations were partially or completely corrected by cobalamin therapy[68]. Similar results have been obtained in other recent studies.[69,70]

Increased HCY levels, positively correlated with serum creatinine, have been consistently reported in patients with varying intensities of chronic renal insufficiency, whether treated by hemodialysis or not[9,71-73]. Since patients with chronic renal failure have higher risk of premature vascular disease of multifactorial pathogenic origin[74], it has been suggested that hyperhomocysteinemia in this clinical condition may be an additional contributing factor which, interestingly, can be lowered by folic acid treatment[75].

Other conditions and agents have been reported to be associated with increased HCY levels, such as zinc deficiency, cancer, psoriasis, several drugs (see ref. 15 for a review), non-insulin-dependent diabetes mellitus (especially the patients with macroangiopathy[76]), and alcoholism[77].

V. MODERATE HYPERHOMOCYSTEINEMIA AND VASCULAR DISEASE

Since 1976, when Wilcken and Wilcken[78] first demonstrated that altered levels of MDS after methionine loading were much more frequent in patients suffering from CAD than in controls, increasing attention has been paid to the association between alterations in HCY metabolism and premature vascular disease. A number of clinical studies have followed (reviewed herein), indicating that congenital or acquired conditions leading to mild/moderate hyperhomocysteinemia are associated with higher risk of premature vascular disease (both arterial and venous).

A. CLINICAL STUDIES ON HYPERHOMOCYSTEINEMIA AND VASCULAR DISEASE: ESTABLISHING AN ASSOCIATION

Overall, these studies can be said to be of an observational type, aimed mainly at providing information on the presence and strength of an association between hyperhomocysteinemia and occurrence of vascular disease. Only one recent study had a prospective design[79], measuring HCY levels in a cohort of US physicians in prospectively collected blood samples, and comparing the results of those suffering myocardial infarction or death from CAD with matched controls. All the others are case-control studies, in which investigations on HCY metabolism were carried out in groups of patients with ascertained vascular disease and compared with control subjects; in a few studies the controls were historical.

The studies differ in several important ways. In many, but not all, the patients examined were relatively young so as to limit the investigation to cases with premature vascular disease. Criteria for the choice of the control subjects are obviously of paramount importance. Controls should have been matched for sex and age, and possibly for other risk factors for vascular disease and atherosclerosis. This was the case in most, though not all, studies. In a few of them, particularly accurate, controls were selected from patients referring for the same clinical symptoms and/or underlying disease in whom the end point thrombotic event was excluded by means of objective criteria (for instance, coronary angiography). HCY was measured with different methodologies. In early studies HCY was determined as mixed disulfide (MDS) or free fraction (in both cases the protein-bound fraction was therefore not considered), while most of the recent studies measured total HCY levels; as mentioned before, greater variability of results should be expected in the former case. Finally, sometimes only fasting HCY levels were measured, whereas many studies also included the response to methionine loading.

Some important features and results of these studies are detailed in Table I, grouped according to the different vascular districts involved. More than 1900 patients with CAD were examined vs more than 1700 controls. Most of these studies (especially those which measured total HCY) showed statistically significant higher baseline HCY in patients than in controls. More than 20% of the patients had abnormally high baseline HCY levels, while an abnormal response to methionine loading was recorded in about 18% of patients. In the prospective study cited above[79], the only one to date designed in this way, HCY levels turned out to be significantly higher ($p<0.03$) in patients presenting outcome events than in controls; abnormally high HCY levels were found in 11% of patients vs less than 5% in controls. The relative risk for the highest 5% vs the bottom 90% of HCY levels was 3.4 (CI 1.3-8.8; $p<0.01$) after adjustment for the other risk factors.

As regards cerebrovascular disease, more than 1100 patients were examined vs about 850 controls. In all studies the mean baseline HCY levels were significantly higher in patients than in controls. Abnormally high basal HCY levels and an abnormal response to methionine loading test were recorded in 26.6% and 24.1% of patients respectively.

Table I : Synopsis of the studies on Homocysteine (HCY) in Patients with
Coronary/Cerebrovascular/Peripheral Arterial Disease or Venous Thromboembolic Disease

Disease (References)	pt/ctl n.	pt/ctl HCY ratio[a]	High baseline HCY [b] n. (%)	Abnormal methionine load[b] n. (%)
Coronary Artery Disease (23,24,78-93)	1911/1763	1.18	187/863 (21.7%)	70/392 (17.9%)
Cerebrovascular Disease (21,23,62,76,81,87,89,94-101)	1124/864	1.40	80/301 (26.6%)	110/457 (24.1%)
Peripheral Arterial Disease (21,23,81,87,89,101-105)	660/601	1.48	139/424 (32.8%)	84/294 (28.6%)
Venous Thromboembolic Disease (106-111)	294/197	1.20	38/275 (13.8%)	51/200 (25.5%)

Number of patients/controls examined (pt/ctl n.), results of patient/control (pt/ctl) HCY
ratio, frequencies of high baseline HCY levels, and of abnormal response to methionine loading
[a] ratio between mean plasma HCY levels in patients and controls
[b] criteria for high baseline HCY levels and abnormal response to methionine loading= higher than control mean plus 2 SD, or above 95th percentile for controls, or higher than any control values (max frequency in control groups = 5% for both tests)

A total of more than 600 patients, most under 55 y and affected by peripheral arterial disease, were examined and compared with a similar number of controls. Even in this type of vascular disease most studies reported significantly higher HCY levels than in controls, and the percentages of patients with abnormally high basal HCY or with methionine intolerance (32.8% and 28.6% respectively) were higher than in CAD and cerebrovascular disease.

Only very recently have patients with venous thromboembolic disease also been investigated; these studies are few (summarized in Table I) and the total number of patients examined relatively small (about 290). Nevertheless, a not negligible percentage of the patients has been found to have either high HCY levels (13.8%) or abnormal methionine loading test (25.5%), thus suggesting that hyperhomocysteinemia may also be involved in venous thrombotic disease.

In summary, almost 4000 patients with arterial or venous disease have so far been examined in various case-control studies. Most studies have reported mean HCY levels higher in patients than in controls; furthermore, in about one fourth of all patients abnormally high fasting HCY levels and/or signs of methionine intolerance have been recorded. From all these studies, it may be concluded that conditions of mild/moderate homocysteinemia are associated with premature vascular disease, both arterial and venous. Results from the only prospective study performed to date are consistent with these conclusions.

B. HYPERHOMOCYSTEINEMIA AND OTHER RISK FACTORS FOR VASCULAR DISEASE

In many studies possible correlations between HCY levels and other risk factors for vascular disease and atherosclerosis were investigated. A significant correlation with age was found in several series[79,91,98,100]. A number of studies showed that HCY correlated positively with uric acid or creatinine levels[76,82,84,91,96,98], indicating a relationship between renal insufficiency and increased HCY levels. Significant correlation was found in some studies with hypertension[79,92,95], fibrinogen[91,100], and plasma viscosity[91]. Homocysteinemia was not correlated with other factors associated with atherosclerosis, such as cholesterol (except in one study[100]), lipoprotein, triglyceride, cigarette smoking, and diabetes.

Most studies, after considering other risk factors, concluded that HCY was an independent risk factor for vascular disease.

VI. PATHOGENIC MECHANISMS

The pathogenic mechanisms linking hyperhomocysteinemia and thrombotic vascular disease have been comprehensively reviewed in recent years by several authors[69,112-114].

A. ENDOTHELIAL CELL DAMAGE

In their pioneering experimental studies in baboons Harker et al.[115] found that HCY infusion produced extended endothelial desquamation, shortened platelet survival, and arterial thrombosis; if infusion was more prolonged, vascular lesions similar to those typical of atherosclerosis in man were detected[116]. Though these findings were not confirmed by studies in animal species[117,118], it was speculated that endothelial cell damage induced by HCY was the initial factor leading to accelerated atherogenesis[119]. In *in vitro* studies, a cytotoxicity of the compound HCY thiolactone on endothelial cells has been demonstrated[120], even though the use of this compound has been questioned[121]. Furthermore, sulfur-containing amino-acids showed a cytotoxic effect on endothelial cells which was much more pronounced when these were derived from subjects with cystathionine β-synthase deficiency than from normal controls[122]. The mechanism of endothelial cell injury has been postulated to be mediated by the H_2O_2 generated by an interaction between the sulfhydryl group of homocysteine, copper, and oxygen[123].

HCY reduces the anticoagulant function of vessel wall by downregulating the endothelial-induced protein C activation[124] and by inhibiting the surface expression of thrombomodulin, a protein C cofactor[125,126]. Moreover, it has been proved that HCY increases the activation of factor V[127], produced by endothelial cells, which should in turn be inhibited by activated protein C, thus contributing to an impairment of the protein C anticoagulation pathway.

An increase in von Willebrand factor antigen (vWFAg) levels from endothelial cells after incubation with HCY has been recently described[128]. The vWFAg is not only a marker of vessel wall damage but plays also a role in atherosclerosis by promoting platelet adhesion to subendothelium. A direct connection between the endothelial injury caused by HCY and activation of blood coagulation has been demonstrated by proving that endothelial-derived tissue factor activity is induced by HCY in a time- and concentration-dependent manner[129]. Finally, it has been proposed that the adverse vascular effect of HCY is mediated by oxides of nitrogen released from damaged endothelial cells[130].

B. COAGULATION FACTOR CHANGES, PLATELET INVOLVEMENT

Though infrequently investigated, some changes in coagulation factors have been reported in patients with homocystinuria (for a review see ref. 41). Low levels of factor VII have been consistently found[50,131-134], as well as reduced antithrombin III activity levels[50,135-137]. These findings seem to be contradictory, since if the low antithrombin III activity is consistent with a thrombotic tendency typical of these patients, this is not the case for the reduced factor VII values; however, it should be considered that occurrence of thromboembolic complications have already been reported in subjects with congenital factor VII deficiency[138,139].

Results of studies on the effects of HCY on platelet survival have been controversial: an increase in platelet turnover was found in some studies[115,140], but not in others[141,142]. Recently, Di Minno et al.[143] have provided results confirming that in patients with homocystinuria there is an enhanced thromboxane biosynthesis, likely reflecting the in vivo platelet activation and sensitive to treatment with low-dose aspirin.

HCY may also affect fibrinolysis through an action on lipoprotein (a), which is known to be associated with vascular disease. It has recently been demonstrated that HCY increases the affinity of lipoprotein (a) for fibrin[144]. The lipoprotein (a) apoprotein has homology with plasminogen, and competes with this for binding to fibrin: the more lipoprotein (a) is linked to fibrin the less plasminogen attaches to fibrin, reducing in this way fibrinolytic activity and promoting thrombosis.

VII. NOTES ON THE TREATMENT

A. HOMOCYSTINURIA

Main aims in treating patients with homocystinuria are: 1) to keep blood HCY levels as low as possible, 2) to treat, and possibly prevent, complications (mainly thromboembolism). Treatment with pyridoxine (vitamin B_6) in patients with cystathionine β–synthase deficiency responsive to vitamin B_6 (approximately 50% of them) proved effective by either reducing HCY levels[3] or avoiding thromboembolic events[4]. A low methionine intake diet is widely recommended, especially in those patients non-responsive to pyridoxine. Another therapeutic approach is to promote remethylation of HCY to methionine. Vitamin B_{12}[145], folic acid[3,146], and betaine[82,147] have been found to be useful for this purpose. Treatment of thromboembolic events is not different from the usual standard; it mainly is based on an indefinitely prolonged oral anticoagulation. Studies with antiplatelet agents have not been conclusive[3]. Prophylaxis of post-operative thromboembolic complications should be routine in these patients.

B. HYPERHOMOCYSTEINEMIA

Several investigators have demonstrated that elevated levels of HCY in adult subjects are almost invariably reduced or even normalized by small doses of folate (1-5 mg/day). This occurs not only in patients with folate deficiency[14], but also in patients with chronic renal insufficiency[75], vascular disease and atherosclerosis[21,148], post-menopausal women[64], and in normal subjects[149]. Combined vitamin treatments, including pyridoxine, folic acid, and vitamin B_{12}, or betaine in varying dosages, proved effective in normalizing the response to methionine loading[21,150], and reducing fasting plasma HCY concentration in patients with vascular diseases[101,150,151] or chronic renal insufficiency[152], as well as in asymptomatic subjects with hyperhomocysteinemia[153].

Combined vitamin treatment is therefore effective in reducing hyperhomocysteinemia and also safe, since no side effects have been reported. However, it should be pointed out that no results of clinical studies are available yet, to determine whether lowering HCY levels is accompanied by any reduction in the incidence of vascular events. Further work is needed in this direction as well as to determine the lowest required dosage of these substances.

REFERENCES

1. **Carson, N. A. J., Neill, D. W.,** Metabolic abnormalities detected in a survey of mentally backward individuals in Northern Ireland, *Arch. Dis. Child.*, 37, 505, 1962.
2. **Mudd, S. H., Finkelstein, J. D., Irreverre, F., Laster, L.,** Homocystinuria: an enzymatic defect, *Science*, 143, 1443, 1964.
3. **Mudd, S. H., Levy, H. L., Skovby, F.,** Disorders of transulfuration, in *The metabolic basis of inherited disease*, Vol. 1, 6th ed., Scriver, C., Beaudet, A.L., Sly, W.S., Valle, D., Eds., McGraw-Hill, New York, 1989, 693.
4. **Mudd, S. H., Skovby, F., Levy, H. L., Pettigrew, K. D., Wilcken, B., Pyeritz, R. E., Andria, G., Boers, G. H. J., Bromberg, I. L., Cerone, R., Fowler, B., Grîbe, H., Schmidt, H., Schweitzer, L.,** The natural history of homocystinuria due to cystathionine ··-synthase deficiency, *Am. J. Hum. Genet.*, 37, 1, 1985.
5. **McCully, K. S., Wilson, R. B.,** Homocystinuria theory of arteriosclerosis, *Atherosclerosis*, 22, 215, 1975.
6. **Perry, T. L., Hansen, S.,** Technical pitfalls leading to errors in the quantitations of plasma amino acids, *Clin. Chim. Acta*, 25, 53, 1969.
7. **Refsum, H., Helland, S., Ueland, P. M.,** Radioenzymic determination of homocysteine in plasma and urine, Clin. Chem., 31, 624, 1985.
8. **Gupta, V. J., Wilcken, D. E. L.,** The detection of cysteine-homocysteine mixed disulfide in plasma of normal fasting man, *Eur. J. Clin. Invest.*, 8, 205, 1978.
9. **Wilcken, D. E. L., Gupta, V.J.,** Sulphur containing amino acids in chronic renal failure with particular reference to homocysteine and cysteine-homocysteine mixed disulphide, *Eur. J. Clin. Invest.*, 9, 301, 1979.
10. **Araki, A., Sako, Y.,** Determination of free and total homocysteine in human plasma by high-performance liquid chromatography with fluorescence detection, *J. Chromatogr.*, 422, 43, 1987.
11. **Mansoor, M. A., Svardal, A. M., Schneede, J., Ueland, P.M.,** Dynamic relation between reduced, oxidized, and protein-bound homocysteine and other thiol components in plasma during methionine loading in healthy men, *Clin. Chem.*, 38, 1316, 1992.
12. **Wilcken, D. E. L,, Gupta, V. J.,** Cysteine-homocysteine mixed disulfide differing plasma concentrations in normal men and women, *Clin. Sci.*, 57, 211, 1979.
13. **Kataoka, H., Tanaka, H., Fujimoto, A., Noguchi, I., Makita, M.,** Determination of sulphur amino acids by gas chromatography with flame photometric detection, *Biomed. Chromatogr.*, 8, 119, 1994.
14. **Stabler, S. P., Marcell, P. D., Podell, E. R., Allen, R. H., Savage, D. G., Lindenbaum, J.,** Elevation of total homocysteine in the serum of patients with cobalamin or folate deficiency detected by capillary gas chromatography-mass spectrometry, *J. Clin. Invest.*, 81, 466, 1988.
15. **Ueland, P. M., Refsum, H.,** Plasma homocysteine, a risk factor for vascular disease - Plasma levels in health, disease, and drug therapy, *J. Lab. Clin. Med.*, 114, 473, 1989.
16. **Ubbink, J. B., Vermaak, W. J. H., Vandermerwe, A., Becker, P. J.,** The effect of blood sample aging and food consumption on plasma total homocysteine levels, *Clin. Chim. Acta*, 207, 119, 1992.
17. **Israelsson, B., Brattström, L., Refsum, H.,** Homocysteine in frozen plasma samples - A short cut to establish hyperhomocysteinaemia as a risk factor for arteriosclerosis, *Scand. J. Clin. Lab. Önvest.*, 53, 465, 1993.
18. **Bittles, A. H, and Carson, N. A. J.,** Homocystinuria: studies on cystathionine ··-synthase, S-adenosylmethionine synthase and cystathionase activities in skin fibroblasts, *J. Inherited Metab. Dis.*, 4, 3, 1981.
19. **Boers, G. H. J., Fowler, B., Smals, A. G. H., Trijbels, F. J. M., Leermakers, A. I., Keijer, W. J., Kloppenborg, P. W. C.,** Improved identification of heterozygotes for homocystinuria due to cystathionine synthase deficiency by the combination of methionine loading and enzyme determination in cultured fibroblasts, *Hum. Genet.*, 69, 164, 1985.
20. **Sandharwalla, I. B., Fowler, B., Robins, A. J., Komrower, G. M.,** Detection of heterozygotes for homocystinuria - Study of sulphur-containing amino acids in plasma and urine after L-methionine loading, *Arch. Dis. Child.*, 49, 553, 1974.
21. **Brattström, L., Israelsson, B., Norrving, B., Bergqvist, D., Thîrne, J., Hultberg, B., Hamfelt, A.,** Impaired homocysteine metabolism in early-onset cerebral and peripheral occlusive arterial disease-effects of pyridoxine and folic acid treatment, *Atherosclerosis*, 81, 51, 1990.
22. **Andersson, A., Brattström, L., Israelsson, B., Isaksson, A., Hultberg, B.,** The effect of excess daily methionine intake on plasma homocysteine after a methionine loading test in humans, *Clin. Chim. Acta*, 192, 69, 1990.
23. **Boers, G. H. J., Smals, A. G. H., Trijbels, F. J. M., Fowler, B., Bakkeren, J. A. J. M., Schoonderwaldt, H. C., Kleijer, W. J., Kloppenborg, P. W. C.,** Heterozygosity for homocystinuria in premature peripheral and cerebral occlusive arterial disease, *N. Engl. J. Med.*, 313, 709, 1985.
24. **Murphy-Chutorian, D. R., Wexman, M. P., Grieco, A. J., Heininger, J. A., Glassman, E., Gaull, G. E., NG, S. K. C., Feit, F., Wexman, K., Fox, A.C.,** Methionine intolerance: a possible risk factor for coronary artery disease, *J. Am. Coll. Cardiol.*, 6, 725, 1985.
25. **Skovby, F.,** Homocystinuria: clinical, biochemical and genetic aspects of cystathionine β−synthase deficiency in man, *Acta Pediatr. Scand.*, Suppl 321, 1985.
26. **Boers, G. H. J., Smals, A. G. H., Drayer, J. I. M., Trijbels, F. J. M., Leermakers, A. I., Kloppenborg, P. W.,** Pyridoxine treatment does not prevent homocystinemia after methionine loading in adult homocystinuria patients, *Metabolism*, 32, 390, 1983.
27. **Wilcken, B., Turner, G.,** Homocystinuria in New South Wales, *Arch. Dis. Child.*, 53, 242, 1978.
28. **Mudd, S. H., Uhlendorf, B. W., Freeman, J. M., Finkelstein, J. D., Shih, V. E.,** Homocystinuria associated with decreased methylenetetrahydrofolate reductase activity, *Biochem. Biophys. Res. Commun.*, 46, 905, 1972.
29. Recently described defects in vitamin B12 metabolism. *Nutr. Rev.*, 44, 236, 1986.
30. **Cooper, B. A., Rosenblatt, D. S.,** Inherited defects of vitamin B12 metabolism, *Annu. Rev. Nutr.*, 7, 291, 1987.
31. **Kang, S. S., Zhou, J., Wong, P. W. K., Kowalisyn, J., Strokosch, G.,** Intemediate homocysteinemia: a thermolabile variant of methylenetetrahydrofolate reductase, *Am. J. Hum. Genet.*, 43, 414, 1988.

32. **Kang, S. S., Wong, P. W. K., Bock, H. G. O., Horwitz, A., Grix, A.**, Intermediate hyperhomocysteinemia resulting from compound heterozygosity of methylenetetrahydrofolate reductase mutations, *Am. J. Hum. Genet.*, 48, 546, 1991.

33. **Kang, S. S., Passen, E. L., Ruggie, N., Wong, P. W. K., Sora, H.**, Thermolabile defect of methylenetetrahydrofolate reductase in coronary artery disease, *Circulation*, 88, 1463, 1993.

34. **Vonsattel, J. P. G., Hedley-Whyte, E. T.**, Homocystinuria, in *Handbook of Clinical Neurology* Vol 11 (55): Vascular Disease, Part III, Toole, J.F., Ed., Elsevier Science Publishers, New York, 1989, 325.

35. **Newman, G., Mitchell, J. R. A.**, Homocystinuria presenting as multiple arterial occlusions, *Q. J. Med.*, 210, 251, 1984.

36. **Monreal, M., Callejas, J. M., Martorell, A., Silveira, P., Gallego, M., Lafoz, E., Casals, A.**, Occlusive arterial disease as a form of presentation of homocystinuria, *J. Cardiovasc. Surg.*, 32, 137, 1991.

37. **Cochran, F. B., Packman, S.**, Homocystinuria presenting as sagittal sinus thrombosis, *Eur. Neurol.*, 32, 1, 1992.

38. **Carson, N. A. J., Dent, C. E., Field, C. M. B., Gaull, G. E.**, Homocystinuria clinical and pathological review of ten cases, *J. Pediatr.*, 66, 565, 1965.

39. **Schimke, R. N., McKusick, V. A., Huang, T., Pollack, A. D.**, Homocystinuria, *JAMA*, 193, 711, 1965.

40. **Schulman, J. D., Agarwal, B., Mudd, S. H., Shulman, N. R.**, Pulmonary embolism in a homocystinuric patient during treatment with dipyridamol and acetylsalicylic acid, *N. Engl. J. Med.*, 299, 661, 1978.

41. **Palareti, G., Coccheri, S.**, Lowered antithrombin-III activity and other clotting changes in homocystinuria - Effects of a pyridoxine-folate regimen, *Haemostasis*, 19 (Suppl. 1), 24, 1989.

42. **Gibson, J. B., Carson, N. A. J., Neill, D. W.**, Pathological findings in homocystinuria, *J. Clin. Pathol.*, 17, 427, 1964.

43. **McDonald, L., Bray, C., Field, C., Love, F.**, Homocystinuria, thrombosis and the blood-platelets, *Lancet*, 1, 745, 1964.

44. **Hopkins, I., Townley, R. R. W., Shipman, R. T.**, Cerebral thrombosis in a patient with homocystinuria, *J. Pediatr.*, 75, 1082, 1969.

45. **Saeed, M., Cohan, R. H., German, D. C., McCann, R. L., Dunnick, N. R.**, Vascular injury and thromboembolism in a young woman, *Invest. Radiol.*, 22, 62, 1987.

46. **Zimmerman, R., Sherry, R. G., Elwood, J. C., Gardner, L.I., Streeten, B.W., Levinsohn, E. M., Markarian, B.**, Vascular thrombosis and homocystinuria, *Am. J. Radiol.*, 148, 953, 1987.

47. **Carey, M. C., Donovan, D. E., Fitzgerald, O., McAuley, F. D.**, Homocystinuria: a clinical and pathological study of nine subjects in six families, *Am. J. Med.*, 45, 7, 1968.

48. **Cusworth, D. C., Dent, C. E.**, Homocystinuria, *Br. Med. Bull.*, 25, 42, 1969.

49. **Almgren, B., Eriksson, I., Hemmingsson, A., Hillerdal, G., Larsson, E., Aberg, H.**, Abdominal aortic aneurysm in homocystinuria, *Acta Chir. Scand.*, 144, 545, 1978.

50. **Palareti, G., Salardi, S., Piazzi, S., Legnani, C., Poggi, M., Grauso, F., Caniato, A., Coccheri, S.**, Blood coagulation changes in homocystinuria: effects of pyridoxine and other specific therapy, *J. Pediatr.*, 109, 1101, 1986.

51. **Rubba, P., Faccenda, F., Pauciullo, P., Carbone, L., Mancini, M., Strisciuglio, P., Carrozzo, R., Sartorio, R., Delgiudice, E., Andria, G.**, Early signs of vascular disease in homocystinuria - A noninvasive study by ultrasound methods in eight families with cystathionine-beta-synthase deficiency, *Metabolism*, 39, 1191, 1990.

52. **James, T. N., Carson, N. A. J., Froggatt, P.**, Coronary vessels and conduction system in homocystinuria, *Circulation*, 49, 367, 1974.

53. **Kanwar, Y. S., Manaligod, J. R., Wong, P. W. K.**, Morphologic studies in a patient with homocystinuria due to 5,10-methylenetetrahydrofolate reductase deficiency, *Pediatr. Res.*, 10, 598, 1976.

54. **Wong, P. W. K., Justice, P., Hruby, M., Weiss, E. B., Diamond, E.**, Folic acid nonresponsive homocystinuria due to methylenetetrahydrofolate reductase deficiency, *Pediatrics*, 59, 749, 1977.

55. **Baumgartner, R., Wick, H., Ohnacker, H., Probst, A., Maurer, R.**, Vascular lesions in two patients with congenital homocystinuria due to different defects of remethylation. *J. Inherited Metab. Dis.*, 3, 101, 1980.

56. **Haan, E. A., Rodgers, J. G., Lewis, G. P., Rowe, P. B.**, 5,10- methylenetetrahydrofolate reductase deficiency. Clinical and biochemical features of a further case, *J. Inherited Metab. Dis.*, 8, 53, 1985.

57. **Brandstetter, Y., Weinhouse, E., Splaingard, M. L., Tang, T. T.**, Cor pulmonale as a complication of methylmalonic acidemia and homocystinuria (Cbl-C-type), *Am. J. Hum. Genet.*, 36, 167, 1990.

58. **Visy, J. M., Lecoz, P., Chadefaux, B., Fressinaud, C., Woimant, F., Marquet, J., Zittoun, J., Visy, J., Vallat, J. M., Haguenau, M.**, Homocystinuria due to 5,10-methylenetetrahydrofolate reductase deficiency revealed by stroke in adult siblings, *Neurology*, 41, 1313, 1991.

59. **Wiley, V. C., Dudman, N. P. B., Wilcken, D. E. L.**, Interrelations between plasma free and protein-bound homocysteine and cysteine in homocystinuria, *Metabolism*, 37, 191, 1988.

60. **Brattström, L., Israelsson, B., LindgÑrde, F., Hultberg, B.**, Higher total plasma homocysteine in vitamin B12 deficiency than in heterozygosity for homocystinuria due to cystathionine -synthase deficiency, *Metabolism*, 37, 175, 1988.

61. **McGill, J. J., Mettler, G., Rosenblatt, D. S., Scriver, C. R.**, Detection of heterozygotes for recessive alleles. Homocyst(e)inemia: paradigm of pitfalls in phenotypes, *Am. J. Med. Genet.*, 36, 45, 1990.

62. **Brattström, L., Israelsson, B., Hultberg, B.**, Plasma homocysteine and methionine tolerance in early-onset vascular disease, *Haemostasis*, 19 (Suppl. 1), 35, 1989.

63. **Andersson, A., Brattström, L., Israelsson, B., Isaksson, A., Hamfelt, A., Hultberg, B.**, Plasma homocysteine before and after methionine loading with regard to age, gender, and menopausal status, *Eur. J. Clin. Invest.*, 22, 79, 1992.

64. **Brattström, L. E., Hultberg, B. L., Hardebo, J. E.**, Folic acid responsive postmenopausal homocysteinemia, *Metabolism*, 34, 1073, 1985.

65. **Boers, G. H., Smals, A. G., Trijbels, F. J., Leermakers, A. I., Kloppenborg, P. W.**, Unique efficiency of methionine metabolism in premenopausal women may protect against vascular disease in the reproduction years, *J. Clin. Invest.*, 72, 1971, 1983.

66. **Nordstrom, M., Kjellstrom, T.**, Age dependency of cystathionine beta-synthase activity in human fibroblasts in homocyst(e)inemia and atherosclerotic vascular disease, *Atherosclerosis*, 94, 213, 1992.

67. **Kang, S. S., Wong, P. W. K., Norusis. M.**, Homocysteinemia due to folate deficiency, *Metabolism*, 36, 458, 1987.

68. **Pennypacker, L. C., Allen, R. H., Kelly, J. P., Matthews, L. M., Grigsby, J., Kaye, K., Lindenbaum, J., Stabler, S. P.**, High prevalence of cobalamin deficiency in elderly outpatients, *J. Am. Geriatr. Soc.*, 40, 1197, 1992.

69. **Ueland, P. M., Refsum, H., Brattström, L.**, Plasma homocysteine and cardiovascular disease, in *Atherosclerotic cardiovascular disease, hemostasis, and endothelial function*, Francis, R.B., Ed., Marcel Dekker Inc., New York, 1992, 183.

70. **Joosten, E., Vandenberg, A., Riezler, R., Naurath, H. J., Lindenbaum, J., Stabler, S. P., Allen, R. H.**, Metabolic evidence that deficiencies of vitamin-B12 (cobalamin), folate, and vitamin-B-6 occur commonly in elderly people, *Am. J. Clin. Nutr.*, 58, 468, 1993.

71. **Wilcken, D. E. L., Gupta, V. J., Reddy, S. G.**, Accumulation of sulphur-containing amino acids including cysteine-homocysteine in patients on maintenance haemodialysis, *Clin. Sci.*, 58, 427, 1980.

72. **Chauveau, P., Chadefaux, B., Coude, M., Aupetit, J., Hannedouche, T., Kamoun, P., Jungers, P.**, Hyperhomocysteinemia, a risk factor for atherosclerosis in chronic uremic patients, *Kidney Int.*, 43, S72, 1993.

73. **Curtis, D., Sparrow, R., Brennan, L., Vanderweyden, M. B.**, Elevated serum homocysteine as a predictor for vitamin B-12 or folate deficiency, *Eur. J. Haematol.*, 52, 227, 1994.

74. **Kaladelfos, G., Edwards, K. D. G**, Increased prevalence of coronary heart disease in analgesic nephropathy: relation of hypertension, hypertriglyceridemia and combined hyperlipidemia, *Nephron*, 16, 388, 1976.

75. **Wilcken, D. E. L., Dudman, N. P. B., Tyrrell, P. A., Robertson, M. R.**, Folic acid lowers elevated plasma homocysteine in chronic renal insufficiency: possible implications for prevention of vascular disease, *Metabolism*, 37, 697, 1988.

76. **Araki, A., Sako, Y., Ito, H.**, Plasma homocysteine concentrations in Japanese patients with non-insulin-dependent diabetes mellitus - Effect of parenteral methylcobalamin treatment, *Atherosclerosis*, 103, 149, 1993.

77. **Hultberg, B., Berglund, M., Andersson, A., Frank, A.**, Elevated plasma homocysteine in alcoholics, *Alcoholism*, 17, 687, 1993.

78. **Wilcken, D. E. L., Wilcken, B.**, The pathogenesis of coronary artery disease. A possible role for methionine metabolism, *J. Clin. Invest.*, 57, 1079, 1976.

79. **Stampfer, M. J., Malinow, M. R., Willett, W. C., Newcomer, L. M., Upson, B., Ullmann, D., Tishler, P. V., Hennekens, C. H.**, A prospective study of plasma homocyst(e)ine and risk of myocardial infarction in United States physicians, *JAMA*, 268, 877, 1992.

80. **Wilcken, D. E. L., Reddy, S. G., Gupta, V. J.**, Homocysteinemia, ischemic heart disease, and the carrier state for homocystinuria, *Metabolism*, 32, 363, 1983.

81. **Boers, G. H. J.**, Carriership for homocystinuria in juvenile vascular disease, *Haemostasis*, 19 (Suppl. 1), 29, 1989.

82. **Kang, S. S., Wong, P. W. K., Cook, H. Y., Norusis, M., Messer, J. V.**, Protein-bound homocyst(e)ine. A possible risk for coronary artery disease, *J. Clin. Invest.*, 77, 1482, 1986.

83. **Israelsson, B., Brattström, L. E., Hultberg, B. L.**, Homocysteine and myocardial infarction, *Atherosclerosis*, 71, 227, 1988.

84. **Malinow, R. R., Sexton, G., Averbuch, M., Grossman, M., Wilson, D. L., Upson, B.**, Homocyst(e)inemia in daily practice: levels of coronary heart disease, *Coronary Artery Dis.*, 1, 215, 1990.

85. **Clarke, R., Daly, L., Robinson, K., Naughten, E., Cahalane, S., Fowler, B., Graham, I.**, Hyperhomocysteinemia - An independent risk factor for vascular disease, *N. Engl. J. Med.*, 324, 1149, 1991.

86. **Genest, J. J., Mcnamara, J. R., Upson, B., Salem, D. N., Ordovas, J. M., Schaefer, E. J., Malinow, M. R.**, Prevalence of familial hyperhomocyst(e)inemia in men with premature coronary artery disease, *Arterioscler. Thromb.*, 11, 1129, 1991.

87. **Ubbink, J. B., Vermaak, W. J. H., Bennett, J. M., Becker, P. J., Vanstaden, D. A., Bissbort, S.**, The prevalence of homocysteinemia and hypercholesterolemia in angiographically defined coronary heart disease, *Klinische Wochenschrift*, 69, 527, 1991.

88. **Williams, R. R., Malinow, M. R., Hunt, S. C.**, Hyperhomocyst(e)inemia in Utah siblings with early coronary disease, *Coronary Artery Dis.*, 1, 681, 1991.

89. **Dudman, N. P. B., Wilcken, D. E. L., Wang, J., Lynch, J. F., Macey, D., Lundberg, P.**, Disordered methionine homocysteine metabolism in premature vascular disease - Its occurrence, cofactor therapy, and enzymology, *Arterioscler. Thromb.*, 13, 1253, 1993.

90. **Murphy Chutorian, D., Alderman, E. L.**, The case that hyperhomocysteinemia is a risk factor for coronary artery disease, *Am. J. Cardiol.*, 73, 705, 1994.

91. **Pancharuniti, N., Lewis, C. A., Sauberlich, H. E., Perkins, L. L., Go, R. C. P., Alvarez, J. O., Macaluso, M., Acton, R. T., Copeland, R. B., Cousins, A. L., Gore, T. B., Cornwell, P. E., Roseman, J. M.**, Plasma homocyst(e)ine, folate, and vitamin-B12 concentrations and risk for early-onset coronary artery disease, *Am. J. Clin. Nutr.*, 59, 940, 1994.

92. **Voneckardstein, A., Malinow, M. R., Upson, B., Heinrich, J., Schulte, H., Schonfeld, R., Kohler, E., Assmann, G.**, Effects of age, lipoproteins, and hemostatic parameters on the role of homocyst(e)inemia as a cardiovascular risk factor in men, *Arterioscler. Thromb.*, 14, 460, 1994.

93. **Wu, L. L., Wu, J., Hunt, S. C., James, B.C., Vincent, G.M., Williams, R. R., Hopkins, P.N.**, Plasma homocyst(e)ine as a risk factor for early familial coronary artery disease, *Clin. Chem.*, 40, 552, 1994.

94. **Brattström. L. E., Hardebo, J. E., Hultberg, B. L.**, Moderate homocysteinemia - A possible risk factor for arteriosclerotic cerebrovascular disease, *Stroke*, 15, 1012, 1984.

95. **Araki, A., Sako, Y., Fukushima, Y., Matsumoto, M., Asada, T., Kita, T.**, Plasma sulfhydryl-containing amino acids in patients with cerebral infarction and in hypertensive subjects, *Atherosclerosis*, 79, 139, 1989.

96. **Coull, B. M., Malinow, M. R., Beamer, N., Sexton, G., Nordt, F., Degarmo, P.**, Elevated plasma homocyst(e)ine concentration as a possible independent risk factor for stroke, *Stroke*, 21, 572, 1990.

97. **Mereau Richard, C., Muller, J. P., Faivre, E., Ardouin, P., Rousseaux, J.**, Total plasma homocysteine determination in subjects with premature cerebral vascular disease [letter], *Clin. Chem.*, 37, 126, 1991.

98. **Brattström, L., Lindgren, A., Israelsson, B., Malinow, M. R., Norrving, B., Upson, B., Hamfelt, A.**, Hyperhomocysteinaemia in stroke - Prevalence, cause, and relationships to type of stroke and stroke risk factors, *Eur. J. Clin. Invest.*, 22, 214, 1992.

99. **Giroud, M., Grosmaire, N., Lemesle, M., Gras, P., Vion, P., Desgres, J., Dumas, R.**, Hyperhomocysteinaemia as a risk factor for cerebral infarction, *Presse Med.*, 22, 35, 1993.

100. **Malinow, M. R., Nieto, F. J., Szklo, M., Chambless, L. E., Bond, G.**, Carotid artery intimal-medial wall thickening and plasma homocyst(e)ine in asymptomatic adults - The atherosclerosis risk in communities study, *Circulation*, 87, 1107, 1993.

101. **Franken, D. G., Boers, G. H. J., Blom, H. J., Trijbels, F. J. M., Kloppenborg, P. W. C.**, Treatment of mild hyperhomocysteinemia in vascular disease patients, *Arterioscler. Thromb.*, 14, 465, 1994.

102. **Malinow, M. R., Kang, S. S., Taylor, L. M., Wong, P. W., Coull, B., Inahara, T., Mukerjee, D., Sexton, G., Upson, B.**, Prevalence of hyperhomocyst(e)inemia in patients with peripheral arterial occlusive disease, *Circulation*, 79, 1180, 1989.

103.   **Taylor, L. M., Defrang, R. D., Harris, E. J., Porter, J. M.,** The association of elevated plasma homocyst(e)ine with progression of symptomatic peripheral arterial disease, *J. Vasc. Surg.*, 13, 128, 1991.

104.   **Molgaard, J., Malinow, M. R., Lassvik, C., Holm, A. C., Upson, B., Olsson, A. G.,** Hyperhomocyst(e)inaemia - An independent risk factor for intermittent claudication, *J. Intern. Med.*, 231, 273, 1992.

105.   **Bergmark, C., Mansoor, M. A., Swedenborg, J., de Faire, U., Svardal, A. M., Ueland, P. M.,** Hyperhomocysteinemia in patients operated for lower extremity ischaemia below the age of 50 - Effect of smoking and extent of disease, *Eur. J. Vasc. Surg.*, 7, 391, 1993.

106.   **Brattström, L., Tengborn, L., Lagerstedt, C., Israelsson, B., Hultberg, B.,** Plasma homocysteine in venous thromboembolism, *Haemostasis*, 21, 51, 1991.

107.   **Bienvenu, T., Ankri, A., Chadefaux, B., Montalescot, G., Kamoun, P.,** Elevated total plasma homocysteine, a risk factor for thrombosis - Relation to coagulation and fibrinolytic parameters, *Thromb. Res.*, 70, 123, 1993.

108.   **David, J. L., Schoos, R. R.,** Homocysteine and venous thromboembolism, *Thromb. Haemost.*, 69, 619 (Abstract 272), 1993.

109.   **Vigano' D'Angelo, S., Fermo, I., Paroni, R., Crippa, L., D'Angelo, A.,** Total plasma homocyst(e)ine in young patients with venous thromboembolic disease, *Thromb. Haemost.*, 69, 625 (Abstract 295), 1993.

110.   **Wenzler, E. M., Rademakers, A. J. J. M., Boers, G. H. J., Cruysberg, J. R. M., Webers, C. A. B., Deutman, A. F.,** Hyperhomocysteinemia in retinal artery and retinal vein occlusion, *Am. J. Ophthalmol.*, 115, 162, 1993.

111.   **Falcon, C. R., Cattaneo, M., Panzeri D., Martinelli, I., Mannucci, P.M.,** High prevalence of hyperhomocyst(e)inemia in patients with juvenile venous thrombosis, *Arterioscler. Thromb.*, 14, 1080, 1994.

112.   **Wilcken, D. E. L., Dudman, N. P. B.,** Mechanisms of thrombogenesis and accelerated atherogenesis in homocysteinaemia, *Haemostasis*, 19 (Suppl. 1), 14, 1989.

113.   **Kang, S. S., Wong, P. W. K., Malinow, M. R.,** Hyperhomocyst(e)inemia as a risk factor for occlusive vascular disease, *Annu. Rev. Nutr.*, 12, 279, 1992.

114.   **Rees, M. M., Rodgers, G. M.,** Homocysteinemia - Association of a metabolic disorder with vascular disease and thrombosis, *Thromb. Res.*, 71, 337, 1993.

115.   **Harker, L. A., Slichter, S. J., Scott, C. R., Ross, R.,** Homocystinemia, vascular injury and arterial thrombosis, *N. Engl. J. Med.*, 291, 537, 1974.

116.   **Harker, L. A., Ross, R., Slichter, S. J., Scott, C. R.,** The role of endothelial cell injury and platelet response in its genesis, *J. Clin. Invest.*, 58, 731, 1976.

117.   **Shane, B.,** Vitamin B12 folate interrelationships, *Annu. Rev. Nutr.*, 5, 115, 1985.

118.   **Jencks, D. A., Matthews, R. G.,** Allosteric inhibition of methylenetetrahydrofolate reductase by adenosylmethionine. Effects of adenosylmethionine and NADPH on the equilibrium between active and inactive forms of the enzyme and on the kinetics of approach to equilibrium, *J. Biol. Chem.*, 262, 2485, 1987.

119.   **Smolin, L. A., Benevenga, N. J., Berlow, S.,** The use of betaine for the treatment of homocystinuria, *J. Pediatr.*, 99, 467, 1981.

120.   **Wall, R. T., Harlan, J. M., Harker, L. A., Striker, G. E.,** Homocysteine-induced endothelial cell injury in vitro: a model for the study of vascular injury, *Thromb. Res.*, 18, 113, 1980.

121.   **Dudman, N. P. B., Hicks, C., Lynch, J. F., Wilcken, D. E. L., Wang, J.,** Homocysteine thiolactone disposal by human arterial endothelial cells and serum invitro, *Arterioscler. Thromb.*, 11, 663, 1991.

122.   **Degroot, P. J., Willems, C., Boers, G. H. J., Gonsalves, M. D., Van Aken, W. G., and Van Mourik, J. A.,** Endothelial cell dysfunction in homocystinuria, *Eur. J. Clin. Invest.*, 13, 405, 1983.

123.   **Starkebaum, G., and Harlan, J. M.,** Endothelial cell injury due to copper-catalyzed hydrogen peroxide generation from homocysteine, *J. Clin. Invest.*, 77, 1370, 1986.

124.   **Rodgers, G. M., Conn, M. T.,** Homocysteine, an atherogenic stimulus, reduces protein C activation by arterial and venous endothelial cells, *Blood*, 75, 895, 1990.

125.   **Lentz, S. R., Sadler, J. E.,** Inhibition of thrombomodulin surface expression and protein-C activation by the thrombogenic agent homocysteine, *J. Clin. Invest.*, 88, 1906, 1991.

126.   **Hayashi, T., Honda, G., Suzuki, K.,** An atherogenic stimulus homocysteine inhibits cofactor activity of thrombomodulin and enhances thrombomodulin expression in human umbilical vein endothelial cells, *Blood*, 79, 2930, 1992.

127.   **Rodgers, G. M., Kane, W. H.,** Activation of endogenous factor V by a homocysteine-induced vascular endothelial cell activator, *J. Clin. Invest.*, 77, 1909, 1986.

128.   **Blann, A. D.,** Endothelial cell damage and homocysteine, *Atherosclerosis*, 94, 89, 1992.

129.   **Fryer, R. H., Wilson, B. D., Gubler, D. B., Fitzgerald, L. A., Rodgers, G. M.,** Homocysteine, a risk factor for premature vascular disease and thrombosis, induces tissue factor activity in endothelial cells, *Arterioscler. Thromb.*, 13, 1327, 1993.

130.   **Stamler, J. S., Osborne, J. A., Jaraki, O., Rabbani, L. E., Mullins, M., Singel, D., Loscalzo, J.,** Adverse vascular effects of homocysteine are modulated by endothelium-derived relaxing factor and related oxides of nitrogen, *J. Clin. Invest.*, 91, 308, 1993.

131.   **Merckx, J., Kuntz, F.,** Deficit en facteur VII et homocystinurie. Association fortuite ou syndrome ?, *Nouv. Presse Med.*, 46, 3796, 1981.

132.   **Charlot, J. C., Haye, C., Chaumien, J.P., Merckx, J. J., Jacob, H.,** Homocystinurie et deficit en facteur VII, *Bull. Soc. Opht. France*, 6-7 (LXXXII), 787, 1982.

133.   **Munnich, A., Saudubray, J. M., Dautzenberg, M. D., Parvy, P., Ogier, H., Girot, R., Manigne, P., Frezal, J.,** Diet-responsive proconvertin (Factor VII) deficiency in homocystinuria, *J. Pediatr.*, 102, 730, 1983.

134.   **Ben Dridi, M. F., Karoui, S., Kastally, R., Gharbi, H. A., Zaimi, I., Ben Osman, R.,** L'homocystinurie, *Arch. Fr. Pediat.*, 43, 41, 1986.

135.   **Hilden, M., Brandt, N. J., Nilsson, M., Schonheyder, F.,** Investigations of coagulation and fibrinolysis in homocystinuria, *Acta Med. Scand.*, 195, 533, 1974.

136.   **Giannini, M. J., Coleman, M., Innerfield, I.,** Antithrombin activity in homocystinuria, *Lancet*, i, 1094, 1975.

137.   **Maruyama, I., Fukuda, R., Kazama, M., Abe, T., Yoshida, Y., Igata, A.,** A case of homocystinuria with low antithrombin activity, *Acta Haem. Jap.*, 40, 267, 1977.

138.   **Gershwin, M. E., Gude, J. K.,** Deep vein thrombosis and pulmonary embolism in congenital factor VII deficiency, *N. Engl. J. Med.*, 288, 141, 1973.

139.   **Shifter, T., Machtey, I., Creter, D.,** Thromboembolism in congenital factor VII deficiency, *Acta Haematol.*, 71, 60, 1984.

140. **Harker, L. A., Scott, C. R.**, Platelets in homocystinuria, *N. Engl. J. Med.*, 296, 818, 1977.

141. **Uhlemann, E. R., TenPas, J. H., Lucky, A. W., Schulman, J. D., Mudd, S. H., Shulman, N. R.**, Platelet survival and morphology in homocystinuria due to cystathionine synthase deficiency, *N. Engl. J. Med.*, 295, 1283, 1976.

142. **Hill-Zobel, R. L., Pyeritz, R.E., Scheffel, U., Malpica, O., Engin, S., Camargo, E. E., Abbott, M., Gutlarte, T. R., Hill, J., McIntyre, P. A., Murhpy, E. A., Tsan, M. F.**, Kinetics and distribution of indium-labeled platelets in patients with homocystinuria, *N. Engl. J. Med.*, 307, 781, 1982.

143. **Di Minno, G., Davi, G., Margaglione, M., Cirillo, F., Grandone, E., Ciabattoni, G., Catalano, I., Strisciuglio, P., Andria, G., Patrono, C., Mancini, M.**, Abnormally high thromboxane biosynthesis in homozygous homocystinuria - Evidence for platelet involvement and probucol-sensitive mechanism, *J. Clin. Invest.*, 92, 1400, 1993.

144. **Harpel, P. C., Chang, V. T., Borth, W.**, Homocysteine and other sulfhydryl compounds enhance the binding of lipoprotein(a) to fibrin - A potential biochemical link between thrombosis, atherogenesis, and sulfhydryl compound metabolism, *Proc. Natl. Acad. Sci. USA*, 89, 10193, 1992.

145. **Schuh, S., Rosenblatt, D. S., Cooper, B. A., Schroeder, M. L., Bishop, A. J., Seargeant, L. E., Haworth, J. C.**, Homocystinuria and megaloblastic anemia responsive to vitamin B12 therapy. An inborn error of metabolism due to a defect in cobalamin metabolism, *N. Engl. J. Med.*, 310, 686, 1984.

146. **Morrow III, G., Barnes, L. A.**, Combined vitamin responsiveness in homocystinuria, *J. Pediatr.*, 81, 946, 1972.

147. **Wilcken, D. E. L., Wilcken, B., Dudman, N. P. B., Tyrrel, P.A.**, Homocystinuria - The effects of betaine in the treatment of patients not responsive to pyridoxine, *N. Engl. J. Med.*, 309, 448, 1983.

148. **Kang, S.S., Wong, P.W.K., Susmano, A., Sora, J., Norusis, M., Ruggie, N.**, Thermolabile methylenetetrahydrofolate reductase - An inherited risk factor for coronary artery disease, *Am. J. Hum. Genet.*, 48, 536, 1991.

149. **Brattström, L. E., Israelsson, B., Jeppsson, J. O., Hultberg, B. L.**, Folic acid - An innocuous means to reduce plasma homocysteine, *Scand. J. Clin. Lab. Invest.*, 48, 215, 1988.

150. **Olszewski, A.J.**, Homocysteine content of plasma in ischemic heart disease, the reducing effect of pyridoxine, folate, cobalamin, choline, riboflavin and troxerutin - Correction of a calculation error, *Atherosclerosis*, 88, 97, 1991.

151. **Franken, D. G., Boers, G. H. J., Blom, H. J., Trjbels, J. M. F.**, Effect of various regimens of vitamin B6 and folic acid on mild hyperhomocysteinaemia in vascular patients, *J. Inherited. Metab. Dis.*, 17, 159, 1994.

152. **Arnadottir, M., Brattström, L., Simonsen, O., Thysell, H., Hultberg, B., Andersson, A., Nilssonehle, P.**, The effect of high-dose pyridoxine and folic acid supplementation on serum lipid and plasma homocysteine concentrations in dialysis patients, *Clin. Nephrol.*, 40, 236, 1993.

153. **Ubbink, J. B., Vermaak, W. J. H., Vandermerwe, A., Becker, P. J.**, Vitamin-B-12, vitamin-B-6, and folate nutritional status in men with hyperhomocysteinemia, *Am. J. Clin. Nutr.*, 57, 47, 1993.

SICKLE CELL DISEASE

E. Verdy and R. Girot
Hématologie , Hôpital Tenon, Paris

I. INTRODUCTION

Sickle cell disease (SCD) is now considered by several authors as an hypercoagulable state.[1-3] This opinion is based on several observations : 1) true embolic events have been reported in patients suffering from stroke[4] and from pulmonary complications sometimes leading to death[5], or during pregnancy.[6] 2) biological markers of hypercoagulability in patients in steady state and/or suffering from acute pain crisis have been pointed out.[1-3,7,8] However, the clinical expression of the SCD differs clearly from the classical thromboembolic disease when considering the symptoms and their evolution, either spontaneously or under conventional therapy with or without anticoagulant treatment. This is particularly the case concerning the painful crisis, the main complication of SCD. The pathophysiology of the crisis is complex and the very term to designate it, "vascular occlusion", means that nobody knows exactly the respective participation of sickled red cells, vessels and the different components of hemostatic system in the genesis of the symptoms

In this paper, we shall look on successively, 1) the molecular and cellular aspects of the pathophysiology of SCD ; 2) the sickle cell adhesion to endothelium and blood vessels abnormalities ; 3) the abnormalities of platelets, coagulation and fibrinolysis and their possible role in the pathophysiology of the disease.

II. MOLECULAR AND CELLULAR ASPECTS OF THE PATHOPHYSIOLOGY OF SCD

SCD is an autosomal genetic disorder resulting from the mutation of the sixth codon of β globin gene. In the abnormal β chain (βS) a valine replaces a glutamic acid (β Glu ==> Val). This chain combines with α-chains to give hemoglobin S (HbS). The main characteristic of HbS molecules is their ability to form polymers in the red cell under deoxygenated condition. Deoxy HbS molecules have a markedly reduced solubility in comparison with oxyHbS molecules. The reduction in solubility induces the polymer fibres within the erythrocyte upon deoxygenation. This polymerisation has been studied "in vitro", in solution of HbS or "in vivo" directly within the cell.[9] Several factors influence the formation of the polymer. The mean cell hemoglobin concentration (MCHC) is one of these critical factors : a high concentration increases the polymer formation, and, on the contrary a low hemoglobin concentration reduces it. Thus, α thalassemia, a very common genetic disorder which decreases MCHC and which is frequently associated with SCD in concerned populations, has a tendency to reduce the polymerisation. Another important factor is hemoglobin F (HbF). This hemoglobin is much more soluble than HbS, even in the deoxy state, and does not enter the polymer. In fact, patients with a high proportion of HbF more than 40-50% of hemoglobin (for example, homozygous SS neonates or sickle cell subjects affected with a hereditary persistence of fetal hemoglobin) are protected against the complications of the disease.

The morphologic changes observed in the red blood cells of SCD patients are due to the polymerisation of HbS within the cell upon deoxygenation. At complete deoxygenation, the polymerisation leads to a morphological deformation and formation of classical sickled forms. The sickle erythrocytes are heterogeneous when considering their mean corpuscular volume, mean cell hemoglobin concentration, density and other biochemical properties. The variations in hemoglobin concentration are reflected in a wide spectrum of cell densities when sickle cells are fractionated on

0-8493-5804-3/96/$0.00+$.50

density gradients.[10] The dense cells are defined by MCHC > 37 g/dl and are considered as deleterious in the circulation. The percentage of dense cells is very different according to the patients (8-40%) and is thought to be a factor of prognosis of the disease.[11] Amongst the various properties of sickle erythrocytes, certain modifications concern the rearrangement of phospholipids and will be studied in detail later (see below). Hemoglobin polymerisation and sickle cell formation are reversible phenomena. However, after repeated cycles of HbS polymerisation-depolymerisation, the sickle erythrocytes remain permanently deformed (irreversible sickle cells - ISCs). ISCs are found predominantly in the dense cell fraction.

The main rheological abnormalities in SCD are a permanent increase of blood viscosity due to a decrease of blood cell deformability. This fact stems from several factors, mainly hematocrit : a low hematocrit (< 20%) decreases its intensity.[12] It has been shown that the many cell populations have different rheological properties. The denser the cells are, the higher their viscosity, and this viscosity is clearly dependent of the number of ISCs.[13]

III. SICKLE CELL ADHESION TO ENDOTHELIUM AND BLOOD VESSEL ABNORMALITIES

A . SICKLE CELL ADHESION TO ENDOTHELIUM

In 1980, HEBBELL et al[14] had shown that sickle erythrocytes adhere to endothelium in cell cultures. This initial feature was confirmed later by other authors in different experimental conditions as perfusion studies in animals.[15-18] It has been shown that oxygenated sickle erythrocytes pass correctly through the microvasculature, but that deoxygenated cells and ISCs can cause obstruction of arterioles, capillaries and vessels, due to adherence of the cells to endothelium. It was established that as the cell density increases, so does their adherence. In the experimental work of KAUL et al,[19] it was demonstrated that the main site of microvasculature concerned with this adherence is the post-veinulary capillary endothelium. This adherence may induce a partial obstruction trapping other sickle dense erythrocytes causing a complete obstruction. The mechanisms of adherence were partially established. They involve both membrane modifications and environmental factors. Amongst red cell membrane modifications, the increased content of sialic acid in glycophorin and phosphatidylserine externalisation has been demonstrated as promoting factors of increased adhesivity in experimental conditions.[20] Regarding plasma proteins, several factors have been studied as potential agents for adhesivity. Fibrinogen and fibronectin can facilitate adherence.[21] Plasma von Willebrand factor (vWF) is a poor promotor to adhesion. High-molecular-weight vWF multimers do not increase adherence to human microvascular or umbilical vein endothelial cells in culture, but increase their adhesion to human arterial endothelial cells. Futhermore, it has been shown recently that the endothelial vascular cell adhesion molecule-1 (VCAM-1) and its ligand, the adhesion molecule VLA-4 expressed by sickle cell reticulocytes, were involved in adhesion to endothelium.[22]

B . BLOOD VESSEL ABNORMALITIES

For a long time, neurologic complications in SCD were thought to be due to vascular obstruction by sickle erythrocytes. Partial or complete stenosis of large cerebral arteries including carotids, anterior and middle cerebral, and vertebral arteries have been observed by angiography.[23] It was subsequently demonstrated that the abnormalities involve the vessel walls. Histological studies of the vessels showed an hyperplasia of the intima due to the proliferation of the fibroblasts and the smooth muscle cells, the destruction of the internal elastic lamina and the fibrosis in the media. Occlusion is the result of this vascular intimal hyperplasia, sometimes complicated by the formation of thrombus. These features demonstrate that all complications in SCD are not exclusively the consequence of microvascular occlusion, but also, the consequence of alterations involving large vessels of neck or cerebral arteries. The mechanisms of the arterial lesions are not known. We can suppose that adhesion of sickle erythrocytes in these regions and subsequent drawing of endothelial cells repeatedly expose the sub-endothelium to platelet adhesion, and perhaps other cells like the leucocytes. Platelets and leucocytes could release mitogenic and chemotactic factors inducing migration and proliferation of smooth muscle cells and fibroblasts. If the mechanism of vascular intimal hyperplasia is not exactly known, it has been clearly established that it is due to the regular perfusion of blood vessels by the sickle erythrocytes because long term transfusion therapy in patients affected with stroke has sometimes been efficient for reducing this abnormality.[24]

IV. ABNORMALITIES OF PLATELETS, COAGULATION AND FIBRINOLYSIS

Platelet, coagulation and fibrinolytic systems are modified in sickle cell disease and the abnormalities seem more important during sickle cell crisis.[1-3,25]

A. PLATELETS[7,8,26]

In the steady state, platelet number is often normal but moderate thrombocytosis, due to functional asplenia, appear in older children and adults in the steady state, while during a crisis, several reports notice a significant decrease in platelet number probably due to increased consumption.

Platelet functions varied according to age, state of disease and conditions in *in vitro* studies. Platelet aggregability appears to be normal in children and increased in adult during the steady state. This function has not been extensively investigated during the crisis : a discordance is observed i.e. normal or decreased aggregation. However, in steady state, since no modification of platelet aggregability is observed using washed platelets, an hyperaggregability is found when platelets are tested in whole blood that is closely related to *in vivo* conditions.

B. COAGULATION

Several coagulation factors have been reported to be modified in sickle cell disease either in the steady state or during crisis in the absence of hepatocellular disease.

The contact system protein levels are always found decreased in SS patients. This drop affects factor XII coagulant, factor XI, prekallikrein and high molecular weight kininogen and is more important during the crisis. Fibrinogen concentration is normal or slightly increased in the steady state while a significant rise is observed during the crisis. Factor VIII complex (factor VIII coagulant and factor von Willebrand) is increased in the steady state and during the crisis. Factor V, VII[27] and XIII may decrease.

Inhibitors of coagulation are more often found to decrease : Anti-thrombin III, Protein C and Protein S. Reduced free protein S is not linked to an increase of C4-binding protein.[28] The mean level of these proteins is sometimes equivalent to heterozygous protein hereditary deficiency. A significant reduction in plasma level of heparine cofactor II is also found.[29]

C. FIBRINOLYSIS

Components of the fibrinolysis have not yet been extensively studied. The euglobulin clot lysis time is reported longer in the steady state and shorter than in normal controls during the crisis but the global test of fibrinolysis is not specific for any component of the fibrinolytic system. Plasminogen, tissue plasminogen activator, plasminogen activator inhibitor have to be studied more to allow conclusions on fibrinolysis in SS disease.

D. BIOLOGICAL MARKERS OF THE ACTIVATION OF THE HEMOSTATIC SYSTEM

In SS disease, an increase of markers of platelet secretion[8,25] and of prothrombin and fibrinogen consumption[1-3] was observed in plasma of children and of adult patients.

Several markers of platelet secretion have been studied. The composants of α granules as β-thromboglobulin and platelet factor 4 are always increased in SS subjects but these modifications are perhaps artifactual *in vitro* release partly due to technical problems.[7,26] The release of dense granules as ADP and ATP seems more specific of *in vivo* platelet activation : a decrease of platelet ADP and a rise of total ATP/ADP ratio is observed during crisis while these two markers are stable during periods free of crisis.[8]

The presence of prothrombin fragments 1+2, thrombin-antithrombin III complexes and fibrinopeptides A are reflected the activation of coagulation since the positivity of the D Dimers gives evidence for the activation of fibrinolysis. An increase of these markers is observed in the steady state in adults and children and, in some reports, their levels are found higher during the crisis than during the steady state.[2,3]

V. POSSIBLE ROLE OF THE HEMOSTATIC SYSTEM IN THE PATHOPHYSIOLOGY OF THE DISEASE

The different modifications of the hemostatic system are concordant with an hypercoagulable state which is partly induced by sickle cells per se, but no data permit conclusion about the role of this "Hypercoagulable State" in the initiation or in the progression of vascular occlusion during the crisis. Nevertheless, this hypercoagulability might promote thrombosis when another situation at risk of thrombosis is associated as for example, in pregnant women.[6]

The pathogenesis of the hypercoagulable state and thrombotic events in SCD is not clearly understood but several mechanisms might be evoked involving sickle erythrocytes, endothelial cells, sub-endothelium and platelets.

1 - The membrane phospholipids of SS cells have lost their asymmetrical configuration which prevents the abnormal activation of the coagulation of the normal erythrocytes. In sickled cells, the outer membrane contains significant amounts of negatively charged amino phospholipids as phosphatidylserine and phosphatidyl-ethanolamine[20,30] which support procoagulant activity. The consequence of this abnormal lipid configuration on the hemostatic system could be explained by the shortening of clotting time using Russell viper venom[31] and enhanced activation of prothrombin by factor Xa in the presence of sickled cell in comparison with normal erythrocytes.[32] Furthermore, an imbalance in the inhibitor system is also linked to the decrease of the protein S concentration. This inhibitor has been reported absorbed to the membrane phospholipids and its decrease might be due to altered phospholipid asymmetry.[33] Thus, in *in vitro* conditions, sickled erythrocytes might enhance thrombin formation. Furthermore, this abnormal membrane phospholipid configuration might perhaps explain the frequent increase of antiphospholipid antibodies often associated with thrombotic events.

2 - An abnormal interaction between sickled cells and endothelial cells has been reported, perhaps due to the abnormal configuration of the phospholipids of the SS cells, and the enhanced erythrocyte adherence seems to correlate with the severity of the disease.[14] The adherent erythrocytes impede the blood flow which permits the process of deoxygenation-induced red cell sickling and, thus, the vascular occlusion. Moreover, these data have led to the hypothesis that SS cells induce an endothelial injury which may contribute to the vasocclusive crisis. In fact, the levels of circulating endothelial cells, a potent marker of endothelial injury, are significantly more increased during crisis than in the steady state.[34] This endothelial injury might lead to the release of cell components. One of them, the Willebrand factor, is a protein involved in adhesion of the platelets to the sub-endothelium.

3 - Adhesion of the platelets to the sub-endothelium initiates the different steps of the primary hemostasis which are potentiated by the increased concentration of the fibrinogen, a protein involved in the platelet aggregation. During this activation, the α granule components are released. The platelet-derived growth factor which stimulates the proliferation of the fibroblasts and smooth muscle cells might be responsible for the vascular stenosis (and consequently thrombosis) in neurologic complications.[23]

4 - Furthermore, tumor necrosis factor and interleukin 1 have been found frequently increased in patients suffering from SS disease even without inflammatory state.[35] These cytokines enhance endothelial adhesiveness, have a procoagulant effect since they increase the procoagulant properties and affect the anticoagulant properties of vascular endothelium.[36]

VI. CONCLUSION

The pathophysiology of SCD is complex. Several factors are involved, sickle erythrocytes, endothelial cells, vessel wall, leucocytes, platelets, plasma proteins including the hemostatic system and cytokines.

Interferences between these biological factors are not clearly understood and have to be further investigated to identify the role of each cellular and humoral component in the genesis of acute complications and/or chronic organ damage in SCD. Some complications are due to thrombotic phenomena, but others are not. In other words, SCD is not a thromboembolic disease "stricto sensu", but it appears to be a disease which can be complicated by thrombotic events. This is the reason why the biological markers of hypercoagulable state in this disease are of considerable interest because they draw attention to the hemostatic system and its potential role in the pathophysiology of SCD.

REFERENCES

1. **Francis, R. B.**, Platelets, coagulation, and fibrinolysis in sickle cell disease : their possible role in vascular occlusion, *Blood. Coag. Fib.*, 2, 341, 1991.
2. **Francis R. B.**, Elevated Fibrin D Dimer Fragment in Sickle cell anemia : Evidence for activation of coagulation during the steady state as well as in painful crisis, *Haemost.*, 19, 105, 1989.
3. **Peters M., Plaat B. E. C., ten Cate H., Wolters H. J., Weening R. S., Brandjes D. P. M.**, Enhanced thrombin generation in children with sickle cell disease, *Thromb. Haemost.*, 71, 169, 1994.
4. **Rothman S. M., Fulling K. H., Nelson J. S.**, Sickle cell anemia and central nervous system infarction : A neuropathological study, *Ann. Neurol.*, 20, 684, 1986.
5. **Thomas A. N., Patison C., Serjeant G. R.**, Causes of death in sickle cell disease in Jamaïca, *Br. Med. J.*, 285, 633, 1982.
6. **Koshy M., Burd L., Wallace D., Moawad A., Baron J.**, Prophylactic red-cell transfusions in pregnant patients with sickle cell disease. A randomized cooperative study, *N. Engl. J. Med.*, 319, 1447, 1988.
7. **Triadou P., Fonty E., Ambrosio A. S., Cottat M. C., Girot R., Cornu P.**, Platelet function in sickle cell disease during steady state, *Nouv. Rev. Fr. Hemat.*, 32, 137, 1990.
8. **Beurling-Harbury C., Schade S. G.**, Platelet activation during pain crisis in sickle cell anemia patients, *Am. J. Hemat.*, 31, 237, 1989.
9. **Hebbel R.P.**, Beyond hemoglobin polymerization : the red blood cell membrane and sickle cell pathophysiology, *Blood*, 77, 214, 1991.
10. **Rodgers G. P., Schechter A. N., Noguchi C.T.**, Cell heterogeneity in sickle cell disease. Quantitation of the erythrocyte density profile, *J. Lab. Clin. Med.*, 106, 30, 1985.
11. **Pajot N., Maier-Redelsperger M., Dode C., Labie D., Girot R.**, Density distribution of red cell and prognostic significance in 50 patients with homozygous sickle cell disease, *Hematologia*, 21, 189, 1988.
12. **Chien S.**, Rheology of sickle cells and erythrocyte content, *Blood Cells*, 3, 283, 1977.
13. **Ballas S. K.**, Sickle cell anemia with few painful crisis is characterized by decrease red cell deformability and increase number of dense cells, *Amer. J. Hematol.*, 36, 122, 1991.
14. **Hebbel R. P., Boogaerts M. A. B., Eaton W. A., Steinberg M. H.**, Erythrocytes adherence to endothelium. A possible determinant of disease severity, *N. Engl. J. Med.*, 302, 992, 1980.
15. **Baez S., Kaul D. K., Nagel R.L.**, Microvascular determinants of blood flow behavior and Hb SS erythrocyte plugging in the microcirculation, *Blood Cells*, 8, 127, 1982.
16. **Lipowsky H. H., Usami S., Chien S.**, Human SS red cell rheological behavior in the microcirculation of cremaster muscle, *Blood Cells*, 8, 113, 1982.
17. **Kaul D. K, Nagel R. L, Baez S.**, Pressure effects on the flow behavior of sickle (Hb SS) red cells in an isolated (ex vivo) microvascular system, *Microvasc. Res.*, 26, 170, 1983.
18. **Kurantsin-Mills J., Jacobs H. M., Klug P. P, Lessin L. S.**, Flow dynamics of human sickle erythrocytes in the mesenteric microcirculation of the exchange-transfused rat, *Microvasc. Res.*, 34, 152, 1987.
19. **Kaul D. K., Fabry M. E., Nagel R. L.**, Microvascular sites and characteristics of sickle cell adhesion to vascular endothelium in shear flow condition : pathophysiological implications, *Proc. Natl. Acad. Sci. USA*, 86, 3808, 1989.
20. **Schlegel R. A., Prendergast T. W., Williamson P.**, Membrane phospholipid asymmetry as a factor in erythrocyte-endothelial cell interactions, *J. Cell. Physiol.*, 123, 215, 1985.
21. **Mohandas N., Evans E.**, Adherence of sickle erythrocytes to vascular endothelial cells : requirement for both cell membrane changes and plasma factors, *Blood*, 64, 282, 1984.
22. **Gee B.E., Platt O.S.**, Sickle reticulocytes adhere to VCAM-1, *Blood*, 85,268,1995.
23. **Stockman J. A., Nigro M. A., Mishkin M. M., Oski F. A.**, Occlusion of large cerebral vessels in sickle cell anemia, *N. Engl. J. Med.*, 287, 846, 1972.
24. **Russel M. O., Goldberg H. I., Hodson A. et al.**, Effect of transfusion therapy on arteriographic abnormalities and on recurrence of stroke in sickle cell disease, *Blood*, 63, 162, 1984.
25. **Green D., Scott J.P.**, Is sickle cell crisis a thrombotic event ? *Am. J. Hemat.*, 23, 317, 1986.
26. **Buchanan G., Holtkamp A.**, Evidence against enhanced platelet activation in sickle cell anaemia, *Br. J. Haemat.*, 54, 595, 1983.
27. **Kurantsin-Mills J., Ofosu F., Safa T., Siegel R., Lessin** L., Plasma factor VII and thrombin-antithrombin III levels indicate increased tissue factor activity in sickle cell patients, *Br. J. Haemat.*, 81, 539, 1992.
28. **Francis R. B.**, Protein S deficiency in sickle cell anemia, *J. Lab. Clin. Med.*, 111, 571, 1988.

29.   **Porter J., Young L., Mackie I., Marshall L., Machin** S., Sickle cell disorders and chronic intravascular haemolysis are associated with low plasma heparin cofactor II, *Br. J. Haemat.*, 83, 459, 1993.

30.   **Lubin B., Chiu D., Bastacky J., Roelofsen B., van Deenen L.,** Abnormalities in membrane phospholipid organization in sickled erythrocytes, *J. Clin. Invest.*, 67, 1643, 1981.

31.   **Chiu D., Lubin B., Roelofsen B., van Deenen L.,** Sickled erythrocytes accelerate clotting in vitro : an effect of abnormal membrane lipid asymmetry, *Blood*, 58, 398, 1981.

32.   **Helley-Ben Amer D., Girot R., Eldor A., Ducrocq R., Guillin MC., Bezeaud** A., Activité procoagulante liée à l'exposition de phosphatidylserine à la face externe de la membrane des erythrocytes de sujets β thalassemiques et drepanocytaires, *Nouv. Rev. Fr. Hemat.*, 36, 145, 1994.

33.   **Lane P. O., Connell J., Marlar R.,** Irreversibly sickled cells bind protein S : an indication of altered membrane phospholipid asymmetry, Blood, 76, 67a, 1990.

34.   **Sowemimo-Coker S. O., Meiselman H. J., Francis R.B.**, Increased circulating endothelial cells in sickle cell crisis, *Am. J. Hemat.*, 31, 263, 1989.

35.   **Francis R. B., Haywood L. J.,** Elevated immunoreactive tumor necrosis factor and interleukin-1 in sickle cell disease, *J. Nat. Med. Ass.*, 84, 611, 1992.

36.   **Bauer K. A., ten Cate H., Barzegar S., Spriggs D. R., Sherman M. L., Rosenberg R. D.,** Tumor necrosis factor infusions have a procoagulant effect on the hemostatic mechanism of humans. *Blood*, 74, 165, 1989.

A LIFE-LONG HYPERCOAGULABLE STATE IN BETA-THALASSEMIA MAJOR PATIENTS

A. Eldor*, J. Maclouf **, A. Goldfarb ***, R. Durst***,
M.C. Guillin**** and E.A. Rachmilewitz***
*Institute of Hematology, Tel-Aviv Sourasky Medical Center, Tel-Aviv University
**INSERM unit 348, Hopital Lariboisière Paris
***Department of Hematology, Hadassah University Hospital, Jerusalem
****Service d'Hematologie Hopital Beaujon, Clichy, France

Increased frequency of thromboembolic events, including recurrent transient ischaemic cerebral attacks and stroke as well as peripheral arterial and venous thrombosis has been recently observed in patients with beta-thalassemia major (TM). Hypoxemia, cor pulmonale and autopsy findings of infarcts in the pulmonary microcirculation suggested that thalassemia may be associated with a chronic hypercoagulable state. Subsequently, various hemostatic anomalies were found both in young and adult patients with TM. Platelet function anomalies which indicate chronic in-vivo activation included: impaired aggregation, increased circulating aggregates, shortened survival and enhanced membrane expression of P-selectin (PADGEM/GMP 140). Continuous platelet activation was also evidenced by the increased urinary excretion of thromboxane A_2 (TXA_2) and prostacyclin metabolites, found both in adult patients and in children 2-8 years old. The hypercoagulable state was also manifested in adult and young TM patients by elevated levels of thrombin-antithrombin III (TAT) complexes and decreased plasma levels of the natural coagulation inhibitors, protein C and protein S. These hemostatic anomalies probably result from the basic pathology of the thalassemic erythrocytes, which were found to enhance the formation of thrombin in a "prothrombinase" assay. This effect is caused by a transbilayer movement of phospholipids in the thalassemic erythrocyte membranes, with the exposure of phosphatidylserine which may initiate intravascular coagulation. In view of these findings, anti-thrombotic therapy may be indicated in severe forms of the thalassemia syndrome. Preliminary trials of aspirin and ticlopidine, administered to patients with TM, resulted in a significant decrease of the urinary excretion of the platelet TXA_2 metabolites. Controlled clinical studies are needed to evaluate the efficacy of antithrombotic therapy in preventing the cardiac and pulmonary complications induced by the life-long hypercoagulable state which exists in thalassemia.

Thalassemia is a congenital hemoglobinopathy affecting many millions of heterozygotes and over 100,000 homozygote individuals born annually. The disease arises because of defective synthesis of one of the pairs of alpha or beta globin chains which constitute hemoglobin A. The imbalanced synthesis of the globin chains results in defective hemoglobinization of the erythrocytes and in chronic hemolysis due to the intracellular precipitation of the normal globin chain which is synthesized in relative excess. **Thalassemia major** (TM) results from the homozygous state of the gene anomaly and is usually manifested by anemia, marked hepatosplenomegaly and cardiac structure and function anomalies due to severe hemosiderosis from iron overload. The disease is usually severe and the majority of patients die of cardiac complications or infections in childhood or adolescence.[1]

Platelet function anomalies in thalassemia

We and others have noticed in patients with beta-TM, hemoglobin H disease and in hemoglobin E disease a significant decrease in platelet aggregation responses to various agonists. It was postulated that these anomalies are responsible for the mild hemorrhagic tendency, manifested by easy bruising and frequent epistaxis.[2-4] However, more recently there are increasing numbers of reports that thalassemic patients suffer from **thromboembolic phenomena** which are associated with significant morbidity and mortality. Among these events are recurrent and transient cerebral ischemic attacks and stroke as well as peripheral arterial and venous thrombosis.[5-9] Sonakul et al. reported autopsy findings in thalassemic patients which showed a high frequency of thrombotic lesions in the pulmonary arteries and the development of early atherosclerotic changes.[10] While the in-vitro platelet aggregation anomalies could be the cause of the mild hemorrhagic tendency, they could also result from a **hypercoagulable state**. The impaired aggregation could reflect an acquired functional defect due to "exhaustion" of the platelets following their in-vivo activation by substances released from lysed erythrocytes[1]. Evidence for this assumption is provided by the significant increase in the number of circulating platelet-aggregates in splenectomized thalassemic patients[12,13] and our study which showed that the mean survival of platelets (platelet life span) was decreased by about 50% in adult patients with beta-TM or beta thalassemia intermedia (TI) with or without prior splenectomy.[14] These kinetic studies, which were performed on patients who had no clinical evidence of thrombosis, indicated the existence of enhanced platelet consumption.

Numerous reports have demonstrated the role of thromboxane A_2 (TXA_2) and prostacyclin (PGI_2) in the interaction of platelets with the vessel wall, in thrombo-embolic and atherosclerotic disorders.[15-18] By estimating the excretion of urinary metabolites of TXA_2 and PGI_2 with an enzyme immunoassay, we found evidence for "continuous platelet activation" in splenectomized patients with beta-TM and non-splenectomized patients with beta-TI.[19] A significant increase ($p<0.001$) was observed in the following urinary metabolites, expressed in ng/mmole creatinine, in TM patients vs controls : 2,3-dinor-TXB_2 (176=75 vs 23=9) ; 11-dehydro-TXB_2 (318=170 vs 29=10); 2,3,-dinor-6-keto-$PGF_{1\alpha}$ (60=32 vs 12=5). No significant differences were found between TM and TI patients.[19]

Excretion of 2,3,-dinor-6-keto-$PGF_{1\alpha}$ is an accurate index of biosynthesis of PGI_2 which reflects alterations in the vascular synthesis of this eicosanoid.[15-17] Enhanced excretion of this metabolite was reported in association with severe atherosclerosis, in unstable angina, peripheral vascular disease and systemic sclerosis. In thalassemia this finding could result from vascular intimal injury due to the hemolytic process or from oxygen radicals catalysed by excess iron deposition in many organs and tissues.[20] An alternative possibility is that increased platelet-vessel wall interaction leads to either physical contact or the release of platelet constituents which are potent stimuli of vascular prostacyclin production.[15-17]

Enhanced urinary excretion of 11-dehydro-TXB_2 and 2,3,- dinor-6-keto-$PGF_{1\alpha}$ was recently found by us also in 6 children between 2-8 years of age, who suffered from beta-TM. The levels of both metabolites were not significantly different compared to those that were found in 17 adult TM patients and were at least two standard deviations above the normal levels in healthy controls.[21] None of these children had any clinical evidence for a thrombotic process and they had only mild symptoms ascribed to thalassemia (liver enlargement, cardiac anomalies or iron overload). Similar findings were observed in seven adolescent thalassemic patients who were between 9-18 years old.[20]

Using flow cytometric analysis, Del-Principe et al. studied the membrane expression of P-selectin (PADGEM/GMP-140) -an activation marker - on intact platelets from thalassemic patients.[23] They found that the number of platelets reactive with a monoclonal anti GMP-140 antibody was significantly higher in thalassemia (38.1% v 5.0%). GMP-140 expression on platelets from patients with spherocytosis did not differ from the controls. No correlation was found between GMP-140 expression and splenectomy, platelet counts, serum ferritin, antithrombin III (AT III) and protein C levels.[23] These results demonstrate the existence of circulating activated platelets in thalassemic patients.

The effect of anti-aggregating agents

Administration of a very low dose of **aspirin** (20 mg/day x 6 days) to adult TM patients resulted in a significant decrease in the excretion of platelet TXA_2 metabolites while the vascular or renal prostaglandin metabolites were not changed.[19] Recently we have completed a trial in which **ticlopidine**, a platelet inhibitor drug which has no direct effect on prostaglandin metabolism, was administered to adult TM patients. Thirteen patients received ticlopidine (250 mg b.i.d) and 7 patients received placebo for 30 days. The results showed a significant decrease in the urinary excretion of 11-dehydro-TXB_2, a platelet thromboxane metabolite, in the ticlopidine treated group while patients who received placebo did not show such effect.[22] Since ticlopidine may affect TXA_2 production only indirectly by inhibiting platelet activation, this study provides an additional support for the existence of chronic platelet activation in thalassemia.

Platelet activation in Sickle Cell Disease

It should be noted that the above platelet anomalies are not unique to patients with thalassemia. An association between hemolytic anaemias and predisposition to a hypercoagulable state has been observed before.[24] Platelet function anomalies, similar to those observed in thalassemia major, were found in patients with sickle cell disease, a hemoglobinopathy associated with thrombotic complications. Impaired platelet aggregation,[25-27] increased number of circulating platelet aggregates,[28] elevated plasma beta-thromboglobulin,[29] and elevated urinary levels of 11-dehydro-TXB$_2$ and 2,3,-dinor-6-keto-PGF$_{1\alpha}$,[30,31] were observed in these patients, who were at a steady state without any clinical evidence of sickle cell crisis. Shortened platelet life span was found during sickle cell crisis[32] and a beneficial effect of aspirin and dipyridamole in preventing crisis pain has been reported.[33]

The role of the pathologic erythrocytes in the hemostatic anomaly

The in-vivo platelet activation in thalassemia or sickle cell disease may be caused by the release of ADP or other thromboplastin-like materials from the pathological erythrocytes which are hemolyzing very rapidly.[20] It may also be induced by the pathological erythrocyte membranes which may provide a catalytic surface to attract activated coagulation factors.

In normal erythrocytes, the membrane phospholipids are organized in an asymmetric fashion.[34] Most of the choline-containing phospholipids (75-80%) are found in the outer monolayer, whereas most of the aminophospholipids (100% of phosphatidylserine and 80% of phosphatidylethanolamine) are localized in the inner monolayer.[34] Coagulation requires a surface containing negatively charged phospholipids, preferably phosphatidylserine, for the attraction of activated coagulation factors and the assembly of the "tenase" and "prothrombinase" complexes.[34,35] Under normal conditions no such surfaces are available in the circulating blood. Following platelet activation, negatively charged surfaces are exposed due to a translocation of phosphatidylserine to the outer platelet membrane (a process which is called "flip-flop") and support the induction of coagulation.[35] A similar abnormal exposure of phosphatidylserine was detected also on sickle cells, which enhanced coagulation in the in-vitro prothrombinase assay.[34-36] The formation of thrombin through the prothrombinase complex serves as a most sensitive tool to assess changes in membrane phospholipid asymmetry and to follow the exposure of phosphatidylserine, which chemical or enzymatic methods cannot detect.[37,38] We used the prothrombinase assay to test the hypothesis that exposure of phosphatidylserine in the outer leaflet exists also in TM erythrocytes.[39] The results showed a significant thrombin formation in the presence of TM or TI erythrocytes similar to that induced by sickle cells. In contrast, thrombin formation was not found with erythrocytes obtained from anemic uremic patients or healthy individuals.[39] Thus the exposure of phosphatidylserine on thalassemic erythrocytes may facilitate platelet activation and thrombus formation via enhanced formation of thrombin.

In-vivo thrombin formation in thalassemia

In a prospective study, we determined the activity of the coagulation system in 22 adults and 8 children (age 2-13 years) with thalassemia major and matched controls. All the thalassemia patients had no clinical evidence for thrombosis and did not receive any medication which might influence coagulation or hemostasis. Significant elevated levels of the thrombin-antithrombin III (TAT) complexes were observed both in the adult and the thalassemic children (Table I).[21] The levels of the prothrombin fragment F1+2 were only slightly elevated in the thalassemic children. Elevated levels of TAT are usually observed in patients with acute thrombosis and reflect enhanced *in-vivo* thrombin formation.[40] Increased levels of both TAT and F1+2 were detected in adults and children with sickle cell disease.[41-42] The clinical findings, together with the above in-vitro observations provide evidence for the existence of *in-vivo* activation of the coagulation system in the two major hemoglobinopathies and suggest that the mechanism is probably related to the abnormal erythrocytes.

Table I: Means (± SD) of various hemostatic parameters in thalassemia major

	Adults (n=18)		Children (n=9)		Control(range)	
TAT (ug/L)	5.7	(3.2)*	5.5	(3.6)*	2.93	(0.8)
F1+2 (nmol/L)	1.3	(0.4)	2.6	(1.4)	1.47	(0.1)
AT-III (%)	93.0	(12.5)	95.1	(11.6)	80-120	
PC act(%)	50.4	(10.6)*	48.8	(15.7)*	65-120	
PC ag(%)	51.8	(10.9)*	46.1	(9.7)*	65-120	
PS tot(%)	65.8	(12.8)	55.0	(9.2)	60-120	
PS free(%)	49.9	(9.7)*	43.4	(8.2)*	60-120	
C4b BP(%)	77.0	(17.4)	66.2	(30.1)	55-130	
F.II (%)	67.0	(10.5)*	61.6	(6.9)*	70-100	
F.V (%)	95.1	(29)	120.3	(31.1)	80-100	
Plg (%)	84.1	(16.3)	74.3	(9.4)	60-120	

SD: Standard Deviation; act-activity; ag-antigen; tot-total; F.II-Factor II; Plg-plasminogen
* Significantly (P<0.01) different from the controls

The role of natural coagulation inhibitors in thalassemia

Chronic activation of the coagulation cascade is frequently related to decreased levels of the natural coagulation inhibitors protein C (PC), protein S (PS) and antithrombin III (AT-III).[43-45] Congenital deficiency of these inhibitors results in a higher risk for developing recurrent thrombo-embolism and is defined as familial thrombophilia.[43-45] Several authors have found significantly decreased levels of PC and PS in sickle cell disease while the levels of AT-III were slightly decreased or normal.[46-48] Low PC levels were also observed in thalassemic patients.[49] Proteins C and S are vitamin K dependent proteins produced by the liver, which in the presence of calcium inhibit the activity of thrombin-stimulated factors Va and VIIIa.[43-44] PS is required for the functioning of PC and acts as a cofactor to form a stoichiometric complex.[44]

We measured the levels of PC, PS and AT-III in adult and young TM patients and correlated the results with various liver function tests and the levels of the coagulation factors II, V and plasminogen.[21] A significant decrease in PC (activity and antigen) and a marked decrease in the free form of PS was observed in almost all the patients studied (Table I). The total PS and the levels of C4b-binding protein which is the complement protein which specifically binds PS, were slightly decreased, while the AT-III levels were within the normal range. There were no significant differences in the levels of these inhibitors between adult or young thalassemic patients.[21] The low PS and PC levels could result from impaired production by the liver and/or increased consumption. However, there was no correlation between the levels of the inhibitors and any of the routine liver function tests assayed.[21] Nor was there any impairment in the level of factor V which is synthesized by the liver. The levels of factor II (prothrombin) and plasminogen were low in the thalassemic patients, but there was no correlation between these proteins and the levels of free PS and the PC activity or antigen.[21] Musumeci et al. found decreased PC levels in thalassemic patients, which correlated with the age of the patients, transfusional iron overload, serum ferritin, prothrombin time, serum transaminase and albumin.[49] It is possible that the Sicilian patients differ from our patients in the degree of iron overload and hepatic dysfunction and therefore their low PC levels may be influenced by impaired liver function.

Since significantly low levels of PC and PS were observed in our study in very young patients, who have not yet developed the characteristic complications of thalassemia, it is difficult to ascribe these findings solely to decreased production by the liver. Moreover, low levels of PS and PC were observed in patients with sickle cell disease, which did not correlate with any of the liver function tests.[42] Hence, it appears that liver dysfunction may not entirely explain the PC and PS deficiency in the two major hemoglobinopathies. An additional explanation could be related to enhanced consumption. Consumption due to disseminated intravascular coagulation (DIC) is unlikely in view of the normal levels of AT- III, factor V and platelet counts. An alternative mechanism of consumption of PS and PC may be related to the pathological erythrocytes. Dahlback et al. have demonstrated the affinity of PS to negatively charged phospholipids.[50] PS was found to bind to platelet microparticles which are formed during platelet activation and display increased levels of phosphatidylserine on their outer membrane leaflet.[50] Intact PS also supported the binding of PC to these platelet microparticles which are known to have a pro-thrombotic effect.[50] Binding of PS to sickle cells was recently reported[51] and therefore it is possible that the pathological thalassemic erythrocytes which display phosphatidylserine in their outer membranes provide a surface which adsorbs the above inhibitors, resulting in decreased plasma levels.

The clinical consequences of the hypercoagulable state in thalassemia

What are the clinical implications of the above findings which provide an objective evidence for the existence of a chronic hypercoagulable state in thalassemia from early childhood ? Unlike the situation in sickle cell desease, vaso-occlusive crises do not occur in thalassemia. However there is more evidence that patients with thalassemia major develop recurrent thrombo-embolic events. In a survey of 138 thalassemia patients, 27 patients suffered from ischemic cerebral manifestations, including transient ischemic attacks and strokes.[6-8] Some of our patients developed arterial thrombotic events, cerebral infarctions and recurrent pulmonary embolism.[9] Furthermore, thrombosis and atherosclerotic changes in the pulmonary arterial tree may be more prevalent in thalassemia than is generally recognized. Autopsy findings in thalassemic patients revealed small fresh and old thrombi in the pulmonary microcirculation as well as hypertrophy of the right ventricle, consistent with a long-standing pulmonary "vascular embarrassment" which culminates in right heart failure.[10]

A recent study of 35 thalassemia major patients, using echocardiography showed that pulmonary dysfunction and right ventricular abnormalities are more frequent than left ventricular dysfunction even in the absence of overt heart failure.[52] Pulmonary function anomalies are frequently observed in thalassemia patients, including: reduced lung volumes, reduced flow rates, a diffusion defect, hypoxemia and pulmonary hypertension.[52-55] These anomalies may be due to thrombosis in the pulmonary microvasculature since iron deposition in the lungs does not occur in thalassemia.[54] The observation that some thalassemic patients responded to treatment with antiaggregating agents (aspirin and dipyridamole) with a rise in their arterial oxygen content supports this idea.[55]

The significant platelet anomalies, the evidence for chronic thrombin formation and the decreased levels of two major coagulation inhibitors suggest that a chronic and life long hypercoagulable state exists in patients with the severe clinical forms of the thalassemia syndrome. This condition may lead to overt events of thrombosis as well as to repeated "silent" pulmonary micro-embolization culminating in cor-pulmonale. Moreover, these findings imply that it may be appropriate to administer antithrombotic therapy to patients with the thalassemia syndromes. Both platelet inhibitor drugs and oral anticoagulants may be indicated.

Consequently, clinical studies to evaluate the efficacy of antithrombotic therapy in preventing the development of the pulmonary and cardiac complications are required. Prolonged antithrombotic therapy is definitely indicated in patients who presented with a thrombotic event, since such events may be regarded as a complication of the underlying chronic hemolytic process which is associated with thrombophilia.

REFERENCES

1. **Weatherall, D.J., Clegg, J.B.,** *The Thalassemia Syndrome,* 3rd Ed. Blackwell Scientific Publications, Oxford 1981
2. **Eldor, A.,** Hemorrhagic tendency in beta-thalassemia major. *Isr. J. Med. Sci.,* 14, 1132, 1978
3. **Eldor, A.,** Abnormal platelet function in beta-thalassemia, *Scand. J. Haem.,* 20, 447, 1978
4. **Houssain, M.A.M., Hutton, R.A., Pavidon, O., Hoffbrand, A.V.,** Platelet function in beta-thalassemia major, *J. Clin. Path.,* 32, 429, 1979
5. **Logothetis, J., Constantoulakis, M., Economidou, J., Stefanis, C., Hakas, P., Angoustaki, O., Sofraniadou, K., Loewenson, R., Bilek, M.S.,** Thalassemia major (homozygous beta-thalassemia). A survey of 138 cases with emphasis on neurologic and muscular aspects, *Neurology,* 22, 294, 1972
6. **Sinniah, D., Vignaendra, V., Kamaruddin, A.,** Neurological complications of beta-thalassemia major, *Arch. Dis. Child.,* 52, 977, 1977

7.   **Paolini, E., Monetti, V.C., Gronieri, E., Boldrini, P.**, Acute cerebrovascular insults in homozygous beta-thalassemia: a case report, *J. Neurol.*, 230, 37, 1983

8.   **Wong, V., Yu, Y.L., Liang, R.H.S., Tso, W.K., Li, A.M.C., and Chan, T.K.**, Cerebral thrombosis in beta-thalassemia/hemoglobin H disease , *Stroke.*, 21, 812, 1990

9.   **Michaeli, J., Mittelman, M., Grisaru, D., and Rachmilewitz, E.A.**, Thromboembolic complications in beta-thalassemia major, *Acta Hemat.*, 87, 71, 1992

10.   **Sonakul, D., Pacharee, P., Laohapand, T., Fucharoen, S., Wasi, P.**, Pulmonary artery obstruction in thalassemia, *Southeast Asian. J. Trop. Med. Pub. Hlth.*, 11, 516, 1990

11.   **O'Brien, J.R., Tulevski, V.G., Etherington, M., Madgwick, T., Alkjaersig, N., Fletcher, A.**, Platelet function studies before and after operation and the effect of post-operative thrombosis, *J. Lab. Clin. Med.*, 83, 342, 1974

12.   **Winichagoon, P., Fucharoen, S., Wasi, P.** Increased circulating platelet aggregates in thalassemia, *Southeast Asian J. Trop. Med. Pub. Hlth.*, 12, 556, 1981

13.   **Isarangkura, P., Pintadit, P., Hathirat, P., Sasanakul, W.** Platelet function tests in thalassemic children, in : Fucharoen, S., Rowly P.T., Paul, N.W., Eds., *Thalassemia Pathophysiology and Management*, Alan, Liss Inc. New York, 1988, 395

14.   **Eldor, A., Krausz, Y., Atlan, H., Snyder, D., Goldfarb, A., Hy-Am, E., Rachmilewitz, E.A., Kotze, H.F., Heyns, A.P.** Platelet survival in patients with beta-thalassemia, *Am. J. Hematol.*, 32, 94, 1989

15.   **Fitzgerald, G.A., Smith, B., Pedersen, A.K., Brash, A.R.**, Increased prostacyclin biosynthesis in patients with severe atherosclerosis and platelet activation, *N. Engl. J. Med.*, 310, 1065, 1984

16.   **Fitzgerald, D.J., Roy, L., Catella, F., Fitzgerald, G.A.** , Platelet activation in unstable coronary disease, *N. Engl. J. Med.*, 315, 983, 1986

17.   **Oates, J.A., Fitzgerald, A., Branch, A., Jackson, E.K., Knapp, H.R., Roberts I.J.**, Clinical implications of prostaglandin and thromboxane A$_2$ *N. Engl. J. Med.*, 319, 689, 1988

18.   **Davi, G., Catalano, I., Averna, M., Notarbartolo, A., Strano, A., Ciabattoni, G., Patrono, C.**, Thromboxane biosynthesis and platelet function in type II diabetes mellitus, *N. Engl. J. Med.*, 322, 1769, 1990

19.   **Eldor, A., Lellouche, F. Goldfarb, A., Rachmilewitz, E.A., Maclouf, J.** In vivo platelet activation in beta-thalassemia major reflected by increased platelet-thromboxane urinary metabolites, *Blood,* 77, 749, 1991

20.   **Shinar, E., Rachmilewitz, A.E.**, Oxydative denaturation of red cells in thalassemia, *Sem. Hem.*, 27, 70, 1990

21.   **Eldor, A., Maclouf, J., Durst, R., Hy-Am, E., Goldfarb, A., Abramov, A., Rachmilewitz, E.A., de Raucourt, E., Guillin M.C.A,** unpublished data, 1994

22.   **Durst, R., Maclouf, J. Hy-Am, E., Goldfarb, A., Abramov, A., Rachmilewitz E.A., Eldor, A.,** Unpublished data, 1994

23.   **Del Principe, D., Menichelli, A., Di Giulio, S., De Matteis, W., Cianciulli, P., and Papa G.**, PADGEM/GMP-140 expression on platelet membranes from homozygous beta-thalassemic patients, *Brit. J. Haem.*, 84, 111, 1993

24.   **Rabiner, S.F., Rosenfeld, S.**, Role of intravascular hemolysis and the reticuloendothelial system in the production of hypercoagulable state, *J. Lab. Clin. Med.*, 62, 1005, 1963

25.   **Stuart, M.J., Stockman, J.A., Oski, F.A.**, Abnormalities of platelet aggregation in the vaso occlusive crisis of sickle-cell anemia, *J. Pediatr.*, 85, 629, 1974

26.   **Gruppo, R.A., Glueck, H.I., Granger, S.M., Miller, M.A.**, Platelet function in sickle cell anemia, *Thromb. Res.*, 10, 325, 1977

27.   **Sarji, K.E., Emenius, K., Fullwood, C.O., Schraibman, H.B., Colwell, J.A.**, Abnormalities of platelet aggregation in sickle cell anemia in presence of a plasma factor inhibiting aggravations by ristocetin, *Thromb. Res.*, 14, 283, 1979

28.   **Mehta, P., Mehta, J.**, Circulating platelet aggregates in sickle cell disease patients with and without vaso-occlusion, *Stroke,* 10, 464, 1979

29.   **Mehta, P.** Significance of plasma beta-thromboglobulin values in patients with sickle cell disease, *J. Pediatr.*, 97, 941, 1980

30.   **Longenecker, G.L., Beyers, B.J., Mankad, V.N.**, Platelet regulatory prostanoids and platelet release products in sickle cell disease, *Am. J. Hematol.,* , 40, 12, 1992

31.   **Foulon, I., Bachir, D., Galacteros, F. and Maclouf, J.**, Increased in vivo production of thromboxane in patients with sickle cell disease is accompanied by an impairment of platelet functions to the thromboxane A$_2$ agonist U46619, *Arteriosclerosis and Thrombosis,* 13, 421, 1993

32.   **Haut, M.J., Cownan, D.H., Harris, J.W.** Platelet function and survival in sickle cell disease, *J. Lab. Clin. Med.*, 82, 44, 1973

33.   **Chaplin, H., Alkjaersig, N., Fletcher, A.P., Michael, J.M., Joist, J.H.**, Aspirin-dipyridamole prophylaxis of sickle cell disease pain crisis, *Thromb. Haemost.*, 43, 218, 1980

34.   **Zwaal, R.F.A., Roelofsen, B., van Deenen, L.L.M.**, Organization of phospholipids in human red cell membranes as detected by the action of various purified phospholipases, *Biochim. Biophys. Acta*, 406, 83, 1975

35.   **Schroit, A.J., Zwaal, R.F.A.**, Transbilayer movement of phospholipids in red cell and platelet membranes, *Biochim. Biophys. Acta*, 1071, 313, 1991

36.   **Hebbel, R.P.**, Beyond hemoglobin polymerization : The red blood cell membrane and sickle disease pathophysiology, *Blood,* 77, 214, 1991

37.   **Comfurius, P., Bevers, E., Zwall, R.F.A.**, Prothrombinase complex as a tool to assess changes in membrane phospholipid asymmetry. In Higgins, J.A. Graton, J.(eds). *Methods in Molecular Biology , Membrane Methods*, New York, Vol 3, Humana Press, 1994

38.   **Connor, J., Bucana, C., Fidler, II., Schroit, A.J.**, Differentiation-dependent expression of phosphatidylserine in mammalian plasma membranes : Quantitative assessment of outer-leaflet lipid by prothrombinase complex formation, *Proc. Natl. Acad. Sci. Usa*, 86, 3184, 1989

39.   **Borenstein, V., Barenholz, Y., Hy-Am, E., Rachmilewitz, E.A., Eldor, A.**, Phosphatidylserine in the outer leaflet of red blood cells from beta-thalasssemia patients may explain the chronic hypercoagulable state and thrombotic episodes, *Am. J. Hematol.,* 44, 33, 1993

40.   **Pelzre, H., Stuber, W.** Markers of hemostatic activation perspectives using immunochemical methods for determination of prothrombin fragment F1+2 and thrombin/antithrombin III complex, *Thromb. Haemost.*, 26, 165, 1989

41.   **Kurantsin-Mills, J., Ofosu, F.A., Safa, T.K., Siegel, R.S., Lessin, L.S.**, Plasma factor VII and thrombin-antithrombin III levels indicates increased tissue factor activity in sickle cell patients, *Br. J. Haematol.*, 81, 539, 1992

42.   **Peters, M., Plaat, B.E.C., Ten Cate, H., Walters, H.J., Weening, R.S., and Brandjes, D.P.M.**, Enhanced thrombin generation in children with sickle cell disease, *Thromb. Haemost.*, 71, 169, 1994

43. **Schwartz, H.P., Fischer, M., Hopmeier, P, Batard, M.A., Griffin, J.H.**, Plasma protein C deficiency in familial thrombotic disease, *Blood*, 64, 1297, 1984

44. **Comp. P.C., Nixon, R.R., Cooper, M.R., Esmon, C.T.**, Familial protein S deficiency is associated with recurrent thrombosis, *J. Clin. Invest.*, 74, 2082, 1984

45. **Mannuci, P.M., Tripodi, A., Botasso, B., Baudo, F., Finazzi, G., de Stefano, V., Palareti, G., Monatti, M.G., Mazzuccono, M.G., Gastama, G.**, Markers of procoagulant imbalance in patients with inherited thrombophilic syndromes, *Thromb. Haemost.*, 67, 200, 1992

46. **Francis, R.B. Jr.**, Protein S deficiency in sickle cell anemia, *J. Lab. Clin. Med.*, 111, 571, 1988

47. **Karayalcin, G., Lanzkowsky, P.**, Plasma protein C levels in children with sickle cell disease, *Am. J. Ped. Hem. Onc.*, 11, 320, 1989

48. **El-Hazmi, M.A.F., Bahakim, H., Warsy, A.S.**, Blood proteins C and S in sickle cell disease, *Acta. Haemat.*, 90, 114, 1993

49. **Musumeci, S., Leonardi, S., Di Dio, R., Fischer, A., Di Costa, G.**, Protein C and antithrombin III in polytransfused thalassemic patients, *Acta Haemat.*, 77, 30, 1987

50. **Dahlback, B., Wiedmer, T., and Sims, P.J.**, Binding of anticoagulant vitamin K-dependent protein S to platelet derived microparticles, *Biochemistry*, 31, 12769, 1992

51. **Lane, P.A., O'Connell, J.L., Marlar, R.A.**, Irreversibly sickled cells bind protein S : an indication of altered membrane phospholipid asymmetry, *Blood*, 76, suppl 1, 67a, 1990

52. **Grisaru, D., Rachmilewitz, E.A., Mosseri, M., Gotsman, M., Lafair, J., Okun, E., Goldfarb A., Hasin, Y.** Cardio-pulmonary assessment in beta-thalassemia major, *Chest*, 98, 1138, 1990

53. **Cooper, D.M., Mansell, A.L., Weiner, M.A.**, Low lung capacity and hypoxemia in children with thalassemia major, *Ann. Rev. Respir. Dis.*, 121, 639, 1980

54. **Grant, G.P., Mansell, A.L., Graziano, J.H., Mellins, R.B.** The effect of transfusion on lung capacity diffusing capacity and material oxygen saturation in patients with thalassemia major, *Pediatr. Res.*, 20, 20, 1986

55. **Fucharoen, S., Youngchaiyud, P., Wasi, P.**, Hypoxaemia and the effect of aspirin in thalassemia, *Southeast. Asian. J. Trop. Med. Pub. Hlth.*, 12, 90, 1981

ARTERIAL THROMBOSIS WITH THROMBOCYTOPENIA

H.L. Messmore*,**, W.H. Wehrmacher* and J. Seghatchian***
*Loyola University Stritch School of Medicine, Maywood.
**Hines Veterans Affairs Hospital, Hines
***North London Blood Transfusion Centre, London

I. INTRODUCTION

Our ability to clinically distinguish non-atherosclerotic arterial occlusion from the atherosclerotic type is based primarily upon probability after a thorough evaluation of the patient's history, physical examination and screening laboratory studies. When the patient has clinical ischemic disease associated with thrombocytopenia, there may or may not be a relationship between the two, but when this set of clinical circumstances occurs, the probability is that they are pathophysiologically related unless some other obvious explanation exists. The longer one of these two has been present without the other, the more probable it is that they are not related. For that reason remote history and medical records are important. Since drugs and chemicals as well as infectious diseases may be a causative factor or a cofactor in such disorders, thoroughness and accuracy of the history and physical examination as well as in the initial laboratory screening tests are critical to making the diagnosis.

There are a number of clinical disorders occasionally associated with arterial, venous and microvascular thrombosis that have to be excluded before the diagnosis of thrombotic thrombocytopenic purpura (TTP), hemolytic uremic syndrome (HUS), heparin induced thrombocytopenia (HIT), or the antiphospholipid antibody (APAS) syndrome can be made. The APAS not infrequently occurs in association with each of the above disorders suggesting that it may be arising from that disorder or that they have a common genetic predisposition for that disorder, or that they are acting synergistically to make that disorder clinically evident. The APAS may have prognostic implication as well.

Each of the above disorders will be briefly reviewed in terms of diagnostic criteria and the features that overlap with the other syndromes. Some of the current concepts of pathogenesis and pathophysiology will be explored. The association of these disorders with a variety of possible causes requires that they be classified as syndromes with the exception of HIT, which is relatively well defined. The occasional encounter with a patient who develops immune mediated thrombocytopenia almost immediately after receiving the first dose of heparin suggests that there could be endogenous HIT of an "autoimmune" type-based upon the fact that heparin and heparan sulfate are normal human constituents and under some circumstances could become antigenic.

II. THROMBOTIC THROMBOCYTOPENIA PURPURA

This relatively rare syndrome was initially reported as a previously undescribed syndrome by Moschovitz in 1925. His description included the five cardinal clinical findings of fever, purpura, red cell fragmentation hemolysis, renal impairment and central nervous system (CNS) signs.[1] Thrombocytopenia is invariably present as is hemolytic anemia. Renal impairment, fever, and CNS signs are less constant findings. The terminal arterioles are occluded in many of the organs including skin, gingiva, spleen, kidney, brain, bone marrow and heart. The onset is relatively abrupt with symptoms of a few hours to a few days before the patient comes for medical evaluation. While it may

0-8493-5804-3/96/$0.00+$.50

occur at any age, when it occurs without an obvious associated disease (infection, malignancy, systemic lupus erythematosis) or drug (chemotherapy-mitomycin C, contraceptive drug), it is usually in a younger person or a female for whom the diagnosis of atherosclerosis as a cause of any ischemic symptoms would be uncommon. Young women during pregnancy or in the puerperium are among those more commonly affected. Not only does the etiology seem to be diverse but there appears to be a hereditary tendency, and a tendency to be acute or chronic and relapsing. The most consistently successful treatment in the primary or idiopathic acute variety is plasma exchange performed vigorously for a week or more.[2,3] Other successful treatments have been whole blood or plasma infusion and splenectomy. Antiplatelet agents and immunosuppressive drugs (corticosteroids, vincristine) appear to be useful as well, but are almost always used as a treatment ancillary to one of the principal modes of therapy (blood or plasma transfusion, plasma exchange or splenectomy). Splenectomy is believed to be inferior to plasma transfusion or plasma exchanges and is reserved for refractory cases.[4,5]

III. ETIOLOGY

The association of this syndrome with infections such as Escherichia coli 0157:H7 and its verotoxin[6] and human immunodeficiency virus[7] suggests that other infectious agents could be involved with the pathophysiology representing a stereotyped host response to a variety of infections. Some that have been reported include tropical dysentery, campylobacter and corynebacterium diphtheria.[8] The factor in common may be a host response modulated by a particular HLA type (DR52, 53),[9] or a special type of immune system abnormality. The simultaneous occurrence of TTP and SLE is uncommon. In a review of reported cases,[10] in eight of eighteen the SLE was inactive at the time of diagnosis of TTP. Approximately half the patients had positive anti-DNA antibodies. Plasmapheresis proved to be an effective therapy for 10 of the 11 patients who received that treatment. Reports on the association of antiphospholipid or anticardiolipin antibodies have been variable in patients with TTP. In one study, no association was found[11] but others have found an association.[12]

IV. PATHOPHYSIOLOGY OF TTP

There is no hard evidence that damage to endothelial cells could, by itself, result in thrombocytopenia and thrombosis that would be benefitted by plasmapheresis and plasma exchange or by plasma infusions. On the other hand, agents that aggregate circulating platelets have not been reported to produce TTP, for example HIT. In fact, HIT is a very different syndrome from TTP in spite of the fact that platelet aggregation occurs in both. It therefore is reasonable to speculate that both the endothelium and the platelets are injured by the same agent in these disorders. The agent may be cytolytic for endothelial cells and an activator of platelets. An example could be immune complex mediated damage to both types of cells analogous to an immune complex vasculitis with simultaneous platelet aggregation. The concept of a plasma factor that is lacking in some patients with TTP is supported by the fact that some patients respond very promptly to plasma infusion. The effect of a single infusion of plasma of 500 ml may last for 2 weeks in some of the familial variants (Upshaw syndrome)[13] that have intermittent or relapsing TTP. The response to plasma infusion is excellent. One patient was symptomatic primarily during pregnancy. Her brother had intermittent severe exacerbations.[14] Both responded to plasma infusions.

Patients with malignancy have been reported to have TTP that responded to chemotherapy of the neoplasm.[15] In other cancer patients a TTP like syndrome has developed during chemotherapy, particularly with mitomycin C.[16] Treatment with vincristine has been reported to be a useful treatment of that complication.[17]

Female hormones have been suspected because a number of women with TTP have been taking oral contraceptives. A recent case report suggests a possible association with levonorgestrel implants and advises that all new cases be reported.[18]

The finding of an association of circulating high molecular weight (HMW) multimers of von Willebrand factor in increased amounts when patients with chronic relapsing TTP are in remission and a decrease in these HMW multimers during relapse has been reported.[19] This could be secondary to endothelial cell injury with production of abnormal multimers which could aggregate the platelets and consume the multimers.

There is a possibility that antibodies or cytokines are acting on endothelial cells to cause release of substances that bind platelets (von Willebrand factor) or they may be impairing the natural production of prostacyclin by endothelial cells which would promote platelet adherence. It was shown many years ago that the platelet rich thrombi in the arterioles of TTP patients are surrounded by a zone of decreased fibrinolytic potential.[20] This is probably secondary to the release of large amounts of plasminogen activator inhibitor by the platelets. Since the thrombotic lesions are frequently only partially occlusive and are covered by endothelium, there has been speculation that this disorder is associated with endothelial disruption and that platelets are deposited beneath it. Nonetheless, it is more probable that the platelet thrombi become rapidly covered by endothelium after they attach to the vessel wall, suggesting that a large amount of growth factor (platelet derived growth factor, endothelial cell derived growth factor) is present. There is little doubt that some thrombin is generated at the site of the thrombus since the platelets are intertwined with fibrin strands; but it is doubtful that either thrombin generated via tissue thromboplastin generation on the surface of the endothelial cell or on leukocytes plays an important role in the platelet thrombus formation. It has been shown in the remote past that heparin is not a useful treatment for TTP (and HUS) and is potentially harmful. The participation of adhesion molecules in this process is highly probable and increased understanding of their role might be useful.

The possibility that the HMW von Willebrand factor multimers are of major importance in the pathophysiology of TTP is questionable. They are likely to be the result of rather than the cause of thrombi in this location. It is of interest that one case of the relapsing type of TTP (heredofamilial variety) had no measurable abnormalities of the von Willebrand factor multimers. The patient responded predictably to fresh frozen plasma infusion.[14] One study of the multimers in primary versus secondary acute TTP showed that abnormal multimer patterns occurred in both and that the abnormal pattern disappeared with chemotherapy in the secondary types due to malignancy.[15] Chemotherapy consisted of a variety of chemotherapeutic agents. Unfortunately we do not have a good animal model for TTP. Although there is an animal model for HUS,[21] it may not reflect what is happening in TTP.

V. HEMOLYTIC UREMIC SYNDROME (HUS)

The hemolytic uremic syndrome is very close to, if not the same as, TTP. Histopathology of the vascular lesions in HUS is indistinguishable from that of TTP,[6] but the clinical manifestation of acute renal failure in children and in pre and post partum females strongly suggests a difference in the two. The preponderance of the renal vascular lesion and the relative lack of neurological symptoms is another important difference. The association of this clinical presentation with an enteric infection with Escherichia coli 0157:H7 is much stronger than is such an association with TTP, but in the absence of a study of TTP patients for this organism or its verotoxin, one cannot be certain that many cases of TTP are not associated with this infection. Since 1988 there has been a greater awareness of this association following an editorial in the JAMA.[22] It is the rule that TTP patients either die or recover with little disability but that chronic renal failure with the need for renal transplant is commonly associated with the hemolytic uremic syndrome. The endothelium of the kidney may be particularly sensitive to one or more etiologic agents. This would provide an explanation for this difference in the two syndromes in terms of clinical manifestations and location of the vascular lesion. Because of recent epidemics of enteric infection with E. coli 0157:H7 due to consumption of incompletely cooked beef, an increased surveillance of raw beef has been instituted, and the food industry as well as the general public has been made aware of the dangers of eating undercooked beef, especially hamburger.[23]

The examination of the blood reveals identical changes as is seen with TTP. Thrombocytopenia, red blood cell fragmentation, high serum LDH and high molecular weight multimers of von Willebrand factor are present.[24] Thus, it seems probable that circulating antibodies, immune complexes, cytokines 25 (interleukin,-1 interleukin-6, tissue necrosis factor) bacterial toxins and direct viral invasion may be damaging to the endothelium, of the renal vasculature in HUS and to the arterioles of many organs in TTP. As mentioned previously,[21] there is an animal model being developed for HUS and possibly for TTP.

VI. HEPARIN INDUCED THROMBOCYTOPENIA/THROMBOSIS

Heparin induced thrombocytopenia has been recognized as a clinical problem only in the last twenty-two years.[26] Since the manufacture of heparin has not substantially changed in the last 40 years, it is probable that clinical recognition was lacking in the earlier years due to lack of platelet counting in patients receiving heparin. Heparin induced thrombosis was described in 1958[27] and has been since recognized to be occurring in association with heparin induced thrombocytopenia. Many excellent reviews of this clinical entity have emphasized that there are two types of heparin induced thrombocytopenia, an immediate mild form that is due to heparin binding directly to platelets and a delayed form occurring five to ten days after the initial exposure to heparin.[28,29] The latter type is immune mediated and in some cases is associated with arterial or venous thrombosis or even disseminated intravascular coagulation. The thrombotic complications are associated with much more morbidity and mortality than is bleeding, even though in many cases the heparin has been continued for several days in the presence of thrombocytopenia. This is analogous to the lack of bleeding in the TTP patients, which is probably due to the fact that many of the platelets are young due to increased platelet production, and many are activated. The endothelium in HIT may be damaged independently of the platelet injury.[30]

VII. PATHOPHYSIOLOGY

Current consensus appears to support the concept that in HIT the patient builds an antibody, usually Ig type, to a heparin-plasma protein complex or a heparin-platelet glycoprotein complex. The most recent studies have shown the antigen to be heparin bound to platelet factor 4, and that the complex formed when the antibody complexed with heparin-PF4 binds to a receptor for immune complex (Fc receptor) on the platelet.[30,31] Such binding has been shown to activate the platelet with release of alpha and delta granule contents and presentation of activation proteins, glycoproteins and phospholipids on its surface. The platelets undergo aggregation and release reaction. Heparin binds to platelets, as do most highly sulfated glycosaminoglycans, but it is only weakly immunogenic unless bound to a protein. There is some question as to whether the antigen is heparin-PF4 in all cases. We have shown that the in-vitro aggregation of platelets using the patient's serum or the IgG antibody from that serum will occur in the presence of heparin but not when the glycoprotein 1b of the platelet has been blocked by a specific antibody (MOAB SZ2). Once the antibody forms, it cross reacts with many sulfated glycosaminoglycans, presumably only those capable of binding to platelet factor 4 or to the platelet surface. The lower molecular weight heparins that have exclusively anti-Xa activity react only weakly, if at all, in in-vitro test systems. Dermatan sulfate is non-reactive with the antibody, but most low molecular weight (LMW) heparins commercially available do react with the antibody. In spite of this, some patients have been successfully managed with LMW heparin after demonstration of the antibody in their serum.[32] It is considered, however, very hazardous to try. Instead, a heparinoid such as Orgaran (ORG 10172), hirudin or a synthetic heparin analogue would be safer. In all cases an in-vitro test to determine reactivity with the antibody is advised. The venom Ancrod has been used successfully as well.[33] While the above seems to be a reasonable explanation for the thrombocytopenia, the real problem is to explain the thrombosis that can in some cases be so devastating.

Heparin induced thrombosis occurs most commonly in medium and large arteries and less commonly in the larger veins. It does not have a tendency to occur in the arterioles as a primary process, but emboli from the larger arteries may occlude them. When heparin induced thrombosis was first described it emphasized thrombosis in the aorta as being commonly found.[27] Reports of this occurring in association with thrombocytopenia are continuing to be published.[33,34]

If platelet activation alone is the immunological injury, it is difficult to understand why larger arteries are so prone to thrombosis. It does appear that many of the thrombi ("white clots"-platelet rich) tend to be found at the sites where atherosclerosis occurs. Perhaps endothelium overlying atherosclerotic plaques is for some reason more likely to bind activated platelets. Another reasonable explanation is that the antibody reacts with heparin-platelet factor 4 bound to endothelium. It is possible that glycosaminoglycans (heparan sulfate) on the surface of the endothelial cell bound to platelet factor 4 can act as a target for the antibody resulting in thrombosis.[30] The character of the clot in HIT (very platelet rich) suggests that endothelial injury alone could be responsible for the lesion but it is more probable that the combination of activated platelets with endothelial injury results in thrombosis. Some studies have shown endothelial cell injury by HIT serum, heparin and complement; others have suggested that platelet factor 4 bound to heparan sulfate on endothelial cells is target for the antibody.[30]

Since deep vein thrombosis and/or disseminated intravascular coagulation sometimes occurs in these patients along with, or independent of the arterial thrombosis, there is reason to consider other factors as well. In one study, it was shown that anticardiolipin antibodies may be found in one third of patients with HIT.[35]

The fact that other drug induced antibodies directed to platelets (quinine or quinidine induced thrombocytopenia) are not associated with thrombosis may be due to the fact that the platelets undergo complement lysis rather than aggregation and release reaction.[36] This increases the probability that the process of platelet aggregation and release could result in binding of activated platelets to endothelium damage as a result of atherosclerosis at the site. Since many of the vascular occlusions that are examined histologically could be emboli rather than primary thrombus sites, the fact that an atheromatous lesion is not present at that site may not be significant. Endothelial injury of other types such as trauma due to catheterization of arteries or veins, or chemical injury by contrast media or medications could be important contributing factors as well.

VIII. ANTIPHOSPHOLIPID ANTIBODY SYNDROMES

Antiphospholipid antibody syndromes including anticardiolipin, lupus anticoagulant and systemic lupus erythematosus may at times be associated with arterial thrombosis and thrombocytopenia. The arterial thrombosis is not specifically confined to arterioles (TTP, HUS) or to medium and large arteries (HIT) but is more heterogeneous in its thrombotic manifestations. Additionally, venous thrombosis is as likely or more likely to occur than is arterial thrombosis in patients with the APAS.

The thrombocytopenia is most frequently mediated by antiplatelet IgG or by immune complex binding to platelets.[37] It has been shown that when arterial thrombosis does occur it is frequently manifested as a cerebrovascular event. This could be cardiac valvular in origin (Libman-Sacks valvular lesions in SLE) with cerebral embolization. Antibody injury to endothelium may also occur, with accompanying interference by the antibody with normal antithrombotic mechanisms (protein C function and fibrinolytic activity).[38] Some patients with human immunodeficiency syndrome induced and some with drug induced antiphospholipid antibodies may manifest thrombosis of arteries or veins but most do not. The presence of these antibodies in patients with systemic lupus (SLE) increases the likelihood of thrombotic complications suggesting that factors such as immune complexes or antiendothelial antibodies and/or vasculitis are necessary for thrombosis to occur. Twenty to thirty percent of patients with SLE have antiphospholipid antibodies, but only a fraction have thromboembolic complications.[39]

IX. SUMMARY

Patients who present with thrombocytopenia, thromboembolism and/or antiphospholipid antibody should be assessed for an underlying problem, which may be SLE, TTP, HUS or even HIT if the patient has been recently treated with or is still on heparin. In the hospital setting heparin may be used in flushes to keep arterial lines open, or it may be bonded to a vascular shunt or to a prosthesis and is therefore not apparent as a clinical cause in some cases. A search for infections particularly E. coli 0157:H7 is indicated in patients with the TTP or HUS syndrome. In elderly patients occult carcinoma might reasonably be considered if the diagnosis appears to be TTP or HUS. In these syndromes the activation of enzymes of the coagulation system rarely occurs to any more than a minor degree. For that reason, anticoagulant drugs are not useful except where thrombosis has occurred in the APAS. Heparin may remove antithrombin III from the endothelium, reducing its natural thromboresistance.

REFERENCES

1. **Moschowitz E** An acute febrile pleiochromic anemia with hyaline thrombosis of the terminal arteriole and capillaries: An undescribed disease, *Arch Int Med*, 36, 89, 1925.
2. **Bukowski RM, Hewlett JS, Harris JW, et al.** Exchange transfusion in the treatment of thrombotic thrombocytopenic purpura, *Semin Hematol*,13, 219, 1976.
3. **Bukowski RM**. Thrombotic thromboytopenic purpura: A review, *Haemost Thromb*, 6, 287, 1982.
4. **Talarico J, Grapski R, Lutz C, et al.** Late postsplenectomy recurrence of thrombotic thrombocytopenia purpura responding to removal of accessory spleen, *Am J Med*, 82,845, 1987.
5. **Thompson HW, McCarthy LJ**. Thrombotic thrombocytopenic purpura: Potential benefit of splenectomy after plasma exchange, *Arch Intern Med*, 143, 2111, 1983.
6. **Richardson SE, Karmali MA, Becker LE, et al.** The histopathology of the hemolytic uremic syndrome associated with verotoxin-producing Escherichia coli infections, *Hum Pathol*, 19, 1102, 1988.
7. **Leaf AN, Laubenstein LJ, Raphael B, et al.** Thrombotic thrombocytopenic purpura associated with human immunodeficiency virus type 1 (HIV-1) infection, *Ann Intern Med*, 109, 194, 1988.
8. **Beck EA, Dejana E**. Thrombohemorrhagic phenomenon associated with infectious disease, *Semin Hemat*, 25, 91, 1988.
9. **Joseph G, Smith KJ, Hadley T, et al.** HLA DR53 protects against TTP- hemolytic uremic syndrome TTP/HUS, *Blood*, 82 (suppl 1), 583a (abst 2315), 1993.
10. **Stricker RB, Davis JA, Gershaw J, et al.** Thrombotic thrombocytopenic purpura complicating systemic lupus erythematosis. Case report and literature review from the plasmapheresis era, *J Rheumatol*, 19, 1469, 1992.
11. **Montecucco C, Di Lauro M, Bobbio-Pallavicini E, et al.** Antiphospholipid antibodies and thrombotic thrombocytopenic purpura. *Clin Exp Rheumatol*, 5, 355, 1987.
12. **Itoh Y, Sekine H, Hosono H, et al.** Thrombotic thrombocytopenic purpura in two patients with systemic lupus erythematosis: Clinical significance of antiplatelet antibodies, *Clin Immunol Immunopathol*, 57, 125, 1990.
13. **Upshaw JD, Reidy TJ, Groshart K**. Thrombotic thrombocytopenic purpura in pregnancy. Response to plasma manipulations, *South Med J*, 78, 677, 1985.
14. **Messmore H**. Unpublished case.
15. **Kyrle PA, Brenner B, Mannhalter R, et al.** Identical von Willebrand factor multimer abnormalities in idiopathic and secondary tumor associated thrombotic thrombocytopenic purpura, *Thromb Haemostas*, 69, 949 (abst 1479), 1993.
16. **Jackson AM, Rose BD, Graff LG, et al.** Thrombotic microangiopathy and renal failure associated with antineoplastic chemotherapy, *Ann Intern Med*, 101, 41,, 1984.
17. **Grem JL, Merritt JA, Carbone PP**. Treatment of mitomycin associated microangiopathic hemolytic anemia with vincristine, *Arch Intern Med*, 146, 566, 1986.
18. **Fraser JL, Millenson M, Malynn ER, et al.** Possible association between Norplant contraceptive system (levonorgestrel) and thrombotic thrombocytopenic purpura (TTP), *Blood*, 82, 4030, 1993.
19. **Moake JL. TTP**- Desperation, empiricism, progress, *N Eng J Med*, 325, 426, 1991.
20. Kwaan H Ed: Thrombotic microangiopathy, *Semin Hematol*, 24, 69, 1987.
21. **Hillyer CD, Duncan A, Ledford M, et al**. Chemotherapy induced hemolytic uremic syndrome. Description of a potential animal model, *Thromb Haemostas*, 69, 1721, 1993.
22. Editorial note: Hemolytic-uremic syndrome associated with Escherichia coli 0157:H7 enteric infection in the United States 1984, *JAMA*, 253, 1541, 1985.
23. Update: multistate outbreak of Escherichia coli 0157:H7 infections from hamburgers-Western United States 1992-1993, *MMWR Morb Mortal Wkly Rep*, 42, 258, 1993.

24. **Patton IF, Manning KR,** Case D, et al. Serum lactic dehydrogenase predicts survival in thrombotic thrombocytopenic purpura, *Blood,* 82, 611a (abst 2427), 1993.
25. **Ware AJ, Heistad DD:** Platelet-endothelium interactions, *N Eng J Med,* 328, 628, 1993.
26. **Bell WR, Tomasulo PA, Alving BM, et al.** Thrombocytopenia occurring during the administration of heparin. A prospective study of 52 patients, *Ann Int Med,* 85, 155, 1976.
27. **Weisman RE, Tobin RW.** Arterial embolism occurring during systemic heparin therapy, *Arch Surg,* 76, 219, 1958
28. **Warkentin TF, Kelton JG.** Heparin induced thrombocytopenia, *Annu Rev Med,* 40, 31, 1989.
29. **Chong PL, Faway I, Chesterman CN, et al.** Heparin induced thrombocytopenia: Mechanism of interaction of the heparin-dependent antibody with platelets, *Br J Haematol*, 73, 235, 1989.
30 **Vistentin GP, Ford SE, Scott JP, Aster RH**. Antibodies from patients with heparin-induced thrombocytopenia/thrombosis are specific for platelet factor 4 complexed with heparin or bound to endothelial cells, *J Clin Invest,* 93, 81, 1994.
31. **Anderson GP.** Insights into heparin-induced thrombocytopenia, *Br J Haematol*, 80, 504, 1992.
32. **Patrassi GM, Luzzatto G.** Heparin induced thrombocytopenia with thrombosis of the aorta, iliac arteries and right axillary vein successfully treated by low molecular weight heparin, *Acta Haematol*, 91, 55, 1994.
33. **Demers C, Ginsberg J, Brill-Edwards P, et al**. Rapid anticoagulation using ancrod for heparin induced thromobcytopenia. *Blood*, 78, 2194, 1991.
34. **Messmore H, Nand S, Godwin G.** Heparin induced thrombocytopenia and platelet activation in cardiovascular surgery. Book chapter in "*Anticoagulation, Hemostasis and Blood Preservation in Cardiovascular Surgery.*" PiFarre R, Editor. Hanley and Belfus Inc. Philadelphia; Mosby St. Louis, 185, 1993.
35. **Gruel Y, Rupin A, Watier H, et al.** Anti cardiolipin antibodies in heparin associated thrombocytopenia, *Thromb Res* 67, 601, 1992.
36. **Visentin G, Newman PJ, Aster RH.** Characteristics of quinine- induced antibodies specific for platelet glycoproteins II b and III a, *Blood*, 77, 2668, 1991.
37. **Karpatkin S**. Autoimmune thrombocytopenic purpura, *Sem hematol,* 22, 260, 1985.
38. **Bingley PJ, Hoffbrand BI,** Antiphospholipid antibody syndrome: A review, *JR Soc Med,* 80, 445, 1987.
39. **Vianna JL, Khamashta MA, Ordi-Ros J, et al.** Comparison of primary and secondary antiphospholipid syndrome : A European multicenter study of 114 patients, *Am J Med,* 96, 3, 1994.

Acquired Disorders and Congenital Thrombophilia

C. Therapeutic Aspects

THE LONG SEARCH TOWARD IDEAL ANTITHROMBOTIC DRUGS

M. Verstraete
Center for Molecular and Vascular Biology, University of Leuven, Leuven, Belgium

The tremendous interest in finding new antiaggregating agents stems from increasing awareness of the role that platelets play, not only in hemostasis and thrombosis, but also, be it less definitive, in atherogenesis and arterial spasm. The remarkable but limited effectiveness of aspirin and ticlopidin in the secondary prevention of cardiovascular disorders has stimulated the search for more potent antiplatelet drugs.

I. INHIBITORS OF PLATELET ADHESION

Platelets do not adhere to normal endothelial cells; this property of nonadhesion is the result of a series of active processes of which the endothelial cells are the seat but which cannot take place unless cells are functioning normally. Disruption of the endothelial lining permits nonactivated platelets to adhere to ligands in the subendothelial extracellular matrix. At low shear rate, the platelet GPIb/IIa binds to subendothelial collagen (platelet adhesion). The resulting activation leads to aggregation mediated by the interaction between fibrinogen and GPIb/IIa. At high shear rates, such as those found in arteries, platelets adhere to surface-bound von Willebrand factor via GPIb/IX and then aggregate by binding of von Willebrand factor to GPIIb/IIIa [1]. Other subendothelial ligands as fibronectin and vitronectin may also bind to other platelet receptors.

Monoclonal antibodies raised against GPIb are effective in experimental thrombosis in different animal models[2]. Similarly, antibodies against multimeric von Willebrand factor also have antithrombotic properties[3,4]. A peptide corresponding to fragment amino acids 445-773 of von Willebrand factor blocks the GPIb receptor[5]. Also, inhibition of the multimerization of von Willebrand factor with aurintricarboxylic acid has moderate antithrombotic properties[6].

Patients lacking GPIb (Bernard Soulier syndrome) have a serious bleeding disorder. Whether complete long-term blocking of the platelet GPIb receptors will be safe is still to be investigated.

II. INHIBITORS OF PLATELET AGGREGATION

A. CYCLOOXYGENASE INHIBITORS: ASPIRIN

Several pathways are leading to platelet aggregation. Aspirin inhibits very selectively the thromboxane (TXA_2) formation but impedes only partially platelet aggregation induced by ADP, collagen and by low concentrations of thrombin. Aspirin does not inhibit the adherence of the initial layer of platelets to the subendothelium or atherosclerotic plaques and the release of granule contents is not opposed[7]. Thus the effects of platelet-derived growth factors and other mitogens on smooth muscle cells are not inhibited[8] (Table I).

Table I : aspirin is not an ideal platelet inhibitor

Inhibits only TXA_2 pathway, much less the platelet activation by thrombin, ADP, collagen and not
    by PAF
No inhibition of platelet adhesion
No effect on smooth muscle cell proliferation
Prolongs the bleeding time
Gastro-intestinal problems
Can induce allergy (rare)

The ideal dose of aspirin for the primary or secondary prevention of cardiovascular disease is not determined but it was shown that doses between 324 and 1,300 mg daily seems to induce a similar reduction of cardiovascular complications while doses between 1 and 2 mg/kg daily produce virtually complete inhibition of cyclooxygenase dependent platelet aggregation [9]. Slow release aspirins are associated with few gastrointestinal side effects, particularly when an enteric-coated preparation is used.

Of note, PGF_2-like compounds (F_2-isoprostanes) are produced in vivo in humans by a noncyclooxygenase mechanism involving free radical catalyzed lipid peroxidation [10] and are thus not inhibited by aspirin. Moreover, two prostaglandin G/H synthase genes encoding for different isoforms of the cyclooxygenase enzyme (constitutive cox-1, inducible cox-2) [11] from extraplatelet sources (a.o. inflammatory stimuli on macrophages) have been discovered [11,12]. Aspirin inhibits only cox-1 in platelets, endothelium, stomach and kidney by acetylation of Ser53.

B. INHIBITION OF ADENOSINE-DIPHOSPHATE-EVOKED SIGNAL TRANSDUCTION: TICLOPIDINE AND CLOPIDOGREL

These two thienopyridine derivatives can be considered as bioprecursors since they are inactive in vitro but potent antiaggregating agents in vivo, indicating the importance of at least one active transient metabolite. The metabolic activation takes place in the liver as a porto-jugular shunt abolishes the antiaggregating effect. Ticlopidine and its chemical analogue clopidogrel are noncompetitive but selective antagonist of ADP-induced platelet aggregation. Since the two compounds are chemically related, their mechanism of action is considered similar. Ex vivo studies indicate that the antiaggregating effect is concentration-dependent; the rate of recovery is linked to platelet survival, suggesting a permanent effect on platelets [13-16]. The two compounds are believed to inhibit ADP mediated direct and indirect actions on platelet aggregation. Both reduce responses to other agonists which require feedback amplification by ADP released from internal storage sites during granule secretion [14,17]. The binding of fibrinogen to glycoprotein IIb/IIIa (GPIIb/IIIa) complex, triggered by ADP, is dramatically inhibited; this inhibition is not due to a direct modification of the glycoprotein complex [18]. Ticlopidin and clopidogrel have no effect on phospholipase A activity or thromboxane A_2 and prostacyclin synthesis. They have no direct effect on either cAMP-phosphodiesterase or adenylate cyclase.

Clopidogrel is approximately 40 to 100 times as active as ticlopidine in inhibiting ADP-induced platelet aggregation in animal models but circa 6 times as potent as ticlopidine in the inhibition of ADP-induced aggregation of human platelets.

Ticlopidin and clopidogrel have been tested in several animal models of platelet-dependent arterial or venous thrombosis and found to be more effective than sulfinpyrazone, dipyridamole and aspirin (reviewed by 13,19,20). Other effects are a reduction in fibrinogen levels and blood viscosity and improvement of decreased erythrocyte deformability [13].

The effectiveness of ticlopidine has convincingly been demonstrated in patients at high risk of arterial thromboembolic events, i.e. those with transient ischemic cerebral attacks and stroke, peripheral arterial disease or ischemic heart disease (for review 21,22). A large trial in more than 3,000 patients has shown that ticlopidine has a more pronounced effect on death from all causes or non-fatal stroke than aspirin [23,24].

The most common adverse effects associated with ticlopidine are gastrointestinal symptoms: diarrhea is the most frequently reported, affecting about 20% of treated patients. Other effects are skin reactions (urticaria, pruritus, erythema), hemorrhagic disorders (epistaxis, ecchymoses, menorrhagia). These effects are generally not severe and resolve after discontinuation of ticlopidine. The most potentially serious problem is bone marrow depression (leucopenia, thrombocytopenia, pancytopenia); close monitoring is therefore essential for at least the first 12 weeks of ticlopidine therapy [20]. Ticlopidine has also been associated with an increase in total cholesterol levels by 9% [23]. Clopidogrel was developed because this compound was not toxic to bone marrow pluripotent stem cells in the mouse (Till and McCullogh test). Also, in phase II studies adverse events with clopidogrel were proportionally less frequent than with ticlopidine and not related to the dose.

C. THROMBOXANE SYNTHASE INHIBITORS

Thromboxane synthase inhibitors have been developed with the expectation of not only suppressing TXA_2 biosynthesis but also sparing or even enhancing the formation of prostacyclin by the vascular endothelium. Thromboxane synthase inhibition offers the advantage over aspirin-type cyclooxygenase inhibitors to reorient the arachidonic cascade toward an overproduction of inhibitory prostanoids (PGI_2, PGD_2) and a reduction of TXA_2 formation. However, specific inhibition of TXA_2 synthase produces an accumulation of cyclic prostaglandin endoperoxides which occupy and activate TXA_2 and endoperoxide receptors on platelets and endothelium and, thus, attenuate the inhibitory effect of PGI_2 and PGD_2 [25-28].

Most thromboxane synthase inhibitors have a moderate potency, a short duration of action, and do not result in a sufficiently sustained inhibition of TXA_2 production. Moreover, some individuals are poor responders to this type of drugs. The increased generation of endoperoxides which share the same receptors as TXA_2 is a further problem which will not be solved by more potent and long-acting drugs of this class [29]. Although thromboxane synthase inhibitors have shown some benefit in experimental models, their effects in clinical trials in patients with coronary artery disease have been disappointing.

D. THROMBOXANE RECEPTOR BLOCKERS

The more recently developed thromboxane receptor blockers specifically impede the action of both TXA_2 and endoperoxides on their presumed common receptors on platelets and prevent vasoconstriction induced by TXA_2. These agents leave the normal pattern of thromboxane and prostacyclin formation unaltered. Thromboxane receptor antagonists prolong bleeding time more than thromboxane synthase inhibitors [30]. As expected, TXA_2 synthesis is not inhibited and PGI_2 generation is not augmented with specific thromboxane/endoperoxide receptor antagonists.

Clinical research with thromboxane receptor antagonists has been slow because the first compounds described had antagonistic effects on platelets but were agonistic on the vessel wall or vice versa [28]. Several of the thromboxane/endoperoxide receptor blockers are also relatively short-acting and the magnitude of their blockade is modest. This is particularly the case for daltroban but not so for vapiprost [31] and BMS 180291-1 [32] which are potent TXA_2 receptor blockers with a long duration of action. Unfortunately, the initial clinical studies with vapiprost have been disappointing. The long plasma elimination half-life of BMS 180291-A is most interesting as well as its antiischemic effects in canine models of pacing-induced ischemia. However, no therapeutic studies with this compound have been published and it remains to be demonstrated that such agents will offer a relevant advantage over aspirin.

E. THROMBOXANE SYNTHASE INHIBITORS AND RECEPTOR BLOCKERS COMBINED

Some compounds have a dual activity. Ridogrel is a potent TXA_2 synthase inhibitor with modest additional TXA_2/prostaglandin endoperoxide receptor antagonist properties (at least 100-fold less) [33]. Although the animal pharmacology was most promising, the preclinical evaluation is deceptive [29]. Picotamide is a rather weak thromboxane synthase inhibitor and receptor blocker [34].

F. BLOCKERS OF THE PLATELET GLYCOPROTEIN IIB/IIIA RECEPTOR

Exposure of GPIIb/IIIa receptors at the platelet surface is the final common endpoint of all pathways leading to platelet aggregation (Figure 1).

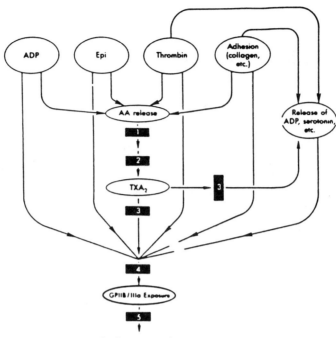

platelet aggregation

1. The first platelet GPIIb/IIIa antagonists to be developed were murine monoclonal antibodies [35,36]. In vitro, these antibodies completely inhibit platelet aggregation and, in animal models of angioplasty injury and thrombolysis, prevent thrombosis and augment the activity of thrombolytic agents [37,38]. Because of concerns about their immunogenicity, the derivative product chimeric monoclonal 7E3Fab (c7E3Fab) was created via genetic recombination. This new molecule consists of the mouse-derived variable regions from the original molecule linked to the constant region derived from human immunoglobulin IgG. Data from a dose-escalation study [39] and a pilot therapeutic trial [40] suggested a c7E3Fab dosing regimen which was evaluated in patients with high-risk PTCA [41,42]. As compared with placebo, a c7E3Fab bolus of 0.25 mg/kg followed by an infusion of 10 µg/kg/hr for 12 hours in 2,099 patients resulted in a 35% reduction in the rate of the primary endpoint (death, nonfatal myocardial infarction, unplanned surgical revascularization, unplanned repeat PTCA, stent or balloon pump for refractory ischemia). However, bleeding episodes and transfusions were more frequent in patients treated with c7E3Fab [41]. At 6 months, the absolute difference in patients with a major ischemic event or elective revascularization was 8.1% between the placebo group and c7E3Fab bolus plus infusion group [42].
    To be effective, over 90% of the GPIIb/IIIa receptors have to be blocked which is associated with a very prolonged bleeding time and risk of bleeding without an antidote being available. Moroever even chimeric monoclonal antibodies contain murine proteins and can be immunogenic.

2. The same drawbacks prevail for cysteine-rich single chain snake venom peptides binding to GPIIb/IIIa which, moreover, have a lower potency than chimeric monoclonal 73EFab. Their shorter half-life may be an advantage in case of bleeding.

3. The synthetic antiplatelet peptides, particularly those in cyclic configuration, are potent antithrombotic agents when tested in platelet-mediated thrombosis in different experimental animals. While short cyclic synthetic peptides have a higher potency they also lack specificity for the GPIIb/IIIa and recognize receptors on several integrins. The most potent compounds, at doses required for effective inhibition of in vivo thrombus formation, also induce a hemorrhagic tendency as witnessed by the marked prolongation of the bleeding time [43]. Structure-activity studies did already resolve in a partial dissociation between the inhibition of ex vivo platelet aggregation and bleeding time prolongation and suggest that it might be possible to obtain GPIIb/IIIa antagonists with an optimized antithrombotic versus hemorrhagic ratio [43].

4. The nonpeptide inhibitors are reversible antagonists and have obvious advantages compared to monoclonal antibodies as their effects is much shorter (3 hours for MK-383 versus 3 days for 7E3Fab, 44), no immunogenicity, and have the potential to be active orally.
    SC-5468A is a prodrug of a nonpeptide mimetic of the tetrapeptide RGDS (Arg-Glyc-Asp-Ser). The active metabolite SC-54701A, is a potent inhibitor of GPIIb/IIIa and exhibits specificity for this receptor with respect to other integrins [45]. More than 50% of the orally administered prodrug are absorbed in dogs and half that amount is converted to the active agent [46]. Platelet aggregation is completely inhibited for more than 8 hours after a single oral dose of 2.5 mg/kg. After intravenous administration, the half-life of the β-phase elimination of the active moiety is 6.5 hours (4.7 ± 0.1 hours) in dogs and the total plasma clearance 0.3 L/h per kilogram. The results of a dose-ranging study show that oral administration of the prodrug gives a dose-dependent inhibition of platelet aggregation which is maintained during a 14-day administration period in dogs without adverse effects [46]. At a dose inhibiting collagen-induced aggregation by 80%, bleeding time was increased 2.5-fold. Whether these results will be translated into less bleeding in a clinical situation is still to be demonstrated.
    BIBU 104XX is the orally available prodrug of the fibrinogen receptor antagonist BIBU 52ZW. Escalating single and multiple oral doses between 10 and 100 mg have been investigated in human volunteers and were well tolerated.

III. VITAMIN K-ANTAGONIST DRUGS

Warfarin sodium and related coumarin congeners are effective antithrombotic compounds which differ in speed in the inhibition of vitamin K-2,3 epoxide within hepatic chromosomes but also of their individual metabolism. These compounds depress the synthesis of vitamin K-dependent procoagulants (factors II, VII, IX and X) and of the natural inhibitor proteins C and S. The plasma concentration of these proteins will decrease in accord with their half-life. The coagulation components with the shortest half-life are the procoagulant factor VII and the endogenous anticoagulant protein C. This may cause a frank imbalance at the start of treatment and lead to thrombosis of skin capillaries and venules with cutaneous necrosis.

The intensity of the effect of warfarin on the synthesis of coagulation factors differs from one patient to another; moreover, in the same individual it may, over a period of time, vary considerably. This explains the need for close monitoring by having daily blood tests in the first week of treatment with warfarin. The test used is the "prothrombin time", a term which leads to confusion because the assay depends in fact on the global activity of five coagulation factors (prothrombin, factors V, VII and X). Among the six coagulation factors factors whose synthesis is inhibited by coumarin derivatives,there are three (prothrombin and factors VII and X) which are effectively measured by this test, but not factor IX and the anticoagulatory proteins C and S. On the other hand, the prothrombin time is also sensitive to factor V, a coagulation protein independent of vitamin K.

Table II : Drawbacks of oral anticoagulants

```
Delayed action
Need for blood monitoring (PT)
PT test does not fully reflect the drug effect
Interaction with many commonly used drugs:
          - potentiation of anticoagulation
          - decreasing anticoagulation level
          - sometimes modifying the activity of the other interacting drug
Anticoagulation level influenced by diet
Annual risk of bleeding      total    6 %
                             major    2 %
                             fatal    0.8 %
Narrow benefit-to-risk ratio
Embryotoxicity during first trimester of pregnancy
```

To perform the prothrombin time a tissue extract (thromboplastin) and calcium are added to citrated plasma and the time to fibrin formation is measured. Commercial thromboplastin reagents which are extracted by different methods from different organs and various species can vary extensively in their sensitivity to reductions in levels of vitamin K-dependent factors. In an effort to standardize prothrombin time determinations, and thus allow direct comparison of results obtained with different thromboplastins, the International Normalized Ratio (INR) is recommended but not yet universally applied.

At the start of warfarin treatment the prothrombin time is prolonged because factor VII has a half-life which is much shorter than the other vitamin K-dependent coagulation factors (II, IX and X). Thus, in the beginning of warfarin treatment, the prothrombin time will be prolonged while the intrinsic and common coagulation pathways are still uninfluenced. This explains why in switching from heparin to warfarin, heparin should be continued unabated for at least one day after the prothrombin time (INR) has reached therapeutic values. Also during long-term warfarin therapy prothrombin times should be checked regularly as many drugs and the diet can enhance or decrease the warfarin effect as do certain intercurrent disease (liver insufficiency, heart failure, hyperthyroidism).

Bleeding is the most important side-effect and the risk may vary from patient to patient, the presence of co-morbid conditions (hypertension, malignancy, older age, recent surgery) and the intensity of anticoagulation. Patients with more intense anticoagulant therapy (INR 2.5 to 4) have over the first three months a risk of clinically important bleeding over two times greater (14% versus 6%)

than those on less intensive anticoagulation (INR 2.0 to 2.5) [47]. In average, the annual risks of total, major and fatal bleeding can be estimated to be 2 and 0.8% [48] (Table II).

A rare, nonhemorrhagic side-effect of warfarin is coumarin-induced skin necrosis, an unexplained complication which occurs on the third to the eighth day of therapy. The rapid decline in protein C level is postulated to play a role in the obscure pathogenesis of thrombosis of skin venules and capillaries within the subcutaneous fat, usually in the lower part of the body [49,50]. Coumarin drugs readily cross the placenta and may be teratogenic, particularly during the first trimester of pregnancy [51].

In conlusion, vitamin K-antagonists are effective antithrombotic drugs with a narrow risk-benefit ratio which require regular monitoring and discipline of the patient (Table II). Their main virtue is that these anticoagulants can be taken orally and are rather unexpensive.

IV. HEPARIN

A. UNFRACTIONATED HEPARIN

The term heparin refers not to a single structure but rather to a family of mucopolysaccharide chains of varying length and composition. Heparin by itself has no anticoagulant property but accelerates the action of two naturally occurring plasma inhibitors by forming a 1:1 stoichiometric complex with antithrombin III (an inhibitor of thrombin and activated factors X, IX and XI) and, at very high doses, to heparin cofactor II which acts only on thrombin decay. Heparin contains a unique pentasaccharide which has a high-affinity binding sequence for antithrombin III [52,53]. This sequence is present in only one third of heparin molecules and is not required for binding to heparin cofactor II [54].

Factor Xa bound to platelets as well as thrombin bound to the endothelium or to fibrin (thrombus) are protected from inactivation by heparin-antithrombin III complex [55,56]. In plasma, approximately 20 times more heparin is needed to inactivate fibrin-bound thrombin than to inactivate free thrombin [55]. This explains that more heparin is needed to prevent the extension of venous thrombosis than its prevention.

Heparin is not adsorbed by the gastrointestinal mucosa. When in the bloodstream after parenteral administration, heparin binds to endothelial cells, mononuclear macrophages and numerous plasma proteins of which some neutralize the anticoagulant activity (e.g. platelet factor 4, vitronectin) and others as von Willebrand factor which thereby looses its function. Elevated levels of these heparin binding proteins explains the different individual dose requirements of heparin to obtain the same antithrombotic effect and the so-called heparin resistance in patients with inflammatory and malignant diseases [56]. Binding of heparin to the endothelium and various plasma proteins contributes to the reduced bioavailability at low concentrations and to the variability of anticoagulant response to fixed doses [56,57] (Table III).

Table III : Drawbacks of unfractionated heparin

Depends on the presence of cofactors (mainly antithrombin III)
Binds to several plasma proteins and endothelial cells
Is inhibited by platelet factor 4 and heparinase
Activates platelets
Can cause thrombocytopenia
Increases vascular permeability
Thrombin bound to fibrin and subendothelial matrix and factor Xa on the platelet surface or in the prothrombinase complex are not accessible to antithrombin III-heparin inhibition
Fibrin monomers protect thrombin from inactivation by heparin-antithrombin III complex
Half-life dose dependent (30 to 150 min)
Unpredictable dose response
Narrow benefit-to-risk ratio

The pharmacokinetics of heparin are complicated; suffice it to say that the anticoagulant response increases disproportionately in intensity and duration as the dose increases [58]. This explains that the anticoagulant effect of heparin has to be closely monitored but at present no completely satisfactory test measuring the generation of thrombin as well as the levels of antithrombin is available. The most commonly used test is the activated partial thromboplastin time (APTT) which is sensitive to the inhibitory effect of heparin on thrombin, factor X and factor IX. Unfortunately, the different commercial APTT reagents vary in their response to heparin [59] in addition to technical variables. The therapeutic level of the APTT should therefore be established in each clinical laboratory to correspond to 0.2 to 0.4 units of heparin per milliliter plasma by protamine titration [56] or to 0.2 to 0.7 units factor Xa per milliliter of plasma by the chromogenic substrate assay for the determination of anti-factor Xa activity [60]. A nomogram may help but should be adapted to the responsiveness of the reagent and APTT test system in use in the local laboratory [60].

The most common and major side effect of heparin is bleeding which is higher when unfractionated heparin is given by intermittent (14.2%) than continuous infusion (6.8%) or subcutaneous route (4.1%). Also the dose of heparin, the patient's anticoagulant response, serious concurrent illness and chronic consumption of alcohol predispose to bleeding [56]. Heparin-induced thrombocytopenia (HIT) occurs in 2.4% for therapeutic heparin and 0.3% for prophylactic heparin with associated vascular occlusions in 0.4% [57]. Rare complications are osteoporosis, alopecia, skin necrosis, urticaria and transient elevation of hepatic transaminases.

B. LOW-MOLECULAR-WEIGHT HEPARINS

Some of the limitations of unfractionated heparin can be overcome with low-molecular-weight (LMW) heparins (mean MW 4,000 to 5,000). These LMW heparins produce their major anticoagulant effect by binding to antithrombin III through the same high-affinity pentasaccharide sequence of unfractionated heparin which, however, is present in only one third of the LMW molecules [53]. A minimum additional chain length of 15 saccharides (MW > 5,400) is required for the inactivation of thrombin but the inactivation of factor X requires only the pentasaccharide. Unfractionated heparin has by definition an antifactor Xa to anti-II ratio of 1:1 which is for the various LMW heparins between 4:1 and 2:1. Drugs with a high anti-factor Xa activity were indeed designed based on the hypothesis that inhibition of earlier steps in the blood coagulation system would be associated with a more potent antithrombotic effect than inhibiting subsequent steps, owing to the amplification process inherent in the coagulation cascade; that is a single factor Xa molecule can lead to the generation of multiple thrombin molecules.

The advantages of LMW heparins over unfractionated heparin are numerous. Factor Xa bound to the platelet membrane in the prothrombinase complex is resistant to inactivation by unfractionated heparin but is not resistant to inactivation by LMW heparins. A further difference is that LMW heparins have lesser binding characteristics to platelet factor 4, other plasma proteins and endothelial cells [61,62] resulting in a higher bioavailability (after subcutaneous injection > 90% versus 30% for unfractionated heparin), reduced plasma clearance which is independent of dose and plasma concentration, a longer half-life (anti-Xa activity between 3 and 4 hours for LMW heparins versus 30 to 150 minutes for unfractionated heparin, 63) and less interindividual variability of the anticoagulant response [64]. LMW heparins have a lower affinity for von Willebrand factor [65], increase vascular permeability less than unfractioned heparin [66] and have a weak effect on platelet function [67]. These differences could explain that LMW heparins produce less bleeding than unfractionated heparin with equivalent or higher antithrombotic effect in experimental animals [64] and in some of the clinical studies [68-72].

The long half-life of LMW heparins and their predictable anticoagulant response to weight-adjusted doses allow a once daily subcutaneous administration without laboratory monitoring [64].

It has been suggested that thrombocytopenia is more common with unfractionated heparin than with low molecular weight heparin [73].

C. MIXTURE OF LOW MOLECULAR WEIGHT SULFATE GLYCOSAMINO-GLYCANS

Danaparoid sodium (Org 10172) is a low molecular weight heparinoid (6 kDa) and consists of a polydispense mixture comprising sulfated glycosaminoglycuronans derived from animal mucosa, heparan sulfate (83% w/w), of which a 4-5% has high affinity for antithrombin III dermatan sulphate (12% w/w) and a minor amount of chondroitin sulfate (5% w/w) [74]. There is uncertainty whether the low affinity fraction of danaparoid sodium has an antithrombotic function [75] or not [76]. Danaparoid sodium is more efficacious than heparin and is associated with less and shorter lasting bleeding than heparin in various animal models of thrombosis. The complex mechanism of the antithrombotic activity of danaparoid sodium can so far only be partially explained. Its anticoagulant profile is characterized by a high ratio of anti-factor Xa/anti-thrombin activity (14 over < 0.5) resulting in an effective inhibition of thrombin generation. The anti-Xa activity is mediated by antithrombin III and is not inactivated by endogenous heparin-neutralizing factors. The low antithrombin activity is mediated by heparin cofactor II and antithrombin III. The heparan sulfate fraction with low affinity for antithrombin III, despite lacking significant effects on coagulation factors Xa and IIa (thrombin) in vitro, has been shown in animal studies to contribute substantially to the antithrombotic activity. In contrast to heparin, danaparoid sodium shows hardly any or no effect on blood platelet function in vitro or in vivo. Danaparoid sodium is essentially free of contaminating heparin, has minimal crossreactivity in in vitro assays for heparin-induced thrombocytopenia (HIT) and had been used successfully in patients with this complication.

Pharmacokinetic studies have been primarily based on the kinetics of relevant anticoagulant activities because no specific chemical assay methods are available. In comparison with heparin, danaparoid sodium has a prolonged elimination half-life of anti-factor Xa activity. After intravenous and subcutaneous administration the antithrombin activity half-life of danaparoid sodium is shorter (1.8 ± 0.6 h) than its anti-factor Xa half-life (17.6 ± 1.1 h). Danaparoid sodium has an absolute bioavailability of 100% after subcutaneous administration. The kidneys play an important role in the elimination of the anti-factor Xa activity of danaparoid sodium, but cellular metabolism seems unlikely since the liver does not affect the anti-factor Xa activity and there is only a slight and reversible binding to the endothelium [77].

Danaparoid sodium has been shown to be effective in the prevention of deep vein thrombosis in patients with thrombotic stroke [78], after elective hip surgery [79-81] or hip fracture [82,83]. Other clinical studies were reviewed by Nurmohamed [84]. The long half-life of danaparoid sodium, which is not effectively neutralized by protamine, has been rather difficult to clinically manage.

V. SPECIFIC THROMBIN INHIBITORS

A. HIRUDIN

Natural hirudin is a single-chain, carbohydrate-free polypeptide containing three intramolecular disulfide bridges and a sulfated tyrosine residue. The polypeptide chain contains 65 amino acids with a molecular weight of approximately 7,000 daltons. Recombinant hirudin has been obtained using E. coli bacteria and yeast. With both methods, hirudin is expressed as desulfatohirudin lacking the sulfate residue on tyrosine 63. The nonsulfated molecules result in about a 10-fold reduction in thrombin affinity [85]. Unlike heparin, which requires endogenous cofactors for activity (mainly antithrombin III, heparin cofactor II), hirudin does not need a cofactor for its anticoagulant activity and therefore is still active in states of deficiency of these proteins (Table IV).

Hirudin is a specific potent inhibitor of thrombin to which it binds near the active center at the substrate recognition site with extraordinary tightness (K_D 2 x 10^{-14} M). In addition, there are multiple other contacts between hirudin and thrombin over an extended area of the molecule forming a highly stable noncovalent complex. All known functions of thrombin are inhibited.

The terminal half-life of r-hirudin in healthy young volunteers is 50-65 min [86,87], with a half-life of its efffect on the APTT of about 2 hours [88,89-91].

Recombinant hirudin appears to be a weak allergen and hirudin-specific IgE antibodies were rarely seen in 163 immunocompetent healthy volunteers receiving recombinant hirudin twice at one month intervals [92].

In contrast to unfractionated and LMW heparins, hirudin penetrates the thrombus and neutralizes thrombin bound to fibrin. Hirudin, but not heparin, reduces platelet deposition and thrombus growth on deep wall injury at both low- and high-shear-rate conditions. As hirudin is not inhibited by plasma proteins and endothelium, while unfractionated heparin is, the anticoagulant effect of hirudin is more predictable. Hirudin being a specific inhibitor of thrombin prevents platelet aggregation induced by thrombin but does not oppose platelet aggregation induced by other agonists. Unfractionated and LMW heparins can induce thrombocytopenia; this untoward effect has not been observed with hirudin.

On the downside, there is no antidote for hirudin. Furthermore, hirudin inhibits all interaction between thrombin and thrombomodulin, a prerequisite for activation of the endogenous coagulation inhibitory proteins C and S.

Table IV : Comparison of some properties of unfractionated LMW heparins and hirudin

UNFRACTIONATED HEPARIN	LWM-HEPARINS	HIRUDIN
Inhibits to the same extent thrombin and factor VII, much lesser IXa and XIa	Inhibits mainly factor Xa, to some extent thrombin	Specific and potent inhibitor of thrombin
Antithrombin III-dependent	Antithrombin III-dependent	Antithrombin III-independent
Neutralized by heparinase several plasma proteins, platelet factor 4 and endothelium	Neutralized by heparinase, weak endothelium binding	Not neutralized by heparinase, endothelium, macrophages, fibrin monomer and plasma proteins
Does not inactivate clot-bound thrombin and factor VII	Does not inactivate clot-bound thrombin and factor VII	Inactivates clot-bound thrombin
Inhibits platelet function	Inhibits platelet function	Prevents thrombin induced aggregation but not other platelet agonists
Induced thrombocytopenia is not rare	Can induce thrombocytopenia	Does not induce thrombocytopenia
Bioavailability after SC injection 30%	Bioavailability after s.c. injection > 90%	Good bioavailability after s.c. injection, circa 85%
Poor dose-effect response	Fair dose-effect response	Fair dose-effect response
Not immunogenic	Not immunogenic	Not or barely immunogenic
Transient increase of liver enzymes is common	Transient increase of liver enzymes possible	No liver toxicity
Increases vascular permeability	No increase of vascular permeability	No increase of vascular permeability

B. HIRULOG

Hirulog is a bifunctional 20-amino acid peptide designed on the structure of hirudin. It combines a fragment of the C-terminus of hirudin (interacting with the anion-binding exosite of thrombin) with an N-terminus fragment [D-Phe-Pro-Arg-Pro(Gly)], which interacts with the catalytic site of thrombin. Its K_D toward thrombin is K_D of 2.3×10^{-9} M (which is much higher than for hirudin (K_D 2×10^{-14} M)[93,94]. This metabolic cleavage contributes to its half-life on the APTT of about 40 min [95,96]. Only 20% of hirulog is excreted in the urine. Newer hirulogs have been synthesized with noncleavable bonds. There is no antidote for hirulog. Further development of hirulog was stopped.

C. ARGATROBAN

Argatroban, an arginine-derivative which binds to thrombin with intermediate affinity (K_D 3.9×10^{-8} M) is a competitive antagonist inhibiting fibrinogen cleavage [97] and platelet activation by thrombin. Compared to heparin, argatroban is significantly more effective in the prevention of platelet-rich thrombi after vascular injury and was effective at APTTs of only 2-3x baseline control [98,99].

In a platelet-rich coronary thrombus model after endothelial injury created by electric current, acceleration of lysis, by alteplase, was observed in dogs pretreated with argatroban at a low dose (41 µg/kg/min). However, abolition of cyclic flow reductions due to intermittent platelet aggregates, required the addition of a thromboxane A$_2$/prostaglandin endoperoxide receptor antagonist [100]. The results with argatroban plus aspirin seem to suggest that additional platelet (thromboxane) inhibition may be necessary, when antithrombins of lower affinity are used to prevent early reocclusion after lysis with alteplase. On the other hand, high-affinity antithrombins like hirudin may be as (or more) effective than antithrombins plus thromboxane blockade, without additional antiplatelet agents [101]. Argatroban combined with aspirin was well-tolerated in humans at a dose yielding a mean APTT 1.6 times baseline. Whether argatroban is effective at this dosage remains unknown as the clinical program of argatroban has been cancelled.

D. DUP 714

This boroarginine tripeptide binds to thrombin with moderately high affinity (K_D $4.1x10^{-11}$ M) and inhibits thrombin-mediated platelet activation and fibrinogen cleavage [102]. DuP 714 reduced the incidence of venous thrombi in rabbits from 100% (controls) to 33%, and arteriovenous shunt thrombosis from 72% to 11% [104]. Its anticipated potential for oral administration has not borne out in experimental or human studies. Because of liver toxicity, presumably related to the boron constituent, human studies were not pursued.

E. OTHER DIRECT ANTITHROMBINS

Other antithrombins still in development are peptides against the thrombin receptor of the platelet membrane [103], and hirudisins, hirudin derivatives combining IIb/IIIa receptor and thrombin inhibition. In the hirudisins, residues 32-35 of hirudin have been replaced by the integrin motif RGDS and KGDS, obtaining a potent thrombin inhibitor (K_D 0.16-0.26 x 10^{-12} M compared to 0.2 x 10^{-12} M for r-hirudin) with additional dysintegrin activity [104]. In addition to inhibiting GP IIb/IIIa receptor-dependent platelet interactions, the platelet-binding integrin motif is expected to target the antithrombin action of hirudin to platelets, possibly allowing lower and safer doses of hirudin in the treatment of thrombotic disease [105]. Similarly, hirudin targeted to fibrin [106] may allow for highly efficient antithrombotic activity at doses lower than presently required for r-hirudin.

VI. FACTOR Xa INHIBITORS

Direct thrombin inhibitors do not affect thrombin generation and may leave some thrombin molecules unaffected. Inhibition of factor X can prevent the thrombus generation and disrupt the thrombin feedback loop that autoamplifies thrombin. The inhibition of coagulation enzymes earlier in the cascade such as factor Xa or tissue factor may be a rewarding approach.

A. FACTOR Xa INHIBITORS
1. Recombinant Tick anticoagulant peptide (TAP)

TAP, originally isolated from the soft tick Ornithodoros moubata, is a slow-binding, specific stoichiometric factor X inhibitor of 6850 dalton. The 60-amino acid peptide has limited homology to the primary sequence of the Kunitz-type inhibitor family and binds tightly, but reversibly, to factor Xa with a K_D of 0.18-0.3 nM [107]. TAP can inhibit factor Xa in the prothrombinase complex as well as free factor Xa. Similar to previous studies with recombinant activated protein C [108], APTT and template bleeding times were only minimally elevated with r-TAP. The observation that procoagulant factor Xa (like thrombin) is adsorbed onto fibrin strands of clots underscores the complexity of prothrombin activation in vivo and provides a further rationale for the efficacy of factor Xa inhibitors as antithrombotic agents [109]. High concentrations of r-TAP (5 μm) were required to prevent fibrinopeptide A generation by clot-bound Xa in vitro. Overall, these studies indicate that r-TAP, which has low immunogenicity, has considerable potential as antithrombotic treatment for the prevention of heparin-resistant arterial thrombosis and as conjunct with thrombolysis. With the emergence of a narrow therapeutic window of the direct thrombin inhibitors, the clinical development of r-TAP, despite its high costs, may become an option for the future.

2. Antistasin

Antistasin is a 119 amino acid protein of 15 kD peptide isolated from the salivary glands of the Mexican leech H. officinalis [110]. Because of its strong immunogenicity, clinical development of r-antistasin is unlikely for the moment.

3. Natural pentasaccharide

The natural pentasaccharide (NP, Org 31540/SR 30107A) is a new sulfated pentasaccharide obtained by total chemical synthesis [52,111]. It is however, chemically identical with the antithrombin III binding site found in heparin and some low molecular weight glycosaminoglucuronans. NP displays antithrombotic activity by virtue of its potentiation of the antifactor-Xa activity of antithrombin III [112]. This compound acts on free factor Xa and not on thrombin decay. NP has been shown to possess antithrombotic efficacy in in vitro thrombosis models [113] and in animal experiments [114,115]. If antithrombotic doses are expressed in anti-Xa units/kg the pentasaccharide is less potent than unfractionated heparin; however, if doses are expressed in mg/kg, pentasaccharide shows more or less the same potency as unfractionated heparin. The duration of action, as measured by anti-Xa levels is longer compared to unfractionated heparin and the duration of the antithrombotic effect parallels the plasma anti-Xa levels.

As yet no satisfactory physico-chemical method is available to evaluate the kinetics of the synthetic pentasaccahride. In human volunteers, plasma peak anti-Xa levels were linearly related to the dose and ranged from 0.12-2.1 U/ml. The elimination half-life is approximately 14 hours, independent of the dose.

4. DX-9065

DX-9065 is a bis-amidinoderivative with highly specific factor Xa inhibitory activity. However, the compound is much less potent than TAP [116]. After intravenous or oral administration this compound rapidly prolongs APTT and prothrombin time and prevents endotoxin and thromboplastin induced disseminated intravascular coagulation in rats. This effect is independent of antithrombin III and not associated with bleeding [117]. The oral absorption is reasonable but the duration of action rather short and associated with hypotension in some species.

B. TISSUE FACTOR PATHWAY INHIBITOR

Tissue Factor (TF) is an integral membrane protein of the vascular endothelium that functions as an essential cofactor for the proteolytic activity of factor VII toward its substrates, factors IX and X [118,119]. Human plasma contains a Tissue Factor Pathway Inhibitor (TFPI). This endogenous multivalant protease inhibitor is a 276-amino acids polypeptide consisting of three Kunitz-type serine protease inhibitor domains. In the first step, which is independent of calcium, TFPI binds to Factor Xa by the second Kunitz domain, presumably through an active arginyl site. This reaction does not involve the Gla-residues on Factor Xa. The bi-molecule then induces a feed-back inhibition of Tissue Factor - Factor VIIa - complex, thereby inhibiting the extrinsic pathway of coagulation. In this second step, the binding occurs through the first Kunitz domain. This reaction requires calcium and the Gla-residues on factor Xa are essential [120].

Recombinant TFPI (TFPI$_{1-161}$) lacking the basic C-terminal region and the third Kunitz domain has been produced in yeast cells [121]. Endothelium and restricted blood flow [122] studies in experimental venous thrombosis revealed that although in the anti-Factor Xa test, APTT and prothrombin time-assays this truncated TFPI displayed a dose dependent increase in activity. APTT and prothrombin time-assays were, for the same antithrombotic effect, much less prolonged compared with LMW heparin. TFPI has no direct effect on thrombin and does not prolong the clotting time in the anti-Factor IIa-assay, even at high dose. No bleeding was observed in rabbits receiving 10 mg/kg TFPI$_{1-161}$, an antithrombotic dose as effective as 60 anti-Factor Xa IU/kg of logiparin.

Full length recombinant TFPI expressed in Escherichia coli [123,124] completely prevented arterial reocclusion after vessel wall injury that yielded platelet-rich thrombi [125].

Administration of recombinant TFPI may become an interesting antithrombotic drug targeted to exposed subendothelium.

C. PROTEIN C

Activated protein C is a natural coagulation inhibitor which plays a key role in the regulation of blood coagulation by selectively degrading coagulation cofactors Va and VIIIa and thereby inhibits thrombin generation [88]. Thus, activated protein C quenches the positive feedback actions of thrombin on the coagulation cascade (thrombin activates factors VIII and V), thereby limiting the coagulation process and thrombus propagation. Protein C is one of the vitamin K-dependent plasma proteins and it is activated on the surface of intact endothelial cells by thrombin bound to thrombomodulin. The anticoagulant effect of activated protein C is enhanced by protein S which is another vitamin K-dependent plasma protein [126]. It has been reported that protein S increases the affinity of activated protein C for thrombogenic phospholipids approximately 10-fold, and that protein S abrogates the protective effect of factor Xa against activated protein C-mediated degradation of factor Va in the prothrombinase complex [126].

Human plasma contains 4 mg/l protein C; the protein can be purified from plasma or obtained by recombinant technology [127]. Because of its endogenous origin and specificity of action, activated protein C is a potentially attractive antithrombotic agent.

VII. THE IDEAL ANTITHROMBOTIC DRUG

It is obvious that commercial antithrombotic drugs currently available for clinical use all have serious drawbacks. Moreover, the assays applied to monitor unfractionated heparin (APTT) and vitamin K antagonist (P.T.) also have serious shortcomings.

Table V : Ideal antithrombotic agent

1.	Oral as well as parenteral effectiveness
2.	Rapid onset of action, < 1 hour
3.	Rapid cessation of effect by non-toxic antidote
4.	Satisfactory therapeutic index, absence of side effects
5.	No cumulative action or toxicity from long-term use
6.	Predictable quantitative relation between dose and anticoagulant action
7.	Antithrombotic effect not requiring laboratory monitoring
8.	No or limited interaction with commonly used drugs
9.	Large benefit-to-risk ratio
10.	Inexpensive

The combination of very low dose oral anticoagulants (targeted INR 1.5) with a potent antiaggregation may be a welcome way out in the prevention of thromboembolic complication in patients at low or medium-high risk. Future drugs or drug combinations will have to be tailored in accord with the pathogenesis of the thrombus (venous versus arterial thrombi, thrombi induced by mechanical trauma as in PTCA, thrombi on foreign surfaces as on stents, platelet rich versus platelet poor thrombi). Local delivery of antithrombotic drugs or targeted to the thrombus may increase their local concentration, where most needed, and allow lower systemic levels, thereby reducing the bleeding risk. With recombinant technology human natural anticoagulants can be obtained in liberal quantities (antithrombin III, thrombomodulin, protein C, tissue factor pathway inhibitor) and allows to make mutants and hybrids.

Table V summarizes what the ideal anticoagulant should be. Hopefully the properties of one of the numerous antithrombotic drugs in development would correspond to this hematologists' dream of obtaining an antithrombotic drug without anticoagulant properties. In the meantime the unabated search for the Holy Grail continues.

REFERENCES

1. **Sakariassen, K.,S., Bolhuis, P.,A., Sixma, J.,J.**, Platelet adherence to subendothelium of human arteries in pulsatile and steady flow. *Thrombosis Res*, 19, 547, 1980.
2. **Miller, J.,L., Thiam-Cisse, M., Drouet, L.,O.**, Reduction in thrombus formation by PG-1 (Fab'), and anti-guinea pig platelet glycoprotein Ib monoclonal antibody. *Arteriosclerosis Thromb*, 11, 1231, 1991.
3. **Bellinger, D.,A., Nichols, T.,C., Read, M.,S.**, Prevention of occlusive coronary artery thrombosis by a murine monoclonal antibody to porcine von Willebrand factor. *Proc Natl Acad Sci USA*, 84, 8100, 1987.
4. **Krupski, W.,C., Bass, A., Cadroy, Y.**, Antihemostatic and antithrombotic effects of monoclonal antibodies against von Willebrand factor in nonhuman primates. *Surgery*, 112, 433, 1992.
5. **Mandle, R., Kenney, D., Bing, D.**, Monitoring functional activity of RG 12986, a novel GPIb receptor antagonist by inhibition of ristocetin-dependent platelet agglutination. In: *Progress in Vascular Biology: Hemostasis and Thrombosis*, Zimmerman Conference, La Jolla (California), February 27, 1992.

6. **Strony, J., Phillips, M., Moake, J., Adelman, B.**, In vivo inhibition of coronary artery thrombosis by aurin tricarboxylic acid. *Circulation*, 80, II, 1989 (Abstract).
7. **Tschopp, T.,B.**, Aspirin inhibits platelet aggregation, but not adhesion to, collagen fibrils: An assessment of platelet adhesion and platelet deposited mass by morphometry and ^{51}Cr-labelling. *Thromb Res*, 11, 619, 1977.
8. **Clowes, A.,W.**, Prevention and management of recurrent disease after arterial reconstruction: a new prospects for pharmacological control. *Thromb Haemostas*, 66, 62, 1991.
9. **Antiplatelet Trialists' Collaborative**, Secondary prevention of vascular disease by prolonged antiplatelet treatment. *Br Med J*, 296, 320, 1988.
10. **Morrow, J., Hill, K., Burk, R., et al**, A series of prostaglandin F2-like compounds are produced in human by a non-cyclooxygenase, free radical-catalyzed mechanism. *Proc Natl Acad Sci USA*, 87, 9383, 1990.
11. **Hla, T., Neilson, K.**, Human cyclo-oxygenase 2 cDNA. *Proc Natl Acad Sci USA*, 89, 7384, 1992.
12. **Picot, D., Loll, P.,J., Garavitto, R.,M.**, The X-ray crystal structure of the membrane protein prostaglandin H2 synthase-1. *Nature*, 367, 243, 1994.
13. **Saltiel, E., Ward, A.**, Ticlopidine: a review of its pharmacodynamic and pharmacokinetic properties, and therapeutic efficacy in platelet-dependent disease states. *Drugs*, 34, 222, 1987.
14. **Defreyn, G., Bernat, A., Delebassee, D., Maffrand, J.,P.**, Pharmacology of ticlopidine: a review. *Thromb Haemostas,* 15, 159, 1989.
15. **Mills, D.,C.,B., Puri, R., Hu, C.,J., Minniti, C., Grana, G., Freedman, M.,D., Freedman, S., Colman, R.,F., Colman, R.,W**, Clopidogrel inhibits the binding of ADP analogues to the receptor mediating inhibiton of platelet adenylate cyclase. *Arterioscler Thromb*, 12, 430, 1992.
16. **Féliste, R., Delebassée, D., Simon, M.,F., Chap, H., Defreyn, G., Vallée, E., Douste-Blazy, L., Maffrand, J.,P.**, Broad spectrum antiplatelet activity of ticlopidine and PCR 4099 involves the suppression of the effects of released ADP. *Thromb Res*, 48, 403, 1987.
17. **Schrör, K.**, The basic pharmacology of ticlopidine and clopidogrel. *Platelets*, 4, 252, 1993.
18. **Gachet, C., Stierlé, A., Cazenave, J.P., Ohlmann, P., Lanza, F., Bouloux, C., Maffrand, J.,P.**, The thienopyridine PCR 4099 selectively inhibits ADP-induced platelet aggregation and fibrinogen binding without modifying the membrane glycoprotein IIb-IIIa complex in rat and in man. *Biochem Pharmacol*, 40, 229, 1990.
19. **Panak, E., Maffrand, J.P., Picard-Fraire, C., Vallée, E., Blanchard, J., et al**, Ticlopidine: a promise for the prevention and treatment of thrombosis and its complications. *Haemostasis*, 13, 1, 1983.
20. **McTavish, D., Faulds, D., Goa, K.,L.**, Ticlopidine. An updated review of its pharmacology and therapeutic use in platelet-dependent disorders. *Drugs*, 40, 238, 1990.
21. **Verstraete, M.**, Risk factors, interventions and therapeutic agents in the prevention of atherosclerotic related ischaemic diseases. *Drugs*, 42, 22, 1991.
22. **Verhaeghe, R.**, Prophylactic antiplatelet therapy in peripheral arterial disease. Drugs, 42, 51, 1991.
23. **Hass, W.,K., Eaton, J.,D., Harold, P., Adams, J.,R., Pryse-Phillips, W., Molonu, B.,A., Anderson, S., Kamm, B., for the Ticlopidine Aspirin Stroke Study,** A randomized trial comparing ticlopidine hydrochloride with aspirin for the prevention of stroke in high-risk patients. *N Engl H Med*, 321, 501, 1989.
24. **Easton, J.,D.**, Antiplatelet therapy in the prevention of stroke. *Drugs*, 42, 39, 1991.
25. **Bertele, V., Schieppati, A., di Minno, G., de Gaetano, G.**, Inhibition of thromboxane synthetase does not necessarily prevent platelet aggrregation. *Lancet*, 1, 1057, 1981.
26. **FitzGerald, G.,A., Brash, A.,R., Oates, J.,A., Pedersen, A.,K.**, Endogenous prostacyclin biosynthesis and platelet function during selective inhibition of thromboxane synthase in man. *J Clin Invest*, 71, 1336, 1983.
27. **FitzGerald, G.,A., Reilly, I.,A., Pedersen, A.,K.**, The biochemical pharmacology of thromboxane synthase inhibition in man. *Circulation*, 72, 1194, 1985.
28. **Gresele, P., Deckmyn, H., Arnout, J., Lemmens, J., Janssens, W., Vermylen, J.**, BM 13.177, a selective blocker of platelet and vessel wall thromboxane receptors, is active in man. *Lancet*, 1, 991, 1984.
29. **Verstraete, M.**, Thromboxane synthase inhibition, thromboxane/endoperoxide receptor blockade and molecules with the dual property. *Drugs Today*, 29, 221, 1993.
30. **Gresele, P., Arnout, J., Deckmyn, H., Huybrechts, E., Pieters, G., Vermylen, J.**, Role of proaggregatory and antiaggregatory prostaglandins in hemostasis: studies with combined thromboxane synthase inhibition and thromboxane receptor antagonism. *J Clin Invest*, 80, 1435, 1987.
31. **Ritter, J.,M., Doktor, H.S., Benjamin, N., Barrow, S.E., Stewart-Long, P.**, On the mechanism of the prolonged action in man of GR32191, a thromboxane receptor antagonist. *Adv Prostagland Thromb Leuk Res*, 21, 351, 1991.
32. **Misra, R.,N., Brown, B.,R., Sher, P.,M., Patel, M.,M., Hall, S.,E., Han, W.,C., Barish, J.,C., Floyd, D.,M., Sprague, P.,W., Morrison, R.,A., Ridgewell, R.,E., White, R.,G., Didonato, G.,C., Harris, D.,N., Hedberg, A., Schumacher, W.,A., Webb, M.,L., Ogletree, M.,L.**, Thromboxane receptor antagonist BMS-180291: a new pre-clinical lead. *Bioorg Med Chem Lett*, 2, 73, 1992.
33. **De Clerck, F., Beertens, J., De Chaffoy de Courcelles, D., Freyne, E., Janssen, P.,A.,J.**, R68070: Thromboxane A$_2$ synthetase inhibition and thromboxane A$_2$/prostaglandin endoperoxide receptor blockade combined in one molecule. I. Biochemical profile in vitro. *Thromb Haemostas*, 61, 35, 1989.
34. **Berrettini, M., De Cunto, M., Parisi, F., Grasselli, S., Nenci, G.,G.**, In vitro and ex vivo effects of picotamide, a combined thromboxane A$_2$-synthase inhibitor and -receptor antagonist, on human platelets. *Eur J Cin Pharmacol*, 39, 495, 1990.
35. **Coller, B.,S.**, A new murine monoclonal antibody reports an activation-dependent change in the conformation and/or microenvironment of the platelet glycoprotein IIb/IIIa complex. *J Clin Invest*, 76, 101, 1985.
36. **Coller, B.,S., Scudder, L.,E.**, Inhibition of dog platelet function by in vivo infusion of F(ab')$_2$ fragments of a monoclonal antibody. *Blood*, 66, 1456, 1985.
37. **Hanson, S.,R., Pareti, F.,I., Fuggeri, Z.,M., Marzac, M., Kunicki, J.,J., Montgomery, P.,R., Zimmerman, T.,S., Harker, L.**, Effects of monoclonal antibodies against the platelet glycoprotein IIb/IIIa complex on thrombosis and hemostasis in the baboons. *J Clin Invest*, 81, 149, 1988.
38. **Gold, H.,K., Coller, B.,S., Yasuda, T., Saito, T., Fallon, J.,T., Guerrero, J.,L., Leinbach, R.,C., Ziskind, A.,A., Collen, D.**, Rapid and sustained coronary artery recanalization with combined bolus injection of recombinant tissue-type plasminogen activator and monoclonal anti-platelet GPIIb/IIIa antibody in a dog model. *Circulation*, 77, 670, 1988.
39. **Tcheng, J.,E., Ellis, S.,G., George, B.,S., Kereiakes, D.,J., Kleiman, N.,S., Talley, D.,J., Wang, A.,L., Weisman, H.,F., Califf, R.,M., Topol, E.,J.**, Pharmacodynamics of chimeric glycoprotein IIb/IIIa integrin antiplatelet antibody Fab 7E3 in high-risk coronary angioplasty. *Circulation*, 90, 1757, 1994.

40.   **Kleiman, N.,S., Ohman, E., Califf, R.,M., George, B.,S., Kereiakes, D., Aguirre, F.,V., Weisman, H., Schaible, T., Topol, E.J.,** Profound inhibition of platelet aggregation with monoclonal antibody 73E Fab after thrombolytic therapy. Results of the Thrombolysis and Angioplasty in Myocardial Infarction (TAMI) 8 Pilot Study. *J Am Coll Cardiol*, 22, 381, 1993.

41.   **The EPIC Investigators,** Use of a monoclonal antibody directed against the platelet glycoprotein IIb/IIIa receptor in high-risk coronary angioplasty. *N Engl J Med*, 330, 956, 1994.

42.   **Topol, E.,J., Califf, R.,M., Weisman, H.,F., Ellis, S.,G., Tcheng, J.,E., Worley, S., Ivanhoe, R., George, B.,S., Fintel, D., Weston, M., Sigmon, K., Anderson, K.,M., Lee, K.,L., Willerson, J.,T., on behalf of the EPIC Investigators,** Randomised trial of coronary intervention with antibody against platelet GPIIb/IIIa integrin for reduction of clinical restenosis: results at 6 months. *Lancet*, 343, 881, 1994.

43.   **Collen, D., Lu, H.,R., Stassen, J.-M., Vreys, I., Yasuda, T., Bunting, S., Gold, H.,K.,** Antithrombotic effects and bleeding time prolongation with synthetic platelet GPIIb/IIIa inhibitors in animal models of platelet-mediated thrombosis. *Thromb Haemostas*, 71, 95, 1994.

44.   **Peerlinck, K., De Lepeleire, I., Goldberg, M., Farrel, D., Barrett, J., Hand, E., Panebianco, D., Deckmyn, H., Vermylen, J., Arnout, J.** MK-383 (L,462), a selective nonpeptide platelet glycoprotein IIb/IIIa antagonist, is active in man. *Circulation* 88: 1512, 1993.

45.   **Nicholson, N.,S., Panzer-Knodle, S.,G., Salyers, A.,K., Taite, B.,B., Haas, N.,F., Szalony, J.,A., Zablocki, J., Keller, B.,T., Broschat, K., Engleman, V.,W., Herin, M., Jacqmin, P., Feigen, L.,P.,** SC-54684-A: an orallyl active inhibitor of platelet aggregation. *Circulation*, 91, 403, 1995.

46.   **Szalony, J., Haas, N., Salyers, A., Taite, B.,B., Nicholson, N.,S., Mehrotra, D.,V., Feigen, L.,P.,** Extended inhibition of platelet aggregation with the orally active platelet inhibitor SC-54684A. *Circulation*, 91, 411, 1995.

47.   **Turpie, A.,G.,G., Gunstenen, J., Hirsh, J., Nelson, H., Gent, M.,** Randomized comparison of two intensities of oral anticoagulant therapy after tissue heart valve replacement. *Lancet*, 1, 1242, 1988.

48.   **Levine, M.,N., Hirsh, J., Landefeld, S., Raskob, G.,** Hemorrhagic complication of anticoagulant therapy. *Chest*, 102, 352, 1992.

49.   **Comp, P.,C.,** Coumarin-induced skin necrosis. Incidence, mechanisms, management and avoidance. *Drug Safety*, 8, 128, 1993.

50.   **Hirsh, J.,** Oral anticoagulant drugs. *N Engl JMed*, 324, 1865, 1991.

51.   **Ginsberg, J.,S., Hirsh, J.,** Anticoagulants during pregnancy. In *Thrombosis in Cardiovascular Disorders*, Fuster V, Verstraete M (eds.), Philadelphia, WB Saunders, pp 485, 1992.

52.   **Choay, J., Lormeau, J.,C., Petitou, M., Sinay, P., Fareed, J.,** Structural studies on a biologically active hexasaccharide obtained from heparin. *Ann NY Acad Sci*, 370, 644, 1981.

53.   **Thunberg, L., Backstrom, G., Lindahl, U.** Further characterization of antithrombin-binding sequence in heparin. *Carbohydr Res*, 180, 393, 1982.

54.   **Lindahl, U., Thunberg, L., Backstrom, G., Riesenfeld, J., Nordling, K., Bjork, I.,** Extension and structural variability of the antithrombin-binding sequence in heparin. *J Biol Chem*, 259, 12368, 1984.

55.   **Weitz, J.,L., Hudoba, M., Massel, D., Maraganore, J., Hirsh, J.,** Clot-bound thrombin is protected from inhibition by heparin-antithrombin III but is susceptible to inactivation by antithrombin III-independent inhibitors. *J Clin Invest* 86, 3619, 1990.

56.   **Hogg, P.,J., Jackson, C.,M.,** Fibrin monomer protects thrombin from inactivation by heparin-antithrombin III: implications for heparin efficacy. *Proc Natl Acad Sci USA*, 86, 3619, 1989.

56.   **Hirsh, J.,** Heparin. *N Engl J Med*, 324: 1865, 1991.

57.   **Glimelius, B., Busch, C., Hook, M.,** Binding of heparin on the surface of cultured human endothelial cells. *Thromb Res*, 12, 773, 1978.

58.   **de Swart, C.,A.,M., Nijmeyer, B., Roelofs, J.,M.,M., Sixma, J.,J.,** Kinetics of intravenously administered heparin in normal humans. *Blood*, 60, 1251-1258.

59.   **Shojania, A.,M., Tetreault, J., Turnbull, G.,** The variations between heparin sensitivity of different lots of acivated partial thromboplastin time reagent produced by the same manufacturer. *Am J Clin Pathol*, 89, 19, 1988.

60.   **Kandrotas, R.J.,** Heparin pharmacokinetics and pharmacodynamics. *Clin Pharmacokinet*, 22, 359, 1992.

61.   **Barzu, T., Molho, P., Tobelem, G., Petitou, M., Caen, J.,P.,** Binding of heparin and low molecular weight heparin fragments to human vascular endothelial cells in culture. *Nouv Rev Fr Hematol*, 26, 243, 1984.

62.   **Barzu, T., Van Rijn, J.,L.,M.,C., Petitou, M., Tobelem, G., Caen, J.,P.,** Heparin degradation in the endothelial cells. *Thromb Res*, 47, 601, 1987.

63.   **Bara, L., Samama, M.,M.,** Pharmacokinetics of low molecular weight heparins. *Acta Chir Scand*, 543, 65, 1988

64.   **Hirsh, J., Levine, M.,N.,** Low molecular weight heparin. *Blood*, 79, 1, 1992.

65.   **Sobel, M., McNeill, P.,M., Carlson, P.,L., Kermode, J.,C., Adelman, B., Conroy, R., Marques, D.,** Heparin inhibition of von Willebrand factor-dependent platelet function in vitro and in vivo. *J Clin Invest*, 87, 1787, 1991.

66.   **Blajchman, M.,A., Young, E., Ofosu, F.,A.,** Effects of unfractionated heparin, dermatan sulfate and low molecular weight on vessel wall permeability in rabbits. *Ann NY Acad Sci*, 556, 245, 1989.

67.   **Holmer, E., Lindahl, U., Backstrom, G., Thunberg, L., Sandberg, H., Sodestrom, G., Andersson, L.,O.,** Anticoagulant activities and effects on platelets of a heparin fragment with high affinity for antithrombin. *Thromb Res*, 18, 861, 1980.

68.   **Hartle, P., Brucke, P., Dienstl, E., Vinazzer, H.,** Prophylaxis of thromboembolism in general surgery: Comparison between standard heparin and Fragmin. *Thromb Res* 57, 577, 1990.

69.   **Eriksson, B.,I., Kalebo, P., Anthmyr, B.,A., Wadenvik, I., Tengborn, L., Risberg, B.,** Comparison of low-molecular weight heparin and unfractionated heparin in the prevention of deep vein thrombosis and pulmonary embolism after total hip replacement. *J Bone Joint Surg*, 73, 484, 1991.

70.   **Albada, J., Nieuwenhuis, H.,K., Sixma, J.,J.,** Treatment of acute venous thromboembolism with low molecular weight heparin (Fragmin): results of a double-blind randomized study. *Circulation*, 80, 935, 1989.

71.   **Simonneau, G., Charbonnier, D., Decousus, H. et al.,** Subcutaneous low-molecular-weight heparin compared with continuous intravenous unfractionated heparin in the treatment of proximal deep vein thrombosis. *Arch Intern Med*, 153, 1541, 1993.

72.   **Hull, R.,D., Raskob, G.,E., Pineo, G.,F., Green, D., Trowbridge, A.,A., Elliot, G., Lerner, R.,G.,, Hall, J., Sparling, T., Bretellini Norton, J., Carter, C.,J., George, R., Merli, G., Ward, J., Mayo, W., Rosenbloom, D., Brant, R.,** Subcutaneous low-molecular-weight heparins compared with continuous intravenous heparin in the treatment of proximal vein thrombosis. *N Engl J Med*, 326, 975, 1992.

73. **Warkentin, T.,E., Levine, M.,N., Roberts, R.,S., Gent, M., Horsewood, P., Kelton, G.,J.,** Heparin induced thrombocytopenia is more common with unfractionated heparin than with low molecular weight heparin. *Thromb Haemost*, 69, 911, 1993 (Abstract).

74. **Van Dedem, G., de Leeuw den Bouter, H.,** The nature of the glucosaminoglycan in Orgaran (Org 10172). *Thromb Haemostas*, 69, 652, 1993 (Abstract).

75. **Meuleman, D.,G.,** Organan (Org 10172): its pharmacological profile in experimental models. *Haemostasis,* 22, 58, 1992.

76. **Zammit, A., Dawes. J.,** Low-affinity material does not contribute to the antithrombotic activity of Orgaran (Org 10172) in human plasma. *Thromb Haemost*, 71, 759, 1994.

77. **Stiekema, J.,C., Wynand, H.,P., Van Danther, Th.,G., Moelker, H.,C.,T., Dawes, J., Vanchenzo, A., Toeberich, H.,** Safety and pharmacokinetics of the low molecular weight heparinoid ORG 10172 administered to healthy elderly volunteers. *Br J Clin Pharmacol*, 27, 39, 1989.

78. **Turpie, A.,G.,G., Levine, M.,N., Hirsh, J., Carter, C.,J., Jay, R.,M., Powers, P.,J., Andrew, M., Magnani, H.,N., Hull, R.,D., Gent, M.,** A double blind randomized trial of Org 10172 low molecular weight heparinoid in the prevention of deep vein thrombosis in patients with thrombotic stroke. *Lancet*, 8532, 523, 1987.

79. **Walker, I.,D., Davidson, J.,F., Cowley, F., Wrobleski, B.,H., Hardinge, K., Murphy, J.,C., Magnani, H.,N.,** The heparanoid Org 10172 in DVT prophylaxis post hip replacement. *Br J Haematol*, 63, 200, 1986 (Abstract).

80. **Leyvraz, P., Bachmann, F., Bohnet, I., Breier, H.,G., Estoppey, D., Haas, S., Hochreiter, J., Jakubek, J., Mair, J., Sorensen, R., Stiekema, J.,** Subcutaneous thromboembolic prophylaxis in total hip replacement: a comparison between the low molecular weight heparinoid Lomoparan and heparin-dihydroergotamine. *Br J Surg*, 79, 911, 1992.

81. **Hoek, J.,A., Nurmohamed, M.,T., Hamelynck, K.,J., Marti, R.,K., Knipscheer, H., Batchelor, D.,A., Büller, H.,R., ten Cate, H., Doets, H.,C., Magnani, H.,N.,** Prevention of deep-vein thrombosis following total hip replacement by a low molecular weight heparinoid. *Thromb Haemostas*, 67, 28, 1992.

82. **Bergqvist, D., Kettunen, K., Fredin, H., Faunø, P., Suomalainen, O., Soimakallio, O., Karjolainen, P., Cederholm, C., Jensen, L.,J., Justesen, T., Stiekema, J.,C.,J.,** Thromboprophylaxis in hip fracture patients - a prospective randomized comparative study between Org 10172 and Dextran 70. *Surgery*, 103, 617, 1991.

83. **Gerhart, T.,N., Yett, H.,S., Robertson, L.,K., Lee, M.,A., Smith, M., Salzman, E.,W.,** Low molecular weight heparinoid (Org 10172) for prophylaxis of deep vein thrombosis in patients with fractures of the hip. *J Bone Joint Surg*, 73, 494, 1991.

84. **Nurmohamed, M.,T., Fareed, J., Hoppensteadt, T.,J.,M., Walenga, J.M., ten Cate, J.,W.,** Pharmacological and clinical studies with Lomoparan, a low molecular weight glycosaminoglycan. *Sem Thromb Hemost,* 17, 205, 1991.

85. **Hofsteenge, J., Stone, S.,R., Donella-Deane, A., Pinna, L.,A.,** The effect of substituting phosphotyrosine for sulphotyrosine on the activity of hirudin. *Eur J Biochem*, 188, 55, 1990.

86. **Markwardt, F., Nowak, G., Stürzebecher, J., Griessbach, U., Walsmann, P., Vogel, G.,** Pharmacokinetics and anticoagulant effect of hiruin in man. *Thromb Haemostas*, 52, 160, 1984.

87. **Bichler, J., Fichtl, B., Siebeck, M., Fritz, H.,** Pharmacokinetics and pharmacodynamics of hirudin in man after single subcutaneous and intravenous bolus administration. *Drug Res*, 38, 704, 1988.

88. **Dahlbäck, B., Stenflo, J.,** A natural anticoagulant pathway. Biochemistry and physiology of proteins C, S, C4b-binding protein and thrombomodulin. In: *Haemostasis and Thrombosis*, third edition. Bloom AL, Forbes CD, Thomas DP, Tuddenham EGD, eds. Churchill Livingstone, London, pp 671, 1993.

89. **Talbot, M.,D.,, Ambler, J., Butler, K.,D., Rindlay, V.,S., Mitchell, K.,A., Peters, R.,F., Tweed, M.,F., Wallis, R.,B.,** Recombinant desulfatohirudin (CGP 39393) anticoagulant and antithrombotic properties in vivo. *Thromb Haemostas*, 61, 77, 1991.

90. **Marbet, G.,A., Verstraete, M., Kienast, J., Graf, P., Hoet, B., Tsakiris, D.,A., Silling-Engelhardt, G., Close, P.,** Clinical pharmacology of intravenously administered recombinant desulfatohirudin (CGP 39393) in healthy volunteers. *J Cardiovasc Pharmacol*, 22, 364, 1993.

91. **Verstraete, M., Nurmohamed, M., Kienast, J., Siebeck, M., Silling-Engelhardt, G., Büller, H., Hoet, B., Bichler, J., Close, P.,** on behalf of the European Hirudin in Thrombosis Group, Biologic effets of recombinant hirudin (CGP 39393) in human volunteers. *J Am Coll Cardiol*, 22, 1080, 1993.

92. **Close, P., Bichler, J., Kerry, R., Ekman, S., Bueller, H.,R., Kienast, J., Marbet, G.,A., Schramm, W., Verstraete, M.,** on behalf of the European Hirudin in Thrombosis Group (HIT Group). Weak allergenicity of recombinant hirudin CGP 39393 (TMRevasc) in immunocompetent volunteers. *Coron Art Dis*, 5, 943, 1994.

93. **Maraganore, J.,M., Bourdon, P., Jablonski, J., Ramachandran, K.,L., Fenton, J.W.** II, Design and Characterization of hirulogs: A novel class of bivalent peptide inhibitors of thrombin. *Biochem*, 29, 7095, 1990.

94. **Skrzypczak-Jankun, E., Carperos, V.,E., Ravichandran, K.,G., Tulinsky, A., Westbrook, M., Maraganore, J.,M.,** Structure of hirugen and hirulog 1 complexes of α-thrombin. *J Mol Biol*, 221, 1379, 1991.

95. **Fox, I., Dawson, A., Loynds, P., Eisner, J., Findlen, K., Levin, E., Hanson, D., Mant, T., Wagner, J., Maraganore, J.,** Anticoagulant activity of hirulog, a direct inhibitor of thrombin. *Thromb Haemost*, 69, 157, 1993.

96. **Cannon, C.,P., Maraganore, J.,M., Loscalzo, J., McAllister, A., Eddings, K., George, D., Selwyn, A.,P., Adelman, B., Fox, I., Braunwald, E., Ganz, P.,** Anticoagulant effect of hirulog, a novel thrombin inhibitor, in patients with coronary artery disease. *Am J Cardiol*, 71, 778, 1993.

97. **Kikumoto, R., Tamao, Y., Tezuka, T., Tonomura, S., Hara, S., Nimomiya, K., Hijikata, A., Okamoto, S.,** Selective inhibition of thrombin by (2R,4R)-4-methyl-1-[N^2-(3-methyl,2,3,4-tetrahydro-8-quinolinyl)sulfonyl]-arginyl]-2-piperidinecarboxylic acid. *Biochemistry* 1984; 23: 85-90.

98. **Imura, Y., Stassen, J.-M., Collen, D.,** Comparative antithrombotic effects of heparin, recombinant hirudin, and argatroban in a hamster femoral vein platelet-rich mural thrombus model. *J Pharmacol Exper Ther*, 261, 895, 1992.

99. **Jang, I., Gold, H.,K., Ziskind, A.,A., Leinbach, R.,C., Fallon, J.,T., Collen, D.,** Prevention of platelet-rich arterial thrombosis by selective thrombin inhibition. *Circulation*, 81, 219, 1990.

100. **Haskel, E.,J., Prager, N.,A., Sobel, B.,E., Abendschein, D.,R,** Relative efficacy of antithrombin compared with antiplatelet agents in accelerating coronary thrombolysis and prevention of reocclusion. *Circulation*, 83, 1048, 1991.

101. **Zoldhelyi, P., Fuster, V., Chesebro, J.,H.,** Antithrombins as conjunctive therapy in arterial thrombolysis. *Coronary Artery Dis*, 3, 1003, 1992.

102. **Kettner, C., Mersinger, L., Knabb, R.,** The selective inhibition of thrombin by peptides of boroarginine. *J Biol Chem*, 265, 18289, 1990.

103. **Hung, D.,T., Vu, T.,K., Wheaton, V.,I., Charo, I.,F,, Nelken, N.,A., Esmon, N., Esmon, C.,T., Coughlin, S.,R.,** "Mirror image" antagonism of thrombin-induced platelet activation based on thrombin receptor structure. *J Clin Invest*, 89, 444, 1992.

104. **Knapp, A., Degenhardt, T., Dodt, J.,** Hirudisins; hirudin-derived thrombin inhibitors with disintegrin activity. *J Biol. Chem*, 267, 24230, 1992.

105. **Bode, C., Hudelmayer, M., Mehwald, P., Bauer, S., Freitag, M., von Hodenberg, E., Newell, J.,B., Kübler, W., Haber, E., Runge, M.,S.,** Fibrin-targeted recombinant hirudin inhibits fibrin depostion on experimental clots more efficiently than recombinant hirudin. *Circulation*, 90, 1956, 1994.

106. **Bode, C., Nordt, T.,K., Runge, M.,S.,** Thrombolytic treatment in acute myocardial infarction-selected recent developments. *Ann Hematol* 69, 35, 1994.

107. **Waxman, L., Smith, D.,E., Arcuri, K.,E., Vlasuk, G.,P.,** Tick anticoagulant peptide (TAP) is a novel inhibitor of blood coagulation factor Xa. *Science*, 248, 593, 1990.

108. **Gruber, A., Hanson, S.,R., Kelly, A.,B., Yan, B.,S., Bang, N., Griffin, J.,H., Harker, L.,A.,** Inhibition of thrombus formation by activatd protein C in a primate model of arterial thrombosis. *Circulation*, 82, 578, 1990.

109. **Eisenberg, P.,R., Siegel, J.,E., Abendschein, D.,R., Miletich, J.,P.,** Importance of factor Xa in determining the procoagulant activity of whole-blood clots. *J Clin Invest*, 91, 1877, 1993.

110. **Dunwiddie, C.,T., Waxman, L., Vlasuk, G.,P., Friedman, P.,A.,** Purification and characterization of inhibitors of blood coagulation factors Xa from hematophageous organisms. *Methods Enzymol. 1993;223:291-312.*

111. **Petitou, M., Duchaussoy, P., Lederman, T., Choay, J., Jacquinet, J.,C., Sinai, P., Torri, G.,** Synthesis of heparin fragments: a methyl-pentaoside with high affinity for antithrombin III. *Crbohydrate Res*, 167, 67, 1987.

112. **Beguin, S., Choay, J., Hemker, C.,H.,** The action of a synthetic pentasaccharide on thrombin generation in whole plasma. *Thromb Haemostas*, 61, 397, 1989.

113. **Lozano, M., Bos, A., de Groot, Ph.,G., Van Willigen, G., Meuleman, D.,G., Ordinas, A., Sixma, J.,J.,** Suitability of low-molecular-weight heparinoids and a pentasaccharide for an in vitro human thrombosis model. *Arterioscl Thromb*, 14, 1215, 1994.

114. **Walenga, J.,M., Fareed, J., Petitou, M., Samama, M., Lormeau, J.,C., Choay, J.,** Intravenous antithrombotic activity of a synthetic heparin polysaccharide in a human serum induced stasis thrombosis model. *Thromb Res*, 43, 243, 1986.

115. **Walenga, J.M., Bora, L., Petitou, M., Samama, M., Fareed, J., Choay, J.,** The inhibition of generation of thrombin and the antithrombotic effect of a pentasaccharide with sole anti-factor Xa activity. *Thromb Res*, 51, 23, 1988.

116. **Hara, T., Yokoyama, A., Ishihara, H., Yokoyama, Y., Nagahara, T., Iwamotov, M.,** DX-9065a, a new synthetic, potent anticoagulant and selective inhibitor for factor Xa. *Thromb Haemostas*, 71, 314, 1994.

117. **Yamazaki, M., Asakura, H., Aoshima, K., Saito, M., Jokaji, H., Uotani, C., Kumabashiri, I., Morishita, E., Ikeda, T., Matsuda, T.,** Effects of DX-9065a, an orally active, newly synthesized and specific inhibitor of factor Xa, against experimental disseminated intravascular coagulation in rats. *Thromb Haemostas*, 72, 393, 1994.

118. **Silverberg, S.,A., Nemerson, Y., Zur, M.,** Kinetics of the activation of bovine coagulation factor X by components of the extrinsic pathway. *J Biol Chem*, 252, 8481, 1977.

119. **Zur, M., Nemerson, Y.,** Kinetics of factor IX activation via the extrinsic pathway. *J Biol Chem*, 255, 5703, 1980.

120. **Broze, G.,J., Jr.,Warren, L.,A., Novotny, W.,F., Higuchi, D.,A., Girard, T.,J., Miletich, J.,P.,** The lipoprotein-associated coagulation inhibitor that inhibits factor VII-tissue factor complex also inhibits Xa: insight into its possible mechanism of action. *Blood*, 71, 335, 1988.

121. **Petersen, J.,G.,L., Meyn, G., Rasmussen, J.,S., Christiansen, L., Petersen, J., Bjørn, S.,E., Jonassen, I., Nordfang, O.,** Characterization of human tissue factor pathway inhibitor variants expressed in Saccharomyces cerevisae. *J Biol Chem*, 268, 13344, 1993.

122. **Holst, J., Lindblad, B., Bergqvist, D., Nordfang, O., Østergaard, P.,B., Petesen, J.,G.,L., Nielsen, G., Hedner, U.,** Antithrombotic effect of recombinant truncated tissue factor pathway inhibitor (TFPI$_{1-161}$) in experimental venous thrombosis - a comparison with low molecular weight heparin. *Thromb Haemostas*, 71, 214, 1994.

123. **Wun, T.,C.,, Kretzmar, K.,K.,, Girard, T.,J., Miletich, J.,P., Broze, G.,J., Jr.,** Cloning and characterization of a cDNA coding for the lipoprotein associated coagulation inhibitor shows that its consists of three tandem Kunitz-type inhibitory domains. *J Biol Chem*, 263, 6001, 1988.

124. **Diaz-Collier, J.,A., Palmier, M.,O., Kretzmer, K.,K., Bishop, B.,F., Combs, R.,G., Obukowicz, M.,G., Frazier, R.,B., Bild, G.,S., Joy, W.,D., Hill, S.,R., Duffin, K.,L., Gustafson, M.,E., Junger, K.,D., Grabner, R.,W., Galluppi, G.,R., Wun, T.,C.,** Refold and characterization of recombinant tissue factor pathway inhibitor expressed in Escherichia coli. *Thromb Haemostas*, 71, 339, 1994.

125. **Haskel, E.,J., Torr, S.,R., Day, K.,C., Palmier, M.,O., Wun, T.,C., Sobel, B., Abendschein, D.,R.,** Prevention of arterial reocclusion after thrombolysis with recombinant Lipoprotein-Associated Coagulation Inhibitor. *Circulation*, 84, 821, 1991.

126. **Dahlbäck, B.,** Protein S and C4b-binding protein. Components involved in the regulation of the protein C anticoagulant system. *Thromb Haemostas*, 66, 49, 1991.

127. **Grinnell, B.,W., Berg, D.,T., Walls, J., Yan, S.,B.,** Trans-activated expression of fully gamma-carboxylated recombinant human protein C, an antithrombotic factor. *Biotechnology*, 5, 1189, 1987.

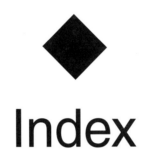

Index

INDEX